Bone Fracture: Evaluation and Treatment

Bone Fracture: Evaluation and Treatment

Edited by Dave Hensley

hayle medical

New York

Hayle Medical,
750 Third Avenue, 9th Floor,
New York, NY 10017, USA

Visit us on the World Wide Web at:
www.haylemedical.com

ISBN: 978-1-63241-720-6

Printed in China.

Cataloging-in-Publication Data

Bone fracture : evaluation and treatment / edited by Dave Hensley.
p. cm.
Includes bibliographical references and index.
ISBN 978-1-63241-720-6
1. Fractures. 2. Fractures--Evaluation. 3. Fractures--Treatment. 4. Bones--Diseases.
5. Orthopedics. I. Hensley, Dave.
RD101 .B66 2019
617.15--dc23

Table of Contents

Preface

A break in the continuity of the bone can be termed as a bone fracture. The break can be both partial or complete. A bone fracture is usually caused by high force impact or minimal trauma injury. Some medical conditions, like osteoporosis, bone cancer and osteopenia can also cause bone fracture. The treatment of bone fractures may involve immobilization, pain management and surgery. Many fractures require the alignment of the bone in the right position and immobilizing the fractured limb using a fibreglass cast, plaster or splint. Radiographic imaging, computed tomography (CT) and magnetic resonance imaging (MRI) are some of the common tests used to diagnose bone fracture. Bone fracture may also be coupled with damage to adjacent muscles, nerves or blood vessels. Some fractures can lead to complications such as compartment syndrome, non-union, mal-union, etc. This book explores all the important aspects of bone fracture in the present day scenario. It is appropriate for students seeking detailed information in this area as well as for doctors and experts.

This book is a comprehensive compilation of works of different researchers from varied parts of the world. It includes valuable experiences of the researchers with the sole objective of providing the readers (learners) with a proper knowledge of the concerned field. This book will be beneficial in evoking inspiration and enhancing the knowledge of the interested readers.

In the end, I would like to extend my heartiest thanks to the authors who worked with great determination on their chapters. I also appreciate the publisher's support in the course of the book. I would also like to deeply acknowledge my family who stood by me as a source of inspiration during the project.

Editor

Risk for Femoral Fractures in Parkinson's Disease Patients with and without Severe Functional Impairment

Petra Benzinger[1]*, Kilian Rapp[1,2], Walter Maetzler[3,4], Hans-Helmut König[5], Andrea Jaensch[2], Jochen Klenk[1,2], Gisela Büchele[2]

1 Department of Clinical Gerontology and Rehabilitation, Robert Bosch Krankenhaus Stuttgart, Stuttgart, Germany, **2** Institute of Epidemiology and Medical Biometry, Ulm University, Ulm, Germany, **3** Hertie-Institute for Clinical Brain Research, University Hospital Tuebingen, Tuebingen, Germany, **4** DZNE, German Center for Neurodegenerative Diseases, Tuebingen, Germany, **5** Department of Health Economics and Health Services Research, Hamburg Center for Health Economics, University Medical Center Hamburg-Eppendorf, Hamburg, Germany

Abstract

Background: Impaired balance is a major problem in patients with idiopathic Parkinson's disease (PD) resulting in an increased risk of falls and fall-related fractures. Most studies which analyzed the risk of femoral fractures in patients with idiopathic PD were performed either in specialized centers or excluded very frail patients. The current study used a large population-based dataset in order to analyze the risk of femoral fractures in patients with idiopathic PD.

Methods: Data from more than 880.000 individuals aged 65 years or older and insured between 2004 and 2009 at a large German health insurance company were used for the analyses. Persons with idiopathic PD were identified by the dispensing of Parkinson-specific medication and by hospital diagnoses, if available. People without PD served as the reference group. Incident femoral fractures were obtained from hospital diagnoses. Analyses were stratified by gender and information on severe functional impairment (care need) as provided by reimbursement claims.

Results: Compared with the reference group, persons with idiopathic PD had a more than doubled risk to sustain a femoral fracture. The risk was higher in men (HR = 2.61; 95%-CI: 2.28–2.98) than in women (HR = 1.79; 95%-CI: 1.66–1.94). The increased risk was only observed in people without severe functional impairment. The sensitivity analysis using a refined definition of idiopathic PD patients yielded similar results.

Conclusion: The findings confirm the increased risk of femoral fractures in patients with idiopathic PD. The relative risk is particularly high in male PD patients and in patients without severe functional impairment.

Editor: Mathias Toft, Oslo University Hospital, Norway

Funding: The analysis was supported by the Bundesministerium für Bildung und Forschung (Förderkennzeichen: 01EC1007A). The funders had no role in study design, data collection and analysis, decision to publish, or preparation of the manuscript.

Competing Interests: The authors have declared that no competing interests exist.

* E-mail: petra.benzinger@rbk.de

Introduction

Parkinson's disease (PD) is the second most common neurodegenerative disorder after Alzheimer's disease [1]. Postural instability and impaired balance is one of the cardinal symptoms of PD posing these patients at an increased risk of falling [2–7]. Fall-related injuries represent the most frequent reason for hospital admission in PD [8]. The occurrence of falls in patients with PD has been shown to be associated with increasing age, severity of symptoms, and use of dopaminergic drugs [3,4,7,9].

The increased risk of falling in combination with a low bone mineral density is putting PD patients at high risk for osteoporotic fractures [10]. In several studies, PD patients were found to have a high rate of fractures [2,11–16]. Among these, femoral fractures are the most common type of non-vertebral fractures [7,12–14,16]. Femoral fractures are associated with high morbidity, mortality, and costs in the general older population [17–19]. In PD patients, femoral fractures are associated with a particularly high risk of unfavorable outcomes such as admission to nursing homes [20]. However, estimates of the magnitude of these patients' increased risk are mainly based on observational studies with a limited number of PD patients and only a low number of femoral fractures [13–16].

PD is characterized by loss of functional abilities as the disease progresses [21–23]. However, the influence of functional limitations on the excess risk for femoral fractures in PD patients has not been explored so far. A large German population-based dataset containing routine data allowed us to identify older individuals with severe functional limitations in activities of daily living. The aim of this study was (1) to estimate the risk of idiopathic PD patients to sustain a femoral fracture and (2) to stratify this estimate for the presence of severe functional impairment.

Materials and Methods

Data Source

The routine data collection systems of the largest health insurance company in Bavaria, the *Allgemeine Ortskrankenkasse Bayern*

(AOK Bavaria), was used to select data on gender, age, long term care need, admission to hospital, admission and discharge diagnosis as well as dispensed medication. Health insurance and long term care insurance is statutory in Germany. The AOK Bavaria covers nearly 50% of the population aged 65 years and over in Bavaria, a federal state with 12.5 million inhabitants.

Data on Medication to Treat PD

Within the stored data of the AOK Bavaria, all prescriptions for medication for the treatment of PD were identified (Tab. 1). Substances were categorized according the Anatomical Therapeutic Chemical Classification System (ATC code) to substance classes. In Germany, outside hospitals Parkinson medication is available only at pharmacies with a written prescription by a physician and is reimbursed by the person's health insurance. For reimbursement, a person's insurance number along with type, dose and amount of drug prescribed, as well as prescription date is transferred to the health insurance. No information on the dosage regime or diagnosis is transferred. Data on reimbursement held by health insurances give complete information on all prescriptions filled in.

Study Population

The dataset consisted of 932,197 people aged 65 years and over who were member at AOK Bavaria between January 1st 2004 and June 30th 2009. Data from the year 2004 (January 1st to December 31st) regarding admission or discharge diagnoses as well as PD medications were used to identify patients with idiopathic PD. Individuals dying in 2004 were not considered (N = 44,333). Identification of the study population and sub-groups is displayed in figure 1.

Table 1. Medication considered as treatment for PD.

	ATC codes
Levodopa	N04BA01/N04BA02
Dopamine agonists	
Apomorphine	N04BC07
Bromocriptine	N04BC01
Cabergoline	N04BC06
Lisurid	N04BC10
Pergolide	N04BC02
Pramipexole	N04BC05
Ropinirole	N04BC04
Rotigotine	N04BC09
Anticholinergics	
Biperiden	N04AA02
Bornaprine	N04AA11
Methixine	N04AA03
Procyclidine	N04AA04
Trihexphenidyl	N04AA01
Budipine	N04BX03
COMT inhibitor	
Entacapone	N04BX02
Tolcapone	N04BX01
MAO B inhibitors	
Rasagiline	N04BD02
Selegiline	N04BD01
Amantadine	N04BB01
Stalevo	N04BA03

Identification of Individuals with Idiopathic PD

Identification of patients with PD using routine data is not straightforward. In our dataset we could use two types of information to identify PD patients: (1) primary hospital admission and discharge diagnoses of hospitalized patients, and (2) information about antiparkinson medication dispensed by pharmacies outside the hospital. Hospital admission and discharge diagnoses covered only a small percentage of PD patients. Therefore, the main information to identify patients with idiopathic PD was the medication to treat PD.

We defined individuals as patients with an idiopathic PD if a) antiparkinson medication was dispensed at least twice in 2004, or once in 2004 and at least once in 2005 or b) idiopathic PD was the primary hospital admission or discharge diagnosis in 2004 (ICD-10: G20) and antiparkinson medication was dispensed at least once in 2004.

Most patients with idiopathic PD are treated with antiparkinson drugs and are covered by the chosen method. However, some other disease entities are also treated by antiparkinson drugs like atypical Parkinsonism, secondary Parkinsonism or restless legs syndrome (RLS). Therefore, these individuals were excluded if they could be identified by hospital admission or discharge diagnoses (ICD-10) (G21/G22/G23/G25.81). The final dataset comprised 323, 404 men and 560, 453 women.

This dataset still included patients with atypical Parkinsonism, secondary Parkinsonism or RLS. Atypical Parkinsonism and secondary Parkinsonism are very rare diseases. RLS, however, has a higher prevalence and might account for a relevant percentage of the dispensed antiparkinson medication. Medically treated RLS is usually treated by monotherapy with dopaminergic drugs. Therefore, we applied two different models to perform a sensitivity analysis. Model I ('possible' idiopathic PD patients) used data of all patients with antiparkinson medication (see above). Most patients with a RLS are still included in this model. Model II ('probable' idiopathic PD patients) excluded all individuals (n = 11,078) from model I who received levodopa only or dopamine agonists only (change of substance within and between substance class possible). In this model most patients with a RLS but also patients with an idiopathic PD treated by monotherapy with dopaminerigic drugs are excluded. Therefore, model II may over-represent patients with an advanced idiopathic PD.

Please note that these terms are not synonymous with the terms for clinical definition of PD [24] and are therefore put in brackets throughout this article.

Reference group: The reference group comprised of individuals without intake of antiparkinson medication and no hospital admission or discharge diagnosis of atypical Parkinsonism, secondary Parkinsonism or RLS in 2004.

Definition of Severe Functional Impairment

The need for long-term nursing care was used as a marker for severe functional impairment and was assessed at the beginning of the observation period (January 1st 2005). In Germany, most persons with a minimum of six months of need for nursing care are eligible to receive reimbursement for long-term care by the long-term care insurance. The long-term care insurance was introduced in the German social insurance system in 1995. All employed citizens are members by law [25]. Experts confirm a person's eligibility to receive long-term care benefit. Long-term care

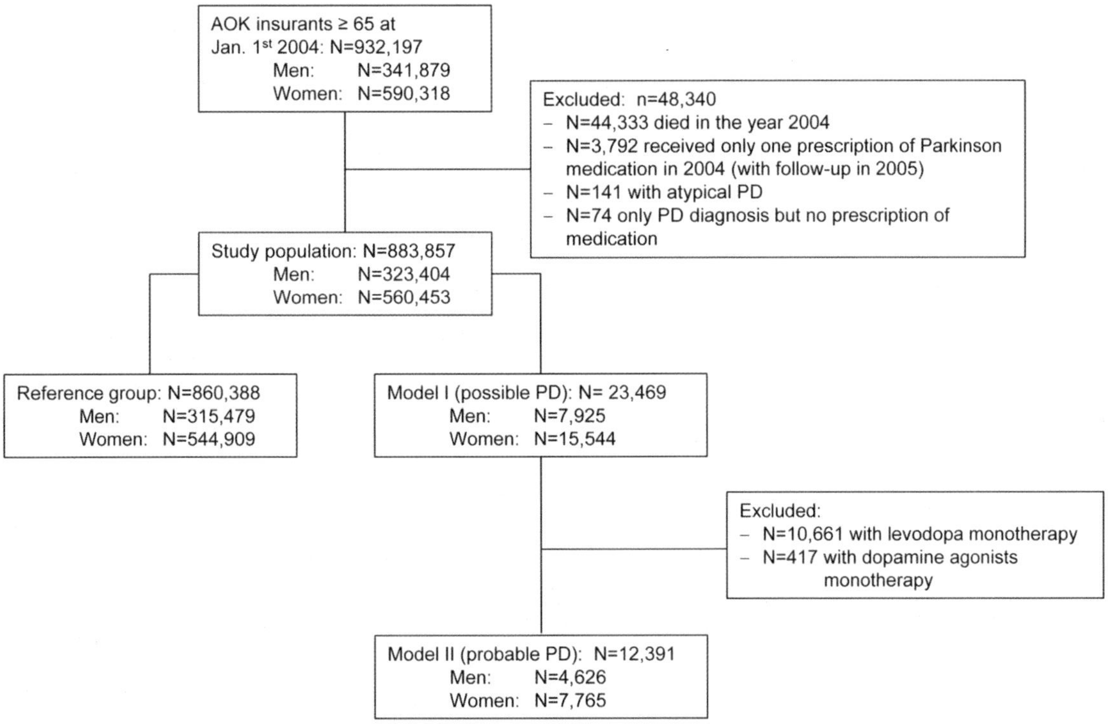

Figure 1. Flow chart of study population and model definitions. Identification was based on characteristics in 2004 as provided by the health insurance company (AOK: Allgemeine Ortskrankenkasse Bavaria) PD: Parkinson's disease; N: number of participants.

benefits are granted for professional, family, and/or informal help. In order to claim long-term care benefits, people must have a daily minimum of 90 minutes of assistance with basic activities of daily living (ADL) such as washing, eating, or dressing, and instrumental activities of daily living (IADL) such as cleaning or shopping. This information thus defines relatively well functional impairment, independent of underlying diseases.

Identification of Femoral Fractures

Hospital discharge diagnoses were used to identify femoral fractures (ICD-10: S72). The observation period started on January 1st 2005 and ended on June 30th 2009. Hospital admissions coding a femoral fracture that occurred within less than 30 days to a previous fracture were excluded in order to avoid double coding.

Table 2. Characteristics of the study population.

	Reference group	PD medication	
		Model I (possible PD)	Model II (probable PD)
Total [N (%)]	860,388 (97.3%)	23,469 (2.7%)	12,391 (1.4%)
Age (y) [Median, IQR]	74.4 (69.7–80.2)	77.9 (72.7–83.1)	76.9 (72.0–82.0)
Women (%)	63.3	66.2	62.7
Follow-up (y) [Median, IQR]	4.50 (4.50–4.50)	4.50 (2.40–4.50)	4.50 (2.47–4.50)
Number of femoral fractures (N)	33,228	1,633	919
Persons with 1 femoral fracture (N)	28,939	1,407	785
Persons with ≥2 femoral fractures (N)	2,104	110	66
Persons without care need [N (%)]	750,806 (87.3%)	12,263 (52.3%)	6,153 (49.7%)
Age (y) [Median, IQR]	73.4 (69.3–78.6)	75.1 (70.7–79.9)	74.5 (70.2–79.0)
Women (%)	61.6	64.9	60.3
Persons with care need [N (%)]	109,582 (12.7%)	11,206 (47.7%)	6,238 (50.3%)
Age (y) [Median, IQR]	83.5 (77.9–89.4)	81.2 (76.0–85.3)	79.6 (74.6–84.0)
Women (%)	75.4	67.7	65.0

PD: Parkinson's disease; N: Number; y: Years, IQR: Inter quartile range.
Characteristics of study population at start of the observation period (January 1st 2005) and number of fractures between January 1st 2005 and June 30th 2009.

Table 3. Frequency of prescribed Parkinson medication of persons identified with 'possible' Parkinson's diseases (PD).

	Number (%)*
Monotherapy	
Levodopa†	10,880 (46.4%)
Dopamine agonists†	425 (1.8%)
Others§	4,249 (18.1%)
Combinations	
Levodopa + dopamine agonists	2,074 (8.8%)
Levodopa + others§	2,951 (12.6%)
Dopamine agonists + others§	136 (0.6%)
Other combinations	2,754 (11.7%)

*percentage refers to all persons included in model I ('possible' PD).
†model II ('probable' PD) excludes persons treated with levodopa only or dopamine agonists only.
§Others: amantadine, MAO B inhibitors, anticholinergic agents, budipine.

Statistics

The accumulation of the individual person-years of individuals with PD and without (reference group) started at beginning of observation period (January 1st 2005) and ended with censoring due to death or at the end of the observation period. Fracture rates and 95% confidence intervals were estimated per 1000 person-years and adjusted for age using negative binomial regression models. To quantify the relative risk for the first femoral fracture during observation time in people with 'possible' or 'probable' idiopathic PD compared to people without PD hazard ratios with 95% confidence intervals were calculated. In the applied proportional hazards models age of participants was used as 'survival time'-variable to adjust for age and to account for the fact that the participants were of different ages at study begin. All models were stratified for sex and considered severe functional impairment by stratification. All statistical calculations were carried out using SAS version 9.3 (SAS Institute Inc., Cary, NC, USA).

Ethics

The study was approved by the Ethical committee of Ulm University.

Results

A total of 883,857 individuals aged 65 years and older were included in our study population. The median follow-up was 4.5 years. As 'possible' PD patients (model I) 23,469 individuals (2.7%) were identified and 12,391 (1.4%) as 'probable' idiopathic PD patients (model II). Table 2 shows baseline characteristics of the reference group as well as of individuals with 'possible' PD (model I) and 'probable' PD (model II). In both models, PD-patients were older than the reference group (77.9, 76.9 years vs. 74.4 years in individuals with 'possible' PD, 'probable' PD, and in individuals of the reference group, respectively). A higher proportion of these individuals had severe functional impairment (47.7, 50.3 and 12.7% of the population with 'possible' PD, 'probable' PD, and of individuals of the reference group, respectively). However, the median age of individuals with severe functional impairment was younger in both models compared to the reference group (81.2/79.6 years vs. 83.5 years, as for individuals with 'possible' PD, 'probable' PD, and for individuals of the reference group, respectively).

As displayed in Table 3, the most commonly prescribed medication of individuals with 'possible' PD was levodopa either

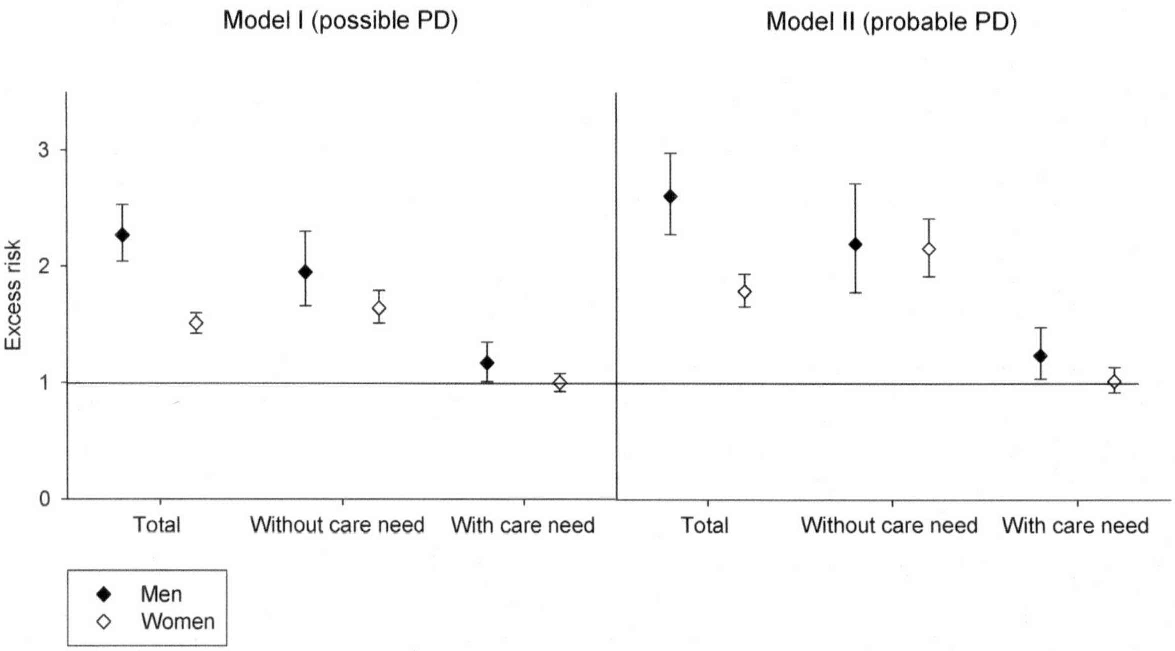

Figure 2. Age-adjusted risk of a first femoral fracture during a median observation period of 4.5 years. Individuals with 'possible' (N = 23,469) or 'probable' (N = 12,391) idiopathic Parkinson's disease (PD, for definition see text) were compared to 860,388 people without PD, stratified by gender and care need.

Table 4. Age-adjusted femoral fracture rates (per 1,000 person-years) of persons aged 65 and older.

	Total			Without care need			With care need		
	No. of femoral fractures	Person-years	Femoral fractures/ 1000 person-years (95% CI†)	No. of femoral fractures	Person-years	Femoral fractures/1000 person-years (95% CI†)	No. of femoral fractures	Person-years	Femoral fractures/1000 person-years (95% CI†)
Reference group									
Men	6,400	1,264,840.91	4.15 (4.03–4.28)	4,871	1,193,887.25	3.35 (3.23–3.46)	1,529	70,953.65	21.59 (20.59–22.74)
Women	26,828	2,202,984.72	9.92 (9.77–10.06)	19,174	1,967,735.28	7.53 (7.39–7.66)	7,654	235,249.44	32.88 (32.14–33.64)
PD treatment									
Model I (possible PD)									
Men	378	26,501.79	13.74 (12.32–15.33)	155	16,949.31	8.07 (6.73–9.68)	223	9,552.48	23.64 (20.67–27.04)
Women	1,255	55,084.97	22.47 (21.17–23.85)	593	33,002.00	15.78 (14.34–17.38)	662	22,082.97	30.40 (28.16–32.83)
Model II (probable PD)									
Men	234	15,701.44	14.47 (12.60–16.62)	92	9,672.50	8.80 (7.00–11.07)	142	6,028.95	23.72 (20.01–28.11)
Women	685	27,588.01	24.72 (22.82–26.78)	327	15,328.23	19.10 (16.81–21.71)	358	12,259.78	29.59 (26.65–32.84)

PD: Parkinson's diseas.

alone or in combination (79.0%). Only 1.8% of individuals received dopamine agonists alone and 9.4% in combination.

Estimates of fracture rates were based on 34,861 femoral fractures overall. Table 4 shows age adjusted fracture rates stratified by severe functional impairment and gender. Rates for femoral fractures are ranging from 3/1000 to 33/1000 person-years. In all strata and models, women had a higher fracture rate than men. The relative difference was less pronounced in individuals with 'possible' or 'probable' idiopathic PD with severe functional impairment. Figure 2 illustrates hazard ratios (HR) using the same strata. Narrowing the criteria from model I to model II increased the HR from 2.27 to 2.61 in men, and from 1.51 to 1.79 in women. The HR was higher in men than in women in both models (HR 2.27 vs. 1.51/2.61 vs. 1.79 in model I/II, respectively). In individuals without severe functional impairment, the relative fracture risk was higher than in those with functional impairment. In fact, women with 'probable' idiopathic PD and severe functional impairment did not have an increased risk to sustain a femoral fracture compared to women of the reference group. Men with 'probable' idiopathic PD and functional impairment had a low risk increase for femoral fractures of 24%. Both models showed similar results (Fig. 2).

Discussion

In this large-scale analysis of population-based data of a health insurance company we compared femoral fracture rates in older individuals with 'possible' or 'probable' PD to a reference group without PD. The rates of femoral fractures found in our analysis are comparable to rates of femoral fractures previously reported [26–28].Our data demonstrate that individuals aged 65 years or older with medically treated idiopathic PD have a more than doubled (men) or almost doubled (women) risk to sustain a femoral fracture compared to the reference group. To test the robustness of our results and the susceptibility to the inclusion and exclusion criteria, two models with refined definitions were used. 'Possible' PD (model I) showed lower hazard ratios compared to 'probable' PD (model II). Both models showed a similar picture with a higher hazard ratio in those PD patients without severe functional impairment compared to PD patients with severe functional impairment and higher hazard ratio in men compared to women.

In PD patients, one out of four falls results in an injury [6]. Falls and fractures represent the leading diagnosis for admission to hospital in PD patients [8]. Our finding of an increased risk for femoral fractures in PD is in line with previous studies that demonstrated an association of PD with an increased risk of falling and a decreased bone mineral density [10]. A meta-analysis pooling data from six prospective studies found 46% of PD patients to fall over a three month period [6]. In addition to known risk factors such as age, female gender and previous falls, various disease-specific risk factors are under discussion such as pathologic gait characteristics [5,29,30], balance problems [5,29], impaired cognition [29,31], and the use of dopaminergic drugs [5,9].

However, the excess risk we found is lower than the values reported previously ranging from a 2.2- to a 4.6-fold risk [12,14–16,32]. Our study is based on an unselected population-based sample of individuals including all stages of PD and including community-dwelling older individuals as well as nursing home residents (in both, PD patients and the reference group). This approach is in clear contrast to a number of studies recruiting from either specialist clinics or cohort studies that excluded the frailest of these patients. Such an example of a non-representative sample would be the Osteoporotic Fractures in Men study (MrOS) that explicitly excluded men unable to walk without personal assistance

[11,33]. A similar approach was chosen for the recruitment of another cohort [14]. Considering the fact that the risk of falling increases with the disease stages [4,6], the advantage of a population-based approach is apparent.

This study introduces an additional approach which may be useful for a better interpretation of the observed risk. We were able to stratify the cohorts according to the need for long-term nursing care as a functional parameter. About every other PD patient in our dataset required long-term nursing care. Stratifying our analyses by this indicator for severe functional impairment, we retrieved a more complex picture. PD patients without severe functional impairment had a more than two fold risk to sustain a femoral fracture, compared to the reference group. In contrast, PD patients with severe functional impairment did not (women) or only slightly (men) differ from the reference group with severe functional impairment. Although we could confirm that PD is a risk factor for femoral fractures, the above data indicate that not the diagnosis per se, but functional impairment as a consequence of PD contributes relevantly to the risk of femoral fractures. Severe functional impairment expressed as care need has been shown to be a risk factor for factures [34,35] The analysis of PD patients versus a reference group presented in this study implies that not the underlying disease is attributable for this risk but the need for help with ADLs.

Our approach has several limitations that need to be considered when interpreting the findings. The dataset used does not allow diagnosis of PD with very high security. However, by introducing a 'possible' and 'probable' PD model (which showed comparable results) and by choosing definitions that make the inclusion of severe atypical Parkinsonism (with an even higher risk of falls) in the PD cohort very probable, we argue that our approach might rather over- than under-estimate the fracture risk in the PD group. Moreover, data from the Rotterdam study indicates that our model approach indeed has a high accuracy to detect the persons of interest: They found 78% of users of Parkinson medication to have clinically confirmed idiopathic PD; intake of more than one substance class yield 100% specificity [36]. The most prevalent other condition treated with dopaminergic drugs is the restless legs syndrome (RLS) [37]. Further arguments for the usefulness of the PD models introduced here are provided by results of epidemiological studies investigating treatment behavior of the most relevant "confounding" disease, i.e. RLS. These studies found that, contrary to what is recommended in the guidelines, only a minority of patients are treated with dopaminergic drugs [38–40].

Another shortcoming of our data is the lack of information on dosage. Data from Denmark demonstrated a dose-dependent association between fracture risk and Parkinson's medication [15]. Reimbursement data in the dataset used in our study did not allow reliable calculation of dosage in the absence of regimes.

We identified persons as 'possible' PD (model I) and 'probable' PD based on medication records in 2004. We could not trace back the duration of dispensing for a longer time period. Hence, this study does not allow any conclusions with respect to the duration of PD.

Our data were derived only from one health insurance company and may not be representative for the whole German population. However, the AOK is the by far largest statutory health care insurance and is open to all people. In Bavaria, the AOK covers almost 50% of the population aged 65 years and older, thus we argue that this is indeed a representative sample.

Conclusions

Our findings confirm the increased risk of femoral fractures in PD patients. However, according to our large population-based dataset it is lower than previously reported. Interestingly, diagnosis-specific differences in fracture risk was observable only in PD patients *without* severe functional impairment, whereas PD patients and the reference group *with* severe functional impairment did not show relevant differences in fracture risk. This may have relevant implications for disease-specific falls prevention programs in PD patients. Such programs may be most effective in early rather than in advanced stages of the disease.

Acknowledgments

We thank Regina Merk-Bäuml, Ralf Brum, Markus Gindl and Stefanie Büttner from the Allgemeine Ortskrankenkasse (AOK) for their support of our analyses.

Author Contributions

Conceived and designed the experiments: PB KR JK AJ GB WM HHK. Performed the experiments: PB GB AJ. Analyzed the data: PB KR JK AJ GB WM. Wrote the paper: PB KR JK AJ GB WM HHK.

References

1. De Lau LML, Breteler MMB (2006) Epidemiology of Parkinson's disease. Lancet Neurol 5: 525–535. doi:10.1016/S1474-4422(06)70471-9.
2. Abou-Raya S, Helmii M, Abou-Raya A (2009) Bone and mineral metabolism in older adults with Parkinson's disease. Age Ageing 38: 675–680. doi:10.1093/ageing/afp137.
3. Balash Y, Peretz C, Leibovich G, Herman T, Hausdorff JM, et al. (2005) Falls in outpatients with Parkinson's disease: frequency, impact and identifying factors. J Neurol 252: 1310–1315. doi:10.1007/s00415-005-0855-3.
4. Bloem BR, Grimbergen YA, Cramer M, Willemsen M, Zwinderman AH (2001) Prospective assessment of falls in Parkinson's disease. J Neurol 248: 950–958.
5. Matinolli M, Korpelainen JT, Sotaniemi KA, Myllylä VV, Korpelainen R (2011) Recurrent falls and mortality in Parkinson's disease: a prospective two-year follow-up study. Acta Neurol Scand 123: 193–200. doi:10.1111/j.1600-0404.2010.01386.x.
6. Pickering RM, Grimbergen YAM, Rigney U, Ashburn A, Mazibrada G, et al. (2007) A meta-analysis of six prospective studies of falling in Parkinson's disease. Mov Disord 22: 1892–1900. doi:10.1002/mds.21598.
7. Wielinski CL, Erickson-Davis C, Wichmann R, Walde-Douglas M, Parashos SA (2005) Falls and injuries resulting from falls among patients with Parkinson's disease and other parkinsonian syndromes. Mov Disord 20: 410–415. doi:10.1002/mds.20347.
8. Temlett JA, Thompson PD (2006) Reasons for admission to hospital for Parkinson's disease. Intern Med J 36: 524–526. doi:10.1111/j.1445-5994.2006.01123.x.
9. Arbouw MEL, Movig KLL, van Staa TP, Egberts ACG, Souverein PC, et al. (2011) Dopaminergic drugs and the risk of hip or femur fracture: a population-based case-control study. Osteoporos Int 22: 2197–2204. doi:10.1007/s00198-010-1455-3.
10. Van den Bos F, Speelman AD, Samson M, Munneke M, Bloem BR, et al. (2013) Parkinson's disease and osteoporosis. Age Ageing 42: 156–162. doi:10.1093/ageing/afs161.
11. Fink HA, Kuskowski MA, Taylor BC, Schousboe JT, Orwoll ES, et al. (2008) Association of Parkinson's disease with accelerated bone loss, fractures and mortality in older men: the Osteoporotic Fractures in Men (MrOS) study. Osteoporos Int 19: 1277–1282. doi:10.1007/s00198-008-0584-4.
12. Genever RW, Downes TW, Medcalf P (2005) Fracture rates in Parkinson's disease compared with age- and gender-matched controls: a retrospective cohort study. Age Ageing 34: 21–24. doi:10.1093/ageing/afh203.
13. Johnell O, Melton LJ 3rd, Atkinson EJ, O'Fallon WM, Kurland LT (1992) Fracture risk in patients with parkinsonism: a population-based study in Olmsted County, Minnesota. Age Ageing 21: 32–38.
14. Schneider JL, Fink HA, Ewing SK, Ensrud KE, Cummings SR (2008) The association of Parkinson's disease with bone mineral density and fracture in older women. Osteoporos Int 19: 1093–1097. doi:10.1007/s00198-008-0583-5.
15. Vestergaard P, Rejnmark L, Mosekilde L (2007) Fracture risk associated with parkinsonism and anti-Parkinson drugs. Calcif Tissue Int 81: 153–161. doi:10.1007/s00223-007-9065-6.

16. Melton LJ 3rd, Leibson CL, Achenbach SJ, Bower JH, Maraganore DM, et al. (2006) Fracture risk after the diagnosis of Parkinson's disease: Influence of concomitant dementia. Mov Disord 21: 1361–1367. doi:10.1002/mds.20946.
17. Bleibler F, Konnopka A, Benzinger P, Rapp K, König H-H (2013) The health burden and costs of incident fractures attributable to osteoporosis from 2010 to 2050 in Germany-a demographic simulation model. Osteoporos Int 24: 835–847. doi:10.1007/s00198-012-2020-z.
18. Ioannidis G, Papaioannou A, Hopman WM, Akhtar-Danesh N, Anastassiades T, et al. (2009) Relation between fractures and mortality: results from the Canadian Multicentre Osteoporosis Study. CMAJ 181: 265–271. doi:10.1503/cmaj.081720.
19. Johnell O, Kanis JA (2006) An estimate of the worldwide prevalence and disability associated with osteoporotic fractures. Osteoporos Int 17: 1726–1733. doi:10.1007/s00198-006-0172-4.
20. Clubb VJ, Clubb SE, Buckley S (2006) Parkinson's disease patients who fracture their neck of femur: a review of outcome data. Injury 37: 929–934. doi:10.1016/j.injury.2005.11.013.
21. Healy GN, Owen N (2010) Sedentary behaviour and biomarkers of cardiometabolic health risk in adolescents: an emerging scientific and public health issue. Rev Esp Cardiol 63: 261–264.
22. Jankovic J, Kapadia AS (2001) Functional decline in Parkinson disease. Arch Neurol 58: 1611–1615.
23. Harrison MB, Wylie SA, Frysinger RC, Patric JT, Huss DS, et al. (2009) UPDRS activity of daily living score as a marker of Parkinson's disease progression. Mov Disord 24: 224–230. doi:10.1002/mds.22335.
24. Hughes AJ, Daniel SE, Kilford L, Lees AJ (1992) Accuracy of clinical diagnosis of idiopathic Parkinson's disease: a clinico-pathological study of 100 cases. J Neurol Neurosurg Psychiatr 55: 181–184.
25. Becker C, Leistner K, Nikolaus T (1998) Introducing a statutory insurance system for long-term care (Pflegeversicherung) in Germany. Michel JP, Rubenstein LZ, Vellas BJ, Albarede JL: Geriatric Programs and departments around the world Serdi-Springer, Paris-New York: 55–64.
26. Icks A, Haastert B, Wildner M, Becker C, Meyer G (2008) Trend of hip fracture incidence in Germany 1995–2004: a population-based study. Osteoporosis International 19: 1139–1145.
27. Icks AIA, Arend WAW, Becker CBC, Rapp KRK, Haastert BHB (2013) Incidence of hip fractures in Germany, 1995–2010. Archives of osteoporosis 8: 1–7.
28. Kanis JA, Odén A, McCloskey EV, Johansson H, Wahl DA, et al. (2012) A systematic review of hip fracture incidence and probability of fracture worldwide. Osteoporosis International 23: 2239–2256.
29. Latt MD, Lord SR, Morris JGL, Fung VSC (2009) Clinical and physiological assessments for elucidating falls risk in Parkinson's disease. Mov Disord 24: 1280–1289. doi:10.1002/mds.22561.
30. Plotnik M, Giladi N, Dagan Y, Hausdorff JM (2011) Postural instability and fall risk in Parkinson's disease: impaired dual tasking, pacing, and bilateral coordination of gait during the "ON" medication state. Exp Brain Res 210: 529–538. doi:10.1007/s00221-011-2551-0.
31. Wood BH, Bilclough JA, Bowron A, Walker RW (2002) Incidence and prediction of falls in Parkinson's disease: a prospective multidisciplinary study. J Neurol Neurosurg Psychiatr 72: 721–725.
32. Bhattacharya RK, Dubinsky RM, Lai SM, Dubinsky H (2012) Is there an increased risk of hip fracture in Parkinson's disease? A nationwide inpatient sample. Mov Disord 27: 1440–1443. doi:10.1002/mds.25073.
33. Fink HA, Kuskowski MA, Orwoll ES, Cauley JA, Ensrud KE (2005) Association between Parkinson's disease and low bone density and falls in older men: the osteoporotic fractures in men study. J Am Geriatr Soc 53: 1559–1564. doi:10.1111/j.1532-5415.2005.53464.x.
34. Benzinger P, Becker C, Kerse N, Bleibler F, Büchele G, et al. (2013) Pelvic Fracture Rates in Community-Living People With and Without Disability and in Residents of Nursing Homes. J Am Med Dir Assoc. doi:10.1016/j.jamda.2013.03.012.
35. Rapp K, Becker C, Cameron ID, Klenk J, Kleiner A, et al. (2012) Femoral fracture rates in people with and without disability. Age Ageing 41: 653–658. doi:10.1093/ageing/afs044.
36. Van de Vijver DA, Stricker BH, Breteler MM, Roos RA, Porsius AJ, et al. (2001) Evaluation of antiparkinsonian drugs in pharmacy records as a marker for Parkinson's disease. Pharm World Sci 23: 148–152.
37. Trenkwalder C, Hening WA, Montagna P, Oertel WH, Allen RP, et al. (2008) Treatment of restless legs syndrome: an evidence-based review and implications for clinical practice. Mov Disord 23: 2267–2302. doi:10.1002/mds.22254.
38. Högl B, Kiechl S, Willeit J, Saletu M, Frauscher B, et al. (2005) Restless legs syndrome: a community-based study of prevalence, severity, and risk factors. Neurology 64: 1920–1924. doi:10.1212/01.WNL.0000163996.64461.A3.
39. Hening W, Walters AS, Allen RP, Montplaisir J, Myers A, et al. (2004) Impact, diagnosis and treatment of restless legs syndrome (RLS) in a primary care population: the REST (RLS epidemiology, symptoms, and treatment) primary care study. Sleep Med 5: 237–246. doi:10.1016/j.sleep.2004.03.006.
40. Cirillo DJ, Wallace RB (2012) Restless legs syndrome and functional limitations among American elders in the Health and Retirement Study. BMC Geriatr 12: 39. doi:10.1186/1471-2318-12-39.

2

DLS 5.0 - The Biomechanical Effects of Dynamic Locking Screws

Stefan Döbele[1]*, Michael Gardner[2], Steffen Schröter[1], Dankward Höntzsch[1], Ulrich Stöckle[1], Thomas Freude[1]

1 BG Trauma Center, Eberhard Karls Universitaet Tuebingen, Tübingen, Germany, **2** Department of Orthopaedic Surgery, Washington University School of Medicine, St. Louis, Missouri, United States of America

Abstract

Introduction: Indirect reduction of dia-/metaphyseal fractures with minimally invasive implant application bridges the fracture zone in order to protect the soft-tissue and blood supply. The goal of this fixation strategy is to allow stable motion at the fracture site to achieve indirect bone healing with callus formation. However, concerns have arisen that the high axial stiffness and eccentric position of locked plating constructs may suppress interfragmentary motion and callus formation, particularly under the plate. The reason for this is an asymmetric fracture movement. The biological need for sufficient callus formation and secondary bone healing is three-dimensional micro movement in the fracture zone. The DLS was designed to allow for increased fracture site motion. The purpose of the current study was to determine the biomechanical effect of the DLS_5.0.

Methods: Twelve surrogate bone models were used for analyzing the characteristics of the DLS_5.0. The axial stiffness and the interfragmentary motion of locked plating constructs with DLS were compared to conventional constructs with Locking Head Screws (LS_5.0). A quasi-static axial load of 0 to 2.5 kN was applied. Relative motion was measured.

Results: The dynamic system showed a biphasic axial stiffness distribution and provided a significant reduction of the initial axial stiffness of 74.4%. Additionally, the interfragmentary motion at the near cortex increased significantly from 0.033 mm to 0.210 mm (at 200N).

Conclusions: The DLS may ultimately be an improvement over the angular stable plate osteosynthesis. The advantages of the angular stability are not only preserved but even supplemented by a dynamic element which leads to homogenous fracture movement and to a potentially uniform callus distribution.

Editor: Bart O. Williams, Van Andel Institute, United States of America

Funding: These authors have no support or funding to report.

Competing Interests: The authors have declared that no competing interests exist.

* E-mail: sdoebele@bgu-tuebingen.de

Introduction

In recent years, extramedullary internal fixation techniques of long bone fractures have evolved from very rigid constructs to more flexible internal fixation constructs [1–3]. This evolution was possible with the introduction of locking plates, as angular stable screw anchorage in the plate eliminated the need for plate compression against the bone [2]. Contrary to absolute stability with primary bone healing, the aim of a less rigid fixation is the stimulation of fracture healing by callus formation [3]. Terms and definitions like "biological plate osteosynthesis" and "bridge plate technique" were introduced and established [1,3,4]. The basic principle of both methods is a minimally invasive reduction and fixation technique preserving fracture vascularity [1–6].

Recent studies have confirmed that axial stiffness of modern locked plating constructs is in some cases too high [3,6–8] which is based on the angular stable plate-screw interface in locked plates. The majority of the fracture motion occurs through bending of the plate under axial load resulting in an asymmetric fracture motion, with greater motion at the far cortex than at the near cortex [8]. This may suppress callus formation, particularly at the near cortex (fig. 1) [5–13].

Several techniques have been described to decrease the stiffness of a locked plating construct [5,6,8,14]. With the introduction of the 3.7 mm Dynamic Locking Screw (DLS 3.7) in 2010, it was demonstrated that the axial stiffness of a locking plate construct was decreased and the interfragmentary motion of the far cortex was increased, while still providing adequate mechanical stability. These changes result in a more symmetrical fracture motion (fig. 2) [8].

The aim of the following study was to determine the biomechanical properties of large fragment 5.0 mm Dynamic Locking Screw (fig. 3, Synthes, Oberdorf, Switzerland) constructs. To achieve this, we used standardized constructs (fig. 4) with Dynamic Locking Screws (DLS) and standard Locking Head Screws (LS) to assess differences in *i*) axial stiffness and *ii*) interfragmentary motion (fig. 5).

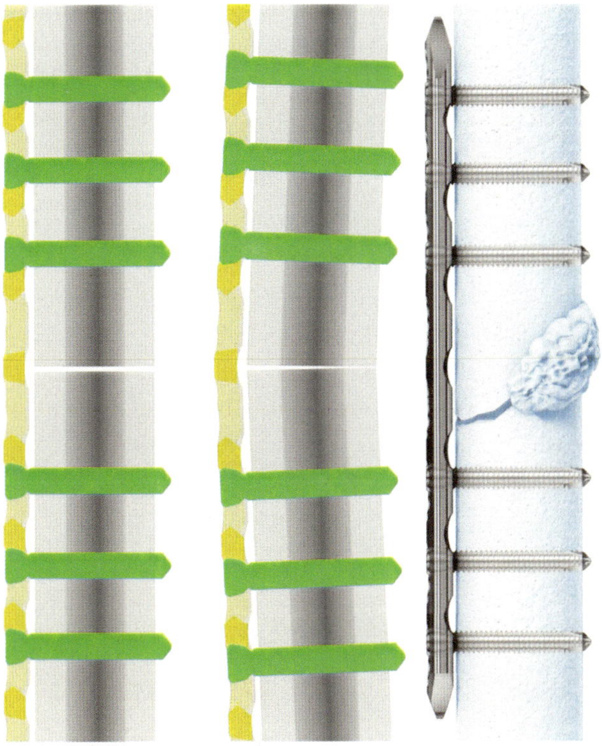

Figure 1. Osteosynthesis with Locking Head Screws without and with axial load and callus formation only at the trans cortex.

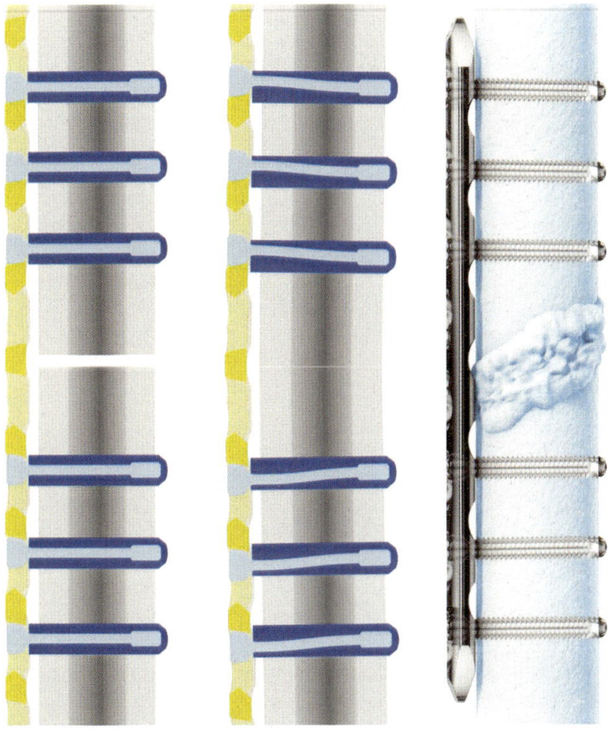

Figure 2. Osteosynthesis with DLS without and with axial load and circumferential callus formation.

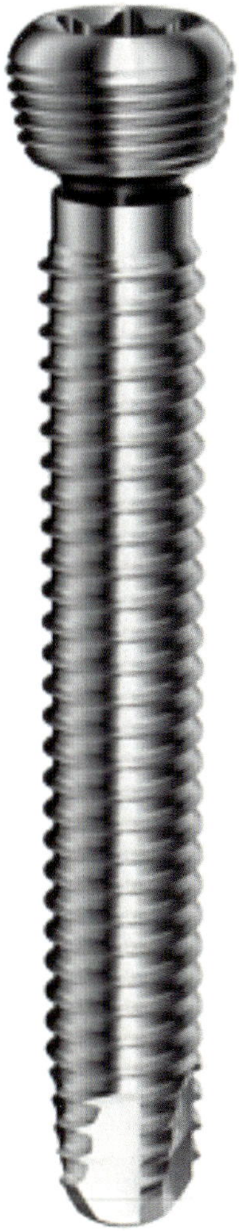

Figure 3. DLS – Dynamic Locking Screw with PIN-Sleeve-Design.

Materials and Methods

1. Specimens

Twelve surrogate bone models were obtained and used for the testing (fig. 4). Two cylinders with a diameter of 27 mm, a wall thickness of 7 mm, a length of 95 mm and a Young's modulus of 16.7 GPa (Sawbones #3403; Pacific Research Laboratories, Vashon, Washington) were used to create a simplified transverse fracture model, according to Bottlang et al. [5]. The holes for the screws were inserted in the cylinders with a computer controlled milling machine. The two cylinders were fixed together using a 6-holes titanium locking compression plates (#426.561 LCP broad 4.5/5.0, L = 116 mm, TiCP, Synthes, Oberdorf, Switzerland). In the first six specimens, DLS (#09.223.038S, 5.0 mm, self-tapping, L38 mm, CoCrMo, Synthes, Oberdorf, Switzerland) screws were tested, while in the second six specimens LS ((#412.213, 5.0 mm, self-tapping, L38 mm, Ti Al6 Nb7, Synthes, Oberdorf, Switzerland) were used. Plates were fixed with three screws per cylinder, which were placed in the first, second and third hole from the fracture site. The fracture gap was 3 mm wide. All screws were tightened to 4.0 Nm with the plate at 2 mm distance from the cylinder surface.

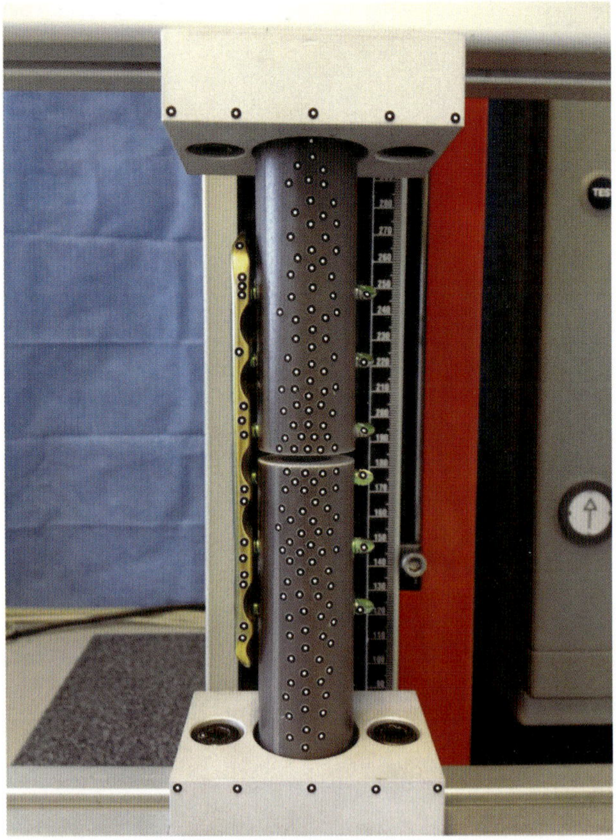

Figure 4. Specimens had a diameter of 27 mm, a wall thickness of 7 mm, a length of 193 mm and a Young's modulus of 16.7 GPa. Passive markers were attached to both cylinders and the LCP to perform the measurement with the optical motion analysis system.

These locked plating constructs, 6 with LS and 6 with DLS, were tested while applying a force-controlled, quasi-static axial load of 0 N to 2.5 kN at 10 mm/min using a mono-axial material testing device (Zwickiline 2.5 kN; Zwick, Ulm, Germany). In this force range (0–2.5 kN), no plastic deformity of the implants was observed. The three-dimensional motion of each osteosynthesis was measured using the optical motion analysis system PONTOS 5M (GOM, Braunschweig, Germany). Using an interface, the force measured by the load cell (testing machine) could be transferred to the optical motion system and processed by the software of the optical motion system. The axial stiffness was calculated using the applied force and the corresponding deviation in the z-axis. Furthermore, motion near the plate (cis-cortex) and far away from the plate (trans-cortex) was calculated. The data was analyzed with Matlab (MathWorks, USA).

2. DLS

The DLS is a new generation of locking screws that allows the surgeon to control the rigidity of plating constructs. The DLS pin-sleeve design combines locking technology with dynamic motion — the threaded sleeve anchors the DLS in the bone, while the pin locks the DLS with its standardized threaded head into Synthes locking plates (fig. 3). The play between the sleeve and the pin determines the amount of motion induced in the fracture gap. Cobalt chromium molybdenum alloy (CoCrMo) ensures the mechanical stability of DLS, while encouraging less ongrowth and facilitating screw removal – similar to stainless steel screws. DLS is fully compatible with all Synthes' titanium and stainless steel locking plates.

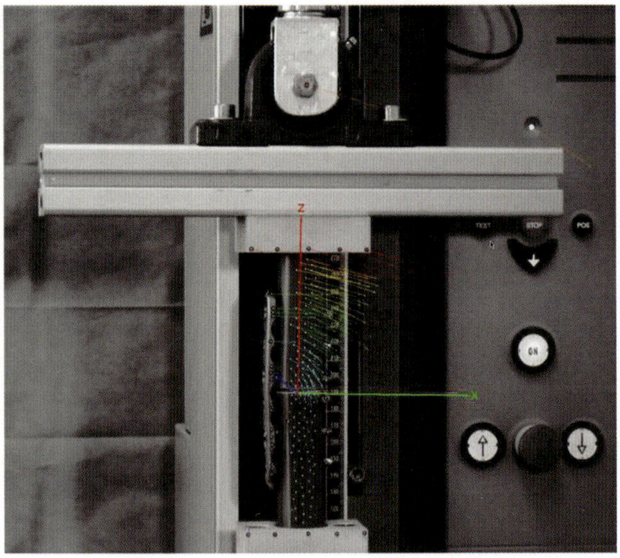

Figure 5. Test set-up. Axial load was applied by a universal testing machine. 3D-motion at the fracture gap was measured with an optical motion analysis system and visualized by vectors. Raw data of the 3D-motion of every passive marker was analyzed using the software MATLAB.

3. Optical motion analysis system

For measuring the 3D fracture motion we used the optical analysis system PONTOS 5 M (GOM - Optical Measuring Techniques, Braunschweig, Germany). The system consists of two CCD (Charge-coupled device) cameras. For the detection of the motion passive markers are required. The points are recorded and tracked by the PONTOS software (fig. 5). The PONTOS 5 M system was set up and calibrated for a measurement volume of 350×280×280 mm according to the manufacturer's documentation. The geometrical setup as well as the optical distortion factors of the lenses were accounted for in the calibration procedure. The frame rate was 4 Hz. White self-adhesive dots with a diameter of 2 mm were used as passive motion markers, with at least 3 points per object. For a higher accuracy, we used about 400 passive markers per specimen. The high number of points allowed fitting two cylindrical geometry elements, which represented the physical cylindrical fracture fragments. The six degrees of freedom motion could, therefore, be directly represented at the location in the center of the fracture gap for each fragment. Relative motion in all six degrees of freedom was analyzed (fig. 5).

4. Statistical analysis

All results were analyzed with a commercial statistical software package (GraphPad Prism, El Camino Real, LaJolla, USA, Version 5.01, t-test, $p \leq 0{,}05$).

Results

In comparison to the LS, the DLS showed a biphasic stiffness distribution with distinct initial - and secondary stiffnesses. As shown in figure 6, the initial axial stiffness of the DLS group was 612.4 N/mm and secondary stiffness was 2301.9 N/mm. In the

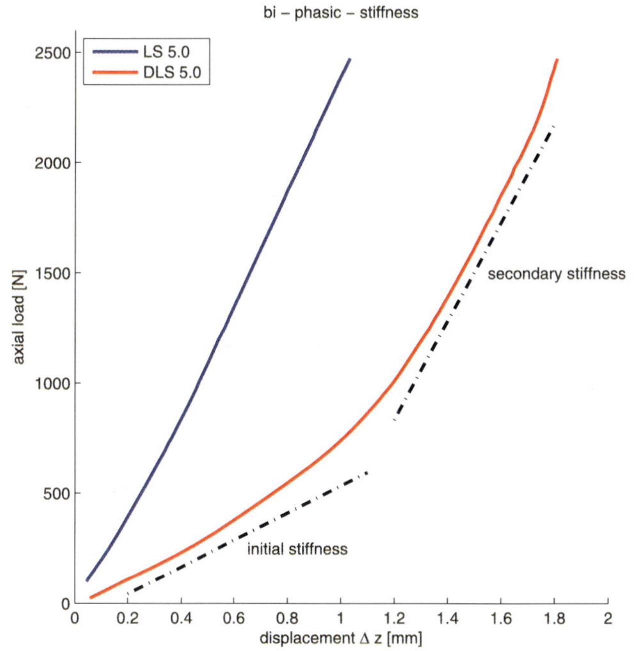

Figure 6. In comparison to the LS, the DLS showed a biphasic stiffness distribution with an initial and a secondary stiffness. The initial axial stiffness of DLS was 612.4 N/mm and secondary stiffness was 2301.9 N/mm. The mean LS axial stiffness was 2394.9 N/mm.

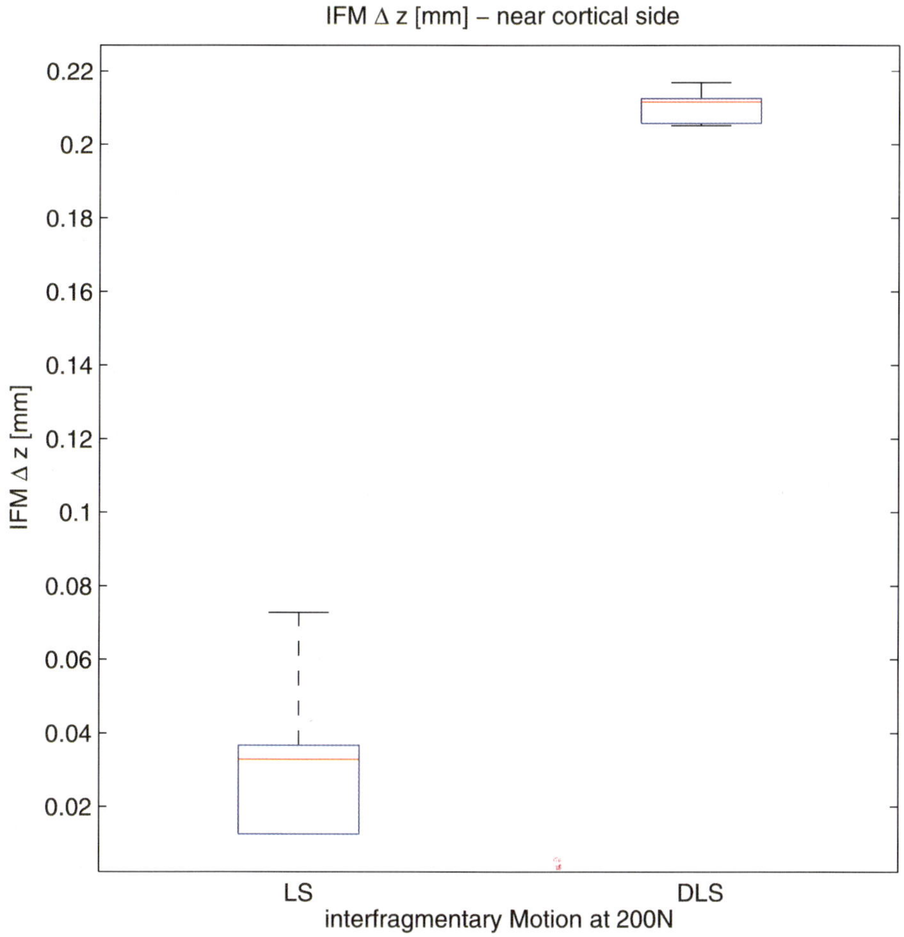

Figure 7. With application of a 200 N axial load, the interfragmentary motion at the near cortex was significantly higher in the DLS group (0.210 mm; SD ± 0,004 mm) (compared to the LS group (0.033 mm; SD ± 0.02 mm).

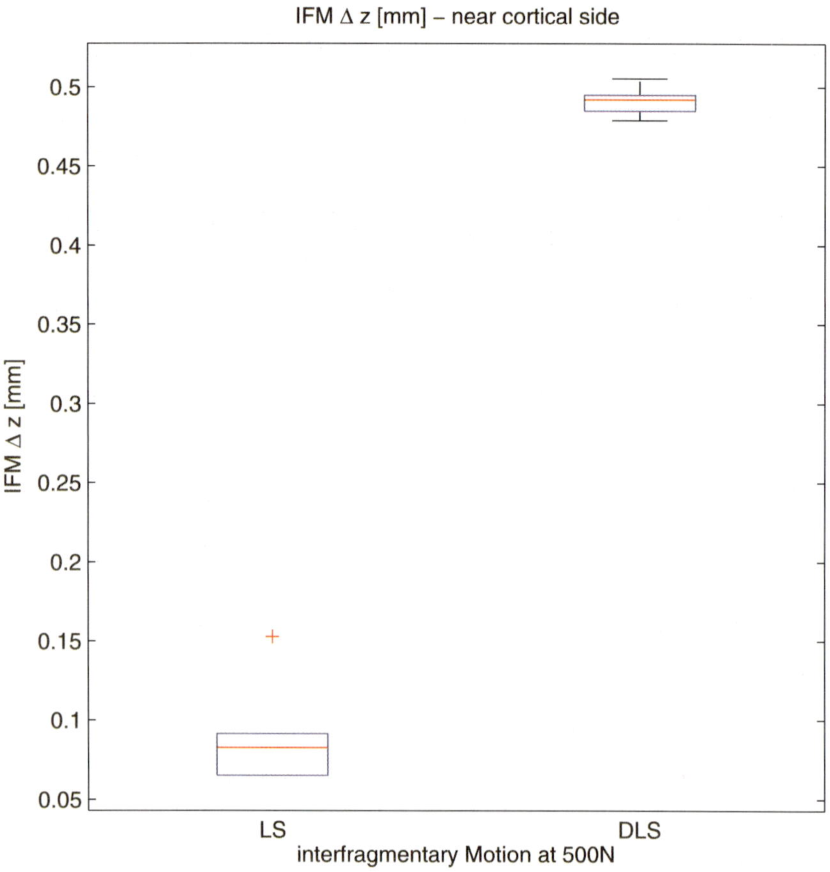

Figure 8. With application of a 500 N axial load, the interfragmentary motion at the near cortex was significantly higher in the DLS group (0.49 mm; SD ± 0,008 mm) compared to the LS group (0.089 mm; SD ± 0,03 mm).

LS group the axial stiffness was generally constant at a mean of 2394.9 N/mm throughout stiffness testing (monophasic stiffness distribution). In the DLS group, the initial stiffness appeared to be a result of the dynamic phase of the screw at low loads. At higher loads, as soon as the pin of the screw has displaced the maximum distance within the sheath, there was a sharp increase stiffness. After the increase there was a secondary stiffness curve, which was similar to the LS. The initial stiffness of the DLS was 74.4% lower than the stiffness of LS. The secondary stiffness of the dynamic construct was 3.4% lower than the stiffness from the non-dynamic construct.

Interfragmentary motion was significantly greater at the near cortex (fig. 7+8) with the DLS compared to the LS (0.089 mm; SD ± 0,03 mm vs 0.491 mm; SD ± 0,008 mm, respectively, $p< 0.001$) under a 500 N load. At an axial load of 200 N, the interfragmentary motion at the near cortex was seven-fold greater with the DLS (0.210 mm; SD ± 0,004 mm) compared to the LS (0.033 mm; SD ± 0.02 mm) ($p<0.001$) (fig. 7).

Discussion

Delayed healing of long bone fractures remains a clinically significant problem. The recent popularity of locking plates has potentially contributed to this problem, as these implants are placed eccentrically and are extremely stiff. The goal of developing a new system with a new screw design was to theoretically retain the advantages of the successful locking screw concept by achieving high stability and bicortical screw bone interface. Additionally, however, this new design is intended to alter the overall axial stiffness of the implant, maintain the bending stiffness of proven plate devices, and increase the near cortex micromovement by more symmetrical axial stress distribution. The aim of our biomechanical investigation was to determine if the new dynamic locking screw was able to meet the functional requirements as theorized. A biomechanical *in vitro* study was performed to assess the differences of a dynamic system using the DLS screws in an osteosynthesis construct compared to standard locking screws. We hypothesized that a dynamic system would result in more balanced fracture motion between the near and far cortices, which could theoretically improve callus formation and equalize callus distribution at the fracture site. To test the hypothesis of the current biomechanical study, two main topics were investigated: the axial stiffness and the interfragmentary motion. We found that stiffness was significantly decreased and near cortex motion was significantly increased in dynamic constructs. The physiological consequence of these altered biomechanics (eg, the callus volume and distribution and the mechanical strength) will be addressed in an ongoing *in vivo* animal study.

In comparison to the non-dynamic screws, the dynamic system provided a significant reduction of the initial axial stiffness up to a certain applied axial load on the construct. While applying a load below 400 N, the axial stiffness of LS and DLS diverge from each other. In the range from 400 N to 2.5 kN however, the axial stiffness of both systems converged again (figure 3). In other words, the dynamic effect of the new screw is more distinctive at lower loads and therefore, would be applicable in a clinical application

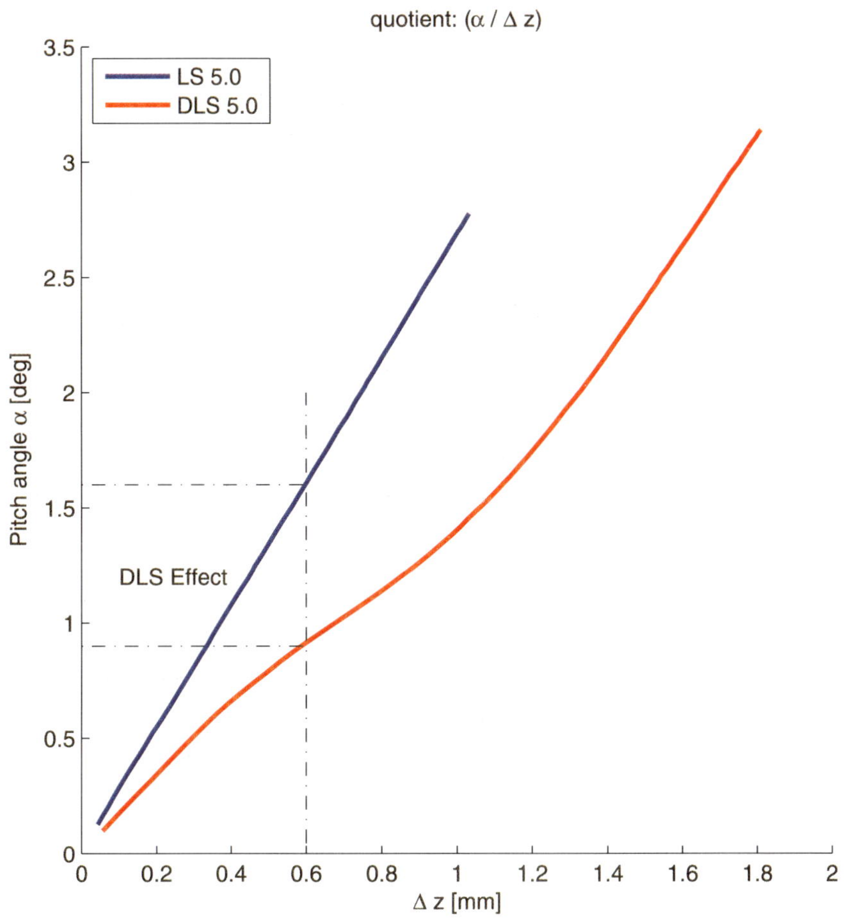

Figure 9. With the same pitch angle of the osteosynthesis plate, interfragmentary motion is higher using the DLS than the LS.

with a partial weight bearing of 25 kg. The pin-sleeve construction was designed in a way that the pin is not only bending as a result of applied axial load on the construct, but that the deformation of the pin is even S-shaped. The length of the pin is always identical and does not depend on the screw length. Therefore the dynamic effect does not depend on the screw length.

After reaching the maximal range of motion limited by pin and sleeve contact, a sharp stiffness increase occurred, which we denoted the "secondary stiffness". The secondary "axial" stiffness of the DLS was in the same range as the LS. In other words, the characteristics of the DLS equal those of the LS when higher loads are applied.

Concerning patient safety, it can be noted that the positive effects of the DLS on fracture motion can be observed when a partial weight bearing of around 25 kg is maintained by the patient. But when higher loads are applied to the osteosynthesis, the DLS reacts like a conventional locking head screw. Because typical postoperative protocols for plated lower extremity fractures involve six to eight weeks of "toe-touch" weight bearing, our data can be extrapolated to being applicable in a clinical setting.

When a conventional LS is used, the fracture motion on the far cortex is much higher than on the near cortex, because the interfragmentary motion is caused essentially by the bending of the plate [2,3,5,6,8].

As is shown in figure 6, the DLS enables the same fracture motion while causing a less bending of the plate. This is called the "DLS-Effect" (fig. 9).

The current biomechanical study was performed in a bone surrogate model. This model was chosen because it enabled reproducible data and allowed for the detection of relatively small differences between the dynamic and the standard system. However, this study also had some limitations. As all tests were carried out with artificial bones, it did not reproduce the human biology. Therefore, we did not simulate the effect of osteoporosis on the two systems, and did not analyze the properties of different fracture types. But this was not in focus of the present study, in which the goal was solely to determine the effect of the DLS in an osteosynthesis construct.

Our testing parameters were chosen deliberately to allow comparisons to previous work in the literature. Several previous studies have examined the biomechanics of "dynamic" locked plating systems. [5,6,8]. Bottlang et al. evaluated the concept of "far cortical locking" (FCL). [5]. This system also showed a biphasic axial stiffness distribution with an initial and a secondary stiffness. Our findings concurred with those authors, in that more balanced fracture motion at the near and far cortices occurred, the axial stiffness was reduced and the distribution of the interfragmentary motion was more homogeneous [5]. The main difference between the DLS and the FCL is the bone fixation of the screws. While FCL allows only for unicortical fixation at the far cortex, DLS functions more like a standard locking screw, allowing bicortical fixation as the sleeve obtains thread purchase at the near cortex [8]. We believe that the bicortical construct likely improves fixation due to more points of bone-screw contact.

Additionally, the dynamic component of the FCL concept relies on the screw shaft toggling against a bone hole at the near cortex, which may cause bone resorption and loss of fixation over time. This is in contrast to the DLS, in which a metal pin toggles against a metal sleeve.

The DLS may ultimately be an improvement over the angular stable plate osteosynthesis. The advantages of the angular stability are not only preserved but even supplemented by a dynamic element which leads to homogenous fracture movement and to a potentially uniform callus distribution. The surgeon has the opportunity to deliberately influence the rigidity of an osteosynthesis through the DLS.

Author Contributions

Conceived and designed the experiments: SD US. Performed the experiments: SD. Analyzed the data: SD MG SS DH US TF. Contributed reagents/materials/analysis tools: SD MG SS DH US TF. Wrote the paper: SD MG TF.

References

1. Perren SM (2002) Evolution of the internal fixation of long bone fractures. The scientific basis of biological internal fixation: choosing a new balance between stability and biology. J Bone Joint Surg Br 84: 1093–1110.
2. Schmal H, Strohm PC, Jaeger M, Sudkamp NP (2011) Flexible fixation and fracture healing: do locked plating 'internal fixators' resemble external fixators? J Orthop Trauma 25 Suppl 1: S15–20.
3. Claes L (2011) Biomechanical principles and mechanobiologic aspects of flexible and locked plating. J Orthop Trauma 25 Suppl 1: S4–7.
4. Perren SM, Perren T, Schneider E (2003) [Are the terms "biology" and "osteosynthesis" contradictory?]. Ther Umsch 60: 713–721.
5. Bottlang M, Doornink J, Fitzpatrick DC, Madey SM (2009) Far cortical locking can reduce stiffness of locked plating constructs while retaining construct strength. J Bone Joint Surg Am 91: 1985–1994.
6. Gardner MJ, Nork SE, Huber P, Krieg JC (2010) Less rigid stable fracture fixation in osteoporotic bone using locked plates with near cortical slots. Injury 41: 652–656.
7. Foux A, Yeadon AJ, Uhthoff HK (1997) Improved fracture healing with less rigid plates. A biomechanical study in dogs. Clin Orthop Relat Res: 232–245.
8. Dobele S, Horn C, Eichhorn S, Buchholtz A, Lenich A, et al. (2010) The dynamic locking screw (DLS) can increase interfragmentary motion on the near cortex of locked plating constructs by reducing the axial stiffness. Langenbecks Arch Surg 395: 421–428.
9. Henderson CE, Bottlang M, Marsh JL, Fitzpatrick DC, Madey SM (2008) Does locked plating of periprosthetic supracondylar femur fractures promote bone healing by callus formation? Two cases with opposite outcomes. Iowa Orthop J 28: 73–76.
10. Uhthoff HK, Poitras P, Backman DS (2006) Internal plate fixation of fractures: short history and recent developments. J Orthop Sci 11: 118–126.
11. Egol KA, Kubiak EN, Fulkerson E, Kummer FJ, Koval KJ (2004) Biomechanics of locked plates and screws. J Orthop Trauma 18: 488–493.
12. Kubiak EN, Fulkerson E, Strauss E, Egol KA (2006) The evolution of locked plates. J Bone Joint Surg Am 88 Suppl 4: 189–200.
13. Smith WR, Ziran BH, Anglen JO, Stahel PF (2008) Locking plates: tips and tricks. Instr Course Lect 57: 25–36.
14. Stoffel K, Dieter U, Stachowiak G, Gächter A, Kuster MS (2003) Biomechanical testing of the LCP – how can stability in locked internal fixators be controlled? Injury 34: 11–19.

The Effect of HIV-Hepatitis C Co-Infection on Bone Mineral Density and Fracture

Tyler J. O'Neill[1]*, Laura Rivera[1], Vladi Struchkov[1,3], Ahmad Zaheen[3], Hla-Hla Thein[1,2]

1 Dalla Lana School of Public Health, University of Toronto, Toronto, Ontario, Canada, **2** Ontario Institute for Cancer Research/Cancer Care Ontario, Toronto, Ontario, Canada, **3** Faculty of Medicine, University of Toronto, Toronto, Ontario, Canada

Abstract

Objective: There is a variable body of evidence on adverse bone outcomes in HIV patients co-infected with hepatitis C virus (HCV). We examined the association of HIV/HCV co-infection on osteoporosis or osteopenia (reduced bone mineral density; BMD) and fracture.

Design: Systematic review and random effects meta-analyses.

Methods: A systematic literature search was conducted for articles published in English up to 1 April 2013. All studies reporting either BMD (g/cm^2, or as a T-score) or incident fractures in HIV/HCV co-infected patients compared to either HIV mono-infected or HIV/HCV uninfected/seronegative controls were included. Random effects meta-analyses estimated the pooled odds ratio (OR) and the relative risk (RR) and associated 95% confidence intervals (CI).

Results: Thirteen eligible publications (BMD N = 6; Fracture = 7) of 2,064 identified were included with a total of 427,352 subjects. No publications reported data on HCV mono-infected controls. Meta-analysis of cross-sectional studies confirmed that low bone mineral density was increasingly prevalent among co-infected patients compared to HIV mono-infected controls (pooled OR 1.98, 95% CI 1.18, 3.31) but not those uninfected (pooled OR 1.47, 95% CI 0.78, 2.78). Significant association between co-infection and fracture was found compared to HIV mono-infected from cohort and case-control studies (pooled RR 1.57, 95% CI 1.33, 1.86) and compared to HIV/HCV uninfected from cohort (pooled RR 2.46, 95% CI 1.03, 3.88) and cross-sectional studies (pooled OR 2.30, 95% CI 2.09, 2.23).

Conclusions: The associations of co-infection with prevalent low BMD and risk of fracture are confirmed in this meta-analysis. Although the mechanisms of HIV/HCV co-infection's effect on BMD and fracture are not well understood, there is evidence to suggest that adverse outcomes among HIV/HCV co-infected patients are substantial.

Editor: Wenyu Lin, Harvard Medical School, United States of America

Funding: These authors have no support or funding to report.

Competing Interests: The authors have declared that no competing interests exist.

* Email: t.oneill@mail.utoronto.ca

Introduction

The success of antiretroviral therapy (ART) and other advanced therapeutics in reducing the mortality of human immunodeficiency virus (HIV)-infected patients has changed the clinical course of this disease. HIV infected patients are less likely to experience death as a result of 'AIDS-related' causes, but are susceptible to 'non-AIDS-related' conditions in the course of their treatment [1] including adverse metabolic outcomes of the skeletal system [2,3]. A common comorbid feature is co-infection with hepatitis C virus (HCV). Studies among HIV patients report hepatic-associated effects of chronic HCV infection, including hepatitis, fibrosis, cirrhosis, and carcinoma, are complicated by HIV co-infection [4]. The effect of non-hepatic outcomes, including mechanisms leading to low bone mineral density (BMD) and fractures associated with hepatic osteodystrophy, remains unclear due to limited evidence of the effects of co-infection [5,6,7].

Osteoporosis is a systemic skeletal disorder characterized by low bone mass. Osteopenia (BMD <1 standard deviations of the mean BMD of a sex-matched, young healthy population below normal BMD, i.e. T-score −1 to −2.5) often precedes osteoporosis (i.e. T-score <−2.5), predisposing affected patients to fracture [8,9,10]. Low BMD is prevalent in HIV patients [11]. Although the incidence of fractures among HIV patients is low, they can be debilitating and potentially life-threatening leading to lower quality of life [12,13,14,15,16,17,18,19,20]. Studies have found higher rates of osteoporotic-associated fractures in HIV patients compared to uninfected controls matched for age [21,22]. The use of ART by HIV mono-patients has also been implicated in exacerbating the severity of adverse skeletal outcomes [3,11,21]. However, it is unclear if it is HIV infection per se, ART, or both that lead to bone loss [10].

Multiple cross-sectional studies have reported an association between chronic HCV infections, reduced BMD [23,24,25,26], and increased risk of fracture [27]. HCV co-infection, compared to HIV mono-infected patients, significantly increases the risk of fractures at many sites [7,28,29]. Low BMD is a recognized complication of HIV infection [11], HIV/HCV co-infection [30], or use of ART [3]. Thus, the risk of fracture in co-infected patients may be greater than that of HIV or HCV mono-infected patients. Not only is co-infection globally prevalent [31], with osteoporotic fractures leading to $12–18 billion USD in direct health care costs annually. Loss of productivity from work because of continual pain, increased absenteeism, and psychological factors add significantly to the total cost of low BMD [32].

Conflicting evidence suggests that adverse bone outcomes are common amongst HIV [2] and HCV [29] mono-infected patients. For example, Lo Re et al. [7] did not find any significant difference in risk of hip fracture between HIV/HCV co-infected and HIV mono-infected patients. While in contrast, Lo Re et al. [30] reported a higher rate of hip fracture was found in co-infected patients compared to HCV mono-infected. However, the suspected synergistic effects of co-infection, including increased inflammation and higher risk of vitamin D deficiency [3], on these outcomes have not been reported as a primary outcome. Therefore, the objective of this systematic review and meta-analysis is to estimate the association of HIV/HCV co-infection on adverse skeletal outcomes (low BMD and risk of fracture). Furthermore, this study intends to generate an estimate for the associations of co-infection with both reduced BMD and bone fracture to stimulate investigation in this important area of growing understanding among HIV patients' comorbidities.

Methods

Search Strategy

Using MEDLINE, EMBASE, Cochrane Library (CENTRAL), and Scopus databases available to the University of Toronto, two investigators (VS and LR) performed a systematic search for relevant literature ever published up to 14 April 2013. The search strategy used MeSH terms ("human immunodeficiency virus" OR "human immunodeficiency virus infection" OR "HIV-1") and ("hepatitis co-infection" OR "hepatitis C" OR "HCV") and ("bone disease" OR "bone density" OR "bone mineral density" OR "osteoporosis" OR "osteopenia" OR "fracture" OR "bone fracture"). In addition, grey literature (e.g. government reports, theses) was searched in The NLM Gateway, The American Society for Bone and Mineral Research, and The Annual Conference on Retroviruses and Opportunistic Infections. The references of identified publications were crosschecked through review of references of relevant publications included in the review (Figure 1).

Study Selection

A Publication was considered eligible for inclusion if it: (1) evaluated the association between HIV-1/HCV co-infection and at least one skeletal outcome (BMD or fracture); (2) reported in English; (3) was a full-length, peer-reviewed observational or randomized control trial (RCTs); (4) reported controls that were either HIV or HCV mono-infected, or uninfected/seronegative; (5) had BMD measured by dual energy X-ray absorptiometry (DXA or DEXA); (6) reported the occurrence of osteoporosis or osteopenia as defined by The World Health Organization (WHO) [10]; and/or (7) reported incident pathologic fracture at any location was reported. Pathologic fractures were defined as fractures possibly due to low BMD (at least osteopenia), typically caused by low energy trauma [28]. Studies in non-human populations, individuals <18 years of age, review articles, case reports or studies that lacked relevant controls, studies on HIV-2 or other HIV strains, and those that did not clearly report the outcomes of interest were excluded from the review.

A two-step procedure was used to screen publications by title and abstract followed by full text review by two investigators (LR and AZ) independently. Any discrepancy concerning a publication's relevancy for inclusion was discussed until consensus was reached. If consensus was not reached, two investigators (HHT and TJO) adjudicated publications.

Data Abstraction

Using a standardized abstraction form, data were extracted by two reviewers (LR and TJO) applying inclusion and exclusion criteria. Information extracted from each study included: (1) study factors: publication status, year of publication, study design, duration of follow-up, inclusion and exclusion criteria, sample size; (2) host factors: age, gender, body mass index (BMI), baseline osteoporotic risk factors, fracture risk factors; (3) infection factors (HIV or HCV): HIV severity as measured by CD4 lymphocyte count and HIV RNA viral load, duration of HIV or HCV infection, clinical symptoms; (4) HCV treatment and ART duration and protocol(s); and (5) outcome factors, relating to BMD and/or fracture. The WHO (1994) criteria were used to define osteopenia (T-score −1.0 to −2.5) and osteoporosis (T-score <−2.5) at any anatomical site. Normal BMD was defined as a T-score greater than −1.0. Fracture could have occurred at any anatomical site. Ascertainments of fracture from radiological confirmation, reports of diagnosis from medical or insurance records, or by patient self-report were included.

Publications were included if they were population-based and reported co-infection as an independent variable and BMD (g/cm^2) or incident fracture as outcome measures. Furthermore, included publication were those in which summary estimates, such as odds ratio (OR) or risk ratio (RR) with 95% confidence interval (CI), were reported or if the publication allowed for the estimation of the summary estimates based on reported data.

Statistical analysis

For case-control and cross-sectional designs, if the adjusted OR of osteopenia or osteoporosis were reported, it was extracted along with covariates controlled for in the model. An unadjusted OR was extracted if an adjusted estimate was not reported. Where necessary, risk was estimated from reported odds according to King and Zeng [33]. The measure of association for cohort studies was summarized using the adjusted RR and 95% CI along with covariates.

Unadjusted measures were estimated where appropriate. For BMD, the mean and its standard deviation (SD) of BMD (g/cm^2) at any location for cases and controls were extracted. The T-score was then calculated comparing to a healthy 30-year old Caucasian female [10] and unadjusted odds were estimated. The odds of having a T-score consistent with osteopenia or osteoporosis were pooled to estimate a dichotomous outcome of low BMD. For publications reporting fracture data (e.g. number of fractures in each group), odds or risk and exact 95% CI were estimated using the reported number of individuals with incident fractures compared to controls.

Pooled analyses, comparing co-infected patients with mono- or uninfected controls, were estimated using random effects models to account for both within- and between-study variability [34]. An inverse variance method was used to weight each estimate. If BMD was measured with more than one control group (e.g. study reported both HIV negative and mono-infected controls) and an average was not reported, data were reported as separate studies within a single publication. If a study evaluated BMD at multiple time points, the value from the first measurement (most reflective of baseline) was selected to avoid dependence. Similarly, only

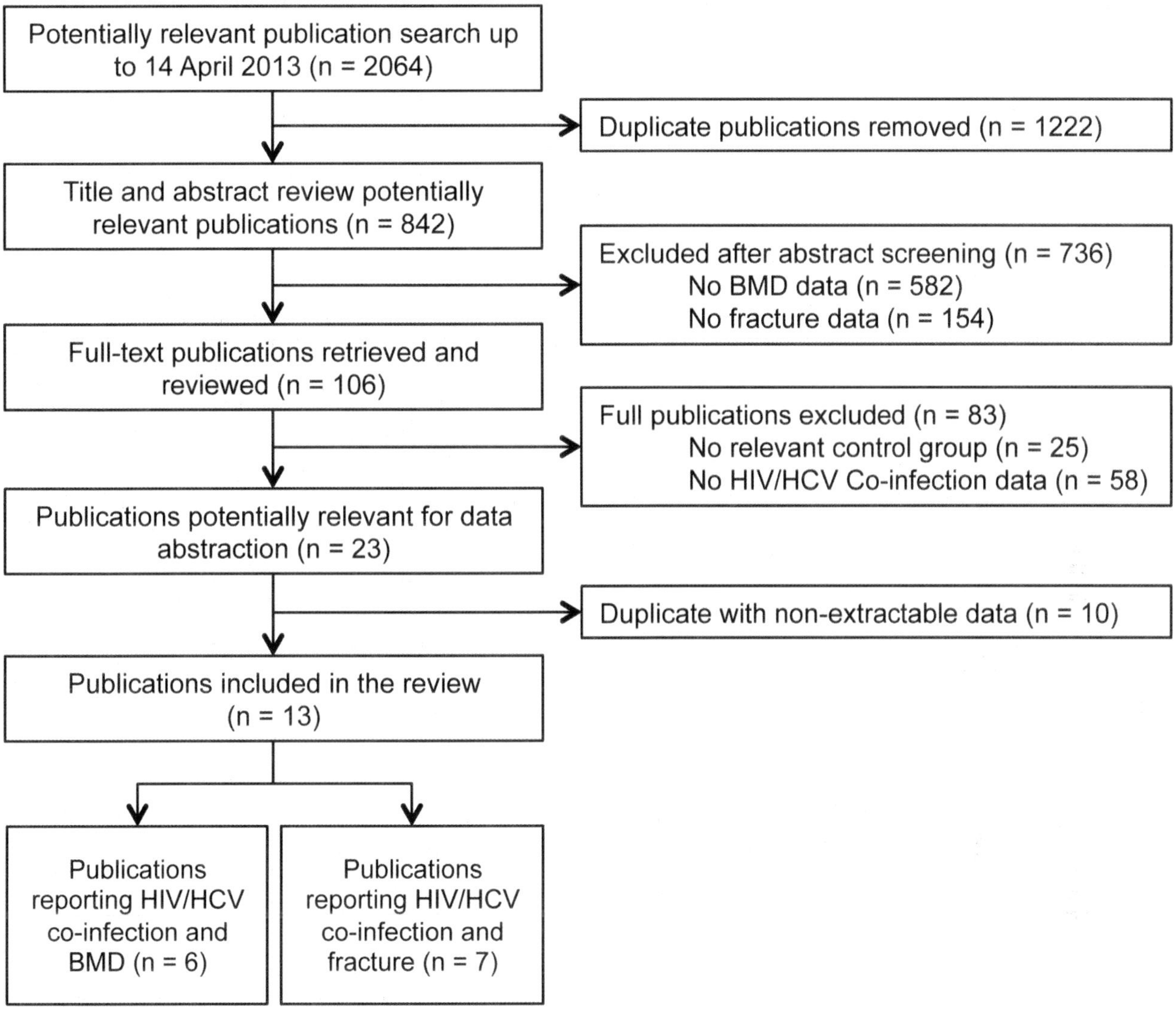

Figure 1. Identification of relevant literature on HIV/HCV co-infection and outcomes of (i) low bone mineral density (BMD) and (ii) fracture. BMD, bone mineral density; HCV, hepatitis C virus; HIV, human immunodeficiency virus.

incident fractures were considered. When sufficient information was provided to stratify data for multiple groups (e.g. gender, age), separate estimates were calculated for each group; again, treating the data as separate studies from a single publication.

The I^2 statistic was estimated as a measure of the total variation in point estimates attributable to between-study heterogeneity [35,36]. The magnitude was interpreted as low ($I^2 \leq 25\%$), medium ($I^2 = 50\%$) and high heterogeneity ($I^2 \geq 75\%$). A χ^2 test was used to assess statistical significance of heterogeneity within each analysis ($\alpha = 0.05$). Sensitivity analyses were employed to determine the causes of heterogeneity by evaluating whether BMD or fracture risk varied significantly based on demographic differences amongst publications. Furthermore, the included publications were selected for step-wise analysis of heterogeneity. Studies were systematically removed and replaced to estimate individual effects on pooled analyses. We evaluated publication bias using Egger regression asymmetry test and Begg's t. The analysis was conducted using Review Manager (RevMan, version 5.2, The Cochrane Collaboration, Copenhagen) and STATA (version 12, StataCorp, College Station, Tx). PRISMA reporting guidelines were adhered to in this publication (Checklist S1).

Results

Selection of Studies

The systematic search identified 2,064 potentially relevant publications (Figure 1). After exclusion of duplicates, and titles and abstracts were screened, 106 independent full-text publications were further evaluated. Studies were subsequently excluded due to lack of relevant control group (n = 25) or no co-infection data reported (n = 58), leaving 23 studies for data abstraction. Ten publications were excluded from abstraction because they did not report BMD or fractures in a co-infected population compared to controls. A total of 13 publications (n = 472,352 subjects) met all inclusion criteria and reported outcome(s) of interest. Manual review of included publication references did not yield any additional articles.

Only one publication required author contact [19] to clarify an adjusted OR point estimate and associated 95% CI due to a clerical error in the original publication. All reported adjusted measures of association were abstracted except one comparison of co- to mono-infected patients from Anastos et al. [19] that required unadjusted estimation of the OR based on reported data.

Demographic and Clinical Characteristics of Included Publications

Published between 2005 and 2012, all included publications reported observational study designs: 7 cohort, 5 cross-sectional, and a single matched case-control (Table 1). Publications were conducted in the United States (n = 7) [7,19,29,38,39,40,41] or Italy (n = 3) [30,37,42], with single publications reporting data from Iran [44], Denmark [28], and Australia [43]. Only effective sample sizes (those used to calculate the measure(s) of interest) were extracted, and ranged from 25 adults from a national multiyear, multicenter cohort [39] to 462,656 individuals in a retrospective cohort analysis of US Medicaid patients [7]. The majority of individuals included were male except for two publications [19,40] with an all-female population. Similar distribution of mean or median ages, BMI, and race was found across publications with no significant differences reported in included publications between cases and controls (Table 1). Lo Re et al. [30] stratified outcomes on gender; Lo Re et al. [7,30] stratified on both age and gender. In the analysis, these were treated as separate studies within each publication.

All studies reported control groups of either HIV mono- [7,19,29,30,39,41,42,43] or uninfected populations [7,19,28,40,44]. Lo Re et al. [7] did not find any significant difference in risk of hip fracture between HIV/HCV co-infected and HIV mono-infected patients. Thus, no data were reported in the publication and were not included in the analysis. In a single publication [30] evaluating rates of incident fracture among co-infected patients and HCV mono-infected controls, a higher rate of hip fracture was found in co-infected patients (HR 1.38, 95% CI 1.25, 1.53). In this study, there were insufficient data for pooled estimates using HCV mono-infection as a comparator.

Details of control selection were reported in all publications selected for pooled analyses. Five studies selected controls from within established cohorts: Lo Re et al. [7,30] used HIV mono- or uninfected controls from the US Medicaid recipients; the ANRS CO8 APROCOC-COPILOTE cohort [39] included HIV mono-infected controls on combination PI-ART; Bedimo et al. [29] used HIV mono-infected patients in the Veterans' Health Administration Clinical Case Registry data; and Anastos et al. [19] and Yin et al. [40] had HIV mono-infected (HAART naïve, non-PI HAART, PI HAART groups) and uninfected female controls, respectively, both from the Women's Interagency HIV Study. ART amongst co-infected patients was also reported in Lo Re et al. [7] compared to antiretroviral treated HIV mono-infected patients. Four publications used population-based controls. The NHANES III cohort in Fausto et al. [42] and Badie et al. [44], described hospital-based controls, matched on age, gender, HBV/HCV infection status, and injecting drug use. The NHAMCS-OPDs cohort in Young et al. [41] obtained controls matched on age and gender. Hansen et al. [28] linked the Danish HIV Cohort study to the Danish Civil Registration System and Danish National Hospital Registry. Hospital-based cohorts were included in three publications with age, gender, and duration of HIV infection individually matched by Yong et al. [43] to mono-infected controls, and HIV mono-infected controls at a single hospital included in Lo Re et al. [7,30].

Individuals on ART at the time of assessment were reported in all publications but one [38] (Table 2). Six publications had an outcome of BMD [19,30,37,38,42,44] whereas 8 reported fracture risk [7,28,29,30,39,40,41,43]. The wrist, hip, and lumbar spine were common locations for assessment of outcomes. All publications used DXA to evaluate BMD. T-scores and Z-scores equivalent to osteopenia or osteoporosis were reported by three [19,42,44] and one [30] publications, respectively. In contrast, less than half of the publications identified incident fracture events by means of International Classification of Disease (ICD) version 9 (ICD-9) [29,43] or 10 (ICD-10) [28]. Diagnosis of fracture was included in the analysis of residents in multiple US states receiving Medicaid [7,30]. Cohort members from the HIV Outpatient Study (HOPS) [43] treated at non-HOPS sites self-reported incident fracture as did Yin et al. [40] and Young et al. [41], who abstracted incident fractures from patient charts similar to Collin et al. [39]. In the meta-analysis of 4 cross-sectional studies, low BMD was increasingly prevalent among co-infected patients compared to those HIV mono-infected (pooled OR 1.98, 95% CI 1.18, 3.31) despite substantial and significant heterogeneity ($I^2 = 83\%$, $p<0.001$) (Figure 2). In contrast, no significant changes in BMD odds or heterogeneity were found by pooling data from two cross-sectional that compared co-infected to uninfected individuals (pooled OR 1.47, 95% CI 0.78, 2.78) ($I^2 = 0\%$, $p = 0.54$). All publications reported adjusted measures.

In the meta-analysis of 5 cohort and 1 case-control study, significant associations between co-infected patients and fracture was estimated compared to HIV mono-infected patients (pooled RR 1.57, 95% CI 1.33, 1.86) with moderate, non-significant heterogeneity ($I^2 = 52\%$, $p = 0.06$) (Figure 3). An increased association with fracture among co-infected individuals compared to those uninfected with HIV or HCV was found from both cohorts (pooled RR 2.46, 95% CI 1.03, 3.88), despite substantial and significant heterogeneity ($I^2 = 94\%$, $p<0.001$), and cross-sectional studies (pooled OR 2.3, 95% CI 2.09, 2.53) with no heterogeneity identified ($I^2 = 1.0\%$, $p = 0.41$). All publications but one [28] reported adjusted measures. There was no evidence of publication bias as indicated by a non-significant Egger test (all $p>0.05$) and Begg's test (all $p>0.05$) in all analyses.

Sensitivity analysis

Moderately attenuated heterogeneity and odds of low BMD (co-infected compared to HIV mono-infected) were found using step-wise publication of a single publication [19] (OR 1.58, 95% CI 1.02, 2.45; $I^2 = 44\%$, $p = 0.17$). Risk of fracture and heterogeneity were substantially attenuated using step-wise publication exclusion of Collin et al. [39] (co-infected compared to HIV mono-infected) (RR 1.51, 95% CI 1.22, 1.71; $I^2 = 31\%$, $p = 0.22$). No significant changes were observed when either analyses were repeated with omission of the total female populations reported in Yin et al. [40] or Anastos et al. [19], or by individual removal of publications from all comparisons.

Discussion

In this meta-analysis, low BMD and fracture was increasingly associated with HIV/HCV co-infection compared to HIV mono-infected and HIV/HCV uninfected or seronegative individuals, suggesting that HCV contributes to a burden a disease greater than HIV infection alone. Despite heterogeneity present in the analysis, the visual trends of the forest plots are suggestive of a positive clinical effect in the population. These findings confirm that co-infection is a risk factor for adverse bone health outcomes. This meta-analysis also confirmed the association between HIV mono-infection and low BMD or fracture as reported in previous studies [2,3]. This is the first attempt to synthesize data across publications to estimate the odds of low BMD or risk of fracture amongst HIV/HCV co-infected patients. Despite significant outcomes, the pooled associations of low BMD or risk of fracture among co-infected patients varied across publications, possibly due to differences in demographics of the study populations.

Table 1. Descriptive characteristics of studies meeting inclusion criteria for low BMD and fracture risk amongst HIV/HCV co-infected patients.

Author	Study Design	Country	N, Total	N, Co-infected (HIV+/HCV+)	Control group(s)		Sex (% Male)		Age (years)	
					N, Monoinfected (HIV+)	N, Uninfected		Ethnicity (% HIV+)		Body Mass Index (kg/m^2, SD)
Anastos 2007	Cross-sectional	USA	387	112	152	123	0	Black (61.3)	36.7 (HIV–)	29.9, 6.72 (HIV–)
									42.1 (HIV+ ART–)	28.9, 6.24 (HIV+ ART–)
								Caucasian (19.7)	40.5 (HIV+ non-PI ART+)	26.8, 5.81 (HIV+ non-PI ART+)
								Hispanic (18.9)	43.8 (HIV+ PI ART+) (median)	28.4, 6.87 (HIV+ PI ART+)
Badie 2011	Cross-sectional	Iran	101	61	40	-	79.2	Middle Eastern (100.0)	39.4, 7.7 (HIV+ ART+)	22.7, 3.40 (HIV+ ART+)
									34.9, 7.3 (HIV+ ART–)	22.7, 3.30 (HIV+ ART–)
									36.6, 10.5 (HIV–) (mean, SD)	22.8, 3.40 (HIV–)
Bedimo 2012	Cohort	USA	951	485	-	466	98.0	Black (56.0)	46 (median)	Not reported
								Caucasian (18.0)		
								Hispanic (23.0)		
								Other (2.0)		
Collin 2009	Cohort	USA	25	13	-	12	77.2	Not reported	36.2 (median)	22.0 (Not reported) (HIV+)
El-Maouche 2011	Cross-sectional	USA	338	Not reported	Not reported	Not reported	55.0	Black (93.8)	42.5, 8 (mean, SD)	23.9, 2.90 (HIV+)*
Fausto 2006	Cross-sectional	Italy	161	55	-	106	64.0	Caucasian (100.0)	38.6, 4.18 (mean, SD)	22.9, 3.16 (HIV+ ART–)
										23.1, 3.47 (HIV+ ART+)
Hansen 2012	Cohort	Denmark	5306	851	Not reported	-	76.0	Caucasian (80.0)	36.7, 30.5–44.5 (mean, 95% CI)	Not reported
Lo Re 2009	Cross-sectional	Italy	1237	625	-	612	62.0	Not reported	43, 10–18 (median, IQR)	23.5, 3.44 (HIV+)*
										23.1, 4.10 (HIV+ HCV+)*
Lo Re 2012	Cohort	USA	462656		366829	95827	63.0	Black (43.1)	39, 33–46 (mean, IQR)	Not reported
								Caucasian (27.4)		
								Hispanic (8.3)		
								Other (21.1)		
Li Vecchi 2012	Cohort	Italy	188	41	76	71	55.9	Caucasian (100.0)	47, 9.7 (HIV+)	22.9, 3.62 (HIV+)*

Table 1. Cont.

Author	Study Design	Country	N, Total	N, Co-infected (HIV+/HCV+)	Control group(s) N, Monoinfected (HIV+)	N, Uninfected	Sex (% Male)	Ethnicity (% HIV+)	Age (years)	Body Mass Index (kg/m^2, SD)
									49, 49, 11.3 (HIV–) (mean, SD)	23.4, 3.81 (HIV–)*
Yin 2010	Cohort	USA	1101	438	663	-	0	Black (56.3)	40.4, 8.8 (HIV+)	28.5, 7.50 (HIV+)
								Caucasian (13.3)		
								Hispanic (27.7)	36.1, 9.9 (HIV–) (mean, SD)	30.0, 8.20 (HIV–)
								Other (3.2)		
Yong 2011	Case-control	Australia	46	16	-	30	88.5	Black (3.0)	49.8 (Case)	24.2, 2.91 (Case)*
								Caucasian (92.0)	49.5 (Control) (mean)	25.6, 3.47 (Control)*
								Asian (5.0)		
Young 2011	Cohort	USA	193	51	-	142	79.0	Black (33.0)	40, 34–46 (median, IQR)	26.7, 4.83 (HIV+)
								Caucasian (51.8)		
								Hispanic (11.7)		
								Other (3.5)		

HIV, Human Immunodeficiency Virus; HCV, Hepatitis C Virus; ART, antiretroviral therapy; CI, confidence interval; IQR, interquartile range; PI, protease inhibitor; SD, standard deviation.
*Mean (SD) estimated from descriptive categorical data reported in publication.

Table 2. Clinical characteristics and reported outcomes of publications included in the HIV/HCV co-infection review.

Author	ART exposure (%)	Reported outcome(s) (classification method)	Location	Co-variates adjusted
Anastos 2007	46.5	BMD (DXA)	Lumbar spine	White, Race, Nadir BMI, HIV+ ART naïve, HIV+ non-PI ART, HIV+ PI ART, post-menopausal
			Femoral neck	
Badie 2011	30.0	BMD (DXA)	Hip	Age, Gender, BMI, Smoking, Alcohol, Exercise, HBV infection, IV drug use, Prison
			Lumbar spine	
Bedimo 2012	69.4	Incident osteoporotic fracture (ICD-9 codes)	Wrist	ART+, CKD, Race, Age, Tobacco use, Diabetes, BMI
			Vertebra	
			Hip	
Collin 2009	100.0	Incident non-stress fracture (patient charts)	Any location	Age, HIV+, HIV-RNA, BMI, Location of birth, PI used first, Alcohol, CD4+ count,
El-Maouche 2011	Not reported	BMD (DXA)	Hip	Gender, Age, BMI, Race, Smoking, Alcohol, IV drug use, Hypogonadal/menopausal, HIV+, Methadone use, ART+, Hormone exposure, Vitamin D
			Femoral neck	
			Lumbar spine	
Fausto 2006	70.2	BMD (DXA)	Hip	Gender, Age, CDC Stage, IV drug use, Lypodistrophy, BMI, CD4+ count, HIV-RNA, HAART+, Length of HIV infection, Bone resorption, Bone formation, Vitamin D
			Lumbar spine	
Hansen 2012	78.0	Incident low energy fracture (ICD-10 codes)	Any location	
Lo Re 2009	79.0	BMD (DXA)	Lumbar spine	Age, Gender, BMI, Length of HIV infection, CD4+ count, ART+, Smoking, Alcohol, Exercise, Amenorrhea, eGFR
			Femoral neck	
Lo Re 2012	100	Incident low energy fracture (Medicaid claim codes)	Hip	Age, Gender, State (location), Propensity score
		BMD (DXA)		
Li Vecchi 2012	93.0	BMD (DXA)	Lumbar spine	Age, Yogurt intake, CD4+, Drug addiction
			Femoral neck	
Yin 2010	65.6	Incident low energy fracture (self-reported)	Hip	HIV+, Age, Race, BMI, Post-menopausal, Fracture before index, Serum creatinine
			Wrist	
			Spine	
Yong 2011	83.6	Incident non-stress fracture (ICD-9 codes)	Any location	HBV status, Previous opportunistic infection, CD4+ count, BMI, HIV-RNA, Duration of viral suppression, Type of DXA performed
Young 2011	72.7	Incident low energy fracture (patient charts; self-reported)	Wrist	Gender, Age, CD4+ count,
			Vertebra	
			Femoral neck	

ART, antiretroviral therapy; BMI, body mass index; CKD, chronic kidney disease; DXA, Dual energy x-ray absorbiometry; eGFR, estimated glomerular filtration rate; HAART, highly active antiretroviral therapy; HBV, hepatitis B virus; ICD, International Classification of Diseases; PI, protease inhibitor.

The inclusion of a co-infected state without regard for the estimated duration of HCV infection relative to HIV infection (and thus, the stage of dynamic fibrosis progression) limits our understanding of infection and its role on either outcome. Although a single study [7] reported significantly greater fracture risk among HCV patients compared to HIV mono-infected patients, we were unable to compare HCV alone to explore the relative contributions of either infection to fractures or BMD. Recent cross-sectional studies have suggested that HCV infected patients with hepatic decompensation have lower BMD than HCV-infected patients with healthy liver function [23,24,30]. The non-hepatic outcomes of HCV remain unclear, including mechanisms leading to low BMD and fractures associated with hepatic osteodystrophy [5,6,7].

Co-infection may have a compounded negative impact on bone strength due to reduced osteoclastic activity and hepatic osteodystrophy leading to increased fractures. This is consistent with findings in this analysis and Lo Re et al. [30], who reported both high odds of low BMD and risk of fracture compared to mono- and uninfected individuals. Unfortunately, no study in this analysis

[A]

Study or Subgroup	Weight	Odds Ratio IV, Random, 95% CI
Anastos, 2007	31.5%	2.93 [2.55, 3.36]
Fausto, 2005	25.0%	1.39 [0.85, 2.27]
Lo Re, 2009 (F)	18.5%	2.99 [1.37, 6.55]
Lo Re, 2009 (M)	25.0%	1.26 [0.77, 2.06]
Total (95% CI)	**100.0%**	**1.98 [1.18, 3.31]**

Heterogeneity: $Tau^2 = 0.21$; $Chi^2 = 17.65$, df = 3 (P = 0.0005); $I^2 = 83\%$
Test for overall effect: Z = 2.59 (P = 0.010)

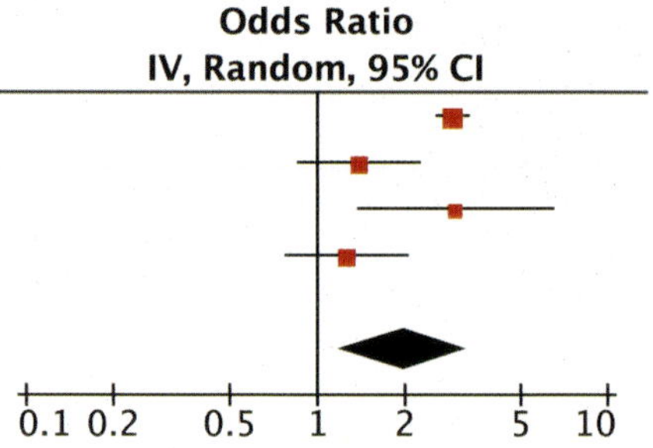

[B]

Study or Subgroup	Weight	Odds Ratio IV, Random, 95% CI
Anastos, 2007	85.5%	1.60 [0.81, 3.18]
Badie, 2011	14.5%	0.91 [0.17, 4.81]
Total (95% CI)	**100.0%**	**1.47 [0.78, 2.78]**

Heterogeneity: $Tau^2 = 0.00$; $Chi^2 = 0.38$, df = 1 (P = 0.54); $I^2 = 0\%$
Test for overall effect: Z = 1.20 (P = 0.23)

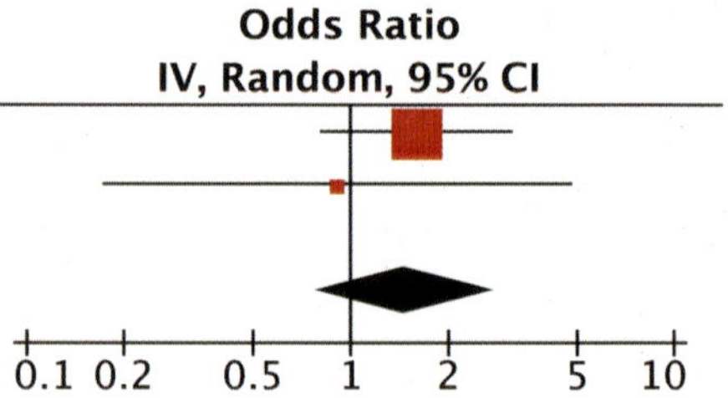

Figure 2. Odds of low bone mineral density between individuals co-infected with HIV and hepatitis C virus compared to HIV mono- (A) or uninfected (B) individuals. HIV, human immunodeficiency virus; HCV, hepatitis C virus.

reported low BMD and risk of fracture as independent outcomes. Therefore, no association between low BMD and fracture risk could be estimated. The theories explaining the causal associations between co-infection and negative skeletal outcomes are reasonable, but require further research into clinical and pathological mechanisms for further clarification.

Risk factors and mechanisms that underlie the increased association between co-infection and low BMD or fracture have not been fully explained. It is likely to be multifactorial, representing complex interactions between infection, traditional osteoporotic risk factors, and ART. It is estimated that up to 9% of all HIV mono-infected patients have low BMD, irrespective of treatment modality [5,54,55] due to chronic inflammation leading to bone resorption [56]. HIV itself may also have direct effects on osteoclastic activity leading to osteoporosis, with the incidence greatly increased among those on ART [56]. Initiation of ART has been associated with 2–6% decrease in BMD over the first two years on therapy [11]. This magnitude in BMD reduction is similar to the first two years of a woman in early menopause. With increased duration of therapy, however, the BMD stabilizes or even improves thereafter. Large subsets of the HIV infected populations (both mono- and co-infected) were on ART of some variation. Insufficient data in the publications on ART duration precluded stratification or adjustment of this potential confounding variable. It is possible that ART patients may have biased the estimates towards a stronger association.

Comparisons between publications are only valid in so far as the groups were demographically similar in other respects. Several studies have reported the prevalence of low BMD in HIV infected patients compared to controls [3,16,50] but few have adjusted for potential confounding variables and heterogeneity of included study groups (e.g. including individuals who acquired HIV through different modes of transmission). No difference of low BMD was estimated between co-infected patients and HIV/HCV uninfected individuals. This may be attributed to the small number of studies included in this analysis of co-infected individuals where the baseline risk of low BMD may have been greater in controls, which lead to conservative estimates.

No association was found when all female populations [19,40] were excluded. It is unlikely that the low BMD was entirely attributed to accelerated bone loss during the menopausal transition given that the reported mean ages were less than the average menopausal woman [52,53] in the United States, where the studies were conducted. Inflammation, leading to bone resorption, and higher risks of vitamin D deficiency have also been reported among mono- and co-infected patients [3,7,8]. Most publications reported a primarily middle-aged (40–55 years) male, Caucasian population. However, non-black race is a known risk factor for osteoporosis as noted in a recent meta-analysis by Shiau et al [2]. It was found that race modified the relationship between HIV infection and fracture, but co-infection was not reported. Although matching was reported in one case control study [43], some publications reported notable differences between HIV-infected individuals that may affect BMD, such as advancing age, menopausal status (estrogen deficiency), smoking history, and alcohol consumption. It is unclear if these potentially modifiable risk factors or other potentially important variables, such as dietary calcium intake, use of medications inducing bone loss (e.g. glucocorticoids), use of antidepressants (e.g. serotonin re-uptake inhibitors), or level of physical activity influenced the results [11,32]. Few publications adequately reported important potential confounding variables (e.g. gender; age; BMI; substance and alcohol consumption; sedentary lifestyle; digestive, renal, and endocrine disorders including diabetes; nadir CD4+ cell count; viral load) that could have potentially biased the measures

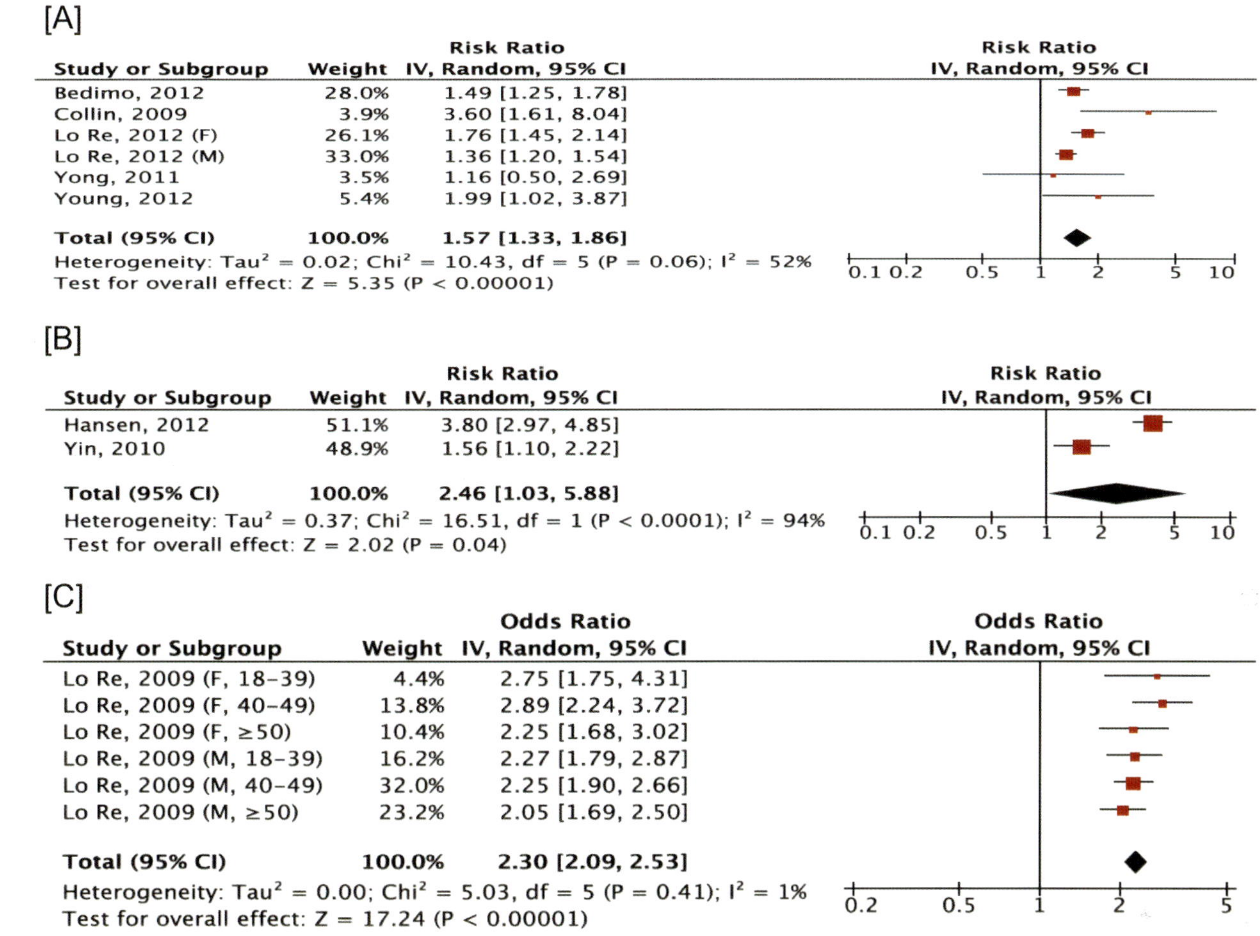

Figure 3. Risk of fracture between individuals co-infected with HIV and hepatitis C virus compared to HIV mono- (A) or uninfected individuals (B), with odds of fracture estimated from cross-sectional studies comparing HIV/HCV co-infected patients to HIV or HCV uninfected individuals (C). HIV, human immunodeficiency virus; HCV, hepatitis C virus.

estimated. Unfortunately, we were unable to adequately adjust in the analysis for this limitation due to inadequate reporting.

Osteopenia is not as sensitive as osteoporosis as a designation of reduced BMD [9]. Developed for post-menopausal women, the T-score has been applied to other adult populations despite controversy around its utility as a metric to quantify bone loss in men and pre-menopausal women [9,48,49]. Thus, age and T-scores are the key predictive factors in determining the BMD testing for screening purposes. The utility of estimating the association of low BMD in co-infected patients relates to the risk of future pathologic fracture. There is a continuous non-linear relationship between BMD and fracture risk [8,46], and measurement of BMD is regarded as the single best predictor of fractures [46,47]. The sensitivity of BMD for fracture prediction is low over most reasonable assumptions, but the specificity is high. Thus, many fractures will occur in individuals with BMD values in the normal range, but fracture risk is quite low. By contrast, fracture risk is very high in individuals with low BMD.

Reporting of fracture diagnosis varied among publications. Studies comparing results of questionnaires and information obtained by medical charts or ICD databases have been inconsistent with both over-reporting and underreporting [51]. The level of misclassification of incident fractures could not be estimated in the included publications and is a limitation of the present study. However, diagnosis of fractures from ICD databases, insurance claims, and charted data for fractures has been reported to be highly valid [45].

This study had several limitations. First, the potential biases of the original studies, methodological issues, and different strategies for adjusting for confounders could affect the results of this meta-analysis. The cross-sectional association may have been confounded by other unadjusted factors or selection bias. Selection bias may also exist in studies using data from electronic records, claims-based, or primary care databases. Second, the number of cohort studies available was limited and the follow-up durations may not be sufficiently long to be able to detect associations. Third, different publications reported different definitions of incident fracture events that would affect the estimates of prevalence/incidence. However, all reported that pathologic fractures were likely due to low BMD [7,28,29,30,40,41,43] or lead to limited activity post-fracture possibly due to osteoporosis [39]. These differences could have also contributed to the observed high heterogeneity seen within some studies [57,58,59]. Last, publication bias may be of concern because studies that report statistically significant results are more likely to be published than studies reporting non-significant results, and this could have distorted the findings in this meta-analysis. Although the Egger's test and Begg's test indicated limited evidence of publication bias, the estimation may not be accurate enough as the number of studies may be insufficient.

The findings in this study add evidence to the importance of monitoring for and informing co-infected patients on the negative outcomes affecting the skeletal system. Increasing studies of multiple morbidities are necessary, as the incidence of co-infection with HIV and viral hepatitis increases and patients live longer. Outcomes will also directly benefit patient health through improved care guidelines (e.g. recommendations to improve physical activity to reduce bone loss once infected). Although the clinical validity of *a priori* chosen measures of association (relative effects) compared to absolute effects (important for interpretation) should be considered, the majority of publications reported adjusted odds or rates with insufficient data to estimate absolute risks. Thus, consideration should be made when interpreting the data as doubling of risk (i.e. 100% greater risk) may only mean an absolute difference of 1% (i.e. from 1 to 2% increase in risk).

In conclusion, this meta-analysis suggests that HIV/HCV co-infection is associated with significantly increased association between HIV/HCV co-infection and low BMD and fractures compared to an uninfected or HIV mono-infected population. The estimated significant cross-sectional and longitudinal associations in the analysis could suggest that there may be an increased risk for adverse bone health outcomes, including pathologic fractures, among co-infected patients. However, the impact of other factors on the estimated outcomes, such as HIV or HCV disease severity and duration, could not be determined. Further controlled, longitudinal studies are necessary to clarify the causal nature of HIV/HCV co-infection according to severity of disease, ART (type or duration), and demographic differences on reduced BMD and risk of fracture. This is especially warranted as the risk of skeletal disease is expected to increase in the future as both HIV and HCV-infected population continue to age. Better understanding of this will provide insight and improvement in screening and early treatment of targeted populations to mitigate fracture risk among aging HIV-infected patients.

Author Contributions

Conceived and designed the experiments: TJO LR HHT. Performed the experiments: TJO LR VS AZ HHT. Analyzed the data: TJO LR HHT. Contributed reagents/materials/analysis tools: TJO LR AZ HHT. Wrote the paper: TJO LR HHT.

References

1. Sackoff JE, Hanna DB, Pfeiffer MR, Torian LV (2006) Causes of death among persons with AIDS in the era of highly active antiretroviral therapy: New York City. Ann Intern Med 145: 397–406.
2. Shiau S, Broun EC, Arpadi SM, Yin MT (2013) Incident fractures in HIV-infected individuals. AIDS 27(12): 1949–57.
3. Brown TT, Qaqish RB (2006) Antiretroviral therapy and the prevalence of osteopenia and osteoporosis: a meta-analytic review. AIDS 20(17): 2165–74.
4. Seef LB (2002) Natural history of chronic hepatitis. Hepatology 36(S1): S35–46.
5. Tebas P, Powderly W, Yarasheski K (2000) Response to 'accelerate bone mineral loss in HIV-infected patients receiving potent antiretroviral therapy' by Drs Weil and Lenhard. AIDS 14(15): 2417.
6. Negredo E, Martinex E, Cinquegrana D, Estany C, Clotet B (2007) Therapeutic management of bone demineralization in the HIV-infected population. AIDS 21(6): 657–63.
7. Lo Re V, Volk J, Newcomb CW, Yang YX, Freeman CP, et al. (2012) Risk of hip fracture associated with hepatitis C virus infection and hepatitis C/human immunodeficiency virus coinfection. Hepatology 56(6): 1699–98.
8. Cummings SR, Nevitt MC, Haber RJ (1985) Prevention of osteoporosis and osteoporotic fractures. West J Med 143(5): 684–7.
9. Kanis JA (1994) Assessment of fracture risk and its application to screening for postmenopausal osteoporosis: synopsis of a WHO report. WHO Study Group. Osteoporosis Int 4(6): 368–81.
10. WHO (World Health Organization) (2000) Prevention and management of osteoporosis: report of the WHO scientific group. WHO Scientific Group on the Prevention and Management of Osteoporosis. Available: http://www.whqlibdoc.who.int/trs/WHO_TRS_921.pdf: Accessed 8 September 2013.
11. McComsey GA, Tebas P, Shane E, Yin MT, Turner Overton E, et al. (2010) Bone disease in HIV infection: a practical review and recommendations for HIV care providers. Clin Infect Dis 51(8): 937–46.
12. Tebas P (2001) Editorial comment: re-emerging infections – implicating the immune reconstitution syndrome. AIDS Read 11(12): 610.
13. Grinspoon SK, Bilesikian JP (1992) HIV disease and endocrine system. N Engl J Med 327(19): 1360–5.
14. Meyer D, Behrens G, Schmidt RE, Stoll M (1999) Osteonecrosis of the femoral head in patients receiving HIV protease inhibitors. AIDS 13(9): 1147–8.
15. Stephens EA, Das R, Madge S, Barter J, Johnson MA (1999) Symptomatic osteoporosis in two young HIV-positive African women. AIDS 13(18): 2605–6.
16. Moore AL, Vashisht A, Sabin CA, Mocroft A, Madge S, et al. (2001) Reduced bone mineral density in HIV-positive individuals. AIDS 15(13): 1731–3.
17. Knobel H, Guelar A, Vallecillo G, Nogues X, Diez A (2001) Osteopenia in HIV-infected patients: is it disease or is it treatment? AIDS 15: 807–8.
18. Thomas J, Doherty SM (2003) HIV infection – a risk factor for osteoporosis. JAIDS 33(3): 281–91.
19. Anastos K, Lu D, Shi O, Mulligan K, Tien PC, et al. (2007) The association of bone mineral density with HIV infection and antiretroviral treatment in women. Antiviral Therapy 12: 1049–58.
20. Paton NIJ, Macallan DC, Griffin GE, Pazianas M (1997) Bone mineral density in patients with Human Immunodeficiency Virus infection. Calcified Tissue Int 61(1): 30–2.
21. Triant VA, Brown TD, Lee H, Grinspoon SK (2008) Fracture prevalence among Human Immunodeficiency Virus (HIV)-infected versus non-HIV-infected patients in a large U.S. healthcare system. Endocrine Care 93(9): 3499.
22. Womack JA, Goulet JL, Gibert C, Brandt C, Chang CC, et al. (2011) Increased risk of fragility fractures among HIV infected compared to uninfected male vetrans. PLoS One 6(2): e17217, doi:10.1371/journal.pone.0017217.
23. Gallego-Rojo FJ, Gonzalez-Calvin JL, Munoz-Torres M, Mundi JL, Fernandez-Perez R, et al. (1998) Bone mineral density, serum insulin-like growth factor I, and bone turnover markers in viral cirrhosis. Hepatology 28(3): 695–9.
24. Gonzalez-Calvin JL, Gallego-Rojo F, Fernandez-Perez R, Casado-Caballero F, Ruiz-Escolano E, et al. (2004) Osteoporosis, mineral metabolism, and serum tumor necrosis factor receptor p55 in viral cirrhosis. J Clin Endocrinol Metab 89: 4325.
25. Leslie WD, Bernstein CN, Leboff MS (2003) AGA technical review on osteoporosis in hepatic disorders. Gastroenterology; 125: 941–66.
26. Rouillard S, Lane NE (2001) Hepatic osteodystrophy. Hepatology 33: 301–7.
27. Cummings SR, Black DM, Nevitt MC (1993) Bone density at various sites for prediction of hip fractures. Lancet 341: 72–5.
28. Hansen ABE, Gerstoft J, Kronborg G, Larsen CS, Pedersen G, et al. (2012) Incidence of low and high-energy fractures in persons with and without HIV infection: a Danish population-based cohort study. AIDS 26(3): 285–93.
29. Bedimo R, Maalouf NM, Zhang S, Drechsler H, Tebas P (2012) Osteoporotic fracture risk associated with cumulative exposure in tenofovir and other antiretroviral agents. AIDS 26(7): 825–31.
30. Lo Re V, Volk J, Newcomb CW, Yang YX, Freeman CP, et al. (2009) Viral hepatitis is associated with reduced bone mineral density in HIV-infected women but not men. AIDS 23: 2191–8.
31. Thein HH, Ti Q, Dore GJ, Krahn MD (2008) Estimation of stage-specific fibrosis progression rates in chronic hepatitis C virus infection: a meta-analysis and meta-regression. Hepatology 48(2): 418–31.
32. USPSTF (U.S. Preventive Services Task Force) (2011) Screening for osteoporosis: U.S. Preventive Services Task Force recommendation statement. Ann Intern Med 154: 356–64.
33. King G, Langche Z (2002) Estimating risk and rate levels, ratios, and difference in case-control studies. Stats Med 21: 1409–27.
34. Hedges LV, Pigott TD (2004) The power of statistical tests for moderators in meta-analysis. Psych Methods 9(4): 426–55.
35. Higgins JPT, Thompson SG (2002) Quantifying heterogeneity in meta-analysis. Stat Med 21(11): 1539–58.
36. Higgins JPT, Thompson SG, Deeks JJ, Altman DG (2003) Measuring inconsistency in meta-analyses. BMJ 327(7414): 557–60.
37. Li Vecchi V, Soresi M, Giannitrapani L, Mazzola G, La Sala S, et al. (2012) Dairy calcium intake and lifestyle risk factors for bone loss in HIV-infected and uninfected Mediterranean subjects. BMC Infect Dis 12: 192.
38. El-Maouche D, Mehta SH, Sutcliffe CG, Higgins Y, Torbenson MS, et al. (2013) Vitamin D deficiency and its relation to bone mineral density and liver fibrosis in HIV-HCV co-infection. Antivir Ther 18(2): 237–42.
39. Collin F, Duval X, Moing VL, Piroth L, Al Kaied F, et al. (2009) Ten year incidence and risk factors of bone fractures in a cohort of treated HIV1-infected adults. AIDS 23: 1021–6.

40. Yin MT, Shi Q, Hoover DR, Anastos K, Young M, et al. (2010) Fracture incidence in HIV-infected women: results from the Women's Interagency HIV Study. AIDS 24: 2678–86.
41. Young B, Dao CN, Baker R, Brooks JT (2011) Increased rates of bone fracture among HIV-infected persons in the HIV Outpatient Study (HOPS) compared with the US general population, 2000–2006. Clin Infect Dis 52: 1061–8.
42. Fausto A, Bongiovanni M, Cicconi P, Menicagli L, Ligabo EV, et al. (2006) Potential predictive factors of osteoporosis in HIV-positive subjects. Bone 38: 893–7.
43. Yong MK, Elliott JH, Woolley IJ, Hoy JF (2011). Low CD4 count is associated with an increased risk in fragility fracture in HIV fracture in HIV-infected patients. JAIDS 57: 205–10.
44. Badie BM, Soori T, Kheirandish P, Izadyar S (2011) Evaluation of bone mineral density in Iranian HIV/AIDS patients. Acta Medica Iranica 49(7): 460–7.
45. Ray WA, Griffin MR, Fought RL, Adams ML (1992) Identification of fractures from computerized medicare files. J Clin Epidemiol 45(7): 703–14.
46. Lofman O, Hallberg I, Berglund K, Wahsltrom O, Kartous L, et al. (2007) Women with low-energy fracture should be investigated for osteoporosis. Acta Orthop 78(6): 813–21.
47. Kanis JA, Melton LJ, Christiansen C, Johnston CC, Khaltaev N (1994) The diagnosis of osteoporosis. J Bone Miner Res 9: 1137–41.
48. Lewiecki EM (2004) Low bone mineral density in premenopausal women. South Med J 97(6): 544–50.
49. Lewiecki EM, Miller PD, Leib ES, Bilezikian JP (2005) Response to "The perspective of the International Osteoporosis Foundation on the Official Positions of the International Society for Clinical Densitometry," by John A. Kanis, et al. J Clin Densitom 8(2): 143–4.
50. Binkley N, Buehring B (2009) Beyond FRAX: It's time to consider "sarco-osteopenia". J Clin Densitom 12(4): 413–6.
51. Siggeirsdottir K, Aspelund T, Sigurdsson G, Mogensen B, Chang M, et al. (2007) Inaccuracy in self-report of fractures may underestimate association with health outcomes when compared with medical record based fracture registry. Eur J Epidemiol 22: 631–9.
52. Hernandez CJ, Beaupre GS, Carter DR (2003) A theoretical analysis of the relative influences of peak BMD age-related bone loss and menopause on the development of osteoporosis. Osteoporos Int 14: 843–47.
53. Palacios S, Henderson VW, Siseles N, Tan D, Villaseca P (2010) Age of menopause and impact of climacteric symptoms by geographical region. Climacentric 13(5): 419–28.
54. Amiel C, Ostertag A, Slama L, Baudoin C, N'Guyen T, et al. (2004). BMD is reduced in HIV-infected men irrespective of treatment. J Bone Min Res 19(3): 402–9.
55. Carr A, Miller J, Eisman J, Cooper D (2001) Osteopenia in HIV-infected men: association with asymptomatic lactic academia and lower weight preantiretroviral therapy. AIDS 15(6): 703.
56. Aukrust P, Haug C, Ueland T, Lien E, Muller F, et al. (1999) Decreased bone formative and enhanced resorptive markers in Human Immunodeficiency Virus infection: indication of normalization of the bone-remodeling process during highly active antiretroviral therapy. J Clinc Endocrin Metab 84(1): 145–50.
57. Egger M (1998) Meta-analysis bias in location and selection of studies. BMJ 316: 61.
58. Stroup DF, Berlin JA, Morton SC, Olkin I, Williamson GD, et al. (2000) Meta-analsysis of observational studies in epidemiology: a proposal for reporting. JAMA 283(15): 2008–12.
59. Huedo-Medina T, Sanchez-Meca J, Marin-Martinez F, Botella J (2006) Assessing heterogeneity in meta-analysis: Q statistic or I2 index? Psychol Methods 11(2): 193–206.

4

Dynamics of Polymer Molecules with Sacrificial Bond and Hidden Length Systems: Towards a Physically-Based Mesoscopic Constitutive Law

Ahmed E. Elbanna[1,2]*, Jean M. Carlson[3]

1 Department of Physics, University of California Santa Barbara, Santa Barbara, California, United States of America, **2** Department of Civil and Environmental Engineering, University of Illinois at Urbana- Champaign, Urbana, Illinois, United States of America, **3** Department of Physics, University of California Santa Barbara, Santa Barbara, California, United States of America

Abstract

We investigate the entropic force-elongation behavior of a polymer chain in the presence of the sacrificial bond and hidden length (SBHL) system observed experimentally in many biomaterials. We show that in most cases the SBHL system leads to a significant increase in toughness. However, the presence of a large number of bonds or relatively strong bonds in the SBHL system can reduce the net gain in toughness. We also incorporate the polymer model into a network of polymers with random properties (e.g., contour length, number and strength of sacrificial bonds, length of hidden loops). This allows us to derive a physically-based mesoscopic force-displacement law that governs the collective behavior.

Editor: Jie Zheng, University of Akron, United States of America

Funding: This work was supported by the David and Lucile Packard Foundation and the Institute for Collaborative Biotechnologies through contract no. W911NF-09-0001 from the U.S. Army Research Office. The content of the information does not necessarily reflect the position or the policy of the Government, and no official endorsement should be inferred. The funders had no role in study design, data collection and analysis, decision to publish, or preparation of the manuscript.

Competing Interests: The authors have declared that no competing interests exist.

* E-mail: elbanna2@uiuc.edu

Introduction

Entropy based energy dissipation mechanisms were shown to play an important role in the dynamics of many physical systems. These include granular materials [1], glassy materials [2], thin film lubricants [3], and hard spheres [4]. Laws of statistical thermodynamics provide a framework for tracking the evolution of entropy and energy flow across different scales in these systems enabling a physically based description of the constitutive response [5–7]. In this paper, we use this framework to construct the force extension law for bone deformation at the scale of mineralized collagen fibrils (~1 μm).

The mineralized collaged fibrils constitute the building blocks of the bone hierarchical structure at the sub micrometer scale. Studies on bone structure show that it is a hierarchical composite of collagen and hydroxyapatite [8–9] with mechanisms to resist fracture at different size scales [10]. These size scales relate to the characteristic structural dimensions in bone, which vary from twisted peptide chains at the nanometer scale to the (secondary) osteon (haversian) structures, which are several hundred micrometers in size. The hierarchical structure at the intermediate scales includes (i) hydroxyapatite-impregnated twisted collagen fibrils at the scale of tens of nanometers; (ii) collagen fibers that are typically a micrometer in diameter and (iii) the lamellar structure of collagen fibers at several micrometer dimensions. It is the simultaneous operation of the fracture-resistance mechanisms at these various length scales that provides bone with its enduring strength and toughness.

Here, we focus on the mechanics of deformation at the scale of the mineralized collagen fibrils. Atomic Force Microscope (AFM) experiments done at this scale [11–12] showed that the fibrils are interconnected by a special type of glue that is composed of polymer chains with sacrificial bonds and hidden length (SBHL) systems. The basic structure and operation mechanism of the SBHL system are shown in Fig. 1. The assembled glue molecule (insert in Fig. 1a) may include more than one polymer chain with sacrificial bonds forming within the chain itself, crosslinking the different chains and connecting the chains to the collagen fibrils. The large scale separation of the collagen fibrils is resisted by an array of parallel gel molecules as shown in Fig. 1a. We use the worm-like chain model [13–15] (WLC) to describe the mechanical response of the glue molecules and to identify the relationship between the SBHL system internal variables and macroscopic observables such as toughness and strength. We also examine the mechanical response of the array of parallel molecules.

The operation of the SBHL system depends on the state of the sacrificial bond. As long as the bond is intact, it shields parts of the polymer length from contributing to the end-to-end distance. This corresponds to a reduction in the chain entropy (the possible number of configurations resulting in the same end-to-end distance) and a corresponding increase in the initial stiffness of the polymer chain. The increased stiffness means that a larger force is required to extend the polymer chain any finite distance, compared to that required in the case of a polymer with no SBHL system. After the sacrificial bond is broken, the shielded loop unfolds and significant energy is dissipated in reducing the chain entropy as it straightens out. Atomic Force Microscope (AFM)

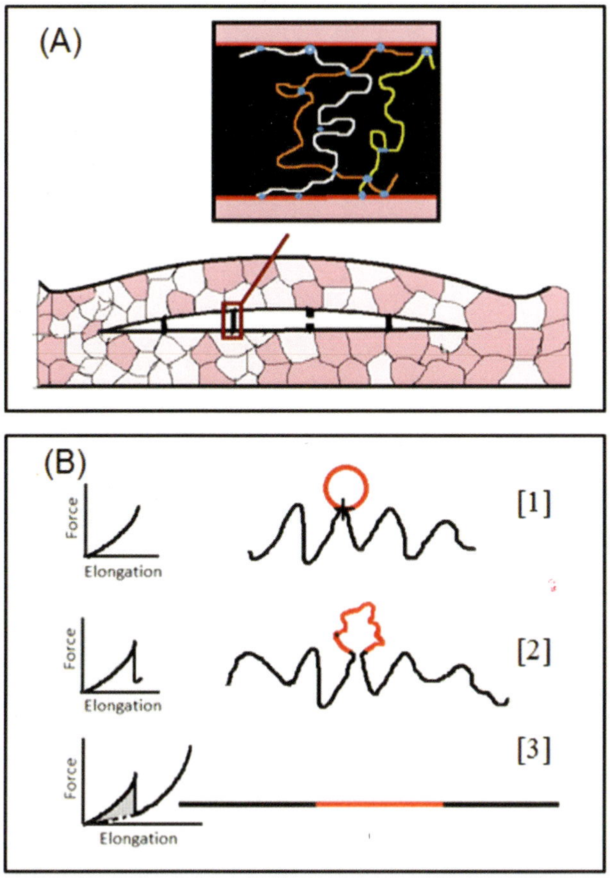

Figure 1. The structure and the basic operation principles of the SBHL system. (A) Hypothesized structures of assembled glue molecules, with sacrificial bonds (represented by blue circles) along the backbone of the polymer molecules resisting rupture of the molecules as they are stretched during microcracking. There are three types of bonds: (i) bonds within the polymer chain, (ii) bonds between different chains, and (iii) bonds connecting the chains to the backbone. (Adapted from Figure 3 in Fantner *et al.* Nature Materials 2005; 4:612–616.) (B) Schematic drawing of the basic principles of the sacrificial bond-hidden length mechanism. [1] Before a sacrificial bond is broken, only the black length of the molecule contributes to the entropic configurations and to the force with which the molecule resists stretching. The red length of the molecule is hidden from the force by the sacrificial bond. [2] When the bond fracture threshold is reached, the bond breaks and the whole length of the polymer (black plus red) contributes to its entropy. The force supported by the polymer molecule abruptly drops in response to this sudden increase in entropy. [3] As the polymer molecule is further stretched the force supported by it increases. This continues until the molecule becomes straight and breaks. The grey area represents the extra work done in stretching a polymer with SBHL system relative to a polymer of the same length but without the SBHL system.
doi:10.1371/journal.pone.0056118.g001

indentation [11], pulling [11], and imaging [16] experiments support this understanding. Moreover, these experimental results suggest that SBHL system, found in gel molecules binding the mineralized collagen fibrils together, may play a substantial mechanical role in bone [12,17–19]. Order of magnitude calculations show that less than 1% by weight of this "glue" can have profound effects on the fracture resistance [12]. This challenges the conventional belief that collagen fibrils and mineral plates are the only components of bone with a strengthening mechanical role [20].

Interestingly, the SBHL system is not limited to bone. Rather, it is widespread in many remarkably tough nano-composite biomaterials such as abalone shell and diatoms [21-27]. Abalone shell, for example, is 97% crystalline calcium carbonate plates by weight, but is 3,000 times more fracture resistant than pure calcium carbonate [21–22]. The other 3% is an interstitial organic matrix, which contains extremely efficient "glue" that incorporates the SBHL system [17]. Adhesive nanofibers from live diatoms exhibit the signature of modular proteins and they show remarkable toughness [27]. The saw-tooth behavior in their force extension response corresponds to unfolding and detachment events similar to the SBHL systems mechanism [27]. A similar behavior has been reported for parallel polyprotein dimers [28] and spider capture silk [29]. A more complete understanding of the SBHL system mechanics may be useful in developing innovative therapeutic procedures as well as designing bio-inspired composite materials with improved strength and toughness.

This paper is organized as follows. In Section II we use the worm like chain model to describe the mechanics of a polymer with the SBHL system and compare the model predictions with AFM experimental observations. In Section III we investigate the influence of the SBHL internal variables, such as the number of bonds and the strength of bonds, on the macroscopic observables such as the increase in toughness. In Section IV we use the polymer force law discussed in Section II in a model of an ensemble of parallel polymers to predict the collective force-elongation behavior at mesoscopic scales. We also examine the effect of the polymer density on the collective behavior. Finally we summarize our conclusions and discuss future directions in Section V.

Review of The Basic Mechanical Properties of Polymers with Sacrificial Bonds and Hidden Length

Polymer elasticity is essentially entropic [30–31]. The relationship between the chain force (f) and its end-to-end distance (x) is controlled by the multiplicity of the number of configurations the chain can take consistent with this given end-to-end distance. The higher the multiplicity, the higher the chain entropy, and the lower the force it can support. As the polymer chain is stretched, its entropy decreases and higher forces are required corresponding to a given end-to-end distance. The end-to-end distance x cannot exceed the contour length of the polymer chain (L_c). (They coincide only when the polymer is completely straight).

The presence of the sacrificial bonds makes the length of the polymer available for entropic fluctuations smaller than the contour length (the difference is the total length of the hidden loops). In this paper, we assume that the bonds break according to a threshold fracture criterion. This is a reasonable assumption in the limit of slow pulling rates [32]. Once a bond breaks, the length of the polymer available for entropic fluctuations increases by an amount equal to the length of the freed loop. This instantaneously increases the chain entropy and leads to an abrupt drop in the force supported by the polymer molecule. With further stretching, the chain entropy decreases and the force in the chain increases.

To quantitatively describe the force-elongation response we use the worm like chain model. We show in Supporting Information Part A in File S1 that this represents a good fit for the experimental data available in the literature on bone glue [11] in the limit of large extension (Fig. S1 in File S1). The force extension relationship is given by:

$$f=\frac{k_BT}{b}\left[\frac{1}{4}\left(1-\frac{x}{L_c}\right)^{-2}-\frac{1}{4}+\frac{x}{L_c}\right], \quad (1)$$

where f is the force, x is the end-to-end distance, b is the persistence length, k_B is Boltzmann' constant and T is the temperature. In the presence of sacrificial bonds, the contour length in Eqn. (1) is replaced by the available length L_a. The available length is the total length of the polymer segments that can contribute to entropic elasticity. The contour and the available lengths are related by:

$$L_a=L_c-\sum_{i=1}^{n}l_i, \quad (2)$$

where l_i is the length of loop i shielded by the sacrificial bond i and n is the number of sacrificial bonds that are not broken yet. Accordingly, Eqn. (1) takes the form:

$$f=\frac{k_BT}{b}\left[\frac{1}{4}\left(1-\frac{x}{L_a}\right)^{-2}-\frac{1}{4}+\frac{x}{L_a}\right]. \quad (3)$$

In this section we review the key features describing the force extension curves observed in AFM experiments on bone glue [11] and discuss their mechanical implications. We follow a computational procedure similar to the one used by Fantner et al., 2006b [19]. In carrying out the numerical simulations, we keep track of the available length. Each time a sacrificial bond is broken, the available length increases by the length of the loop segment that is freed after the bond breakage.

We assume that a bond breaks when it is subjected to a force that exceeds a threshold value taken to be the bond strength. From the AFM experiments, the bond strength is estimated to be of the order of few 100 pN [33]. Several factors can affect this estimate including the bond chemical composition, its interaction with the surrounding solution, and other environmental and loading conditions such as the thermodynamic temperature and the pulling rate. Moreover, a given hidden loop may be shielded by more than one bond. Models based on the transition state theory can be used to account for some of these factors. They have been used to describe unfolding of polymer molecules [34] and strength of molecular adhesion bonds [32].

In this paper we do not account for such details explicitly. Instead, we will make the assumption that the bond strength is a random variable drawn from a uniform distribution between 1 pN and 1 nN (to account roughly for the different sources of variability). This should be a good approximation within the quasistatic loading limit we are considering here. The current framework can be extended to account for the effects of higher loading rates where the details of bond dynamics become significant.

An example of the force-extension behavior generated by Eqn. (2) for a polymer with a single sacrificial bond is shown in Fig. 2. The figure also defines several key concepts including chain stiffness, ductility, and toughness.

The chain stiffness indicates the ability of the chain to resist deformation. It is given by the slope of the tangent to force-extension curve. By differentiating Eqn. (2) with respect to x, we obtain the following expression for the chain stiffness:

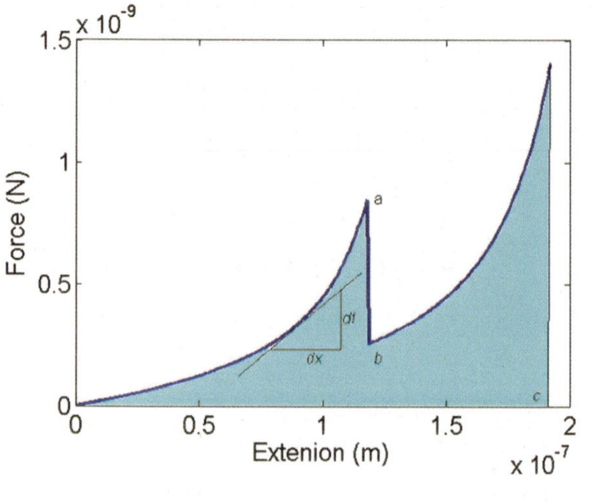

Figure 2. The force-extension behavior of an idealized polymer chain with a single sacrificial bond. The grey-filled area represents the work done in stretching the polymer to its fullest. This is equal to the polymer toughness. Point *a*, corresponding to the first force peak, represents the strength of the sacrificial bond. Point *b* represents the force supported by the chain just after the bond has broken. Point *c* represents the maximum extension to which the polymer chain can be stretched. This is the measure of the chain ductility. The stiffness of the chain at any given displacement is given by the slope of the straight line tangential to the force-extension curve at that displacement ($k=df/dx$).
doi:10.1371/journal.pone.0056118.g002

$$k=df/dx=\frac{k_BT}{b}\left[\frac{1}{2L_a}\left(1-\frac{x}{L_a}\right)^{-3}+\frac{1}{L_a}\right]. \quad (4)$$

That is (i) the chain stiffness decreases as the available length increases, and (ii) the chain stiffness increases as the chain extension x increases. The presence of a sacrificial bond reduces the available length and hence increases the chain stiffness, making the chain stronger at smaller extensions. The saw tooth shape in Fig. 2 is characteristic of sacrificial bond breakage. The peak a corresponds to the bond strength. The magnitude of the force drop Δf is readily computed as:

$$\Delta f=f(x_b,L_a^o)-f(x_b,L_a^o+l_i), \quad (5)$$

where $f(x_b,L_a^o)$ and $f(x_b,l_a^o+l_i)$ are the forces in the chain (Eqn. (2)) just before and after the breakage of the sacrificial bond respectively, x_b is the displacement at which the bond breaks, L_a^o is the available length before the sacrificial bond breakage and l_i is the length of the loop freed by the breakage of the sacrificial bond i.

Two other important concepts, ductility and toughness, are introduced in Fig. 2. The ductility of the polymer is indicative of its ability to deform and stretch without breakage. It is measured by the maximum end-to-end distance the polymer can be stretched to before its failure or detachment from the back bone. The end-to-end distance is always less than or equal to the contour length (the equality holds only when the polymer chain becomes fully straight). Hence, the ductility of the chain cannot exceed its contour length. On the other hand, the toughness represents the work done in stretching the polymer to its maximum end-to-end distance. It is measured by the area under the force-extension line (the hatched area).

Figure 3(a) shows an example force-elongation curve from an AFM experiment [11]. In these experiments, two pieces of the fibril plates placed in a solution are used. One piece is glued to the AFM cantilever tip and the other one is kept fixed at the base. The two pieces are connected together by the polymeric gel filaments. The pieces can be pressed together and then pulled apart to simulate the molecular interactions that occur during the separation of mineralized fibrils within bone. Experiments can be carried out either under displacement-controlled conditions or force-controlled conditions. Figure 3a shows an example from a displacement- controlled AFM experiment. After the two pieces of bone are put in contact, a force is required to separate them. The force as a function of distance during the separation phase is given by the upper line in Fig. 3(a) which consists of a number of smooth increases of the force interrupted by sudden drops. Each force drop corresponds to the breakage of a sacrificial bond or the detachment of a polymer chain from the backbone. The maximum force reported is typically of the order of nanonewtons and the maximum extension is of the order of hundreds of nanometers. As the two ends approach each other, the force in the chain relaxes and the response is described by the smoother lower line in Fig. 3(a). (No bond breakage or polymer detachment occurs during retraction).

Figures 3(b) and 3(c) illustrate our corresponding numerical results for the model when multiple sacrificial bonds and hidden loops are included. The arrangement of the force peaks in the plots depends on the topology of the polymer chain (shown to the right of the plots). In particular, we identify two cases:

Case 1 illustrates the response of a polymer with the SBHL system in which the force peaks are monotonically increasing (Fig. 3(b)). This occurs when each sacrificial bond shields only one hidden loop. With the strength of sacrificial bonds drawn from a random distribution, the weakest sacrificial bonds in this case breaks first.

Case 2 illustrates a situation in which the force peaks are not arranged monotonically (Fig. 3(c)). This latter case is more consistent with AFM experiment (Fig. 3(a)). Possible mechanisms for this non-monotonic variability in the force peaks within the force-elongation response include: (i) weak bonds contained within hidden loops [shown here] and (ii) more than one polymer chain is pulled simultaneously. We will further discuss the case of having multiple parallel connections between the fibrils in Section IV.

The discussion in this section reveals the mechanical role of the SBHL system which improves both the polymer stiffness and toughness. This leads to two key contributions to the intrinsic mechanical response of the bio-material in which the SBHL system exists:

1) Increased resistance to crack initiation: The strength of the polymer chain with sacrificial bonds is always higher at low and intermediate values of displacement. Hence, larger forces will be required to initiate a tear or increase a crack opening in the presence of the SBHL system.

2) Improved energy dissipation: The SBHL system increases polymer toughness. Tougher materials are more ductile and more resistant to brittle (catastrophic) failure. This is particularly important in cases of impact loading where the presence of sacrificial bonds will facilitate the dissipation of the impact energy in inelastic deformation and will reduce the probability of bone breakage.

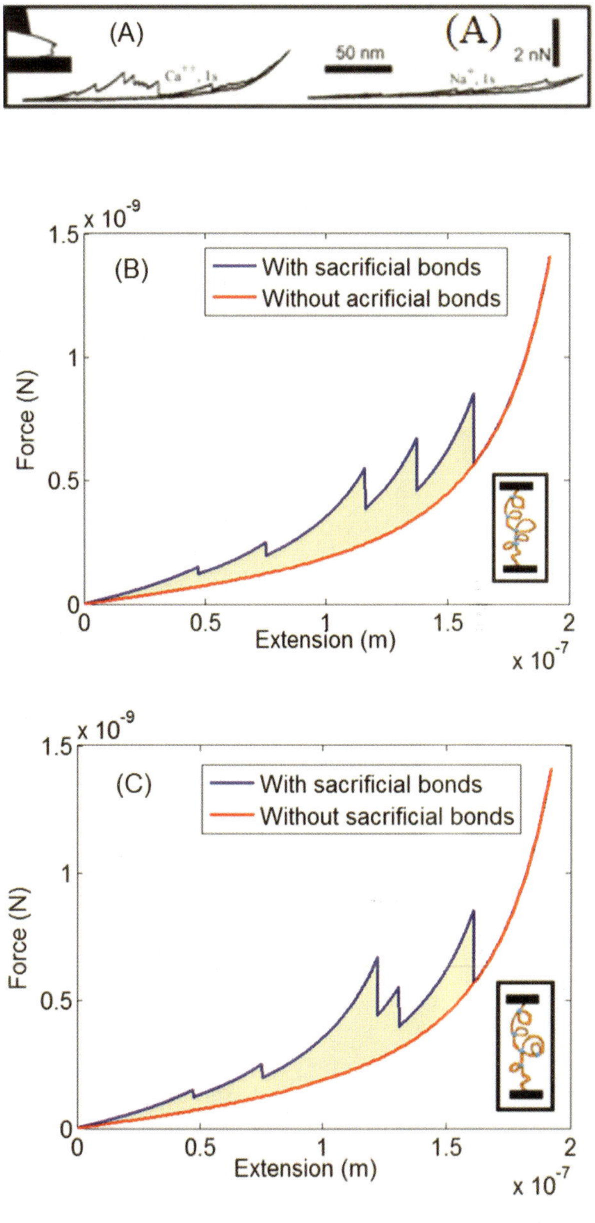

Figure 3. Experimental and numerical results for the force-extension response of polymer chains with SBHL system. (a) The force-extension response typically observed in AFM experiments (Reprinted with permission from [33]), (b) The force-extension response generated by the WLC model Eqn. (2) showing force peaks that are monotonically increasing (Case 1). In this case the weakest sacrificial bond breaks first. (c) The force-extension response generated by the WLC model Eqn. (2) showing force peaks that are non-monotonic (Case 2). This is consistent with the AFM experimental results (shown in Fig. 3(a)). A possible mechanism is that the weaker bond (bond no. 4 from the top) is shielded within a stronger bond loop (bond no.3 from top) and will become exposed only if the third bond breaks and its attached loop unfolds. In both Figs. 3(b) and 3(c), the blue lower line represents a polymer chain with the same contour and persistence length but with no SBHL system. The filled area between the lower blue and upper red lines represents the increase in toughness due to the presence of the SBHL system. ($L_c = 235\,nm$, $b = 0.02$ nm. It is more probable in these experiments that a single connection between the fibrils consist of a number of polymers interconnected with each other and pulled simultaneously. In this case, our model could be understood as being representative of the equivalent polymer chain with the same peak force and maximum extension).

Limitations of The Sacrificial Bonds and Hidden Length System

In this section, we investigate the relationship between the SBHL system internal variables (bond strength and density) and the macroscopic response of the polymer chain in terms of its strength, ductility, and toughness. These factors are expected to play a key role in designing bio-inspired composite materials and in developing therapeutic interventions for improving bone health.

To investigate the effect of the number of sacrificial bonds (i.e. bond density per polymer) on the polymer toughness, we consider a polymer chain with a given contour lengthL_c and n sacrificial bonds. Each bond hides a loop with length l. For the purpose of this estimate, we consider an idealized case in which $l = L_c/(2n+1)$(i.e. all loops have the same length). The available length of the polymer is then readily calculated as

$$L_a = L_c - nl = L_c - \frac{nL_c}{2n+1}. \tag{6}$$

The increase in toughness is the difference in the work done to extend the polymer chain with and without the sacrificial bonds. We calculate the increase in toughness for different values of n. The results are shown in Fig. 4 ($L_c = 240\,nm$and$b = 0.02\,nm$).

In generating the numerical results, each point represents the average of 5000 realizations with randomly varying bonds strength. As the number of bonds increases there is a large increase in the toughness after which the curve eventually levels off.

One of the factors affecting the number of sacrificial bonds is the type of the solution in which the polymer is placed. Negative charges on the chains can combine with free cations in the solution to form sacrificial bonds [35]. Fig. 3a suggests that during the separation of fibrils, more energy is dissipated when filaments are pulled in Ca^{2+} solutions than in Na^{+} solutions. A possible explanation for this difference, in the light of the curves in Fig. 4, is that more sacrificial bonds are formed in the former (with the divalent calcium ion in the solution combining with two negative

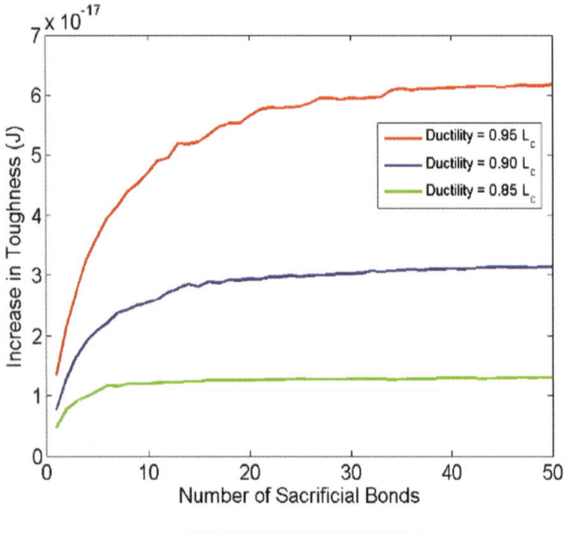

Figure 4. Effect of varying the number of sacrificial bonds on the increase in toughness of the polymer chain. Different curves correspond to different ductility values.

ions on the polymer backbone) than in the latter enabling a larger increase in toughness.

The asymptotic results represented by the curves in Fig. 4 can be understood from the continuum limit of the SBHL system chain as the number of bonds becomes large. For a fixed contour length, as the number of sacrificial bonds increases, the initial value of the available length approaches$L_c/2$asymptotically (Eqn. (6)).In this limit, the instantaneous stiffness of the chain varies weakly with the breakage of sacrificial bonds (Supporting Information Part B in File S2) and the force-extension curves become indistinguishable from each other (Fig. S2 in File S2). Since toughness is measured by the area under the force-extension curve, this implies that there will be little or no change in toughness due to the change in the number of bonds.

The number of bonds at which the increase in toughness levels off depends on the ductility of the polymer chains. As the ductility increases, the increase in toughness for each additional (extra) bond decreases at a smaller rate. The ductility depends on the strength of the bonds connecting the chain to the collagen fibrils as we shortly discuss.

Another important control parameter for the SBHL system is the strength of the sacrificial bonds. Two types of sacrificial bonds are considered: sacrificial bonds within the polymer chain (internal bonds) and sacrificial bonds connecting the polymer to the collagen fibrils (end bonds). This distinction between the two types of bonds is important as they can be structurally different and hence can have different values of strength.

In order for the SBHL system to enhance the polymer toughness, the strength of both types of sacrificial bonds must be such that the polymer can extend to its fullest length. This implies that the strength of end bonds should be, at least, larger than the strength of all the internal sacrificial bonds. This can be explained as follows.

The force in the polymer chain (Eqn. (3)) depends on the x/L_aratio (where x is the end-to-end distance and L_a is the available length). Sacrificial bonds reduce the available length and hence higher forces develop in the chain at smaller extensions. If the internal bond is stronger than the polymer, the polymer breaks first. On the other hand, if the end bonds are weaker than the polymer, this leads to the premature detachment of the polymer chain from the collagen fibrils (Section IV). In both cases, the system fails before the polymer achieves its full extension (corresponding to its contour length). Accordingly, both the ductility and toughness are reduced.

Efforts to enhance the bone mechanical response, whether by stimulating the bone production of or by injecting the bone with gel molecules, must account for these effects. Our results suggest density of internal bonds and constraints on the strength of the internal and end bonds will be factors affecting the SBHL system performance.

A Mesoscopic Cohesive Law for The Polymeric System

AFM experiments [12] suggest that the force supported by a fibril is of the order of a few micronewtons whereas the strength of the single polymer is of the order of several hundred piconewtons to a few nanonewtons. This means that on average 1000 polymers per fibril are required, in a healthy individual, to assure the full transfer of the force by the fibril plate.

We incorporate this in our models of the mechanical response by analyzing a group of polymer chains placed parallel to each other and constrained by the same displacement-controlled loading conditions considered previously. This setup is relevant to a wide range of applications. For example, the mechanical signature of modular proteins in diatoms [27] and parallel polyprotein dimers [28] have been previously identified in AFM experiments. Another example is quasi-brittle cracking in crystalline solids. There, the crack proceeds by breaking arrays atomic bonds intersecting with its path [36].

For the purpose of the current investigation, we consider the contour length of different polymer chains as an additional variable that is drawn from a uniform random distribution. The length of a single polymer is typically 200–350 nm. In reality, however, polymers connect with each other to form chains of much longer length enabling end-to-end extension of the order of micrometers. We assume that the total length of the chain is a random variable with a maximum value of 5 μm.

The strength of sacrificial bonds is drawn from the same random variable distribution used in Sections II and III. Each individual polymer chain deforms according to the worm like chain model (Eqn. (3)). We investigate the collective behavior of the group of polymer chains represented by the overall force-displacement response and how this response changes as a function of the number of polymer chains (N_p).

At any given instant of time, all surviving polymers are constrained by the same end-to-end distance. This is achieved by envisioning a loading apparatus of infinite rigidity. In this limit, the stress disturbance, resulting from the detachment of individual polymers, equilibrates instantaneously and does not affect the force distribution on neighboring polymers.

The force-extension response for different number of polymer chains is shown in Fig. 5. A representative pulling curve observed in AFM experiments on dintin molecules [35] is illustrated in Fig. 5a The case of small number ($N_p = 5$, 10, 20) is shown in Fig. 5(b) while that for the large number ($N_p = 50$, 100, 200) is shown in Fig. 5(c).

For small number of chains ($N_p < 20$) the discrete effects of sacrificial bond breakage and polymer detachment are pronounced. In this range, the results are intrinsically stochastic and sample dependent. These features have been observed in AFM experiments on blobs of dentin molecules (Fig. 5a) suggesting that a small number of chains (~10 molecules) is being pulled in such experiments. On the other hand, when the number of polymer chains becomes sufficiently large ($N_p > 50$) the response is increasingly well approximated by relatively smooth force-extension curves, similar to the cohesive laws routinely used in fracture mechanics [36–37].

We identify two distinct regimes in the force-extension plots shown in Fig 5. For small displacements, the force peaks tend to increase in magnitude as the extension increases. This is the displacement-strengthening regime which is expected to play a significant role in resisting crack initiation and controlling stable crack growth. On the other hand, for large displacements the force peaks tend to decrease with increasing extension corresponding to failure of end bonds and the detachment of polymer chains. This is the displacement-weakening regime which is expected to allow for the growth of instabilities and dynamic crack propagation. This displacement weakening instability is a collective effect of the polymer network and is qualitatively different from the continuing upward trend observed for a single polymer in Fig. 3(b) and 3(c).

The magnitude of the force drops in Fig. 5(b) relative to the overall force scale is large compared to the force fluctuations in Fig. 5(c) where the curves are much smoother. While small scale roughness persists in Fig. 5(c), these irregularities are in most cases of the order of 5% of the maximum force.

Another important difference is the variability in size of the force drops of significantly in Fig. 5(b) compared with Fig. 5(c) or

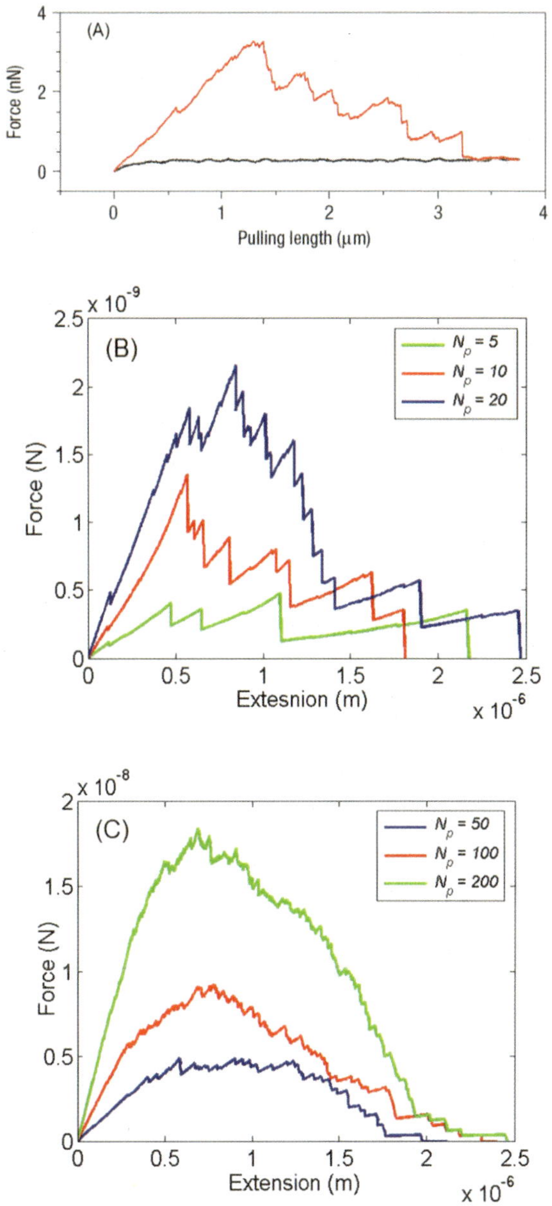

Figure 5. The force-extension response for different number of polymers under controlled displacement loading conditions. (a) Representative pulling curve observed in AFM experiments on dentin molecules (reprinted with permission from [35]) (b) Representative curves illustrating force-extension response for 5, 10 and, 20 polymers. The smaller force drops correspond in most cases to the breakage of sacrificial bonds while the larger force drops typically represent the detachment of polymer chains. The curve shows similar features to the plot in (a) suggesting that only a few chains are being pulled simultaneously during the AFM experiment. (c) The force extension plot for the polymeric gel when the number of polymer chains is large. The curves look much smoother than the curves in (b).

Fig 3(b) and 3(c). The force drops of smaller magnitude correspond in most cases to the breakage of individual sacrificial bonds and unfolding of the hidden loops, whereas the force drops of larger magnitude typically represent detachment of polymers from the backbone. This is because the breakage of an internal sacrificial bond leads to the unfolding of a single hidden loop. This only reduces the stiffness of the system slightly and causes a small force drop. However, once the polymer chain detaches, the force supported by it drops to zero. The force drop in this case is usually bigger especially if the chain is close to its maximum extension.

The detachment of the polymer chain can occur either because the bond connecting it to the fibril breaks (weak end bond) or because the force in the polymer chain exceeds the polymer strength. While polymers also detach from the backbone in Fig. 5(c), the number of polymers is large enough that detachment of single polymer does not significantly impact the system as a whole.

If the number of polymers contributing to the polymeric gel system is small, the accuracy of large-scale models of fracture in mineralized collagen fibrils may depend critically on modeling these discrete effects characteristic of the force-extension curves. However, if the number of polymers is sufficiently large, the interfacial description may be greatly simplified. Our results suggest that the quasi-static cohesive law in this case may be represented by a smooth curve parameterized by three variables: (i) the magnitude of the maximum force that the interface can resist ($F_{\max}$), (ii) the magnitude of the maximum displacement at complete separation ($\delta_{\max}$) and (iii) the displacement corresponding to $F_{\max}$. The self-similarity of the force extension curves (in the limit of large number of polymers) enabled such parameterization. We have found that an expression of the form $F = A\sin(b\delta)\exp(-c\delta)$, fits the results fairly well ($R > 0.97$). In this expression$F$and δ are the force and displacement normalized by their maximum values respectively. A,b,and$c$ are fitting constants. For a good approximation: $b = \delta_c^{-1}$, $c = 2\delta_c^{-1}$ and $A = \sin(1)\exp(-1/2)$. δ_c is the normalized displacement at maximum force.

Examination of the trends in Figs. 5(b) and 5(c) suggest that the maximum force F_{max} is proportional to the number of polymers while the maximum displacement $\delta_{\max}$ is weakly dependent on the number of polymers. This is verified quantitatively in Fig. 6 which illustrates statistical results for these parameters as a function of the number of polymers N_p. For each value of N_p the numerical experiment was repeated for 1500 realizations. The distribution of the maximum force, for a fixed value of N_p , is non-Gaussian. It can be represented, however, by a finite sum of Gaussian functions. On the other hand, the maximum extension distribution was found to be approximately Gaussian.

The increase in the maximum force with the increase in the number of polymers follows directly from the parallel arrangement of the polymers. At any given displacement x the total force supported by the system is given by:

$$F(x) = \sum_{i}^{N \leq N_p} f_i(x), \tag{7}$$

where$F$is the total force, f_i is the force in the ith polymer chain computed by Eqn.(3) and N is the number of unbroken polymer chains at displacement x. In the displacement strengthening regime,$N\tilde{N}_p$, so that the largerN_p the higher the maximum force F.

On the other hand, the approximate independence of the maximum extension on the number of polymers follows from the fact that the maximum displacement depends only on the contour length of the last surviving polymer chain. This is taken to be a random variable independent of the number of polymers.

Finally we examine the effect of the strength of the end bonds on the macroscopic properties of the polymeric system. End bonds may have different structure from internal bonds and hence the two groups might differ in their strength. The distinction is then important as it impacts the dynamics of the SBHL and could have potential therapeutic implications.

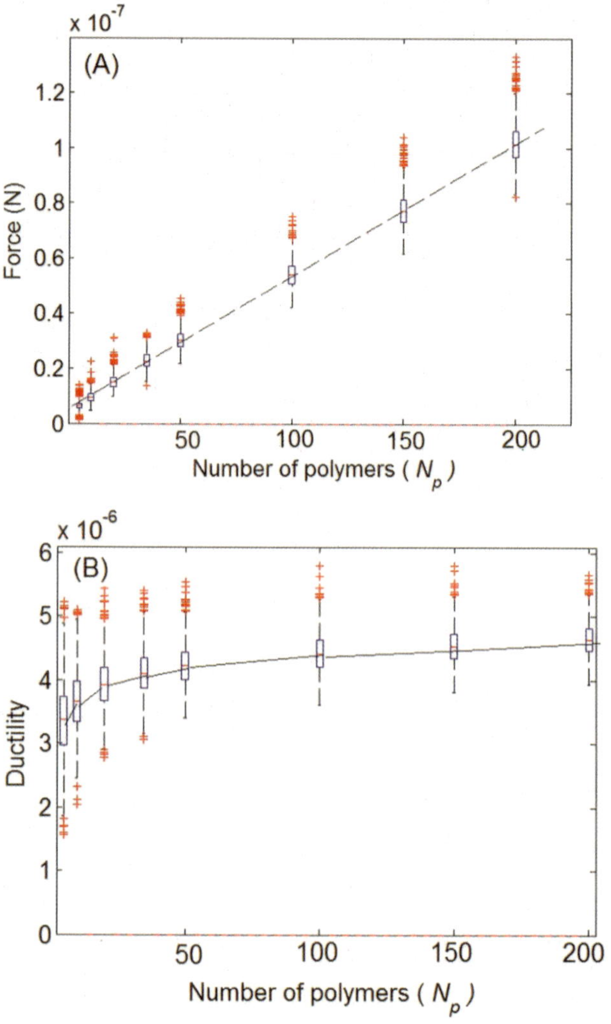

Figure 6. The effect of the number of polymers (N_p) on the maximum force and ductility (maximum extension) of the polymer group. On each box, the central mark is the median, the edges of the box are the 25th and 75th percentiles, the whiskers extend to the most extreme data points not considered outliers, and outliers are plotted individually. (a) The maximum force increases linearly with increasing the number of polymers and (b) the maximum extension is weakly dependent on the number of polymers.

Following the discussion in Section III, if the strength of the end bonds is less than the polymer chain strength, the bonds will break and the polymers will prematurely detach before the SBHL system is fully utilized. This lowers both the strength and toughness of the system. On the other hand, if the end bonds are stronger than the polymer, all the internal sacrificial bonds in each chain will break before detachment and each polymer will extend to its fullest. This, in turn, enables maximal contribution of each polymer to the overall system strength and toughness.

We investigated the two scenarios of weak and strong end bonds by simulating 1500 realizations of polymers with the SBHL system. In both cases, the geometric properties of the polymer chains, such as the contour length and the length of the hidden loops, are drawn from the same random distribution. In one group of simulations, the strength of the end bonds is chosen from the same probability distribution governing the bonds. In this case, the strength of both types of bonds is drawn from a uniform distribution of force thresholds ranging from a minimum value of 1pN to a maximum value of 1nN. In another group of simulations, the strength of the end bonds is chosen greater than the strength of the polymer chain (> 1nN) so that only when the polymer is fully extended it detaches by breaking internally. The results of the numerical investigation are shown in Fig. 7. The cases with strong end bonds (circles) attain on average higher maximum forces, longer extensions and larger toughness values than the cases with nominal (weak) end bonds (squares).

By preventing premature detachment of the polymer chains, the mechanical performance of the polymer group, as measured by strength, ductility and toughness, is significantly enhanced. This suggests that development of therapies which target enhancement of end bonds may play an important role in reducing bone health problems, especially in the elderly.

Conclusion

Problems involving dynamics of cohesively held interfaces arise broadly in biological [Martin *et al.*, 1998] as well as in Engineering [36,38] and geophysical [39–40] applications. Common to all of these applications are fundamental physical processes involving deformation, rupture nucleation, propagation and arrest. In strongly nonlinear problems, like dynamic fracture, small scale instabilities can lead to large scale system fragilities [1,41–43] and it is imperative to understand how the microscopic processes influence the crack macroscopic response. In the case of bone, the internal interfaces between the mineralized collagen fibrils may fail under different loading conditions, and the details of the resulting dynamic rupture can determine whether only a part or the whole of the body part (e.g. knee) will fracture.

The separation of the mineralized collagen fibrils under shear or tension is resisted by a special type of polymeric glue that is composed of polymers with sacrificial bonds and hidden length (SBHL) system. The constitutive response of this glue controls the strength and ductility of the fibril plates.

Several mathematical models have been proposed to explain polymer nonlinear elasticity. Of these models, the worm like chain (WLC) and the freely jointed chain (FJC) models are the most widely used [13–15,36]. The two models differ in their idealization of the polymer chain and their prediction of the force extension response.

In this paper we investigated the mechanics and implications of entropy-based energy dissipation in polymer chains with SBHL system using the worm like chain model. Our primary focus was on the influence of the SBHL system on the larger scale mechanical observables such as toughness, ductility and mesco-sopic constitutive response.

Our numerical results indicate that the SBHL system generally enhances the toughness and the strength of the polymeric system and this should allow for better resistance to crack initiation and propagation as well as better performance under dynamic loading. These properties can be used in designing base isolators to damp vibrations in structures subjected to ground motions [44].

Investigation of the dependence of polymer toughness and ductility on the internal variables of the SBHL system reveals constraints on the optimum number of sacrificial bonds as well as the strength of the bonds in order for the SBHL system to be fully utilized. In particular, the net gain in toughness may not increase in the presence of a larger number of bonds. Moreover, we show that the presence of strong internal sacrificial bonds can reduce the polymer ductility and toughness. Unlike the strength requirements

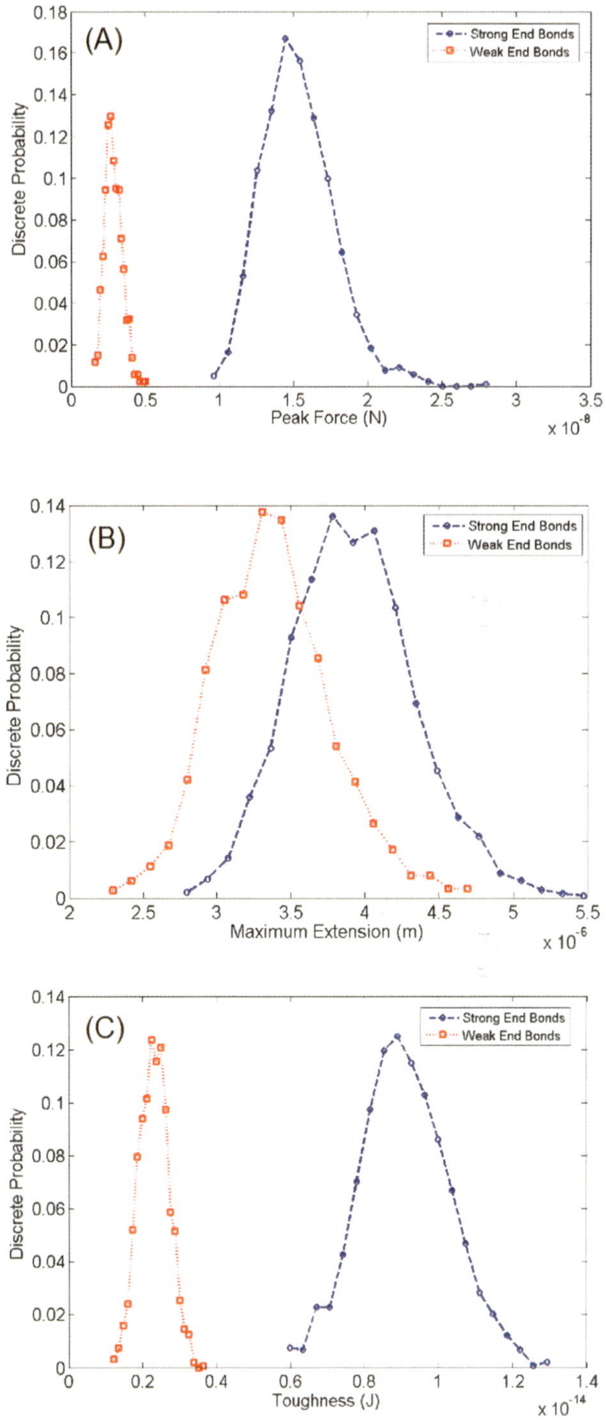

Figure 7. Effect of the strength of the bonds connecting the polymer chains to the mineralized collagen fibrils. Polymers with strong end bonds (blue circles) lead systematically to (a) higher strength, (b) ductility, and (c) toughness, compared to cases where the end bonds are weaker than the polymer itself (red squares). [Depicted probabilities are discrete].

for the internal bonds, strong end bonds are required to prevent premature detachment of the polymer chain and to allow the SBHL system to fully operate. These observations must be taken into account in developing therapeutic procedures that aim to enhance bone mechanical behavior or in designing bio-inspired composites with improved fracture resistance properties.

We also investigated the collective behavior of a system of parallel polymers constrained by the same displacement controlled loading. In real elastomeric networks, polymers can develop crosslinks with each other. This crosslinking will definitely affect the force distribution and ductility in the polymeric system [45]. The study of the parallel setup, however, acts as a starting point for understanding the constitutive response at larger scales. It is also relevant to a wide range of applications such as modeling diatoms [27], and parallel polyprotein dimers [28]. Moreover, it serves as a good approximation for the glue between the bone fibrils in young healthy individuals. Aging increases the crosslinking between polymers and reduces their toughness and ductility. This effect will be investigated further in our future work.

For a small number of polymer chains, we show that the cohesive law describing the force- extension response carries a clear signature of the microscopic processes of bond breakage and polymer detachment. This is manifested in the existence of force drops of magnitude comparable to the magnitude of the maximum force supported by the system. The implementation of these details in any large scale model of fracture is required because they can significantly affect crack initiation and propagation. We also showed that these details agree with observations from AFM experiments done on dentin molecules [35].

For a large number of polymer chains, however, the force fluctuations due to these microscopic processes are small compared to the amplitude of the maximum forces achieved in the system. The cohesive law in this case is greatly simplified and can be approximated by a smooth curve characterized by two numbers: the maximum force and the maximum extension.

Our results show that the maximum force supported by the polymeric system is proportional to the polymer density (number of polymer chains per unit area) and so is the system toughness. These results are relevant for understanding changes in the bone mechanical response with aging. Since the number of polymers produced by the osteocytes may decrease as the individual ages, this investigation reveals possible mechanisms for bone toughness degradation with age other than loss of bone density. It also suggests that therapeutic interventions that stimulate the production of the polymeric gel can help enhance bone health especially in the elderly [9,20].

A future extension of this study will involve use of the derived cohesive law as a boundary condition for individual elements in large scale dynamical models of bone hierarchal structure. These models will ultimately incorporate the structural complexity of the human bone at different scales to determine the combined effects of microscopic mechanisms of the SBHL system with material and geometric heterogeneities in resisting fracture. Multiscale modeling is a critical ingredient in understanding the fracture toughness in bone as well as in designing new composite materials with high levels of strength and toughness.

Supporting Information

File S1 Supporting Information Part A and Figure S1. Representative Force extension data (dots) from AFM experiments on bone glue. Different colors correspond to retraction curves in Calcium ion solutions after different delay [Source: Thompson et al., 2001]. The data is fitted by the worm like chain model (smooth curves). [Force is normalized by 70 pN and extension is normalized by 2.35 nm].

File S2 Supporting Information Part B and Figure S2. Force-extension plots of a polymer chain ($L_c = 240nm, b = 0.02nm$) with different numbers of sacrificial bonds *n*.

Acknowledgments

The authors are grateful for the comments of two anonymous reviewers that were very useful in improving the manuscript. They are also grateful to Paul Hansma, Jim Langer and Dan Morse for numerous, insightful discussions.

Author Contributions

Conceived and designed the experiments: AE JC. Performed the experiments: AE. Analyzed the data: AE JC. Wrote the paper: AE.

References

1. Daub E, Carlson JM (2010) Friction, Fracture and Earthquakes. Ann. Rev. Cond. Mat. Phys. 1: 397–418.
2. Falk M, Langer JS (1998) Dynamics of viscoplastic deformation in amorphous solids. Phys. Rev. E 57: 7192–7205.
3. Lieou CKC, Langer JS (2012) Nonequilibrium thermodynamics in sheared hard-sphere materials. Phys. Rev. E 85: 061308.
4. Lemaitre A, Carlson JM (2004) Boundary lubrication with a glassy interface. Physical Review E 69: 61611.
5. Bouchbinder E, Langer JS (2009a) Nonequilibrium thermodynamics of driven amorphous materials. Phys. Rev. E. 80, 031131.
6. Bouchbinder E, Langer JS (2009b) Nonequilibrium thermodynamics of driven amorphous materials. II. Effective-temperature theory. Phys. Rev. E. 80, 031132.
7. Bouchbinder E, Langer JS (2009c) Nonequilibrium thermodynamics of driven amorphous materials. III. Shear-transformation-zone plasticity. Phys. Rev. E. 80, 031133.
8. Koester KJ, Ager JW, Ritchie RO (2008) The true toughness of human cortical bone measured with realistically short cracks. Nature Materials 7: 672–677.
9. Nallaa RK, Kruzica JJ, Kinney JH, Ritchie RO (2004) Effect of aging on the toughness of human cortical bone: evaluation by R-curves. Bone 35:1240–1246.
10. Ritchie RO, Beuhler M, Hansma P (2009) Plasticity and toughness in bone. Physics Today: 41–47.
11. Thompson JB, Kindt JH, Drake B, Hansma HG, Morse DE, et al. (2001) Bone Indentation Recovery Time Correlates with Bond Reforming Time. Nature 414:773–775.
12. Fantner GE, Hassenkam T, Kindt JH, Weaver JC, Birkedal H (2005) Sacrificial bonds and hidden length dissipate energy as mineralized fibrils separate during bone fracture. Nature Materials 4: 612–616.
13. Wang MD, Yin H, Landick R, Gelles J, Block SM (1994) Stretching DNA with optical tweezers. Biophys. J. 72:1335–1346.
14. Marko JF, Siggia ED (1995) Stretching DNA. Macromolecules 28: 8759–8770.
15. Bouchiat C, Wang MD, Allemand JF, Strick T, Block SM, et al. (1999) Estimating the Persistence Length of a Worm-Like Chain Molecule from Force-Extension Measurements. Biophys J. 76, No. 1, 409–413.
16. Hassenkam T, Fantner GE, Cutroni JA, Weaver JC, Morse DE, et al. (2004) High-resolution AFM imaging of intact and fractured trabecular bone. Bone 35: 4–10.
17. Smith BL, Schaeffer TE, Viani M, Thompson JB, Frederick NA, et al. (1999) Molecular mechanistic origin of the toughness of natural adhesives, fibres and composites. Nature 399: 761–763.
18. Fantner GE, Oroudjev E, Schitter G, Golde LS, Thurner P, et al. (2006a) Sacrificial Bonds and Hidden Length: Unraveling Molecular Mesostructures in Tough Materials. Biophysical Journal 90 (4): 1411–1419.
19. Fantner GE, Rabinovych O, Schitter G, Thurner P, Kindt JH, et al., (2006b) Hierarchical interconnections in the nano-composite material bone: Fibrillar cross-links resist fracture on several length scales. Composites Science and Technology 66: 1205–1211.
20. Gass M, Dawson-Hughes B (2006) Preventing osteoporosis-related fractures: an overview. Am. J. Med. 119, S3–S11.
21. Currey JD (1977) Mechanical Properties of Mother of Pearl in Tension. Proceedings of the Royal Society of London Series B-Biological Sciences 196: 443–463.
22. Jackson AP, Vincent JFV, Turner RM (1988) The Mechanical Design of Nacre. Proceedings of the Royal Society of London Series B-Biological Sciences 234: 415–440.

23. Gebeschuber IC, Kindt JH, Thompson JB, Del Amo Y, Stachelberger H, et al. (2003) Atomic force microscopy study of living diatoms in ambient conditions. J. Microsc 212: 292–299.
24. Higgins MJ, Crawford SA, Mulvaney P, Wetherbee R (2002) Characterization of the adhesive mucilages secreted by live diatom cells using atomic force microscopy. Protist 153: 25–38.
25. Higgins MJ, Sader JE, Mulvaney P, Wetherbee R (2003) Probing the surface of living diatoms with atomic force microscopy: the nanostructure and nanomechanical properties of the mucilage layer. J. Phycol. 39: 722–734.
26. Higgins MJ, Molino JP, Mulvaney P, Wetherbee R (2003) The structure and nanomechanical properties of the adhesive mucilage that mediates diatom: substratum adhesion and motility. J. Phycol. 39: 1181–1193.
27. Dugdale TM, Degastine R, Chiovitti A, Mulvaney P, Wetherbee R (2005) Single adhesive nano-fibers from a live diatom have the signature fingerprint of modular proteins. Biophysical Journal 89: 4252–4260.
28. Sarkar A, Caamano S, Fernandez J (2007) The Mechanical Fingerprint of a Parallel Polyprotein Dimer. Biophysical Journals, L36-L38, doi: 10.1529/biophysj.106.097741.
29. Becker N, Oroudjev E, Mutz S, Cleveland JP, Hansma PK, et al. (2003) Molecular nanosprings in spider capture-silk threads. Nature Materials 2, no. 4: 278–283.
30. Bustamante C, Marko JF, Siggia ED, Smith S (1994) Entropic elasticity of lambda-phage DNA. Science 265: 1599–1600.
31. Rubenstein M (2003) Polymer Physics. Oxford University Press, USA.
32. Evans E, Ritchie K (1997) Dynamic strength of molecular adhesion bonds. Biophysical Journal 72(4): 1541–1555.
33. Hansma PK, Fantner GE, Kindt JH, Thurner PJ, Schitter G, et al. (2005) Sacrificial bonds in the interfibrillar matrix of bone. J. Musculoskelet Neuronal Interact 5(4): 313–315.
34. Rief M, Fernandez JM, Gaub HE (1998) Elastically Coupled Two-Level Systems as a Model for Biopolymer Extensibility. Phys. Rev. Lett. 81: 4764–4767.
35. Adams J, Fantner GE, Fisher LW, Hansma PK (2008) Molecular energy dissipation in nanoscale networks of Dentin Matrix Protein 1 is strongly dependent on ion valence. Nanotechnology 19: 384008.
36. Barenblatt GI (1962) Mathematical theory of equilibrium cracks in brittle fracture. Advances in Applied Mechanics VII: 55–129.
37. Xu XP, Needleman A (1993) Void nucleation by inclusion debonding in a crystal matrix. Materials Science and Engineering A129: 111–132.
38. Xia K, Chalivendra VB, Rosakis AJ (2006) Spontaneous Mixed-Mode Fracture in Bonded Similar and Dissimilar Materials. Experimental Mechanics 46:163–171.
39. Scholz C (2002) Earthquakes and faulting. Cambridge University Press 2nd edition.
40. Lapusta N (2009) Seismology: The roller coaster of fault friction. Nature Geoscience 2: p. 676–677.
41. Kolmogrov AN (1991) The Local Structure of Turbulence in Incompressible Viscous Fluid for Very Large Reynolds Numbers. Proceedings of the Royal Society of London, Series A: Mathematical and Physical Sciences 434: 9–13.
42. Rice JR (1983) Constitutive Relations for Fault Slip and Earthquake Instabilities. Pure and Applied Geophysics 121: 443–475.
43. Carlson JM, Langer JS (1989) Properties of earthquakes generated by fault dynamics. Phys. Rev. A. 40: 6470–6484.
44. Yang HT, Lin CH, Bridges D, Randall CJ, Hansma PK (2010) Bio-inspired passive actuator simulating an abalone shell mechanism for structural control. Smart Materials and Structures 19(10), 105011.
45. Sbrana F, Lorusso M, Canale C, Bochicchio B, Vassalli M (2011) Effect of chemical cross-linking on the mechanical properties of elastomeric peptides studied by single molecule force spectroscopy. Journal of Biomechanics 44(11): 2118–2122.

5

Immunohistochemical Localization of Key Arachidonic Acid Metabolism Enzymes during Fracture Healing in Mice

Hsuan-Ni Lin[1], J. Patrick O'Connor[1,2]*

1 Department of Biochemistry & Molecular Biology, Graduate School of Biomedical Sciences, Rutgers, The State University of New Jersey, Newark, New Jersey, United States of America, **2** Department of Biochemistry & Molecular Biology, New Jersey Medical School, Rutgers, The State University of New Jersey, Newark, New Jersey, United States of America

Abstract

This study investigated the localization of critical enzymes involved in arachidonic acid metabolism during the initial and regenerative phases of mouse femur fracture healing. Previous studies found that loss of cyclooxygenase-2 activity impairs fracture healing while loss of 5-lipoxygenase activity accelerates healing. These diametric results show that arachidonic acid metabolism has an essential function during fracture healing. To better understand the function of arachidonic acid metabolism during fracture healing, expression of cyclooxygenase-1 (COX-1), cyclooxygenase -2 (COX-2), 5-lipoxygenase (5-LO), and leukotriene A_4 hydrolase (LTA4H) was localized by immunohistochemistry in time-staged fracture callus specimens. All four enzymes were detected in leukocytes present in the bone marrow and attending inflammatory response that accompanied the fracture. In the tissues surrounding the fracture site, the proportion of leukocytes expressing COX-1, COX-2, or LTA4H decreased while those expressing 5-LO remained high at 4 and 7 days after fracture. This may indicate an inflammation resolution function for 5-LO during fracture healing. Only COX-1 was consistently detected in fracture callus osteoblasts during the later stages of healing (day 14 after fracture). In contrast, callus chondrocytes expressed all four enzymes, though 5-LO appeared to be preferentially expressed in newly differentiated chondrocytes. Most interestingly, osteoclasts consistently and strongly expressed COX-2. In addition to bone surfaces and the growth plate, COX-2 expressing osteoclasts were localized at the chondro-osseous junction of the fracture callus. These observations suggest that arachidonic acid mediated signaling from callus chondrocytes or from callus osteoclasts at the chondro-osseous junction regulate fracture healing.

Editor: Daotai Nie, Southern Illinois University School of Medicine, United States of America

Funding: This research was supported by the National Institute of Dental & Craniofacial Research of the National Institutes of Health under award number R01DE019926 and by the Department of Defense Peer Reviewed Orthopaedic Research Program under award number W81XWH-10-1-0944 to JPOC. The content is solely the responsibility of the authors and does not necessarily represent the official views of the National Institutes of Health, the United States Army, or the Department of Defense. The funders had no role in study design, data collection and analysis, decision to publish, or preparation of the manuscript.

Competing Interests: The authors have declared that no competing interests exist.

* E-mail: oconnojp@njms.rutgers.edu

Introduction

Genetic ablation or pharmacological inhibition of cyclooxygenase-2 (COX-2) or 5-lipoxygenase (5-LO) significantly affects bone regeneration during fracture healing. Loss of COX-2 activity impairs fracture healing, while loss of 5-LO activity accelerates healing in rodent models [1–5]. COX-2 and 5-LO catalyze critical steps in the conversion of arachidonic acid into prostaglandins and leukotrienes, respectively [6,7]. Prostaglandins and leukotrienes are eicosanoids, which are 20 carbon lipid signaling molecules that regulate many physiological processes including inflammation and pain.

Arachidonic acid metabolism is complex and involves many enzymes, receptors, oxidative mechanisms, and even transcellular synthetic pathways to produce prostaglandins, leukotrienes, lipoxins, resolvins, and other lipid signaling molecules [8]. Prostaglandins and leukotrienes appear to be the most abundant bioactive lipids produced from arachidonic acid. Typically, arachidonic acid is released from cellular membrane stores by the calcium-dependent, cytoplasmic phospholipase ($cPLA_2$ or PLA2G4A) and converted into prostaglandin H_2 (PGH_2) by cyclooxygenase-1 (COX-1) or COX-2 or into leukotriene A_4 (LTA_4) by 5-LO. PGH_2 and LTA_4 are intermediates. Specific synthase enzymes convert PGH_2 into thromboxane A_2 (TXA_2), PGD_2, PGE_2, $PGF_{2\alpha}$, or PGI_2 which are then secreted to activate receptors specific for each prostaglandin or thromboxane. Similarly, LTA_4 is converted into LTB_4 by leukotriene A_4 hydrolase (LTA4H) or into LTC_4 by leukotriene C_4 synthase. LTC_4 is further modified to produce the cysteinyl leukotrienes (LTD_4 and LTE_4). Typically, these arachidonic acid metabolizing enzymes are abundantly expressed in leukocytes, consistent with the role of prostaglandins and leukotrienes in mediating inflammation [9]. However, these enzymes are expressed in many cell types to mediate other physiological processes [10].

The mechanisms through which COX-2 and 5-LO regulate fracture healing are not understood. In mice lacking COX-2, bone fracture healing is impaired and is characterized by formation of a small, cartilaginous callus [4,11]. In contrast, fracture healing is accelerated in mice lacking 5-LO in which there is an early, large cartilaginous callus that is rapidly replaced by bone through endochondral ossification [1]. Pharmacological inhibition of COX-2 or 5-LO produces similar effects in rats [2–4]. Loss of COX-1 activity does not appear to affect the early stages of healing [4]. Genetic ablation of COX-1, COX-2, or 5-LO alters the levels of PGE_2, $PGF_{2\alpha}$, and LTB_4 produced at the fracture site, indicating that these enzymes function at the fracture site [1]. However, which cells express COX-2 or 5-LO during fracture healing has not been determined. Identifying which cells express these enzymes could significantly improve our understanding of the role of COX-2 and 5-LO in bone regeneration.

To address this, we performed an immunohistochemical analysis of time-staged fracture callus specimens from normal mice to identify which cells express COX-1, COX-2, 5-LO, and LTA4H. As expected, all the enzymes localized to leukocytes. We failed to observe consistent expression of these enzymes in osteoblasts. In contrast, COX-1, COX-2, 5-LO, and LTA4H expression was detected in chondrocytes. Interestingly, COX-2 was abundantly expressed in osteoclasts. These data indicate that arachidonic acid metabolism may be regulating the later regenerative stage of fracture healing when endochondral ossification is occurring through an osteoclast, chondrocyte, or osteoclast-chondrocyte mediated mechanism.

Materials and Methods

Animal Model

Female ICR mice that were 8–10 weeks old and weighed 28.9±2.6 g (mean ± standard deviation) were used in this study (Taconic Farms, Inc. Germantown, NY). Eight mice were used in each group. Mice were anesthetized by intraperitoneal injection of ketamine and xylazine (0.1 and 0.01 mg/g body weight, respectively). A closed, diaphyseal fracture was created in the right femur using a custom-made, three-point bending device (BBC Specialty Automotive Center, Linden, NJ) as described previously except the mice were allowed to recover for 7 days between insertion of the intramedullary pin and production of the fracture or euthanization [12]. Mice were euthanized at 0 (before fracture but 7 days after intramedullary pin insertion), 6 hours and 1, 2, 4, 7, 10, and 14 days after fracture. Tissues were quickly resected, fixed in Streck Tissue Fixative (Streck, Inc., Omaha, NE) for one day, and then decalcified in 10% EDTA for a week. After decalcification, tissues were embedded in paraffin. All experimental procedures were approved by the University of Medicine and Dentistry of New Jersey-New Jersey Medical School Institutional Animal Care and Use Committee (protocol 10075).

Histology

Five um thick serial sections were cut, then deparaffinized in three changes of xylene and rehydrated in a graded alcohol series. Osteoclasts were detected by tartrate-resistant acid phosphatase (TRAP) staining as described previously [13]. TRAP stained sections were counterstained with hematoxylin (Sigma-Aldrich). Cartilage was identified by safranin-O staining, then counterstained with Fast Green (Sigma-Aldrich) and hematoxylin. Sections were mounted using Permount mounting medium (Fisher Scientific).

Immunohistochemistry

COX-1, COX-2, 5-LO, and LTA4H were detected in the paraffin sections by immunohistochemistry using antibodies from Cayman Chemicals (Ann Arbor, MI; rabbit polyclonal anti-COX-1 catalog no. 160109 and rabbit polyclonal anti-COX-2 catalog no. 160126), Cell Signaling Technologies (Danvers, MA; anti-5-LO rabbit monoclonal antibody clone C49G1 catalog no. 3289), and Epitomics, Inc. (Burlingame, CA, anti-LTA4H rabbit monoclonal antibody clone EPR5713, catalog no. 3911-1). For COX-2, antigen retrieval was performed at 70°C for 3 hours in 10 mM sodium citrate buffer, pH 9.5. For COX-1, 5-LO, and LTA4H, antigen retrieval was done at 60°C overnight in 0.2 M boric acid buffer, pH 7.0. After antigen retrieval, the paraffin sections were immersed in SuperBlock buffer (ThermoScientific, Waltham, MA) for 5 minutes to reduce non-specific binding of antibody. Sections were then incubated with primary antibodies overnight at 4°C using an Antibody Amplifier tray (Pro-Histo, LLC, Columbia, SC). Primary antibodies were used at the following dilutions: 1:700 for anti-COX-1 and for anti-COX-2, 1:15,000 for anti-LTA4H, and 1:100 for anti-5-LO and for the rabbit IgG negative control (rabbit DA1E monoclonal IgG, Cell Signaling Technologies). All antibodies were diluted in Amplifying Antibody Dilution Buffer (Pro-Histo, LLC). After incubation with the primary antibody, sections were treated with 3% H_2O_2 for 15 minutes to quench endogenous peroxidase activity. Primary antibodies were detected using the Polink-2 Plus HRP with DAB kit (IHC World, LLC, Woodstock, MD), counterstained with methyl green (Sigma-Aldrich), and mounted on glass slides using Permount. Antibody specificity was verified using bone marrow cell extracts prepared from COX-1, COX-2, 5-LO, and LTA4H knockout mice (Figure S1).

Image Collection and Analysis

Histological specimens were examined using a Nikon Eclipse E800 microscope with a Nikon DS-Fi1 digital camera and Nikon NIS-Elements BR 3.0 imaging software (Nikon Instruments Inc., Melville, NY).

When periosteal leukocytes, periosteal fibroblasts, intramedullary fracture site cells, intramedullary canal cells, external callus leukocytes, or muscle interstitial cells were the target cell populations for counting, five different fields of view were captured as digital images for each specimen using a 20X objective lens. Within each digital image, a 75×75 um (5,625 um^2) area was selected that contained the appropriate target cell type. The number of target cells and the number of target cells that were positive for enzyme expression as detected by secondary antibody reactivity were manually counted. Counts from the five images collected for each specimen were averaged. For every time point, one specimen (section) from each of the eight mice was examined by immunohistochemistry for each target enzyme. Thus, 4 specimens from each mouse callus were used to detect COX-1, COX-2, 5-LO, and LTA4H, respectively. However, specimens from only 2–8 mice were counted as described above depending upon the presence of the target cell population and quality of the histological specimen. In total, 352 time point, cell type, and target enzyme combinations were examined. Of those combinations, only 2 combinations (Day 4, COX-2, Callus Leukocytes and Day 7, COX-2, Callus Leukocytes) used 2 specimens for cell counting, 5 combinations used 3 specimens, 4 combinations used 4 specimens, 5 combinations used 5 specimens, and the remaining combinations used 6 or more specimens (Tables S3–S13 in File S1). The mean number of enzyme positive cells and total cells were calculated from the counted specimens for each target enzyme and cell type.

When chondrocytes, external callus osteoclasts, or internal callus osteoclasts were the target cell populations for counting, cells were counted as described above except cells were counted within a 200×200 um (40,000 um^2) area.

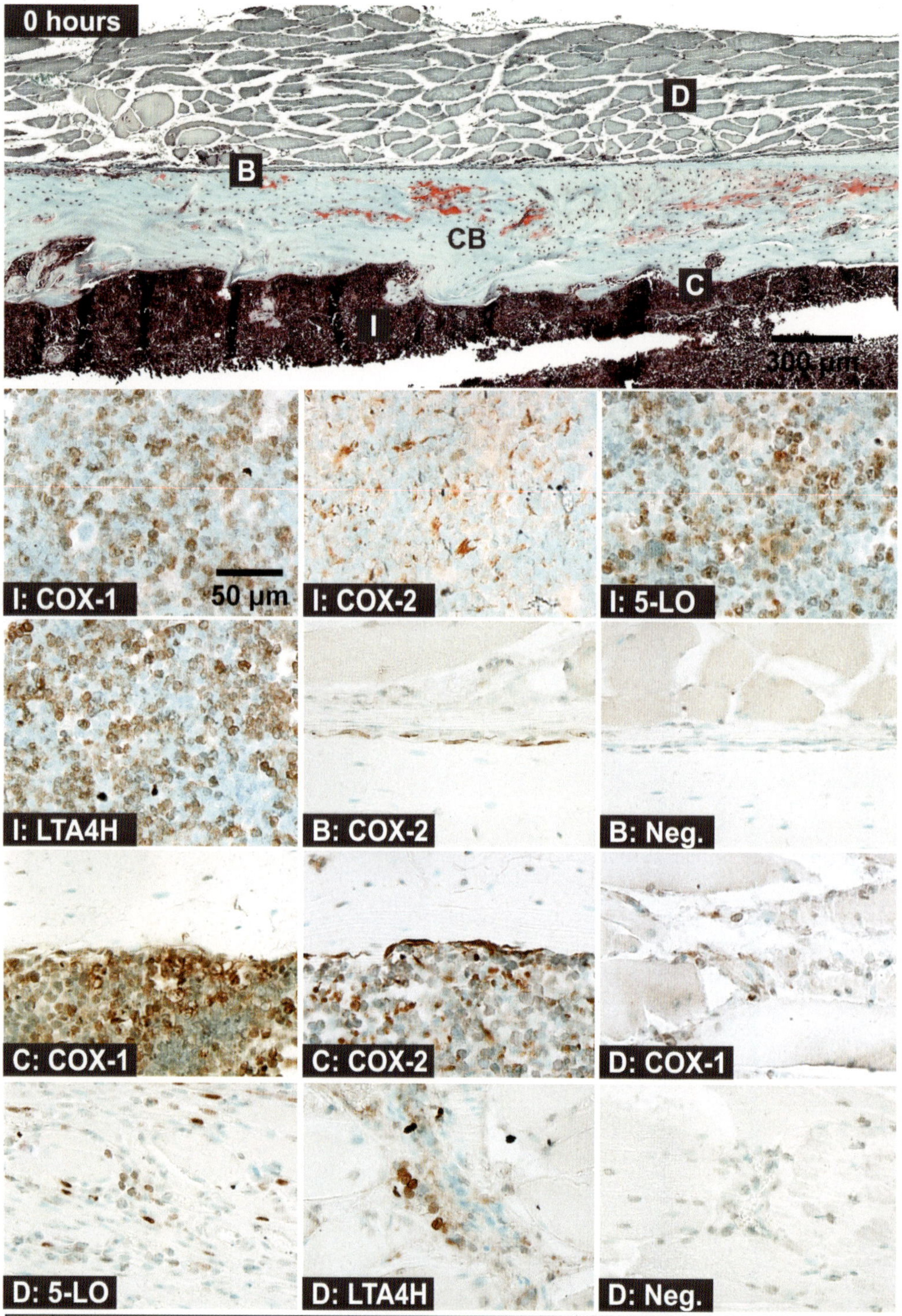

A	Intramedullary fracture site	E	Leukocytes in periosteum	I	Marrow cells
B	Periosteum	F	Chondrocytes	J	Leukocytes in callus
C	Endosteum	G	Internal callus osteoclasts	K	External callus osteoblasts
D	Muscle interstitial cells	H	External callus osteoclasts	L	Fibroblasts

Figure 1. Immunolocalization of Enzyme Positive Cells before Fracture. Top image shows a mouse femur stained with safranin-O (orange) and counter stained with fast green (green) and hematoxylin (black; CB: cortical bone; scale bar: 300 um). Bottom images show immunohistochemical staining of different cell types with antibodies to COX-1, COX-2, 5-LO, or LTA4H (brown; scale bar: 50 um). Rabbit IgG was used as a negative control (Neg.). Immunohistochemistry specimens were counter stained with methyl green. The higher magnification images are labeled with the primary antibody target (COX-1, COX-2, 5-LO, LTA4H, or Neg.) and with a letter indicating cell type and location as listed in the bottom of the figure.

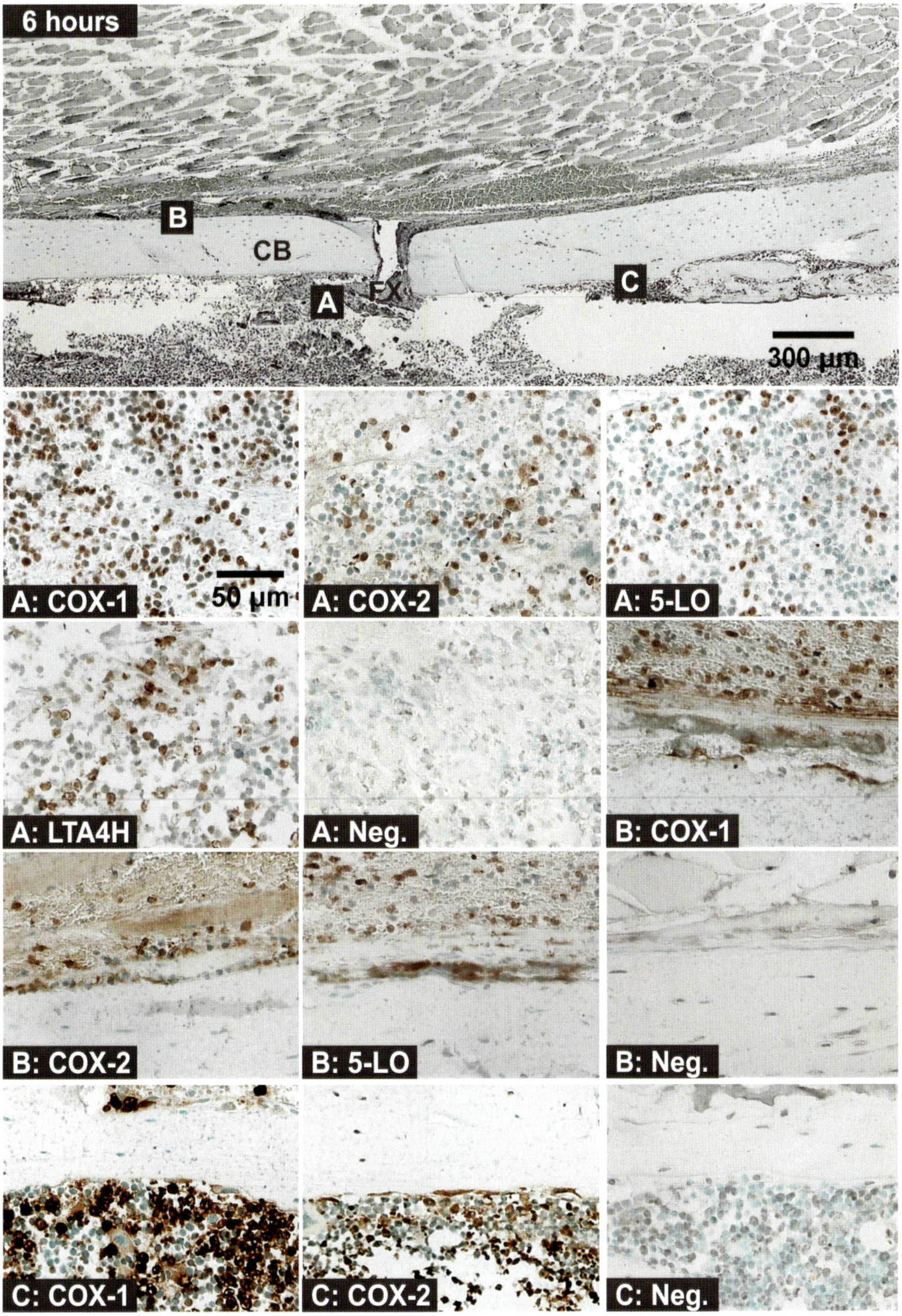

Figure 2. Immunolocalization of Enzyme Positive Cells at 6 hours after Fracture. The top image shows a fractured mouse femur stained with safranin-O (orange) and counter stained with fast green (green) and hematoxylin (black; CB: cortical bone; FX: fracture site; scale bar: 300 um). Bottom images show immunohistochemical staining of different cell types with rabbit IgG (Neg.) or with antibodies to COX-1, COX-2, 5-LO, or LTA4H (brown; scale bar: 50 um). Immunohistochemistry specimens were counter stained with methyl green. The higher magnification images are labeled with the primary antibody target (COX-1, COX-2, 5-LO, LTA4H, or Neg.) and with a letter indicating cell type and location as listed in Figure 1.

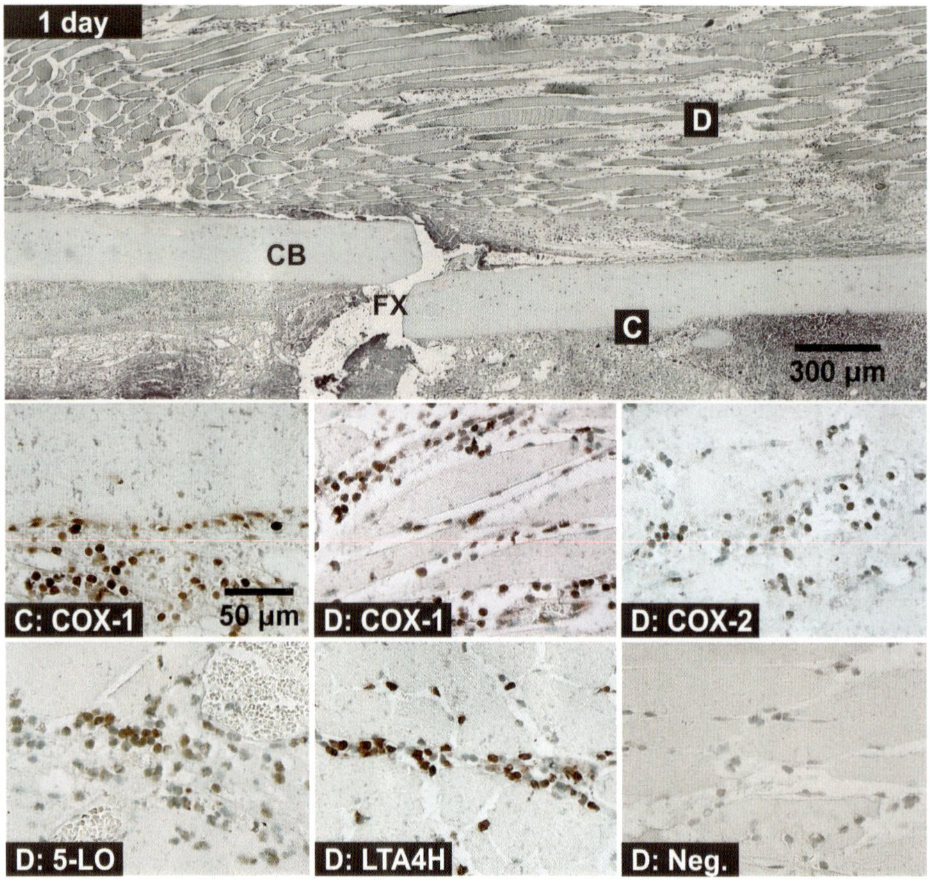

Figure 3. Immunolocalization of Enzyme Positive Cells at 1 day after Fracture. The top image shows a fractured mouse femur stained with safranin-O (orange) and counter stained with fast green (green) and hematoxylin (black; CB: cortical bone; FX: fracture site; scale bar: 300 um). Bottom images show immunohistochemical staining of different cell types with rabbit IgG (Neg.) or with antibodies to COX-1, COX-2, 5-LO, or LTA4H (brown; scale bar: 50 um). Immunohistochemistry specimens were counter stained with methyl green. The higher magnification images are labeled with the primary antibody target (COX-1, COX-2, 5-LO, LTA4H, or Neg.) and with a letter indicating cell type and location as listed in Figure 1.

When periosteal and endosteal bone lining cells were the target cell population for counting, cells were counted using a set of continuous images captured using the 10X objective lens that covered the entire periosteum or endosteum. Enzyme positive cells, TRAP positive cells, and total cells were identified and counted. The length of the periosteum and endosteum was measured using Image Pro Premier version 9.0 software (Media Cybernetics, Inc., Rockville, MD). Percent positive cells and cells per mm of bone lining were calculated. Data from 2–8 specimens at each time point were averaged. The cell counting methodology is summarized in Table S1 in File S1.

Image collection and cell counting was performed by a single investigator at all times points for all target enzymes. Two additional investigators counted cells for all target enzymes and cell types in the day 7 post-fracture specimens to assess observer-related cell counting variation. No significant differences in cell counts between observers were found and intraclass correlation coefficients were 0.95, 0.87, 0.99, and 0.96 for counting COX-1, COX-2, 5-LO, and LTA4H positive cells, respectively (Figure S2 and Table S2 in File S1). Data were statistically analyzed using SigmaPlot version 12.5 software (Systat Software, Inc. Chicago, IL) or MedCalc version 12.7 software (MedCalc Software bvba, Ostend, Belgium). The statistical analyses are summarized in Tables S3–S23 in File S1.

Results

1. Intact Bone

Specimens were collected 7 days after intramedullary rod placement and before any fracture production to assess cellular expression of COX-1, COX-2, 5-LO, and LTA4H in the femur (Figure 1). Cells positive for COX-1, 5-LO, and LTA4H were abundant in the marrow and appeared to be neutrophils based upon morphology (Figure 1I). Cells expressing COX-2 were abundant in the marrow but had a morphology distinct from the COX-1, 5-LO, and LTA4H expressing cells and appeared to be macrophage-like cells (Figure 1I). COX-2 positive cells were present in the periosteum (Figure 1B) and on the endosteal surface (Figure 1C) and appeared flattened, elongated, and associated with sites of bone resorption, suggesting that these COX-2 positive cells are osteoclasts. Some of the endosteal cells also appeared to express COX-1 (Figure 1C). Within the muscle, interstitial leukocytes appeared to be positive for COX-1, 5-LO, and LTA4H (Figure 1D). Endothelial cells did not appear to consistently express 5-LO, though 5-LO positive cells were adjacent to capillaries (Figure 1D). Osteocytes appeared to inconsistently express COX-1 and COX-2 (Figure 1B and 1C).

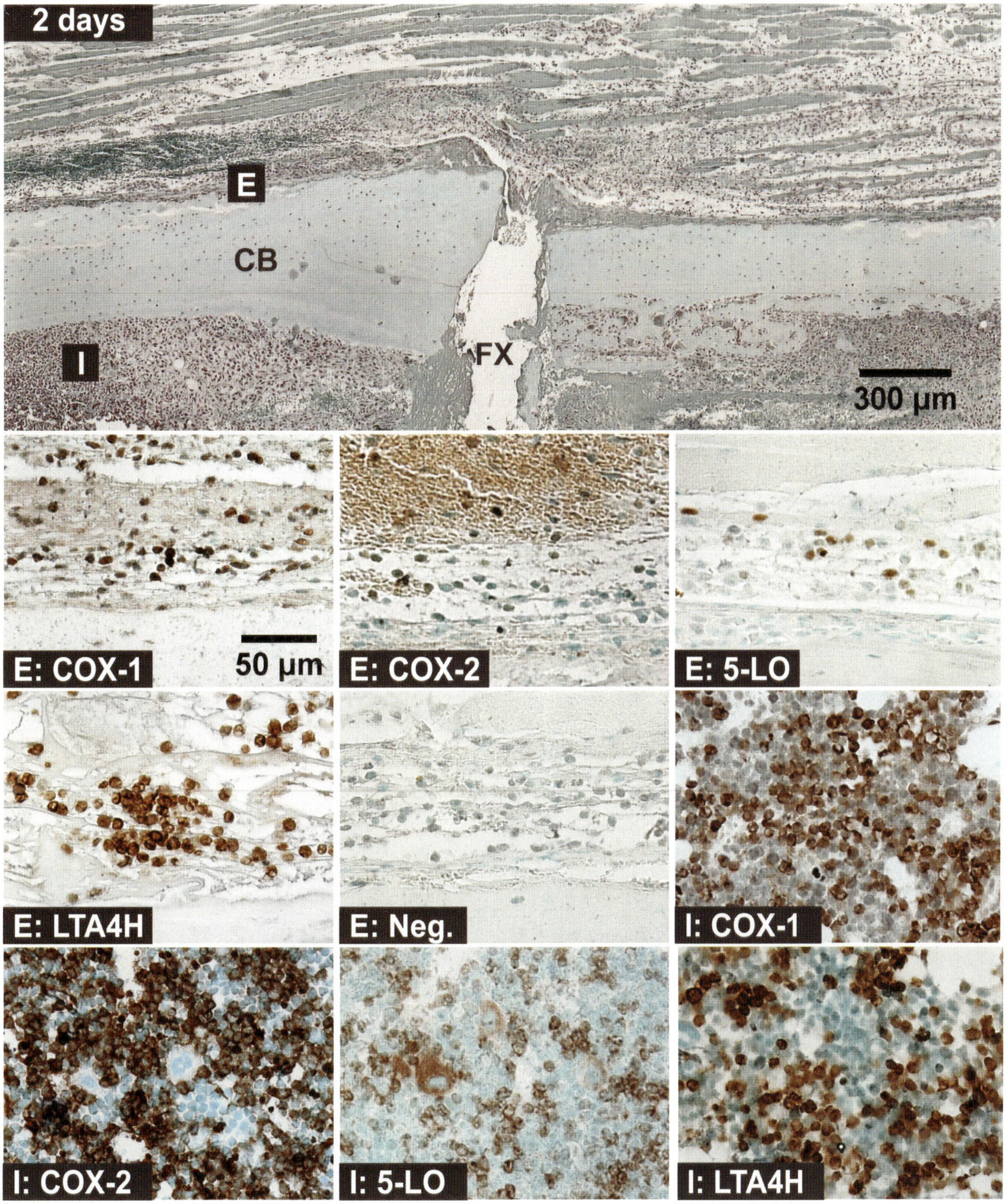

Figure 4. Immunolocalization of Enzyme Positive Cells at 2 days after Fracture. The top image shows a fractured mouse femur stained with safranin-O (orange) and counter stained with fast green (green) and hematoxylin (black; CB: cortical bone; FX: fracture site; scale bar: 300 um). Bottom images show immunohistochemical staining of different cell types with rabbit IgG (Neg.) or with antibodies to COX-1, COX-2, 5-LO, or LTA4H (brown; scale bar: 50 um). Immunohistochemistry specimens were counter stained with methyl green. The higher magnification images are labeled with the primary antibody target (COX-1, COX-2, 5-LO, LTA4H, or Neg.) and with a letter indicating cell type and location as listed in Figure 1.

2. Stages of Fracture Healing

In this mouse femur fracture model, healing occurs through 4 temporally and spatially overlapping phases which are the immediate response (6 hours and 1 day after fracture), inflammation (days 1 through 7), regeneration (days 4–21), and remodeling (day 14 onward) [12,14]. In this model, fractures bridge with new

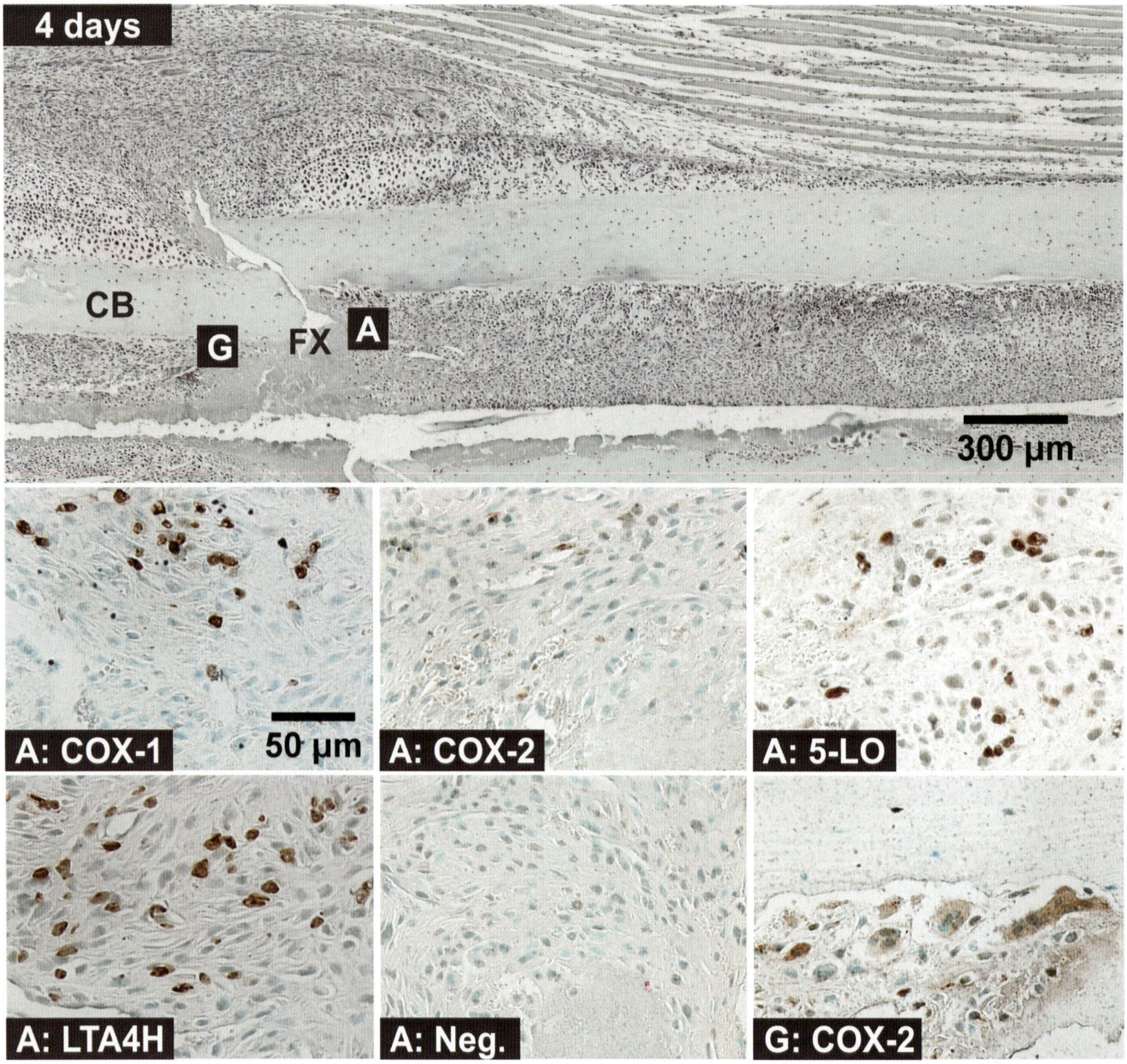

Figure 5. Immunolocalization of Enzyme Positive Cells at 4 days after Fracture. The top image shows a fractured mouse femur stained with safranin-O (orange) and counter stained with fast green (green) and hematoxylin (black; CB: cortical bone; FX: fracture site; scale bar: 300 um). Bottom images show immunohistochemical staining of different cell types with rabbit IgG (Neg.) or with antibodies to COX-1, COX-2, 5-LO, or LTA4H (brown; scale bar: 50 um). Immunohistochemistry specimens were counter stained with methyl green. The higher magnification images are labeled with the primary antibody target (COX-1, COX-2, 5-LO, LTA4H, or Neg.) and with a letter indicating cell type and location as listed in Figure 1.

bone at approximately 21 days after fracture. This study focused on the immediate, inflammatory, and regenerative stages of healing and so healing was not assessed after day 14.

Hematoma, leukocytic invasion, tissue swelling, and thickening of the periosteum and endosteum at the fracture site were evident at 6 hours and 1 day after fracture and are consistent with the immediate response to fracture and inflammation initiation (Figures 2 and 3). Mesenchymal cell migration to the intramedullary (internal) and external callus as well as muscle fiber degeneration and more extensive leukocytic infiltration of the soft tissues were evident 2 days after fracture (Figure 4). By 4 days after fracture, a distinct, external callus morphology was evident which included newly formed periosteal bone at the periphery of the fracture callus, mesenchymal cells at the center of the callus, and chondrocytes between the newly formed bone and centrally located mesenchymal cells (Figure 5). Apparent endochondral ossification was evident at days 7, 10, and 14 after fracture and was associated with increased callus size that appeared to peak at day 10, cartilage formation based upon safranin-O staining, and bone formation from the peripheral edges of the callus towards the centrally located fracture site (Figures 6–8). Also evident was reduced swelling, intact muscle fibers, and reduced leukocytic infiltration as healing progressed.

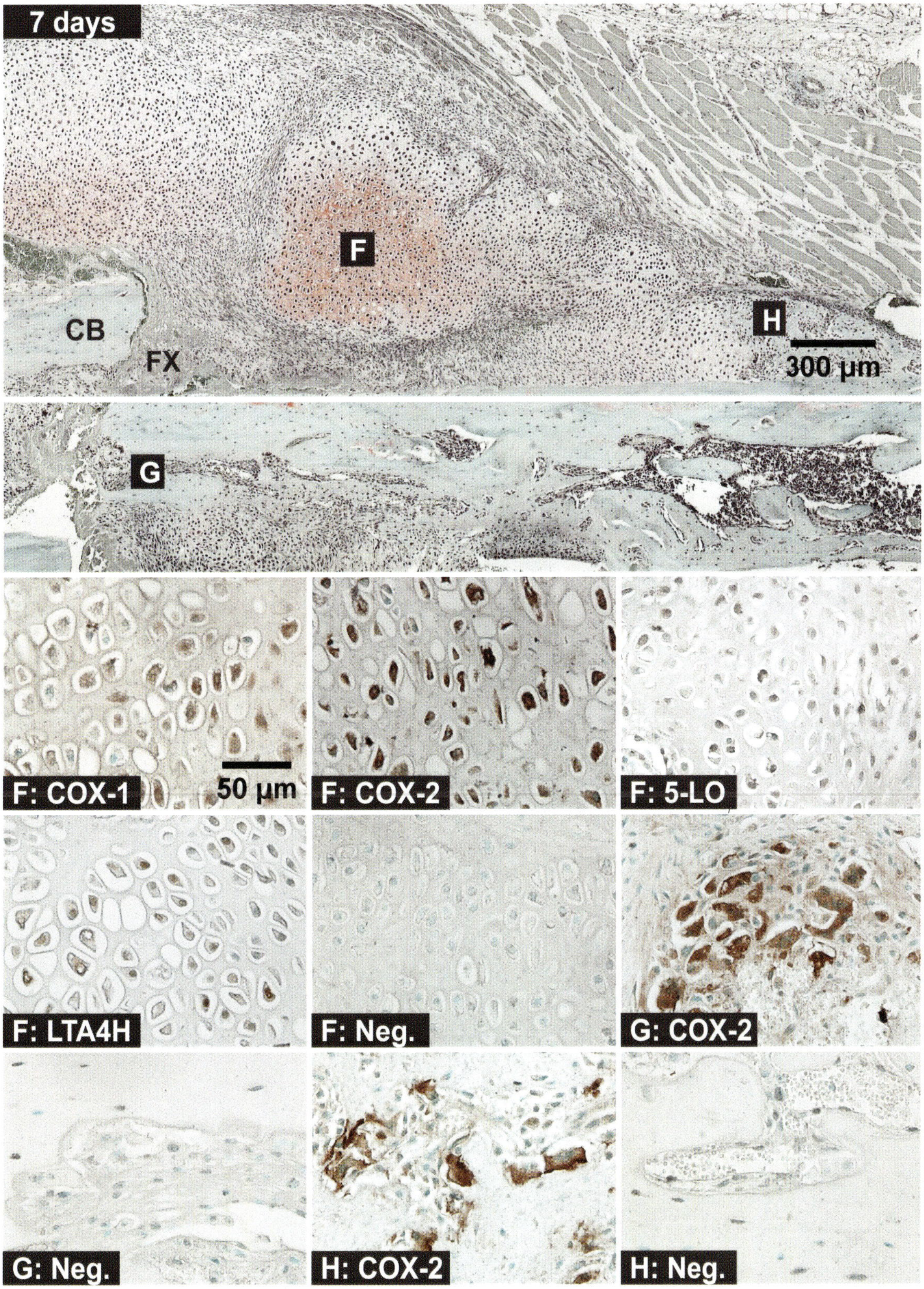

Figure 6. Immunolocalization of Enzyme Positive Cells at 7 days after Fracture. The top image shows the external callus and the image immediately below shows the internal callus of a fractured mouse femur stained with safranin-O (orange) and counter stained with fast green (green) and hematoxylin (black; CB: cortical bone; FX: fracture site; scale bar: 300 um). Bottom images show immunohistochemical staining of different cell types with rabbit IgG (Neg.) or with antibodies to COX-1, COX-2, 5-LO, or LTA4H (brown; scale bar: 50 um). Immunohistochemistry specimens were counter stained with methyl green. The higher magnification images are labeled with the primary antibody target (COX-1, COX-2, 5-LO, LTA4H, or Neg.) and with a letter indicating cell type and location as listed in Figure 1.

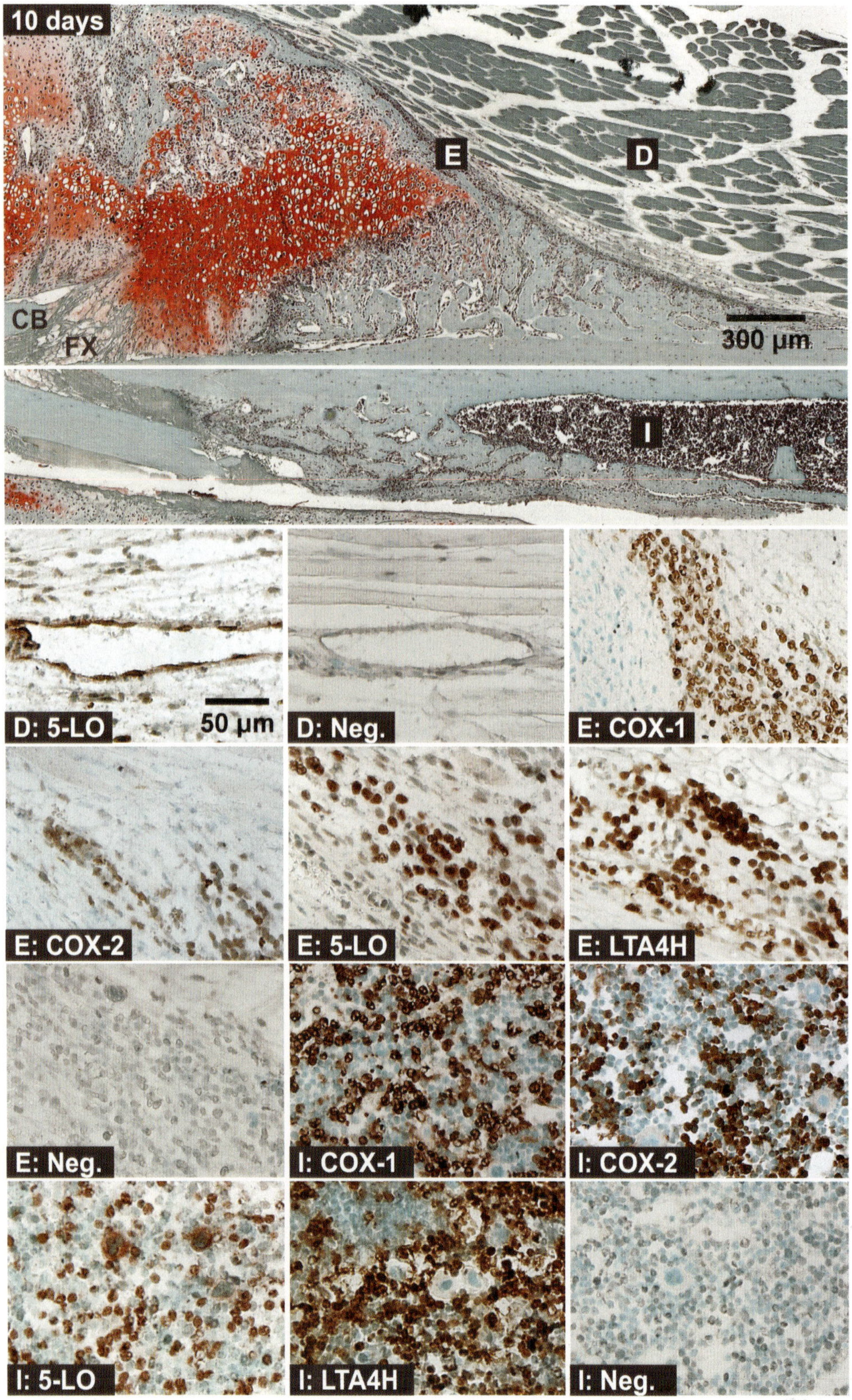

Figure 7. Immunolocalization of Enzyme Positive Cells at 10 days after Fracture. The top image shows the external callus and the image immediately below shows the internal callus of a fractured mouse femur stained with safranin-O (orange) and counter stained with fast green (green) and hematoxylin (black; CB: cortical bone; FX: fracture site; scale bar: 300 um). Bottom images show immunohistochemical staining of different cell types with rabbit IgG (Neg.) or with antibodies to COX-1, COX-2, 5-LO, or LTA4H (brown; scale bar: 50 um). Immunohistochemistry specimens were counter stained with methyl green. The higher magnification images are labeled with the primary antibody target (COX-1, COX-2, 5-LO, LTA4H, or Neg.) and with a letter indicating cell type and location as listed in Figure 1.

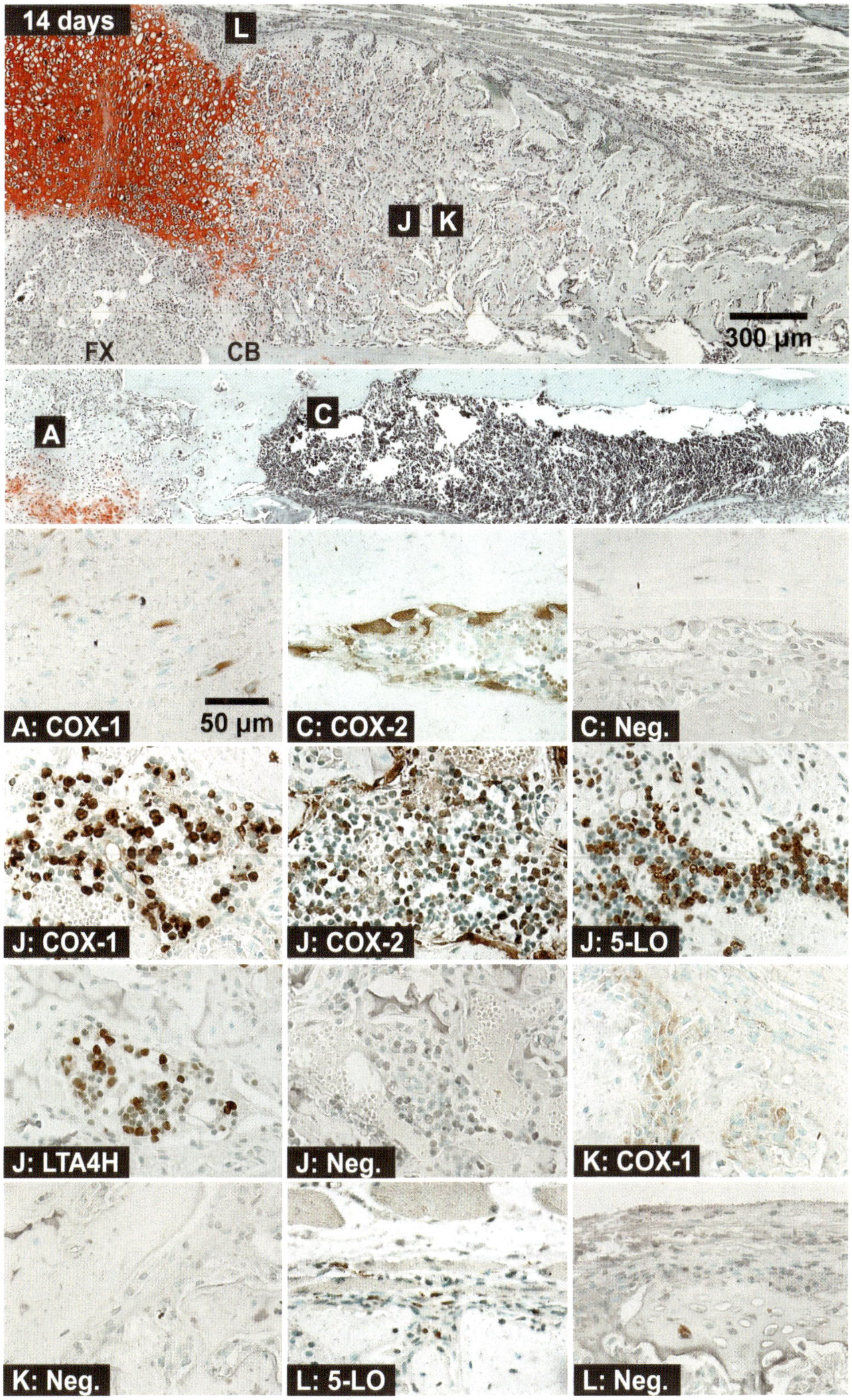

Figure 8. Immunolocalization of Enzyme Positive Cells at 14 days after Fracture. The top image shows the external callus and the image immediately below shows the internal callus of a fractured mouse femur stained with safranin-O (orange) and counter stained with fast green (green) and hematoxylin (black; CB: cortical bone; FX: fracture site; scale bar: 300 um). Bottom images show immunohistochemical staining of different cell types with rabbit IgG (Neg.) or with antibodies to COX-1, COX-2, 5-LO, or LTA4H (brown; scale bar: 50 um). Immunohistochemistry specimens were counter stained with methyl green. The higher magnification images are labeled with the primary antibody target (COX-1, COX-2, 5-LO, LTA4H, or Neg.) and with a letter indicating cell type and location as listed in Figure 1.

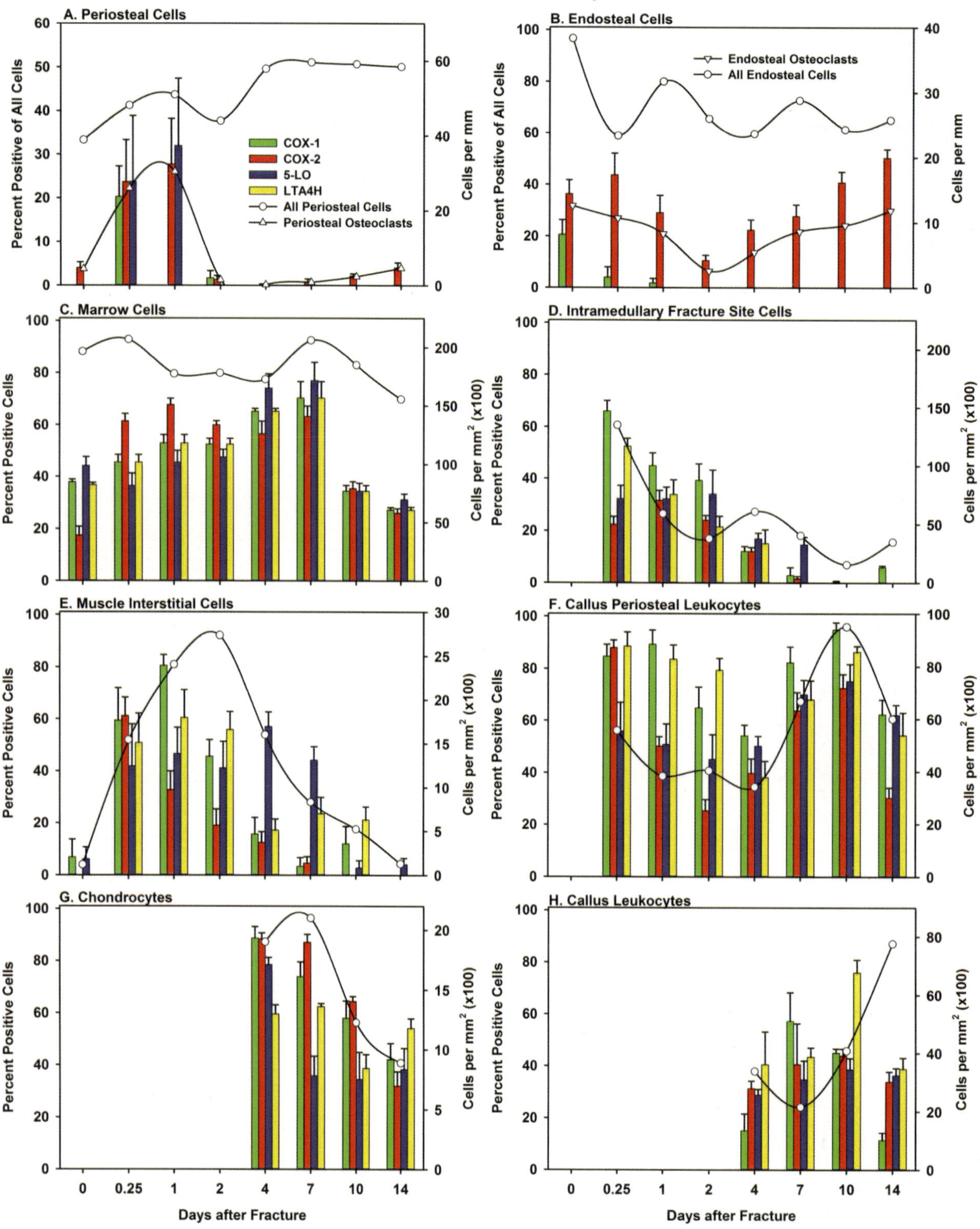

Figure 9. Quantitation of Enzyme Positive Cells during Fracture Healing. The total number of each cell type was counted from before till 14 days after fracture as described in the Materials and Methods and are shown as cells per mm or cells per mm^2 (circles; right axis). The number of periosteal (triangles, right axis) and endosteal (inverted triangles, right axis) osteoclasts were also counted (Panels A and B, respectively). The percentage of cells positive for COX-1 (green), COX-2 (red), 5-LO (blue), or LTA4H (yellow) was calculated and mean values (+S.E.M) are shown (left axis). Cell types are indicated for each panel. For Panel D: Intramedullary Fracture Site Cells and Panel F: Callus Periosteal Leukocytes, no data were available before fracture. For Panel G: Chondrocytes and Panel H: Callus Leukocytes, no chondrocytes or external callus marrow containing leukocytes were present prior to day 4 after fracture and so no values were entered for earlier time points. Note that the X-axis scales (Days after Fracture) are not linear with respect to time.

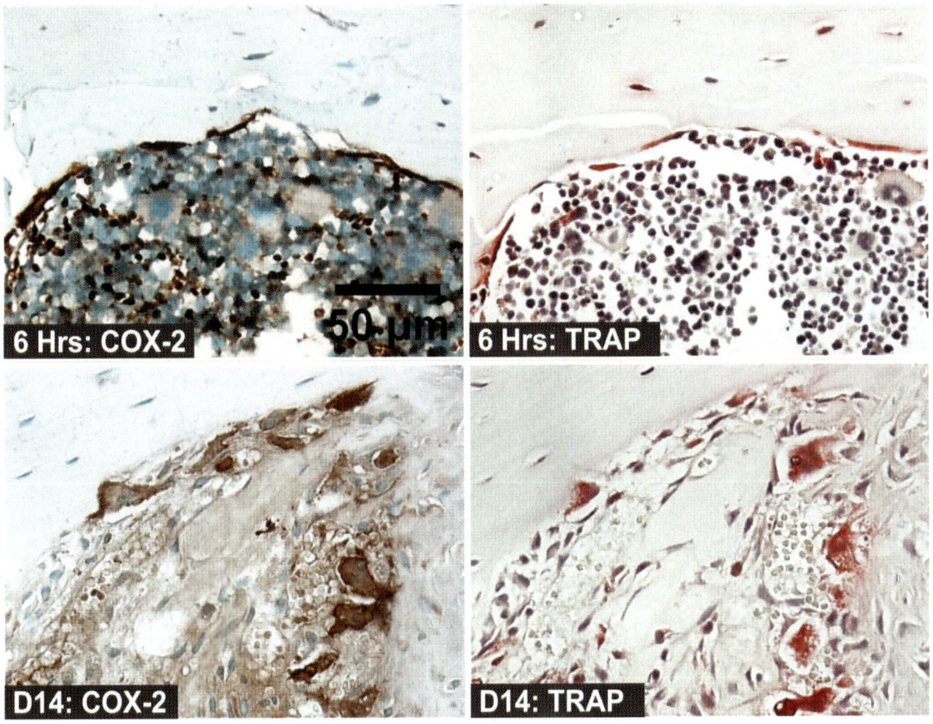

Figure 10. Co-localization of TRAP and COX-2 Positive Cells. Serial sections from mouse femurs at 6 hours (top images) and 14 days (bottom images) after fracture were used for immunohistochemical detection of COX-2 expressing cells (left images; brown staining) and for tartrate-resistant acid phosphatase staining (right images; red staining; scale bar: 50 um).

3. Cell-Type Specific Expression

The expression of COX-1, COX-2, 5-LO, and LTA4H in the major cell types present during fracture healing are described below.

3a: Leukocytes. Inflammation is mediated by leukocytes and bone marrow is rich with leukocytes. In this study, we did not attempt to distinguish different populations of leukocytes using immunohistochemical methods. Cells were considered leukocytes based upon their morphology and locations within the tissues.

Following fracture, leukocytes were evident in the marrow of the intramedullary canal and external fracture callus, the periosteum, and surrounding muscle at the fracture site. The number of leukocytes in the surrounding muscle increased and decreased in a pattern consistent with inflammation amplification and resolution (Figure 9E). The leukocytes were positive for COX-1, COX-2, 5-LO, or LTA4H at all sites and times after fracture. Further, leukocytes present in the bone marrow at a significant distance from the fracture site were positive for COX-1, COX-2, 5-LO, or LTA4H suggesting that these enzymes are normally expressed in these cells (Figures 1I, 4I and 7I).

After fracture, the periosteum typically thickens into multiple cell layers near the fracture site as osteoprogenitor cells within the periosteum proliferate [15,16]. The periosteum also appeared to be invaded by leukocytes that were positive for COX-1, COX-2, 5-LO, or LTA4H expression (Figure 4E). As healing progressed, the periosteum appeared as a layer of cells between the external surface of the callus and the surrounding muscle. Leukocytes positive for COX-1, COX-2, 5-LO, or LTA4H expression were present within the callus periosteum 14 days after fracture, even though inflammation had subsided and significant amounts of cartilage and bone had already formed (Figures 7E, 8, and 9F).

3b: Osteoblasts. For these experiments, osteoblasts were identified by morphology and localization next to bone. At one day after fracture, some endosteal cells with the appearance of osteoblasts were positive for COX-1 in one of six specimens (Figure 3C). Additional COX-1 expression was not observed in osteoblasts until day 14 after fracture. In all the 14 day fracture callus specimens, COX-1 expression was observed in some of the external callus osteoblasts (Figure 8K). COX-2 expression was observed in endosteal, periosteal, and external fracture callus osteoblasts at different time points (Figure 2B). However, the staining was faint compared to other COX-2 positive cell types and was not consistently observed between specimens. Expression of 5-LO and LTA4H was not observed in osteoblasts.

3c: Chondrocytes. For these experiments, chondrocytes were identified based upon morphology, position within the fracture callus, and staining with safranin-O. Chondrocytes were evident by day 4 after fracture (Figure 5). Chondrocytes positive for COX-1, COX-2, 5-LO, or LTA4H were observed at 4, 7, 10, and 14 days after fracture (Figure 6F). The percentage of COX-1, COX-2, 5-LO, or LTA4H positive chondrocytes decreased as healing progressed (Figure 9G). However, there was a sharp decline in the proportion of 5-LO positive chondrocytes between days 4 (79%) and 7 (40%; Figure 9G).

3d: Osteoclasts. Osteoclasts were identified based upon morphology and localization on mineralized tissue surface. In early time points after fracture (6 hours to 2 days), cells on the bone surface with morphology similar to osteoclasts or osteal macrophages were positive for COX-1, COX-2, or 5-LO, but not for LTA4H (Figures 2B and 2C) [17]. At all subsequent time points, osteoclasts were negative for COX-1, 5-LO, and LTA4H. Osteoclasts positive for COX-2 expression were observed at all time points and locations within the fracture callus and growth

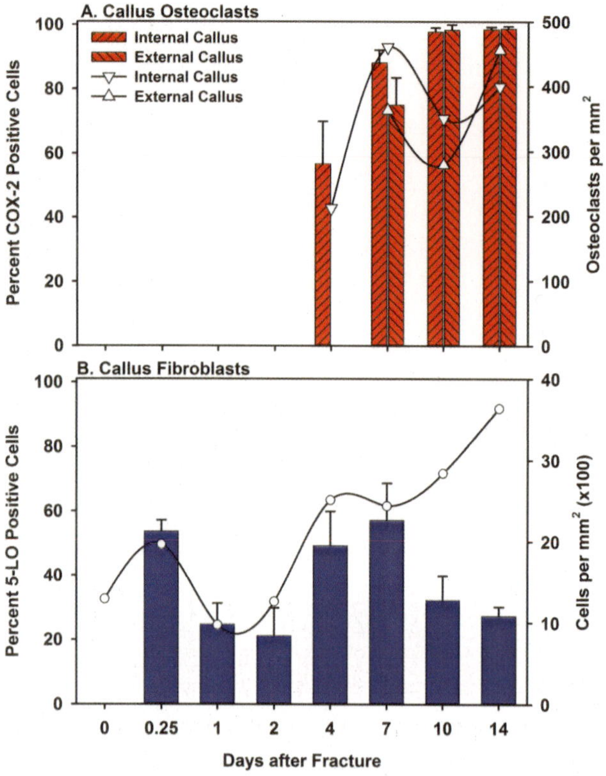

Figure 11. Quantitative Analysis of Fracture Site COX-2 Positive Osteoclasts and 5-LO Positive Fibroblasts. The number of external callus osteoclast (triangles), internal callus osteoclast (inverted triangles), and callus fibroblasts (circles) were counted (right axis). The percentage of osteoclast that also were positive for COX-2 by immunohistochemical detection were calculated for the external (right bars)and internal callus (left bars) at each time point and are shown as mean values (+ S.E.M.; Panel A; left axis). The percentage of fibroblasts positive for 5-LO by immunohistochemistry were calculated at each time point and are shown as mean values (+S.E.M.; Panel B; left axis). Note that the X-axis scales (Days after Fracture) are not linear with respect to time.

plate (data not shown). COX-2 positive osteoclasts were readily observed in the intramedullary canal at the fracture site by 4 days after fracture and in the external callus by 7 days after fracture (Figures 5G, 6G, 6H, and 8C).

To confirm that these COX-2 positive cells were indeed osteoclasts, serial sections were examined for COX-2 expression by immunohistochemistry and for tartrate-resistance acid phosphatase (TRAP) activity by histochemical staining. As shown in Figure 10, COX-2 positive cells on the bone surface were also TRAP positive. In the internal and external callus, the percentage of osteoclasts that were COX-2 positive varied as healing proceeded (Figure 11A). In the internal callus, the percentage of TRAP positive cells that were also COX-2 positive increased from about 55% on day 4 to almost 100% on day 14. In the external callus, the number of COX-2 positive TRAP cells increased from 75% on day 7 to almost 100% on day 14.

3e: Endothelial cells. Angiogenesis is essential for fracture healing and capillaries were evident in the fracture callus and surrounding muscle. The endothelial cells of the capillaries were positive for 5-LO expression from day 7 onward (Figure 7D). Endothelial cells positive for COX-1 were also observed in one of six samples on day 4 (not shown).

3f: Fibroblasts. Some spindle-shaped cells in the periosteum were positive for 5-LO expression at all time points after fracture (Figure 8L). Approximately 50% of these callus fibroblasts were positive for 5-LO at 6 hours and 4 and 7 days after fracture with lesser amounts at days 1,2, 10, and 14 (Figure 11B).

4. The Chondro-Osseous Junction

A striking feature of fracture callus morphology and COX-2 expression is shown in Figure 12. The interface between the cartilage stained with safranin-O and the zone of calcified cartilage and bone formation was highly enriched with cells that co-express TRAP and COX-2 and appeared to be osteoclasts.

5. Quantitative Analysis of Enzyme Positive Cells

The percentage of enzyme positive cells within different regions of the callus was determined. The total number of cells with the same morphology was also counted in that tissue region to derive the proportion of enzyme positive cells. The data are summarized in Figures 9 and 11. These data were analyzed using ANOVA and post-hoc Holm-Sidak tests to identify differences in the percent of enzyme positive cells with time after fracture (Tables S3–S13 in File S1). The percentage of periosteal cells that expressed COX-1, COX-2, or 5-LO peaked by day 1 after fracture before rapidly declining (Figure 9A). In contrast, endosteal cells preferentially expressed COX-2 throughout healing (Figure 9B). The COX-2 positive bone lining cells appeared to be osteoclasts and the number of apparent osteoclasts (TRAP positive cells identified in serial sections) was highly correlated to the number of COX-2 positive cells on the periosteal ($R = 0.997$) and endosteal surfaces ($R = 0.916$) using a Gaussian peak fit curve. The total number of muscle interstitial cells peaked at day 2 after fracture and showed an early preference for expressing COX-1 and COX-2 and a later preference for expressing 5-LO (Figure 9E). Conversely, 5-LO expression in chondrocytes occurred early while COX-1 and COX-2 expression continued into later times (Figure 9G). Callus periosteal leukocytes peaked at day 10 after fracture, which coincides with peak callus volume (Figure 9F). Osteoclasts were observed at the intramedullary fracture site by day 4 after fracture and in the external callus by day 7 (Figure 11A). By day 10 after fracture, over 95% of callus osteoclasts were positive for COX-2 and negative for the other target enzymes.

Discussion

We performed an immunohistochemical analysis of time-staged mouse fracture callus specimens to identify cells that express COX-1, COX-2, 5-LO, and LTA4H with the goal of identifying potential mechanisms through which arachidonic acid metabolism regulates fracture healing. We used morphological observations to identify cell types rather than performing additional experiments to confirm each cell type except for using TRAP or safranin-O staining to aid in identifying osteoclasts and chondrocytes, respectively. This is a limitation of the study particularly with the leukocytes as we cannot precisely assign enzyme expression to specific leukocyte types, such as neutrophils, T-cells, or macrophages. Additional experiments will be needed to refine assignment of COX-1, COX-2, 5-LO, or LTA4H expression to cell type subpopulations. It also should be noted that expression of COX-1, COX-2, 5-LO, or LTA4H does not equate with enzyme activity. Rather the presence of these enzymes indicates that a cell has the potential capacity to produce prostaglandins or leukotrienes when appropriately stimulated.

As expected, COX-1, COX-2, 5-LO, and LTA4H were expressed in multiple cell types over the time course examined.

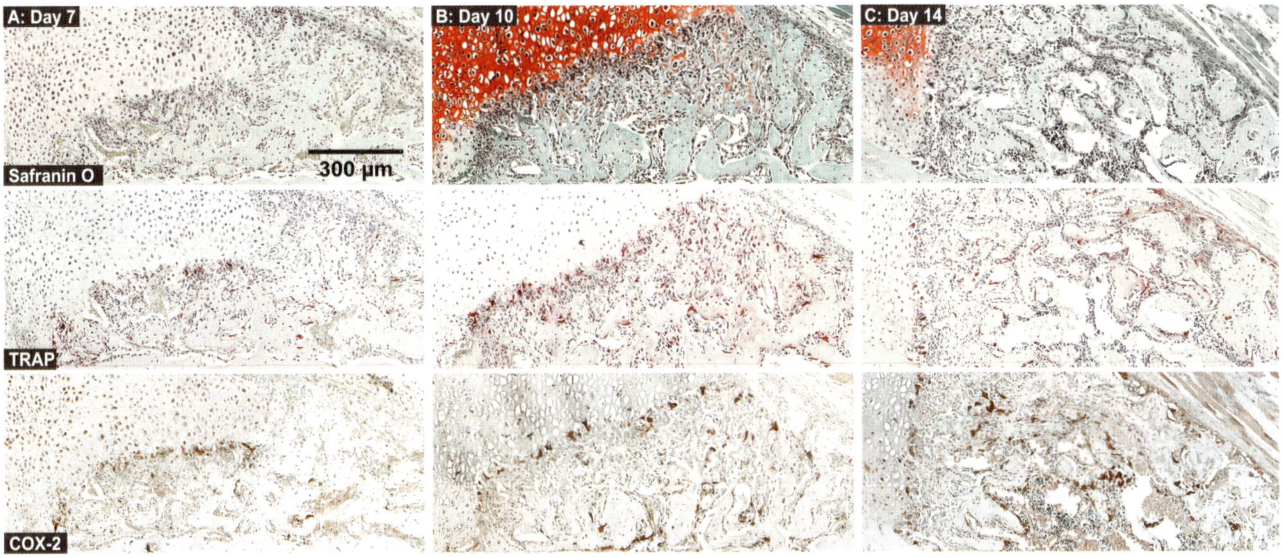

Figure 12. Osteoclasts at the Chondro-Osseous Junction during Fracture Healing. Serial sections from mouse femur fractures collected at 7 (A), 10 (B), and 14 days (C) after fracture were stained with safranin-O (top images), TRAP (middle images), or stained for COX-2 using immunohistochemistry (bottom images; scale bar: 300 um). The images show that COX-2 expressing osteoclasts appear to preferentially localize at the junction between callus cartilage and the zone of active new bone formation during fracture healing.

Enzyme positive leukocytes increased at the fracture site and surrounding muscle during the early stages of healing and then decreased. Osteoblasts in the periosteum and in the newly formed bone of the callus did not appear to express COX-2, 5-LO, or LTA4H to an extent that could be reliably detected using these immunohistochemical methods. COX-1 expression was detected in osteoblasts of newly formed callus bone. This was unexpected since COX-1 and COX-2 expression had been detected in rat tibia osteoblasts and induction of COX-2 expression in cultured osteoblasts has been repeatedly observed [18–24]. In contrast, callus chondrocytes expressed COX-1, COX-2, 5-LO, and LTA4H. Osteoclasts and osteal macrophages appeared to abundantly express COX-2 and transiently express COX-1 and 5-LO during the early stages of healing (6 hours, 1, and 2 days). Previous studies found that COX-2 mRNA levels were elevated immediately after fracture during the inflammation phase, declined, and then peaked again [2,25]. The basis for the second increase in COX-2 expression was never fully explained. However, the data presented here indicate that the second peak in COX-2 mRNA correlates with COX-2 expression in the callus chondrocytes and an abundance of COX-2 positive osteoclasts present in the callus during endochondral ossification.

The continued presence of enzyme positive leukocytes and 5-LO positive fibroblasts at the interface of the callus and surrounding muscle (callus periosteum), even at the later stages of healing suggests that these 5-LO positive cells could be secreting eicosanoids to regulate the healing process. In support of this concept, chondrocytes can utilize leukotriene A_4 synthesized from polymorphonuclear leukocytes to produce leukotriene B_4 and C_4 through a transcellular process [26]. The 5-LO positive cells also could be aiding in additional functions known to be mediated by 5-LO, including angiogenesis and the resolution of inflammation [28–31].

Osteoblasts are necessary for bone formation and consequently for fracture healing. Numerous studies have demonstrated that COX-2 expression can be induced in cultured osteoblasts [18,19,22,23,32–37]. Many other studies have shown that COX-2 activity in cultured osteoblasts or prostaglandin treatment of osteoblasts can promote proliferation or differentiation [38–44]. In vivo, treatment with prostaglandins or prostaglandin analogs can promote bone formation and enhance fracture healing [45–49]. In contrast, leukotrienes can inhibit osteoblast proliferation and impair bone formation [50,51]. In vivo, COX-1 and COX-2 expression was previously detected in endosteal osteoblasts and cortical bone osteocytes of the rat tibiae with little apparent expression of either enzyme in periosteal osteoblasts [24]. In this study, COX-2 was not consistently detected in bone-surface osteoblasts (Figure 2B). A previous study concluded that fracture healing is impaired in COX-2 null mice because loss of COX-2 function impairs osteoblast differentiation in vitro [11]. However, lack of COX-2 expression in osteoblasts in vivo, as shown here, and the ability of COX-2 null, as well COX-1, 5-LO, or LTA4H null mice to develop normally sized and growing skeletons indicates that expression of these enzymes in osteoblasts is not essential for osteoblast function [52–54]. Indeed, a femur segment from a wild-type mouse transplanted into a COX-2 null mouse fails to heal while a femur segment from a COX-2 null mouse transplanted into a wild-type mouse does heal indicating that COX-2 null osteoblasts can participate in healing within a COX-2 sufficient environment [55]. We suggest that eicosanoids synthesized by leukocytes, chondrocytes, and osteoclasts that are in close proximity to osteoblasts and mesenchymal cells during fracture healing may be regulating the proliferation and differentiation of osteoblasts through cell dependent signaling. Such a mechanism could be mediated by osteal macrophages (osteomacs) that organize as a cellular network or canopy over bone surface osteoblasts [17]. While it is possible that expression of COX-1, COX-2, 5-LO, or LTA4H was not consistently detected in osteoblasts for technical reasons, the positive expression of the target enzymes in other cell types of the same specimen indicates that this possibility is unlikely.

The significance of the COX-1, COX-2, 5-LO, and LTA4H expression in the callus chondrocytes is not yet known. Expression of these enzymes in growth plate and in normal or pathological articular chondrocytes has been detected previously [26,56–59]. In rat tibia growth plates, COX-1 was strongly expressed in the reserve zone, while only moderate COX-2 expression was detected in the reserve zone [57]. In cultured rat growth plate chondrocytes, cell proliferation was inhibited by treatment with SC-236, a COX-2 selective inhibitor, but not with SC-560, a COX-1 selective inhibitor [57]. Proliferation of the cultured rat growth plate chondrocytes could be stimulated with PGE_2 or with a selective EP1 agonists [57]. Consistent with a COX-2 proliferative effect on growth plate chondrocytes, treatment of chicken growth plate chondrocytes with PGE_2 inhibited Type X collagen, VEGF, and MMP-13 expression indicating that PGE_2 treatment was inhibiting chondrocyte differentiation [60]. Similarly, treatment of osteoarthritic chondrocytes with butaprost, a PGE_2 analog that specifically activates the EP2 receptor, also reduced MMP-13 expression [61]. Less is known of leukotriene effects on chondrocyte functions. Treatment of articular chondrocytes with IL-1ß reduced synthesis of LTB_4 while inducing synthesis of PGE_2 [62]. In contrast, treatment of human osteoarthritic articular chondrocytes with naproxen, a non-selective COX-1 and COX-2 inhibitor, caused a significant increase in chondrocyte LTB_4 synthesis [59]. Expression of COX-2 can be induced in articular chondrocytes by treatment with IL-1ß while expression of 5-LO and its essential co-factor five lipoxygenase activating protein (FLAP) can be induced with TGF-ß and 1, 25-dihydroxy vitamin D_3 [56,59]. In fracture calluses, inhibition of 5-LO appears to accelerate chondrocyte differentiation during endochondral ossification and increases COX-2 expression, while inhibition of COX-2 appears to prevent chondrocyte differentiation leading to impaired endochondral ossification [2]. These prior observation show that chondrocyte proliferation and differentiation are affected by prostaglandins. In addition, chondrocytes can interact with other cell types to produce leukotrienes through transcellular pathways [26]. However, additional experiments are needed to determine whether callus chondrocytes behave similarly to growth plate or articular chondrocytes with respect to eicosanoid treatment, whether callus chondrocyte expression of these enzymes signifies a response to the local growth factor milieu, or whether callus chondrocyte expression of these enzymes underlies a regulatory role for chondrocytes in the regenerative process.

Of the 4 enzymes, only COX-2 expression was detected consistently in osteoclasts at the fracture site. Osteoclasts within the growth plate of the fractured femurs or in control, unfractured femurs were also positive for COX-2 (data not shown) and immunohistochemical detection of COX-2 expression was severely reduced in mice in which COX-2 was deleted in osteoclasts (Figure S3). A previous report also demonstrated expression of COX-2 in osteoclasts by immunohistochemical detection in rat tibiae [24]. Not all the TRAP and COX-2 positive cells appeared to be multinucleated in our specimens and some of the COX-2 and TRAP positive cells may be macrophages, dendritic cells, monocytes differentiating into osteoclasts, or macrophages or dendritic cells transdifferentiating into osteoclasts [63–67]. The proportion of TRAP positive cells in the fracture callus that were also COX-2 positive increased to almost 100% over time (Figure 11A). This suggests that either a population of TRAP positive, COX-2 negative cells are present early in healing and then disappear or that COX-2 expression increases as TRAP positive cells mature into osteoclasts.

The importance of COX-2 in osteoclast biology is well established [68–71]. Stimuli that induce COX-2 expression and activity in osteoblasts or bone marrow cells in turn enable the osteoblasts or bone marrow cells to promote osteoclast differentiation [33]. Thus, COX-2 has been thought to regulate osteoclast biology only through the activity of other cell types. However, the clear demonstration that COX-2 is expressed in osteoclasts themselves suggests that COX-2 may have a cell-autonomous function in osteoclasts. One role may be directly related to osteoclast development since prostaglandins produced by osteoclasts may aid in osteoclast formation and function through an autocrine signaling mechanism. Spleen or bone marrow cells from COX-2 null mice have a reduced capacity to form osteoclasts which can be rescued by exogenous PGE_2 treatment [68]. Further, COX-2 expression can be induced by a variety of stimuli including RANKL in osteoclast precursors such as monocytes or macrophage-like cell lines that can be induced to differentiate into osteoclasts [70,72,73]. This suggests a direct role for COX-2 in osteoclastogenesis in which stimuli, such as, RANKL induces COX-2 expression in osteoclast precursors and the prostaglandins produced by that COX-2 act in an autocrine feedback mechanism to promote osteoclastogenesis.

Parallel observations between effects of impaired osteoclast activity and impaired COX-2 activity indicate that osteoclast COX-2 activity may be regulating fracture healing. The localization of COX-2 positive osteoclasts at the interface of callus cartilage and active endochondral ossification (chondro-osseous junction) suggests that the osteoclasts may be the critical regulatory cell controlling the regenerative phase of fracture healing (Figure 12). Classically, these osteoclasts have also been referred to as chondroclasts [74]. Osteoclast activity is necessary to resorb the calcified cartilage produced by the hypertrophic chondrocytes and to provide calcified tissue surfaces for new bone formation [75–77]. Osteoclasts may also promote chondrocyte hypertrophy and calcified cartilage formation necessary for endochondral ossification to proceed. In mice treated with zoledronate to inhibit osteoclast activity, expression of Type X collagen was delayed in tibia fracture calluses [78]. Similarly, in rats treated with celecoxib to inhibit COX-2 activity, fracture callus Type X collagen expression was significantly reduced [2]. Finally, macrophage-like cells present in the periosteum (osteomacs) which could potentially differentiate into osteoclasts have been shown to enhance osteoblast activity and bone formation [17]. Indeed, prostaglandins produced by COX-2 can promote osteoblast activity [78]. Together, the observations support a model in which COX-2 exerts its regulatory functions on fracture healing through the osteoclast.

Supporting Information

Figure S1 Antibody Specificity. The specificity of the antibodies used to detect COX-1, COX-2, 5-LO, and LTA4H was verified be using bone marrow derived cells and macrophages. Total protein extracts prepared from the bone marrow of COX-1, COX-2, 5-LO, and LTA4H knockout mice were analyzed for COX-1, 5-LO, and LTA4H expression by immunoblot analysis (Bone Marrow Cells). Expression of ß-tubulin was used as a control. The antibodies for COX-1, 5-LO, and LTA4H failed to detect any protein in their corresponding knockout bone marrow cell extracts but did detect proteins of the correct size (markers not shown) in the other bone marrow cell extracts. To detect COX-2 expression, bone marrow cells from wild-type and COX-2 knockout mice were cultured in DMEM with 10% FBS and 20% L929 conditioned media to promote macrophage development (Macrophages). The cultures were then induced to express COX-2 by treating with 100 ng/ml of LPS overnight followed by protein extract preparation and immunoblot analysis for COX-2 expression. The COX-2 antibody detected a protein of the correct size in the LPS-treated wild-type cells but failed to detect any protein in the COX-2 knockout cells. Antibodies were detected by chemiluminescence using appropriate horseradish peroxidase conjugated secondary antibodies and a Proteinsimple Fluorchem M imaging system.

Figure S2 Inter-Observer Variation for Each Antibody. Consistency between observers for the percentage of antibody positive cells counted in each sample was determined using intraclass correlation coefficient tests. The cumulative frequency distribution for each observer (or rater) and each antibody (A: COX-1, B: COX-2, C: 5-LO, and D: LTA4H) are shown with maximum 100% positive target cells.

Figure S3 Expression of COX-2 in Osteoclasts. Mice homozygous for a floxed allele of COX-2 (COX-2 f/f; generously provided by T. Ishikawa and H. Herschman, UCLA) and with or without a Lyz2-Cre transgene (Lyz2$^{tm1(cre)Ifo}$, Jackson Laboratory) were used to obtain femur samples for immunohistochemical detection of COX-2 and identification of osteoclasts by TRAP staining in serial sections. The Lyz2-Cre transgene expresses Cre recombinase in monocyte-derived cells and should therefore create a null allele of COX-2 in osteoclasts. Bone surface, TRAP-positive cells were detected in samples from mice of both genotypes. However, COX-2 expression was diminished in the apparent osteoclasts but not in the bone marrow leukocytes of the COX-2 f/f; Lyz2-Cre mice.

File S1 Tables S1–S23 summarize cell counting methods, immunohistochemistry cell counting results, inter-observer variation analysis of Day 7 specimens, and statistical analyses.

Acknowledgments

We thank Ashley Mitchell, Sangeeta Subramanian, and Marcus Meyenhofer for their technical assistance.

Author Contributions

Conceived and designed the experiments: JPOC. Performed the experiments: HNL. Analyzed the data: HNL JPOC. Wrote the paper: HNL JPOC.

References

1. Manigrasso MB, O'Connor JP (2010) Accelerated fracture healing in mice lacking the 5-lipoxygenase gene. Acta Orthop 81: 748–755.
2. Cottrell JA, O'Connor JP (2009) Pharmacological inhibition of 5-lipoxygenase accelerates and enhances fracture-healing. J Bone Joint Surg Am 91: 2653–2665.
3. Simon AM, O'Connor JP (2007) Dose and time-dependent effects of cyclooxygenase-2 inhibition on fracture-healing. J Bone Joint Surg Am 89: 500–511.
4. Simon AM, Manigrasso MB, O'Connor JP (2002) Cyclo-oxygenase 2 function is essential for bone fracture healing. Journal of Bone and Mineral Research 17: 963–976.
5. Cottrell J, O'Connor JP (2010) Effect of Non-Steroidal Anti-Inflammatory Drugs on Bone Healing. Pharmaceuticals 3: 1668–1693.
6. Smith WL, Urade Y, Jakobsson PJ (2011) Enzymes of the cyclooxygenase pathways of prostanoid biosynthesis. Chem Rev 111: 5821–5865.
7. Haeggstrom JZ, Funk CD (2011) Lipoxygenase and leukotriene pathways: biochemistry, biology, and roles in disease. Chem Rev 111: 5866–5898.
8. Brown HA, Marnett LJ (2011) Introduction to lipid biochemistry, metabolism, and signaling. Chem Rev 111: 5817–5820.
9. Shimizu T (2009) Lipid Mediators in Health and Disease: Enzymes and Receptors as Therapeutic Targets for the Regulation of Immunity and Inflammation. Annu Rev Pharmacol Toxicol 49: 123–150.
10. Funk CD (2001) Prostaglandins and leukotrienes: advances in eicosanoid biology. Science 294: 1871–1875.
11. Zhang X, Schwarz EM, Young DA, Puzas JE, Rosier RN, et al. (2002) Cyclooxygenase-2 regulates mesenchymal cell differentiation into the osteoblast lineage and is critically involved in bone repair. J Clin Invest 109: 1405–1415.
12. Manigrasso MB, O'Connor JP (2004) Characterization of a closed femur fracture model in mice. Journal of Orthopaedic Trauma 18: 687–695.
13. Tay BK, Le AX, Gould SE, Helms JA (1998) Histochemical and molecular analyses of distraction osteogenesis in a mouse model. J Orthop Res 16: 636–642.
14. Manigrasso MB, O'Connor JP (2008) Comparison of fracture healing among different inbred mouse strains. Calcif Tissue Int 82: 465–474.
15. Iwaki A, Jingushi S, Oda Y, Izumi T, Shida J-i, et al. (1997) Localization and quantification of proliferating cells during rat fracture repair: detection of proliferating cell nuclear antigen by immunohistochemsitry. Journal of Bone and Mineral Research 12: 96–102.
16. Beam HA, Parsons JR, Lin SS (2002) The effects of blood glucose control upon fracture healing in the BB Wistar rat with diabetes mellitus. J Orthop Res 20: 1210–1216.
17. Chang MK, Raggatt LJ, Alexander KA, Kuliwaba JS, Fazzalari NL, et al. (2008) Osteal tissue macrophages are intercalated throughout human and mouse bone lining tissues and regulate osteoblast function in vitro and in vivo. J Immunol 181: 1232–1244.
18. Onoe Y, Miyaura C, Kaminakayashiki T, Nagai Y, Noguchi K, et al. (1996) IL-13 and IL-4 inhibit bone resorption by suppressing cyclooxygenase-2-dependent prostaglandin synthesis in osteoblasts. J Immunol 156: 758–764.
19. Maciel FM, Sarrazin P, Morisset S, Lora M, Patry C, et al. (1997) Induction of cyclooxygenase-2 by parathyroid hormone in human osteoblasts in culture. J Rheumatol 24: 2429–2435.
20. Tai H, Miyaura C, Pilbeam CC, Tamura T, Ohsugi Y, et al. (1997) Transcriptional induction of cyclooxygenase-2 in osteoblasts is involved in interleukin-6-induced osteoclast formation. Endocrinology 138: 2372–2379.
21. Koide M, Murase Y, Yamato K, Noguchi T, Okahashi N, et al. (1999) Bone morphogenetic protein-2 enhances osteoclast formation mediated by interleukin-1alpha through upregulation of osteoclast differentiation factor and cyclooxygenase-2. Biochem Biophys Res Commun 259: 97–102.
22. Warden SJ, Favaloro JM, Bennell KL, McMeeken JM, Ng KW, et al. (2001) Low-intensity pulsed ultrasound stimulates a bone-forming response in UMR-106 cells. Biochem Biophys Res Commun 286: 443–450.
23. Chikazu D, Li X, Kawaguchi H, Sakuma Y, Voznesensky OS, et al. (2002) Bone morphogenetic protein 2 induces cyclo-oxygenase 2 in osteoblasts via a Cbfa1 binding site: role in effects of bone morphogenetic protein 2 in vitro and in vivo. Journal of Bone and Mineral Research 17: 1430–1440.
24. Forwood MR, Kelly WL, Worth NF (1998) Localisation of prostaglandin endoperoxide H synthase (PGHS)-1 and PGHS-2 in bone following mechanical loading in vivo. Anat Rec 252: 580–586.
25. Gerstenfeld LC, Thiede M, Seibert K, Mielke C, Phippard D, et al. (2003) Differential inhibition of fracture healing by non-selective and cyclooxygenase-2 selective non-steroidal anti-inflammatory drugs. Journal of Orthopaedic Research 21: 670–675.
26. Amat M, Diaz C, Vila L (1998) Leukotriene A4 hydrolase and leukotriene C4 synthase activities in human chondrocytes: transcellular biosynthesis of Leukotrienes during granulocyte-chondrocyte interaction. Arthritis Rheum 41: 1645–1651.
27. Serhan CN, Petasis NA (2011) Resolvins and protectins in inflammation resolution. Chem Rev 111: 5922–5943.
28. Hulth A, Johnell O, Lindberg L, Paulsson M, Heinegard D (1990) Demonstration of blood-vessellike structures in cartilaginous callus by antilaminin and antiheparin sulfate proteoglycan antibodies. Clin Orthop Relat Res: 289–293.
29. Gubitosi-Klug RA, Talahalli R, Du Y, Nadler JL, Kern TS (2008) 5-Lipoxygenase, but not 12/15-lipoxygenase, contributes to degeneration of retinal capillaries in a mouse model of diabetic retinopathy. Diabetes 57: 1387–1393.
30. Finkensieper A, Kieser S, Bekhite MM, Richter M, Mueller JP, et al. (2010) The 5-lipoxygenase pathway regulates vasculogenesis in differentiating mouse embryonic stem cells. Cardiovasc Res 86: 37–44.
31. Talahalli R, Zarini S, Sheibani N, Murphy RC, Gubitosi-Klug RA (2010) Increased synthesis of leukotrienes in the mouse model of diabetic retinopathy. Invest Ophthalmol Vis Sci 51: 1699–1708.
32. Xu J, Cissel DS, Varghese S, Whipkey DL, Blaha JD, et al. (1997) Cytokine regulation of adult human osteoblast-like cell prostaglandin biosynthesis. J Cell Biochem 64: 618–631.
33. Li L, Pettit AR, Gregory LS, Forwood MR (2006) Regulation of bone biology by prostaglandin endoperoxide H synthases (PGHS): a rose by any other name. Cytokine Growth Factor Rev 17: 203–216.
34. Pavalko FM, Chen NX, Turner CH, Burr DB, Atkinson S, et al. (1998) Fluid shear-induced mechanical signaling in MC3T3-E1 osteoblasts requires cytoskeleton-integrin interactions. Am J Physiol 275: C1591–1601.

35. Wadleigh DJ, Herschman HR (1999) Transcriptional regulation of the cyclooxygenase-2 gene by diverse ligands in murine osteoblasts. Biochemical and Biophysical Research Communications 264: 865–870.
36. Klein-Nulend J, Burger EH, Semeins CM, Raisz LG, Pilbeam CC (1997) Pulsating fluid flow stimulates prostaglandin release and inducible prostaglandin G/H synthase mRNA expression in primary mouse bone cells. J Bone Miner Res 12: 45–51.
37. Pilbeam C, Rao Y, Voznesensky O, Kawaguchi H, Alander C, et al. (1997) Transforming growth factor-beta1 regulation of prostaglandin G/H synthase-2 expression in osteoblastic MC3T3-E1 cells. Endocrinology 138: 4672–4682.
38. Feyen JH, Di Bon A, van der Plas A, Lowik CW, Nijweide PJ (1985) Effects of exogenous prostanoids on the proliferation of osteoblast- like cells in vitro. Prostaglandins 30: 827–840.
39. Centrella M, Casinghino S, McCarthy TL (1994) Differential actions of prostaglandins in separate cell populations from fetal rat bone. Endocrinology 135: 1611–1620.
40. Ho ML, Chang JK, Chuang LY, Hsu HK, Wang GJ (1999) Effects of nonsteroidal anti-inflammatory drugs and prostaglandins on osteoblastic functions. Biochem Pharmacol 58: 983–990.
41. Kajii T, Suzuki K, Yoshikawa M, Imai T, Matsumoto A, et al. (1999) Long-term effects of prostaglandin E_2 on the mineralization of a clonal osteoblastic cell line (MC3T3-E1). Archives of Oral Biology 44: 233–241.
42. Kaneki H, Takasugi I, Fujieda M, Kiriu M, Mizuochi S, et al. (1999) Prostaglandin E2 stimulates the formation of mineralized bone nodules by a cAMP-independent mechanism in the culture of adult rat calvarial osteoblasts. Journal of Cellular Biochemistry 73: 36–48.
43. Yoshida K, Oida H, Kobayashi T, Maruyama T, Tanaka M, et al. (2002) Stimulation of bone formation and prevention of bone loss by prostaglandin E EP4 receptor activation. Proc Natl Acad Sci U S A 99: 4580–4585.
44. Quarles LD, Haupt DM, Davidai G, Middleton JP (1993) Prostaglandin F2 alpha-induced mitogenesis in MC3T3-E1 osteoblasts: role of protein kinase-C-mediated tyrosine phosphorylation. Endocrinology 132: 1505–1513.
45. Miller SC, Marks SC Jr (1993) Local stimulation of new bone formation by prostaglandin E1: quantitative histomorphometry and comparison of delivery by minipumps and controlled-release pellets. Bone 14: 143–151.
46. Ueda K, Saito A, Nakano H, Aoshima M, Yokota M, et al. (1980) Cortical hyperostosis following long-term administration of prostaglandin E_1 in infants with cyanotic congenital heart disease. Journal of Pediatrics 97: 834–836.
47. Li M, Ke HZ, Qi H, Healy DR, Li Y, et al. (2003) A novel, non-prostanoid EP2 receptor-selective prostaglandin E2 agonist stimulates local bone formation and enhances fracture healing. J Bone Miner Res 18: 2033–2042.
48. Paralkar VM, Borovecki F, Ke HZ, Cameron KO, Lefker B, et al. (2003) An EP2 receptor-selective prostaglandin E2 agonist induces bone healing. Proc Natl Acad Sci U S A 100: 6736–6740.
49. Li M, Healy DR, Li Y, Simmons HA, Crawford DT, et al. (2005) Osteopenia and impaired fracture healing in aged EP4 receptor knockout mice. Bone 37: 46–54.
50. Ren W, Dziak R (1991) Effects of leukotrienes on osteoblastic cell proliferation. Calcif Tissue Int 49: 197–201.
51. Traianedes K, Dallas MR, Garrett IR, Mundy GR, Bonewald LF (1998) 5-Lipoxygenase metabolites inhibit bone formation *in vitro*. Endocrinology 139: 3178–3184.
52. Langenbach R, Morham SG, Tiano HF, Loftin CD, Ghanayem BI, et al. (1995) Prostaglandin synthase 1 gene disruption in mice reduces arachidonic acid-induced inflammation and indomethacin-induced gastric ulceration. Cell 83: 483–492.
53. Morham SG, Langenbach R, Loftin CD, Tiano HF, Vouloumanos N, et al. (1995) Prostaglandin synthase 2 gene disruption causes severe renal pathology in the mouse. Cell 83: 473–482.
54. Chen XS, Sheller JR, Johnson EN, Funk CD (1994) Role of leukotrienes revealed by targeted disruption of the 5-lipoxygenase gene. Nature 372: 179–182.
55. Xie C, Ming X, Wang Q, Schwarz EM, Guldberg RE, et al. (2008) COX-2 from the injury milieu is critical for the initiation of periosteal progenitor cell mediated bone healing. Bone 43: 1075–1083.
56. Geng Y, Blanco FJ, Cornelisson M, Lotz M (1995) Regulation of cyclooxygenase-2 expression in normal human articular chondrocytes. J Immunol 155: 796–801.
57. Brochhausen C, Neuland P, Kirkpatrick CJ, Nusing RM, Klaus G (2006) Cyclooxygenases and prostaglandin E2 receptors in growth plate chondrocytes in vitro and in situ - prostaglandin E2 dependent proliferation of growth plate chondrocytes. Arthritis Res Ther 8: R78.
58. Welting TJ, Caron MM, Emans PJ, Janssen MP, Sanen K, et al. (2011) Inhibition of cyclooxygenase-2 impacts chondrocyte hypertrophic differentiation during endochondral ossification. Eur Cell Mater 22: 420–436; discussion 436–427.
59. Martel-Pelletier J, Mineau F, Fahmi H, Laufer S, Reboul P, et al. (2004) Regulation of the expression of 5-lipoxygenase-activating protein/5-lipoxygenase and the synthesis of leukotriene B(4) in osteoarthritic chondrocytes: role of transforming growth factor beta and eicosanoids. Arthritis Rheum 50: 3925–3933.
60. Li TF, Zuscik MJ, Ionescu AM, Zhang X, Rosier RN, et al. (2004) PGE2 inhibits chondrocyte differentiation through PKA and PKC signaling. Exp Cell Res 300: 159–169.
61. Sato T, Konomi K, Fujii R, Aono H, Aratani S, et al. (2011) Prostaglandin EP2 receptor signalling inhibits the expression of matrix metalloproteinase 13 in human osteoarthritic chondrocytes. Ann Rheum Dis 70: 221–226.
62. Tawara T, Shingu M, Nobunaga M, Naono T (1991) Effects of recombinant human IL-1 beta on production of prostaglandin E2, leukotriene B4, NAG, and superoxide by human synovial cells and chondrocytes. Inflammation 15: 145–157.
63. Janckila AJ, Parthasarathy RN, Parthasarathy LK, Seelan RS, Hsueh YC, et al. (2005) Properties and expression of human tartrate-resistant acid phosphatase isoform 5a by monocyte-derived cells. J Leukoc Biol 77: 209–218.
64. Janckila AJ, Slone SP, Lear SC, Martin A, Yam LT (2007) Tartrate-resistant acid phosphatase as an immunohistochemical marker for inflammatory macrophages. Am J Clin Pathol 127: 556–566.
65. Nishida T, Emura K, Kubota S, Lyons KM, Takigawa M (2011) CCN family 2/connective tissue growth factor (CCN2/CTGF) promotes osteoclastogenesis via induction of and interaction with dendritic cell-specific transmembrane protein (DC-STAMP). J Bone Miner Res 26: 351–363.
66. Speziani C, Rivollier A, Gallois A, Coury F, Mazzorana M, et al. (2007) Murine dendritic cell transdifferentiation into osteoclasts is differentially regulated by innate and adaptive cytokines. Eur J Immunol 37: 747–757.
67. Udagawa N, Takahashi N, Akatsu T, Tanaka H, Sasaki T, et al. (1990) Origin of osteoclasts: mature monocytes and macrophages are capable of differentiating into osteoclasts under a suitable microenvironment prepared by bone marrow-derived stromal cells. Proc Natl Acad Sci U S A 87: 7260–7264.
68. Okada Y, Lorenzo JA, Freeman AM, Tomita M, Morham SG, et al. (2000) Prostaglandin G/H synthase-2 is required for maximal formation of osteoclast-like cells in culture. Journal of Clinical Investigation 105: 823–832.
69. Igarashi K, Woo J-T, Stern PH (2002) Effects of a selective cyclooxygenase-2 inhibitor, celecoxib, on bone resorption and osteoclastogenesis *in vitro*. Biochemical Pharmacology 63: 523–532.
70. Han SY, Lee NK, Kim KH, Jang IW, Yim M, et al. (2005) Transcriptional induction of cyclooxygenase-2 in osteoclast precursors is involved in RANKL-induced osteoclastogenesis. Blood 106: 1240–1245.
71. Dominguez JH, Mundy GR (1980) Monocytes mediate osteoclastic bone resorption by prostaglandin production. Calcif Tissue Int 31: 29–34.
72. Lee SH, Soyoola E, Chanmugam P, Hart S, Sun W, et al. (1992) Selective expression of mitogen-inducible cyclooxygenase in macrophages stimulated with lipopolysaccharide. J Biol Chem 267: 25934–25938.
73. Cuetara BL, Crotti TN, O'Donoghue AJ, McHugh KP (2006) Cloning and characterization of osteoclast precursors from the RAW264.7 cell line. In Vitro Cell Dev Biol Anim 42: 182–188.
74. Savostin-Asling I, Asling CW (1975) Transmission and scanning electron microscope studies of calcified cartilage resorption. Anat Rec 183: 373–391.
75. Uusitalo H, Hiltunen A, Soderstrom M, Aro HT, Vuorio E (2000) Expression of cathepsins B, H, K, L, and S and matrix metalloproteinases 9 and 13 during chondrocyte hypertrophy and endochondral ossification in mouse fracture callus. Calcif Tissue Int 67: 382–390.
76. Mackie EJ, Ahmed YA, Tatarczuch L, Chen KS, Mirams M (2008) Endochondral ossification: how cartilage is converted into bone in the developing skeleton. Int J Biochem Cell Biol 40: 46–62.
77. Kosaki N, Takaishi H, Kamekura S, Kimura T, Okada Y, et al. (2007) Impaired bone fracture healing in matrix metalloproteinase-13 deficient mice. Biochem Biophys Res Commun 354: 846–851.
78. Chyun YS, Raisz LG (1984) Stimulation of bone formation by prostaglandin E_2. Prostaglandins 27: 97–103.

6

Cortical Bone Mechanical Properties Are Altered in an Animal Model of Progressive Chronic Kidney Disease

Christopher L. Newman[1], Sharon M. Moe[2,3], Neal X. Chen[2], Max A. Hammond[4], Joseph M. Wallace[4,5], Jeffry S. Nyman[6,7], Matthew R. Allen[1]*

1 Department of Anatomy and Cell Biology, Indiana University School of Medicine, Indianapolis, Indiana, United States of America, **2** Division of Nephrology, Department of Medicine, Indiana University School of Medicine, Indianapolis, Indiana, United States of America, **3** Roudebush VA Medical Center, Indianapolis, Indiana, United States of America, **4** Weldon School of Biomedical Engineering, Purdue University, West Lafayette, Indiana, United States of America, **5** Department of Biomedical Engineering, Indiana University—Purdue University, Indianapolis, Indiana, United States of America, **6** Department of Orthopaedic Surgery and Rehabilitation and Vanderbilt Center for Bone Biology, Vanderbilt University Medical Center, Nashville, Tennessee, United States of America, **7** Department of Veterans Affairs, Tennessee Valley Healthcare System, Nashville, Tennessee, United States of America

Abstract

Chronic kidney disease (CKD), which leads tocortical bone loss and increasedporosity,increases therisk of fracture. Animal models have confirmed that these changes compromise whole bone mechanical properties. Estimates from whole bone testing suggest that material properties are negatively affected, though tissue-level assessmentshavenot been conducted. Therefore, the goal of the present study was to examine changes in cortical bone at different length scales using a rat model with theprogressive development of CKD. At 30 weeks of age (~75% reduction in kidney function), skeletally mature male Cy/+ rats were compared to their normal littermates. Cortical bone material propertieswere assessed with reference point indentation (RPI), atomic force microscopy (AFM), Raman spectroscopy,and high performance liquid chromatography (HPLC). Bones from animals with CKD had higher (+18%) indentation distance increase and first cycle energy dissipation (+ 8%) as measured by RPI.AFM indentation revealed a broader distribution of elastic modulus values in CKD animals witha greater proportion of both higher and lower modulus values compared to normal controls. Yet, tissue composition, collagen morphology, and collagen cross-linking fail to account for these differences. Though the specific skeletal tissue alterations responsible for these mechanical differences remain unclear, these results indicate that cortical bone material properties are altered in these animals and may contribute to the increased fracture risk associated with CKD.

Editor: Damian Christopher Genetos, University of California Davis, United States of America

Funding: National Institutes of Health grants AR58005 (SM) and DL100093 (CN); Indiana Clinical Translational Science Institute grant TR000162 (CN). The funders had no role in study design, data collection and analysis, decision to publish, or preparation of the manuscript.

Competing Interests: The authors have declared that no competing interests exist.

* E-mail: matallen@iupui.edu

Introduction

Chronic kidney disease—mineral and bone disorder (CKD-MBD) is characterized by hyperphosphatemia, secondary hyperparathyroidism, and an increased risk offractures[1–3].Unlike osteoporosis, CKD-MBD appears to have a preferential impact on cortical bone, leading to reduced bone mass and increased porosity [4–6].These effects likely underlie the increased fracture risk observed in patients with CKD[7–9].

Whole bone (structural)mechanical properties are dependent upon a number of variables [10–11]. While bone mass is a major determinant, both the distribution of bone and its material properties (inherent physical and chemical properties) also play crucial roles. Most biomechanical studies in rodent models of CKD have focused on structural mechanical properties, employing three-point bending or dynamic mechanical analysis (DMA) [12–18]. These studies indicate that the bending and viscoelastic properties of bone are compromised in animals with CKD. Specifically, DMA indicates that diseased animals have lower storage modulus (a measure of stiffness) and tan delta (a measure of energy dissipation) [14–15], while three point bending studies indicate that ultimate load, stiffness, and energy to failure are lower in CKD animals [12].

While there is an increasing awareness of the importance of bone quality in CKD [19], few studies have explicitly examined material properties in animal models[14–15,20]. Material properties can be estimated from whole bone mechanical tests using standardengineering equations that account for whole bone structure and geometry.Because these estimates assume that skeletal tissue is homogeneous, isotropic, and linearly elastic, direct measures ofmaterial properties in bone would provide additionalinsight into how the disease is affecting fracture resistance. Therefore, the goal of the present study was to examine material-level changes in cortical bone at several length scales using a rat model with the progressive development of CKD. Specifically, we hypothesized that CKD adversely impacts cortical bone material properties as determined by material-level mechanical testing and assessments of bone composition and collagen morphology.

Materials And Methods

Animal Model

The current study utilized a slowly progressive animal model of CKD, the Cy/+ rat. Cy/+ ratsare characterized by autosomal dominant polycystic kidney disease [21]. These animals have a mutation (R823W) in *Anks6*, a gene that codes for the protein SamCystin. Currently, the function of this protein is unknown, and the specific role of this mutation in the development of polycystic kidney disease is unclear. Aside from its expression in the kidney, however, little is known about its role in the cell [22].Unlike most other PKD-related proteins, though, SamCystin does not localize to the primary cilia of kidney cells [23]. While there is no known human disease associated with this gene, thespontaneous onset of disease provides a helpful phenotypic model of human CKD [21].Unlike the more common surgical models[24], Cy/+ rats display a gradual onset of disease.And unlike most genetic models[25–26], they exhibit a slow enough progression that bone disease does not begin to occur until after skeletal maturity.

Skeletal tissuefrom animals in a previous study wasutilized [12]. All animals were fed a casein diet (Purina AIN-76A; 0.7% Pi) to increase phosphorus availability in order to produce a more consistent kidney disease phenotype.Fresh frozen tibiaefrom 30-week-old male Cy/+ ratsand their age-matched non-affected littermates were assessed mechanically, compositionally, and morphologically at several length scales.Fresh frozen femora were used for collagen cross-linking analyses. Blood was collected at the end of the experiment for biochemical analyses (previously reported in [12]).All procedures were conducted under the approval of Indiana University School of Medicine Institutional Animal Care and Use Committeeprotocol # 10479.

Reference Point Indentation

Tibiae were thawed to room temperature and soaked overnight in phosphate-buffered saline. The anteromedial surface of the proximal diaphysis of the tibia was assessed using reference point indentation (RPI) (Biodent Hfc, Active Life Scientific, Santa Barbara, CA). The reference probe, which housed a BP2 test probe, waslowered vertically, normal to the surface, until itrested on the surface of the bone.In order to stabilize the unit, a reference force of ~13 N was applied before each measurement was initiated.Each test included a series of 10 cycles at 2 Hz to a force of 10 N. Bones were maintained in a hydrated state throughout the test. Five locations per sample, each ~2 mm apart, were indented. Raw data from the RPI analysis software (version 2.0) were imported into a customized MATLAB code (Mathworks) designed to provide cycle-by-cycle data for each test [27], from which first cycle unloading slope, indentation distance increase, first cycle energy dissipation, creep indentation distance, first cycle indentation distance, total indentation distance, and total energy dissipation were calculated for each test. All five tests from each animal were averaged to produce a single value for each variable.

Tissue Composition

Raman spectroscopy was performed using a LabRAM HR 800 Raman Spectrometer (HORIBA JobinYvon, Edison, NJ) connected to a BX41 microscope (Olympus, Tokyo, Japan). A 660 nm laser was focused on the bone surface using a 50X objective to a spot size of ~10 μm. Five locations were imaged ~1 mm apart on the anteromedialmid-diaphysiswith five 20 second acquisitions at each location as previously published [28]. A five point linear baseline correction was applied in LabSpec 5 (HORIBA JobinYvon). Using OriginPro 8.6 (OriginLab, Northampton, MA), a single Gaussian peak was fit to the PO_4^{3-}ν1 peak, and the areas under the PO_4^{3-}ν1, CO_3^{2-}ν1, and Amide I peaks were calculated at each location. Type B carbonate substitution was found by the band area ratio of CO_3^{2-}ν1/PO_4^{3-}ν1. The degree of matrix mineralization was determined by the band area ratios of PO_4^{3-}ν1/Amide I. Mineral maturity (crystallinity) was determined by the inverse of the full width at half maximum (FWHM) of the PO_4^{3-}ν1 peak.

AFM Indentation

The anteromedial portion of the mid-diaphysis used above was polished with a 3 μm polycrystalline water-based diamond suspension in order to create a flat region for testing. Nanoindentation was performed using a BioScope Catalyst atomic force microscope (Bruker, Santa Barbara, CA), operating in peak force tapping mode using previously published methods [29]. Indentations were performed using a polycrystalline diamond probe (NaDia ND-DYC series; Advanced Diamond Technologies, Inc.) with a measured spring constant of 29.25 N/m. Four locations per sample were indented and, at each location (20 μm×20 μm grid), 49 indentationswere performed. Samples were loaded to 200 nN with force-separation curves acquired from each indentation. Within each location, indentations were spaced about 2 μm apart in order to avoid interactions from neighboring indentations. In total, 196 indentations were performed for each sample. The indentation elastic modulus was calculated from 5% to 95% of the withdrawal curve using the classic Hertz model of contact between a rigid sphere and an elastic half space because the indentation depth is much smaller than the radius of curvature of the probe [29]. The indentation elastic modulus was determined from the following equation: E = 3F(1-v^2)/(4r^(1/2) δ^(3/2)) where E is the indentation elastic modulus, F is the indentation force, v is the Poisson's ratio of the sample (assumed to be 0.35), r is the tip radius (nominal radius of 50 nm, with the same probe used for all samples), and δ is the indentation depth. All of the individual indentations were averaged to produce a single value for each animal, though individual tests were used for distribution comparisons among the groups.

Collagen Morphology

Following AFMindentation, the polished surface was partially decalcified by soaking the bones in 0.5 M EDTA for 25 minutes followed by five minutes of sonication in a water bath. This process was repeated five times for each sample. For imaging, RTESPA probes were used (Bruker; radius nominally 8 nm, spring constant = 40 N/m). The scan size was set at 3.5 μm with 512×512 pixels and a scan rate of 0.5 lines/s. For measurements of collagen morphology, four locations were imaged per sample, and 10 to 15 fibrils were measured at each location. 40 to 50 fibrils per sample were averaged to produce a single value for each animal, though the individual tests were used for distribution comparisons. Using SPIP 5.1.10 (Image Metrology, Hrsholm, Denmark),D-periodic spacing was calculated using2D Fast Fourier Transformations (2D FFTs) as previously described [28].

Collagen Cross-Linking

Segments of bone (~3 mm in length) from the proximal femoral diaphysis were fully demineralized in 20% EDTA (0.68 M, pH 7.4). Approximately 10 mg of demineralized bonewerehydrolyzedin6 N HCl (~10 μL per 1 mg) at 110°C for 20 to 24 hours. After evaporating the acidusing a SpeedVAC centrifuge with coldtrap, each hydrolysate was resuspended in ultrapure water, split into two equal portions, and dried. Half the residue was resuspended in ultrapure water with an internal standard

(5×10^{-6} g/L pyridoxine). The solution was filtered and diluted with 0.05% heptafluorobutyric acid in 10% acetonitrile, and 50 μL of each hydrolysate were assayed by a high performance liquid chromatography (HPLC) system (Beckman-Coulter System Gold 168) with a silica-based column (Waters Spherisorb). Standards with varying concentrations of pyridinoline (Pyd) (Quidel),deoxypyridinoline (Dpd) (Quidel),pentosidine(PE) (International Maillard Reaction Society), and a constant amount of pyridoxinewere also assayed. Using a Waters 2475 fluorescence detector (excitation/emission of295/400 nm for Pyd and Dpd and 328/378 nm for PE), chromatograms were recorded to determine the amount of each crosslink. These amounts were then normalized by collagen content, which was determined from the other half of each hydrolysate by another HPLC assay [30]. Briefly, withα-amino-butyric acid (α-ABA) included as an internal standard, the amino acids were subjected to derivatization withphenyl isothiocyanate (PITC). Along with standards of varying concentrations of hydroxyproline (Sigma) and proline (Sigma)and a constant amount of α-ABA, the derivatized samples were resuspendedin a buffer solution of 5% acetonitrile in 5 mM disodium phosphate. Upon injecting 50 μLof this sample, chromatograms were generated with a UV detector (Beckman-Coulter System Gold 168). The calculated mass of hydroxyproline was then multiplied by 7.5 (assuming 13–14% of type I collagen by mass) and divided by the molecular weight of collagen (30,000 Da) [31], thereby giving crosslink concentration as mol/mol of collagen.

Statistical Analysis

All analyses were performed using SPSS software. Comparisons between groups were made with Student's t-tests (assumptions validated by Shapiro-Wilk and Levene tests). When non-normal distributions or unequal variances were present, comparisons were made using Wilcoxon ranked-sum tests and unequal variance t-tests, respectively. Distributions included all measures from each individual, and comparisons were made using Kolmogorov-Smirnov tests. *A priori* α-levels were set at 0.05 to determine significance.

Results

Animal Model

Details about the phenotype of these animals have been previous published [12]. Briefly, measures of kidney function, including BUN (+116%) and the albumin-to-creatinine ratio (+ 301%), weresignificantly higher in Cy/+ animals compared to the normal controls. Similar to what is observed in humans with CKD, there were no differences between groups for phosphorus or calcium levels, but both serum PTH (+240%) and FGF23 (+195%) weredrastically higher(**FIGURE 1**).Cy/+ animals had higher numbers of osteoclasts and higher levels of bone remodeling. Using three-point bending, they exhibited lower ultimate load (−28%), stiffness(−17%), and energy to fracture (−46%). Estimates of material properties indicate that they had lower ultimate stress (−20%) and toughness (−47%) (**FIGURE 2**)[12].

Reference Point Indentation

Indentation distance increase (IDI)provides an assessment of the change in depth between the first cycle and the final cycle. Cy/+ animals had significantly higher IDI (+18%), indicating that the tissue ismore prone to damage under the same applied load (**FIGURE 3**). The amount of energy dissipated during the first cycle was also significantlyhigher in animals with CKD (+8%). While the first cycle creep indentation distance (+18%) was higher in Cy/+ animals, there was no difference in microstructural stiffness (first cycle unloading slope)between the two groups.No differences were noted in first cycle indentation distance, total indentation distance, or total energy dissipation (**Table 1**).

AFM-based indentation

There was no difference in the indentation elastic modulus between the groups (**FIGURE 4a**). However, when all indentations within each groupwere considered as a population, the distribution of elastic modulus values did differ between the two groups. Animals with CKD had a greater proportion of both high and low values of elastic modulus than their normal counterparts (**FIGURE 4b**).

Tissue Composition

Raman spectroscopy revealed no differences between animals with CKD and their normal counterparts with regard to overall compositionof the mineral and organic matrices (**Table 2**). Specifically, there were no differences between the groups in the phosphate-to-amide I ratio (the mineral-to-matrix ratio), mineral crystallinity, or the carbonate-to-phosphate ratio (a reflection of type B carbonate substitution).

Collagen Morphology and Cross-Linking

There were no mean differences in D-periodicity between the two groups (**Table 2**). There were also no differences in the distribution of D-periodicity when all fibrils were considered. In addition, both enzymatic and non-enzymatic cross-linksas assessed by HPLC were similar between groups (**Table 2**).

Discussion

The mechanical integrity of skeletal tissue is determined by the amount of tissue present, its distribution, and its quality. Compromises in any of these factors can lead to an increased fracture risk. The notable loss of cortical bone mass associated with CKD is assumed to be primarily responsible for the increased fracture risk seen in patients [5]. The current study advances our understanding of bone fragility in CKD by showing that microscale and nanoscale mechanical properties are alteredindependently of changes in bone mass and porosity.

Our lab has previously documented reductions in both structural and estimated materialproperties in Cy/+ rats, animals with progressive CKD [12,32]. But, whole bone testing only provides indirect estimates of material properties, which is why wedirectly assessedmicroscale mechanical propertiesusing reference point indentation (RPI).RPI data from the present study indicate that animals with CKD had higher IDI, higher first cycle creep indentation distance, and first cycle energy dissipation. Taken together, these results indicatethat the tissue in animals with CKD is less resistant to indentation and more prone to damage. Indentation distance increase was nearly 20% higher in CKD animals compared to their normal counterparts. Similar differences in IDI have been previously reported in diabetic rats[33]. These data have two important implications. First, they show that CKD negatively affects skeletal tissue independently of bone mass, which means that estimates of bone massalone likely underestimate the overall mechanical effects of CKD.These differences in bone quality may explain the conflicting data available on BMD and fracture risk in CKD patients[6,34–40]. Second, our data provide a basis for considering *in vivo* applications of RPI in the clinical setting of CKD. RPI has been used to successfully differentiate patients with and without hip fractures[41] as well as those with and without atypical femoral fractures [42]. A related

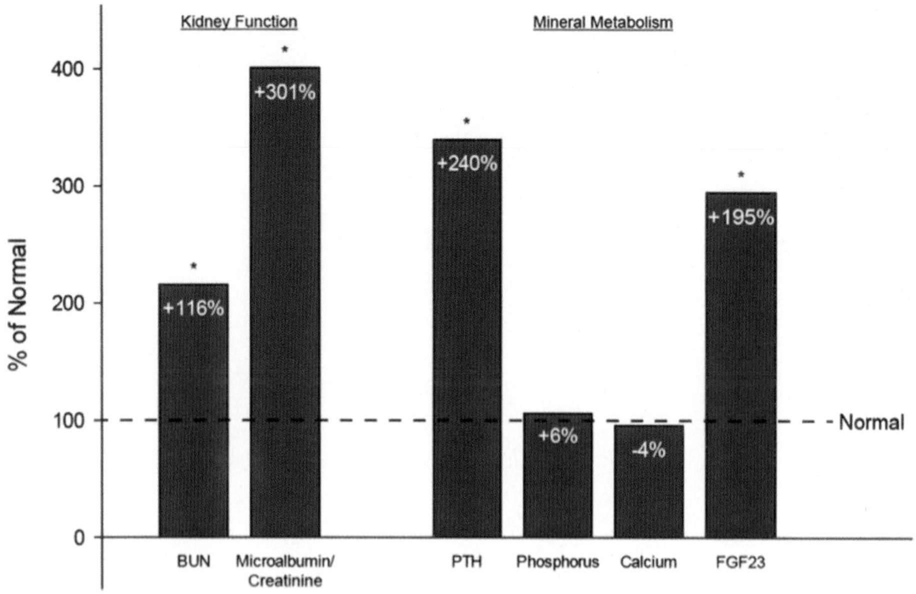

Figure 1. Biochemical assessment of kidney function and mineral metabolism. These previously published data (Allen *et al.*, 2013) show abnormalities in kidney function and mineral metabolism resulting from hyperparathyroidism in the animals utilized in the current work. Data are presented as a percentage of non-affected normal animals with (*) representing statistical significance.

indentation device has also been shown to discriminate patients with diabetes from their normal counterparts[43]. Assessment of tissue-level mechanical properties, combined with standard imaging modalities to measure bone mass, cortical geometry (especially porosity), and trabecular architecture, may prove to be an ideal combination by which to assess the overall mechanical integrity of bones in patients with CKD.

The current study also employed a hierarchical approach by examining nanoscale mechanical properties with atomic force microscopy. AFM indentation provides a direct assessment of the nanoscale stiffness produced by the collagen and mineral composite. Consistent with measurements of microscale stiffness (first cycle unloading slope), these results show that the average indentation elastic modulus was not significantly different between the two groups.Yet, the distribution of elastic modulus values was different. Animals with CKD displayed a greater degree of heterogeneity in nanoscale elasticity. Because increased material heterogeneity is often considered advantageous [44], these results may reflect an adaptive response to declining integrity at larger length scales. Alternatively, extreme variations in nanoscale properties maylead to localized stress concentrations that result in damage accumulation from lower forces[45]. Although heterogeneity is likely necessary for normal mechanical integrity, extreme heterogeneity may be problematic from a mechanical

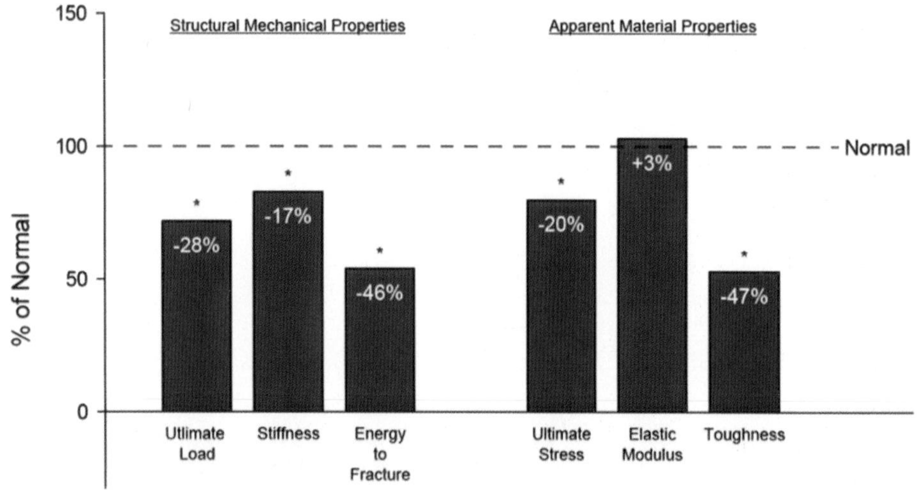

Figure 2. Structural mechanical properties and estimated material properties. These previously published data (Allen *et al.*, 2013) show compromised whole bone mechanical properties from femoral 3-point bending and apparent material-level mechanical properties derived from standard beam bending equations in the animals utilized in the current work. Data are presented as a percentage of non-affected normal animals with (*) representing statistical significance.

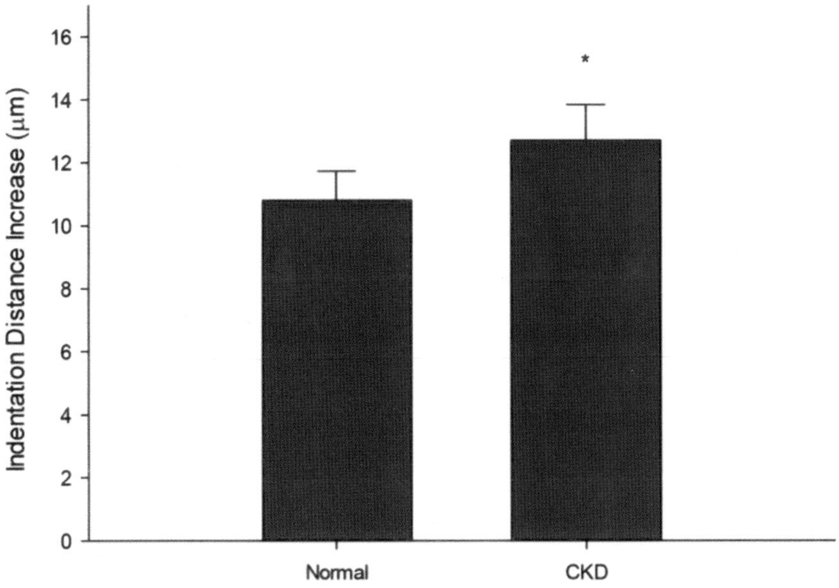

Figure 3. Microindentation reveals that CKD skeletal tissue is less able to resist damage. Using reference point indentation (RPI), the indentation distance increase (IDI) was found to be significantly higher in CKD animals compared to normal. These data indicate that the mechanical integrity of the bone is less able to resist microscale damage formation and propagation. Data are presented as mean and standard deviation. *$p < 0.05$ versus normal controls.

standpoint [46]. Future studies should attempt to better understand the role of material heterogeneity in CKD in order to specifythe contributionofmicroscale and nanoscalepropertiesto whole bone mechanical properties.

While whole bone, microscale, and nanoscale mechanical differences are present in animals with CKD, tissue composition, collagen morphology, and collagen cross-linking fail to account for the differences. These data conflict with studiesshowing higher mineral-to-matrix ratios, lower mineral crystallinity, increased advanced glycationendproducts (AGEs), and decreased gene expression of lysyl oxidase in alternative models of CKD [14–15,47]. One potential explanation for these disparate results is that these previous studies utilized younger animals that developed advanced CKD during skeletal growth. Teasing apart the interaction between growth and disease is difficult, which is why the present study employed the use of a model in which kidney disease occurs after skeletal maturity.

Previous studies have demonstrated that non-enzymatic cross-links (pentosidine, specifically) are increased in the circulation of patients with CKD[48–51]. These findings coincide with the accumulation of AGEs in soft tissues detected by fluorescence methods[52]. Because high levels in the circulation are associated with the deposition of AGEs in other tissues, this may be true of skeletal tissue as well. To date, this has only been confirmed in one small clinical study in patients on dialysis [53]. Currently, there are few data in animal models, and clinical trials examining predialysis patients are lacking. Using a low turnover 5/6 nephrectomy model, two studies have reported increased pentosidineusing

Table 1. Mechanical properties from microindentation and nanoindentation.

RPI	**Normal (n = 6)**	**Cy/+ (n = 6)**	**p-values**
First Cycle Indentation Distance (μm)	83.38±3.15	88.24±5.45	*0.088
First cycle Energy Dissipation (μJ)	275.53±14.00	297.94±19.35	***0.044**
First Cycle Unloading Slope (N/μm)	0.47±0.02	0.45±0.03	*0.113
First Cycle Creep Indentation Distance (μm)	6.08±0.43	7.17±0.95	***0.028**
Indentation Distance Increase (μm)	10.81±0.92	12.71±1.13	***0.009**
Total Indentation Distance (μm)	89.39±2.73	95.21±5.13	#0.080
Total Energy Dissipation (μJ)	663.06±43.53	712.30±89.19	*0.252
AFM	**Normal (n = 5)**	**Cy/+ (n = 4)**	**p-values**
Indentation Elastic Modulus (MPa)	962.99 345.98	996.73 588.99	0.920

Values are presented as mean ± standard deviation.
*equal variance t-test.
#Wilcoxon ranked-sum test.
p-values less than 0.05 are in bold.

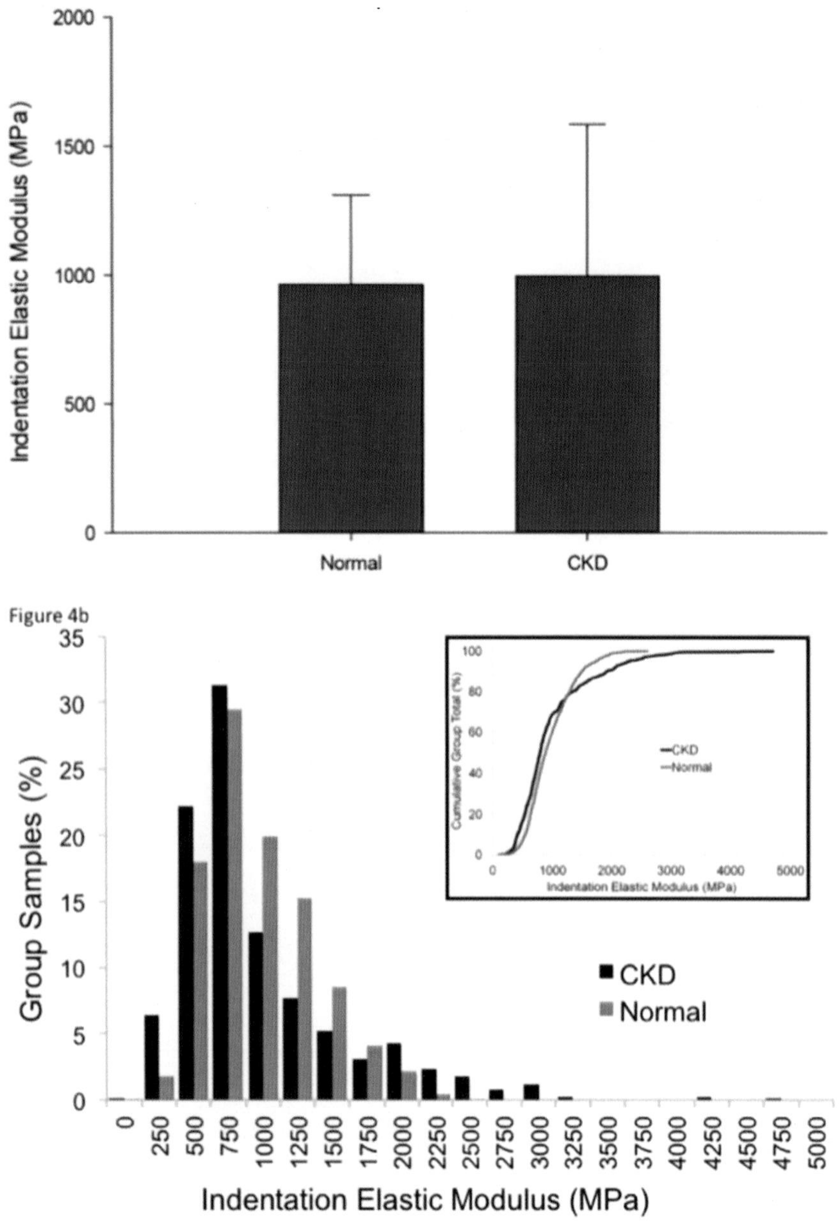

Figure 4. Nanoindenation reveals that CKD skeletal tissue has increased heterogeneity in the elastic modulus compared to normal bone. There was no significant difference in the average elastic modulus (A), but the distribution of elastic modulus values was significantly broader (B), with a greater proportion of both high and low values in CKD relative to normal ($p<0.0001$).

Raman spectroscopy[14–15]. While Raman spectroscopy has been utilized to detect AGEs in ocular tissue[54], its ability to detect changes in bone is unknown as HPLC is the standard method used to measure AGEs in skeletal tissue[53,55–58]. Here, having employed HPLC, thehypothesized increases in AGE content were not observed. While increases may occur with more advanced disease in theseanimals, the relationship between circulating pentosidineand its accumulation in bone collagen in CKDremains unresolved.

At present, clinical data on bone quality in CKD are minimal. Aside from the aforementioned dialysis study [53], CKD patients with high bone turnover had reduced stiffness and a decreased mineral-to-matrix ratio as assessed on iliac crest biopsies [59]. As these data are from cancellous bone, though, direct comparison with the current work on cortical bone is difficult. Connecting these dots by examining cortical bone properties in patients (which is possible with iliac crest biopsies) and cancellous properties in rats will be an essential step in moving forward.

Limitations to the current study should also be recognized. First, because tissue from a previous study was used, the sample sizes used here were small. Hence, any applications to other animal models or patients should occur with a measure of caution. Second, the mechanical assessments were localized to the periosteal surface, which may not be fully representative of the entire cortex. As such, the assessed parameters may differ at other cortical sites. Finally, this study assessed material properties in 30-week-old animals. As the disease progresses, differences in composition and morphologymay arise.Nevertheless, the advan-

Table 2. Tissue composition and collagen morphology.

Raman	Normal (n=6)	Cy/+ (n=6)	p-values
Crystallinity (1/FWHM PO_4^{3-}v1)	0.054±0.001	0.055±0.001	*0.4421
Carbonate Substitution (CO_3^{2-}v1/PO_4^{3-}v1)	0.618±0.037	0.608±0.019	#0.5375
Relative Mineralization (PO_4^{3-}v1/Amide I)	2.539±0.253	2.699±0.317	*0.9372
AFM	**Normal (n=6)**	**Cy/+ (n=5)**	**p-values**
D-Periodicity (nm)	65.641±0.646	65.864±0.838	*0.631
HPLC	**Normal (n=8)**	**Cy/+ (n=6)**	**p-values**
Pyridinoline per Collagen (mol/mol)	0.60±0.17	0.54±0.10	**0.252
Deoxypyridinoline per Collagen (mol/mol)	0.37±0.07	0.37±0.04	**0.974
Pentosidine per Collagen (mol/mol)	878± 153	921±148	*0.523

Values are presented as mean ± standard deviation.
*equal variances t-test.
**unequal variances t-test.
#Wilcoxon ranked-sum test.

tage of using 30-week-old animals is that these animals are skeletally mature but do not yet exhibit the rampant increase in cortical porosity present at 35 weeks [32].

In conclusion, these data show that both microscale and nanoscale cortical bone material properties are altered in an animal model of CKD. The specific skeletal tissue alterations responsible for these mechanical differences remain unclear. Nevertheless, in addition to bone loss and cortical porosity, defects in material-level mechanical properties may also contribute to the increased fracture risk associated with CKD.

Acknowledgments

We would like to thank Mr. Drew Brown for his assistance with analysis and tissue harvesting. We would also like to acknowledge the late Dr. Vincent H. Gattone II, who was instrumental in developing this animal model.

Author Contributions

Conceived and designed the experiments: CLN SMM JMW MRA. Performed the experiments: CLN NXC MAH JMW JSN. Analyzed the data: CLN MAH JMW JSN. Contributed to the writing of the manuscript: CLN SMM JMW JSN MRA.

References

1. Levey AS, Eckardt KU, Tsukamoto Y, Levin A, Coresh J, et al. (2005). Definition and classification of chronic kidney disease: a position statement from Kidney Disease Improving Global Outcomes (KDIGO). Kidney Int 67:2089–2100.
2. Levin A, Bakris GL, Molitch M, Smulders M, Tian J, et al. (2007) Prevalence of abnormal serum vitamin D, PTH, calcium, and phosphorus in patients with chronic kidney disease: results of the study to evaluate early kidney disease. Kidney Int 71:31–38.
3. KDIGO Working Group (2009) KDIGO clinical practice guideline for the diagnosis, evaluation, prevention, and treatment of Chronic Kidney Disease-Mineral and Bone Disorder (CKD-MBD). Kidney Int 76: S1–S130.
4. Cejka D, Patsch JM, Weber M, Diarra D, Riegersperger M, et al. (2011) Bone microarchitecture in hemodialysis patients assessed by HR-pQCT. Clin J Am Soc Nephrol 6:2264–71.
5. Nickolas TL, Stein E, Cohen A, Thomas V, Staron RB, et al. (2010) Bone mass and microarchitecture in CKD patients with fracture. J Am Soc Nephrol 21:1371–1380.
6. Nickolas TL, Cremers S, Zhang A, Thomas V, Stein E, et al. (2011) Discriminants of prevalent fractures in chronic kidney disease. J Am Soc Nephrol 22:1560–1572.
7. Fried LF, Biggs ML, Shlipak MG, Seliger S, Kestenbaum B, et al. (2007) Association of kidney function with incident hip fracture in older adults. J Am Soc Nephrol 18:282–286.
8. Nickolas TL, McMahon DJ, Shane E (2006) Relationship between moderate to severe kidney disease and hip fracture in the United States. J Am Soc Nephrol 17:3223–3232.
9. Nitsch D, Mylne A, Roderick PJ, Smeeth, Hubbard R, et al. (2009) Chronic kidney disease and hip-fracture-related mortality in older people in the UK. Nephrol Dial Transplant 24:1539–1544.
10. Cole JH, van der Meulen MCH (2011) Whole bone mechanics and bone quality. ClinOrthopRelat Res 469:2139–2149.
11. Seeman E, Delmas PD (2006) Bone quality: the material and structural basis of bone strength and fragility. N Engl J Med 354:2250–2261.
12. Allen MR, Chen NX, Gattone II VH, Chen X, Carr AJ, et al. (2013) Skeletal effects of zoledronic acid in an animal model of chronic kidney disease. OsteoporosInt 24:1471–1481.
13. Iwamoto J, Seki A, Sato Y, Matsumoto H (2012) Vitamin K2 improves renal function and increases femoral bone strength in rats with renal insufficiency. Calcif Tissue Int 90:50–59.
14. Iwasaki Y, Kazama JJ, Yamato H, Fukagawa M (2011) Changes in chemical composition of cortical bone associated with bone fragility in rat model with chronic kidney disease. Bone 48:1260–1267.
15. Iwasaki Y, Kazama JJ, Yamato H, Shimoda H, Fukagawa M (2013) Accumulated uremic toxins attenuate bone mechanical properties in rats with chronic kidney disease. Bone 57:477–483.
16. Jokihaara J, Porsti I, Pajamaki I, Vuohelainen T, Jolma P, et al. (2006) Paracalcitol [19-nor-1,25-(OH)2D2] in the treatment of experimental renal bone disease. J Bone Miner Res 21:745–751.
17. Moe SM, Radcliffe JS, White KE, Gattone VH II, Seifert MF, et al. (2011) The pathophysiology of early-stage chronic kidney disease–mineral bone disorder (CKD-MBD) and response to phosphate binders in the rat. J Bone Miner Res 26:2672–2681.
18. Sabbagh Y, Graciolli FG, O'Brien S, Tang W, dos Reis LM, et al. (2012) Repression of osteocyte Wnt/β-catenin signaling is an early event in the progression of renal osteodystrophy. J Bone Miner Res, 27:1757–1772.
19. Malluche HH, Porter DS, Pienkowski D (2013) Evaluating bone quality in patients with chronic kidney disease. Nat Rev Nephrol 9:671–680.
20. Kadokawa S, Matsumoto T, Naito H, Tanaka M (2011) Assessment of trabecular bone architecture and intrinsic properties of cortical bone tissue in a mouse model of chronic kidney disease. J Hard Tissue Biol 20: 79–86.
21. Moe SM, Chen NX, Seifert MF, Sinders RM, Duan D, et al. (2009) A rat model of chronic kidney disease-mineral bone disorder. Kidney Int 75:176–184.
22. Nagao S, Kugita M, Yoshihara D, Yamaguchi T (2012) Animal models for human polycystic kidney disease. Exp Anim Tokyo 61:477–488.
23. Stagner EE, Bouvrette DJ, Cheng J, Bryda EC (2009) The polycystic kidney disease-related proteins Bicc1 and SamCystin interact. BiochemBioph Res Co 383:16–21.
24. Shobeiri N, Adams MA, Holden RM (2010) Vascular calcification in animal models of CKD: a review. Am J Nephrol 31:471–481.
25. Gattone VH II, Tourkow BA, Trambaugh CM, Yu AC, Whelan S, et al. (2004)Development of multiorgan pathology in the *wpk* rat model of polycystic kidney disease. Anat Rec 277A:384–395.

26. Nagao S, Morita M, Kugita M, Yoshihara D, Yamaguchi T, et al. (2010) Polycystic kidney disease in Han:SPRD Cy rats is associated with elevated expression and mislocalizationof SamCystin. Am J Physiol Renal Physiol 299:F1078–F1086.
27. Aref M, Gallant MA, Organ JM, Wallace JM, Newman CL, et al. (2013) *In vivo* reference point indentation reveals positive effects of raloxifene on mechanical properties following 6 months of treatment in skeletally mature beagle dogs. Bone 56:449–53.
28. Hammond MA, Gallant MA, Burr DB, Wallace JM (2014) Nanoscale changes in collagen are reflected in physical and mechanical properties of bone at the microscale indiabetic rats. Bone 60:26–32.
29. Wallace JM (2012) Applications of atomic force microscopy for the assessment of nanoscale morphological and mechanical properties of bone. Bone 50:420–427.
30. Buckley A, Hill KE, Davidson JM (1988) Collagen metabolism. In:Colowick SP, Kaplan NO, Di SabatoG, editors. Methods in Enzymology: Immunochemical Techniques, Part M: Chemotaxis and inflammation. London: Academic Press. pp. 674–693.
31. Saito M, Marumo K, Fujii K, Ishioka N (1997) Single-column high-performance liquid chromatographic-fluorescence detection of immature, mature, and senescent cross-links of collagen. Anal Biochem 253:26–32
32. Moe SM, Chen NX, Newman CL, Gattone VH II, Organ JM, et al. (2014) A comparison of calcium to zoledronic acid for improvement of cortical bone in an animal model of CKD. J Bone Miner Res 29:902–910.
33. Gallant MA, Brown DM, Organ JM, Allen MR, Burr DB (2013) Reference-point indentation correlates with bone toughness assessed using whole-bone traditional mechanical testing. Bone 53:301–305.
34. Iimori S, Mori Y, Akita W, Kuyama T, Takada S, et al. (2012) Diagnostic usefulness of bone mineral density and biochemical markers of bone turnover in predicting fracture in CKD stage 5D patients—a single-center cohort study. Nephrol Dial Transplant 27:345–351.
35. Jamal SA, Hayden JA, Beyene J (2007) Low bone mineral density and fractures in long-term hemodialysis patients: a meta-analysis. Am J Kidney Dis 49:674–681.
36. Jamal SA, Cheung AM, West SL, Lok C (2012) Bone mineral density by DXA and HR pQCT can discriminate fracture status in men and women with stages 3 to 5 chronic kidney disease. OsteoporosInt 23:2805–2813.
37. Jassal SK, von Muhlen D, Barrett-Connor E (2007) Measures of renal function, BMD, bone loss, and osteoporotic fracture in older adults: the Rancho Bernardo study. J Bone Miner Res 22:203–210.
38. Klawansky S, Komaroff E, Cavanaugh PFJr, Mitchell DY, Gordon MJ, et al. (2003) Relationship between age, renal function and bone mineral density in the US population. OsteoporosInt 14:570–576.
39. Piraino B, Chen T, Cooperstein L, Segre G, Puschett J (1988) Fractures and vertebral bone mineral density in patients with renal osteodystrophy. ClinNephrol 30:57–62.
40. Yamaguchi T, Kanno E, TsubotaJ, Shiomi T, Nakai M, et al. (1996) Retrospective study on the usefulness of radius and lumbar bone density in the separation of hemodialysis patients with fractures from those without fractures. Bone 19:549–555.
41. Diez-Perez A, Güerri R, Nogues X, Caceres E, Pena MJ, et al. (2010)Micro-Microindentationfor in vivo measurement of bone tissue mechanical properties in humans. J Bone Miner Res 25:1877–1885.
42. Güerri-Fernández RC, Nogués X, Quesada Gómez JM, Torres Del Pliego E, Puig L, et al. (2013)Microindentation for in vivo measurement of bone tissue material properties in atypical femoral fracture patients and controls. J Bone Miner Res 28:162–168.
43. Farr JN, Drake MT, Amin S, Melton LJ III, McCready LK, et al. (2014) *In Vivo* assessment of bone quality in postmenopausal women with type 2 diabetes. J Bone Miner Res 29:787–795.
44. Tai K, Dao M, Suresh S, Palazoglu A, Ortiz C (2007) Nanoscale heterogeneity promotes energy dissipation in bone. Nat Mater 6:454–462.
45. Phelps JB, Hubbard GB, Wang X, Agrawal CM (2000) Microstructural heterogeneity and the fracture toughness of bone. J Biomed Mater Res 51:735–741.
46. Currey J (2005) Structural heterogeneity in bone: good or bad? J MusculoskeletNeuronal Interact 5:317.
47. Aoki C, Uto K, Honda K, Kato Y, Oda H(2013) Advanced glycation end products suppress lysyl oxidase and induce bone collagen degradation in a rat model of renal osteodystrophy. Lab Invest 93:1170–1183.
48. Galli F (2007) Protein damage and inflammation in uraemia and dialysis patients. Nephrol Dial Transplant 22 (Suppl 5):v20–36.
49. Miyata T, Ueda Y, Shinzato T, Iida Y, Tanaka S, et al. (1996) Accumulation of albumin-linked and free-form pentosidine in the circulation of uremic patients with end-stage renal failure: renal implications in the pathophysiology of pentosidine. J Am Soc Nephrol 7:1198–1206.
50. Sakata N, Noma A, Yamamoto Y, Okamoto K, Meng J, et al. (2003) Modification of elastin by pentosidine is associated with the calcification of aortic media in patients with end-stage renal disease. Nephrol Dial Transplant 18:1601–1609.
51. Zoccali C, Mallamaci F, Asahia K, Benedetto FA, Tripepi G, et al. (2001) Pentosidine, carotid atherosclerosis and alterations in left ventricular geometry in hemodialysis patients. J Nephrol 14:293–298.
52. Arsov S, Graaff R, van Oeveren W, Stegmayr B, Sikole A, et al. (2014) Advanced glycation end-products and skin autofluorescence in end-stage renal disease: a review. ClinChem Lab Med 52:11–20.
53. Mitome J, Yamamato H, Saito M, Yokoyama K, Marumo K, et al. (2011)Nonenzymaticcross-linking pentosidine increase in bone collagen and are associated with disorders of bone mineralization in dialysis patients. Calcif Tissue Int 88:521–529.
54. Glenn JV, Beattie JR, Barrett L, Frizzell N, Thorpe SR, et al. (2007) Confocal Raman microscopy can quantify advanced glycation end product (AGE) modifications in Bruch's membrane leading to accurate, nondestructive prediction of ocular aging. FASEB J 21:3542–52.
55. Nyman JS, Roy A, Acuna RL, Gayle HJ, Reyes MJ, et al. (2006). Age-related effect on the concentration of collagen crosslinks in human osteonal and interstitial bone tissue. Bone 39:1210–1217.
56. Odetti P, Rossi S, Monacelli F, Poggi A, Cirnigliaro M, et al. (2005) Advanced glycationend products and bone loss during aging. Ann NY AcadSci 1043:710–717.
57. Saito M, Fujii K, Mori Y, Marumo K (2006) Role of enzymatic and glycation induced cross-links as a determinant of bone quality in spontaneously diabetic WBN/Kob rats. Osteoporosis Int 17: 1514–1523.
58. Silva MJ, Brodt MD, Lynch MA, McKenzie JA, Tanouye KM, et al. (2009) Type 1 diabetes in young rats leads to progressive trabecular bone loss, cessation of cortical bone growth, and diminished whole bone strength and fatigue life. J Bone Miner Res 24: 1618–1627.
59. Malluche HH, Porter DS, Monier-Faugere M, Mawad H, Pienkowski D (2012)Differences in bone quality in low- and high-turnover renal osteodystrophy. J Am Soc Nephrol 23:525–532.

7

Plasminogen Activator Inhibitor-1 Is Involved in Impaired Bone Repair Associated with Diabetes in Female Mice

Li Mao[1], Naoyuki Kawao[1], Yukinori Tamura[1], Katsumi Okumoto[2], Kiyotaka Okada[1], Masato Yano[1], Osamu Matsuo[1], Hiroshi Kaji[1]*

1 Department of Physiology and Regenerative Medicine, Kinki University Faculty of Medicine, Osaka, Japan, **2** Life Science Research Institute, Kinki University, Osaka, Japan

Abstract

Previous studies suggest that fracture healing is impaired in diabetes; however, the underlying mechanism remains unclear. Here, we investigated the roles of plasminogen activator inhibitor-1 (PAI-1) in the impaired bone repair process by using streptozotocin (STZ)-induced diabetic female wild-type (*PAI-1*$^{+/+}$) and PAI-1-deficient (*PAI-1*$^{-/-}$) mice. Bone repair and the number of alkaline phosphatase (ALP)-positive cells at the site of a femoral bone damage were comparable in *PAI-1*$^{+/+}$ and *PAI-1*$^{-/-}$ mice without STZ treatment. Although the bone repair process was delayed by STZ treatment in *PAI-1*$^{+/+}$ mice, this delayed bone repair was blunted in *PAI-1*$^{-/-}$ mice. The reduction in the number of ALP-positive cells at the site of bone damage induced by STZ treatment was attenuated in *PAI-1*$^{-/-}$ mice compared to *PAI-1*$^{+/+}$ mice. On the other hand, PAI-1 deficiency increased the levels of ALP and type I collagen mRNA in female mice with or without STZ treatment, and the levels of Osterix and osteocalcin mRNA, suppressed by diabetic state in *PAI-1*$^{+/+}$ mice, were partially protected in *PAI-1*$^{-/-}$ mice. PAI-1 deficiency did not affect formation of the cartilage matrix and the levels of types II and X collagen and aggrecan mRNA suppressed by STZ treatment, although PAI-1 deficiency increased the expression of chondrogenic markers in mice without STZ treatment. The present study indicates that PAI-1 is involved in the impaired bone repair process induced by the diabetic state in part through a decrease in the number of ALP-positive cells.

Editor: Luc Malaval, INSERM U1059/LBTO, Université Jean Monnet, France

Funding: This study was supported in part by a grant-in-aid (24590289) from the Ministry of Science, Education to H. Kaji and Japan China Sasakawa Medical Fellowship to L. Mao. The funders had no role in study design, data collection and analysis, decision to publish, or preparation of the manuscript.

Competing Interests: The authors have declared that no competing interests exist.

* E-mail: hkaji@med.kindai.ac.jp

Introduction

The risk of fracture is increased in diabetic patients mainly due to impairment of the bone formation process [1,2]. It is well accepted that type 1 diabetes is associated with a significant decrease in skeletal mass and an increase in fracture risk [1,2]. The detrimental skeletal effects of glucose toxicity, insulin deficiency and diabetic complications might partly explain the association between type 1 diabetes and osteoporosis [3–5]. Previous findings suggest that a decrease in osteoblastic bone formation is a major contributor to diabetic osteoporosis [4,6]. However, the pathogenesis of this skeletal fragility and impaired bone formation in type 1 diabetic patients remain to be fully clarified.

The recruitment of bone marrow-derived mesenchymal stem cells to the site of injury is impaired in diabetic patients [7]. Impaired mobilization and a reduced number of endothelial progenitor cells in diabetic patients prevent vasculogenesis and delay the healing process [8]. Cells that are critical to wound healing, such as fibroblasts, keratinocytes, and endothelial cells, become functionally impaired when exposed to a diabetic high-glucose environment *in vitro* [9,10]. In human studies, hematopoietic stem cell and proangiogenic cell mobilization in response to granulocyte colony-stimulating factor is impaired in diabetes, which might be related to the impaired tissue repair [11]. Several studies indicate that diabetes leads to impaired fracture healing [12–16], and this abnormal repair is insulin-dependent, because it was reversed by insulin treatment [13,17]. More recent studies have shown that the impaired fracture healing observed in diabetic state might be due to the loss of cartilage caused by increased apoptosis and osteoclastogenesis, which is followed by a reduction in the cartilaginous template for endochondral bone formation [13–15]. Increased chondrocyte and osteoblast apoptosis is tumor necrosis factor (TNF)-α-mediated, along with increased osteoclast survival, leading to destruction of early callus tissue and impeding fracture healing [13–15]. However, the details in mechanism of impaired bone repair and fracture healing in diabetic state still remain unclear.

Plasminogen activator inhibitor-1 (PAI-1) is the principal inhibitor of plasminogen activator, and hence fibrinolysis. Several reports have shown that circulating PAI-1 levels are elevated in type 1 and type 2 diabetic patients and animals [18–20]. PAI-1 has various functions, including regulation of extracellular matrix (ECM) degradation, cell migration, and apoptosis [21]. Daci *et al.* previously reported that PAI-1 deficiency partially protects against bone loss in estrogen-deficient mice [22]. Our recent study also showed that PAI-1 deficiency protects against diabetic bone loss in female mice [20]. Clarifying the mechanism of bone repair and regeneration is important to meet the clinical demand for bone reconstruction. We recently showed that plasminogen is crucial for bone repair in mice [23], indicating that the tissue fibrinolytic system is important for bone repair and fracture healing. These findings suggest that PAI-1 may play a crucial role in the bone repair process. However, the role of PAI-1 in impaired bone repair process observed in diabetes is unknown.

In the present study, we therefore examined the effects of PAI-1 deficiency on the impaired bone repair in diabetes by using a mouse model of diabetes induced by streptozotocin (STZ) in female wild-type (*PAI-1*$^{+/+}$) and PAI-1- deficient (*PAI-1*$^{-/-}$) mice.

Materials and Methods

Ethics statement

All mouse experiments were performed according to the Guide for the Care and Use of Laboratory Animals from the National Institutes of Health and the institutional guidelines for the use and care of laboratory animals at Kinki University. The protocol was approved by the Experimental Animal Welfare Committee of Kinki University (permit numbers: KAME-23-023 and KAME-24-009). All surgeries and the collection of quantitative computed tomography (qCT) images were performed under 2% isoflurane. The mice were euthanized with pentobarbital sodium (over 50 mg/kg, intraperitoneally). All efforts were made to minimize suffering.

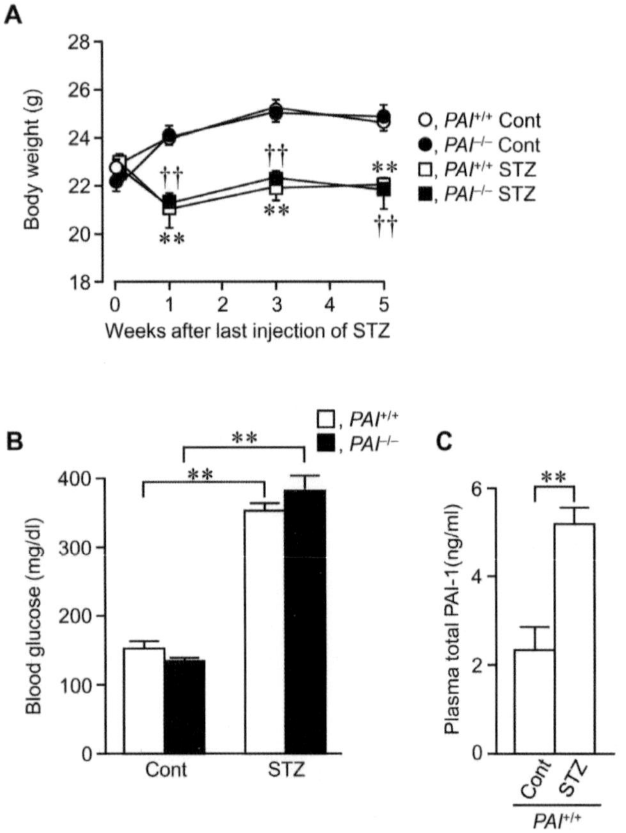

Figure 1. Effects of streptozotocin (STZ) treatment on body weight, blood glucose, and plasma PAI-1 levels in female mice. (A) Growth curve during experiments in control (Cont) and STZ-treated female *PAI-1*$^{+/+}$ and *PAI-1*$^{-/-}$ mice. Results are expressed as the means ± SEM. **$p<0.01$ vs. the *PAI-1*$^{+/+}$ control group, ††$p<0.01$ vs. *PAI-1*$^{-/-}$ control group. (n = 5 in each group). (B) Blood glucose in control and STZ-treated female *PAI-1*$^{+/+}$ and *PAI-1*$^{-/-}$ mice. Results are expressed as means ± SEM. **$p<0.01$ (n = 5 in each group). (C) Plasma total PAI-1 levels in control and STZ-treated female *PAI-1*$^{+/+}$ mice. Results are expressed as means ± SEM. **$p<0.01$ (n = 5 in each group).

Animals

Female *PAI-1*$^{+/+}$ and *PAI-1*$^{-/-}$ mice, 10 weeks old, with a mixed C57BL/6J (81.25%) and 129/SvJ (18.75%) background, were used. These mice were kindly provided by Professor D. Collen (University of Leuven, Belgium).

Diabetic mouse model

Diabetes was induced in female *PAI-1*$^{+/+}$ and *PAI-1*$^{-/-}$ mice by daily intraperitoneal injections of STZ (50 mg/kg body weight, in saline) (Sigma, St Louis, MO, USA, # S0130), a pancreatic β-cell cytotoxin, for 4 days, as previously described [20]. Controls were injected with saline. Four days after the last injection (day 4), non-fasting blood glucose levels were measured with a glucometer (Glutest Ace, Sanwa Kagaku Kenkyusyo, Nagoya, Japan) by using blood obtained from the tail vein. Mice with blood glucose levels greater than 300 mg/dl were considered diabetic. At 2 weeks after induction of diabetes, a bone defect surgery was performed in the right femur of the mice. Animals were maintained in metabolic cages on a 12-h light/dark cycle, and they received food and water *ad libitum*.

Blood measurements

Blood was obtained from mice at 4 weeks after induction of diabetes. Plasma total PAI-1 was measured using a Murine Total PAI-1 ELISA kit (Molecular Innovations, MI, USA, # MPAIKT-TOT).

Bone defect model

A bone defect was induced in the mice according to a previously described method [23]. Briefly, under anesthesia induced by 2% isoflurane, the anterior skin over the mid-femur of the right leg was incised longitudinally for 5 mm in length. After splitting the muscle, the surface of femoral bone was exposed. Then, a hole was made using a drill with a diameter of 0.9 mm during the saline irrigation to prevent thermal necrosis of the margins. The incised skin was then sutured in a sterile manner, and anesthesia was discontinued. Body temperature was maintained at 37°C during surgery by a heating pad.

In vivo quantitative computed tomography (qCT) analysis

The mice were anesthetized using 2% isoflurane, and the femur was scanned using an X-ray CT system (Latheta LCT-200; Hitachi Aloka Medical, Tokyo, Japan). Parameters for the CT scans were as follows: tube voltage, 50 kVp; tube current, 500 μA; integration time, 3.6 ms; axial field of view, 48 mm, with an isotropic voxel size of 48 μm. Images were generated by integration of 2 signal averages for the femur. Total scan time was approximately 5 min. Volume-rendered 3-dimensional CT pictures were reconstructed using the VGStudio MAX2.2 software (Nihon Visual Science, Tokyo, Japan). The area of the bone defect in the femur was quantified using an image processing program (ImageJ, http://rsbweb.nih.gov/ij/download.html).

Histological analysis

Mice were anesthetized using pentobarbital sodium (50 mg/kg, intraperitoneally) on day 7 after surgery. The femur was removed, fixed in 4% paraformaldehyde, demineralized in 22.5% formic acid and 340 mM sodium citrate solution for 24 h, and then embedded in paraffin. Thereafter, 4-μm-thick sections were obtained. Immunostaining was performed as described previously [23]. Briefly, the sections were incubated with an anti-alkaline phosphatase (ALP) antibody (Abnova, Taipei, Taiwan, # PAB12279) at a dilution of 1:100 followed by incubation with

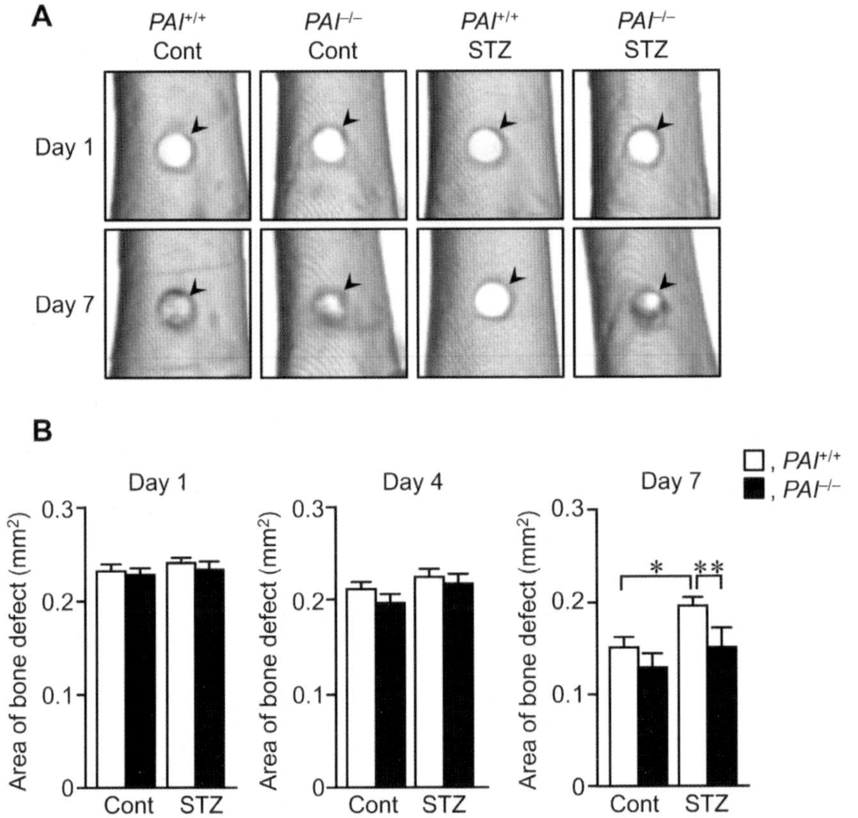

Figure 2. Bone repair after a femoral bone defect. (A) Three-dimensional images of the damaged site on days 1 and 7 after a femoral bone defect in female *PAI-1*$^{+/+}$ and *PAI-1*$^{-/-}$ mice with or without STZ treatment, as assessed by qCT. The arrowheads indicate the damaged site. (B) Quantification of the area at the damaged site on days 1, 4, and 7 after a femoral bone defect in female *PAI-1*$^{+/+}$ and *PAI-1*$^{-/-}$ mice with or without STZ treatment. Data represent the mean ± SEM of 5-6 mice. **p*<0.05, ***p*<0.01. Cont, control.

the appropriate secondary antibody conjugated with horseradish peroxidase (Nichirei Biosciences Inc., Tokyo, Japan, # 414341). Positive signals were visualized using a tyramide signal amplification system (PerkinElmer, Waltham, MS, USA, # NEL744B001KT). The number of ALP-positive cells per 0.1 mm^2 in the microscopic fields of the damaged site of femur was quantified in a blinded evaluation, as described previously [23]. The number of ALP-positive osteoblast-like cells per 1 mm of bone surface (N.Ob/BS) and osteoblast surface per bone surface (Ob.S/BS) were measured according to the guidelines of the American Society of Bone and Mineral Research [24]. The sections were stained with tartrate-resistant acid phosphatase (TRAP) by using a TRAP staining kit (Wako Pure Chem., Osaka, Japan, # 294-678001). The number of TRAP-positive multinucleated cells per 1 mm of bone surface was measured at the damaged site of the femur in a blinded evaluation. The sections were processed for Alcian blue and toluidine blue staining. The areas of the cartilage matrices that included proteoglycans and glycosaminoglycans were quantified by measuring the Alcian blue-positive areas and the metachromatic areas in the sections stained with toluidine blue using image processing software (Mac SCOPE; Mitani Co., Fukui, Japan) in a blinded evaluation.

Real-time polymerase chain reaction (PCR) analysis

Bone samples were crushed in liquid nitrogen, and total RNA was extracted from the homogenized samples using an RNeasy mini kit (Qiagen, Tokyo, Japan, # 74104). Real-time PCR was performed with a StepOne Plus cycler using Fast SYBR GREEN PCR Master Mix (Life Technologies Japan, Tokyo, Japan, # 4385610). The primer sets used are shown in Table S1. The mRNA levels of target genes in the mouse tissues were normalized relative to the levels of glyceraldehyde-3-phosphate dehydrogenase (GAPDH) mRNA.

Statistical analysis

Data are expressed as means ± SEM. Statistical significance was assessed using unpaired 2-tailed *t*-tests and one-way ANOVA. Differences with *p* values less than 0.05 were considered statistically significant. All statistical analyses were performed using StatView version 5.0 software (SAS Institute; Cary, NC, USA).

Results

Effects of STZ treatment in female mice

STZ treatment decreased the body weight of *PAI*$^{+/+}$ and *PAI*$^{-/-}$ mice from 7 days after the last injection of STZ (Fig. 1A). Four days after the final STZ injection, blood glucose levels were markedly elevated in *PAI*$^{+/+}$ and *PAI*$^{-/-}$ mice (Fig. 1B), indicating that STZ induced diabetes in the mice. Consistent with the elevation in blood glucose levels, circulating PAI-1 levels were elevated by STZ treatment in *PAI*$^{+/+}$ mice (Fig. 1C). These data were compatible with those obtained in our previous study [20].

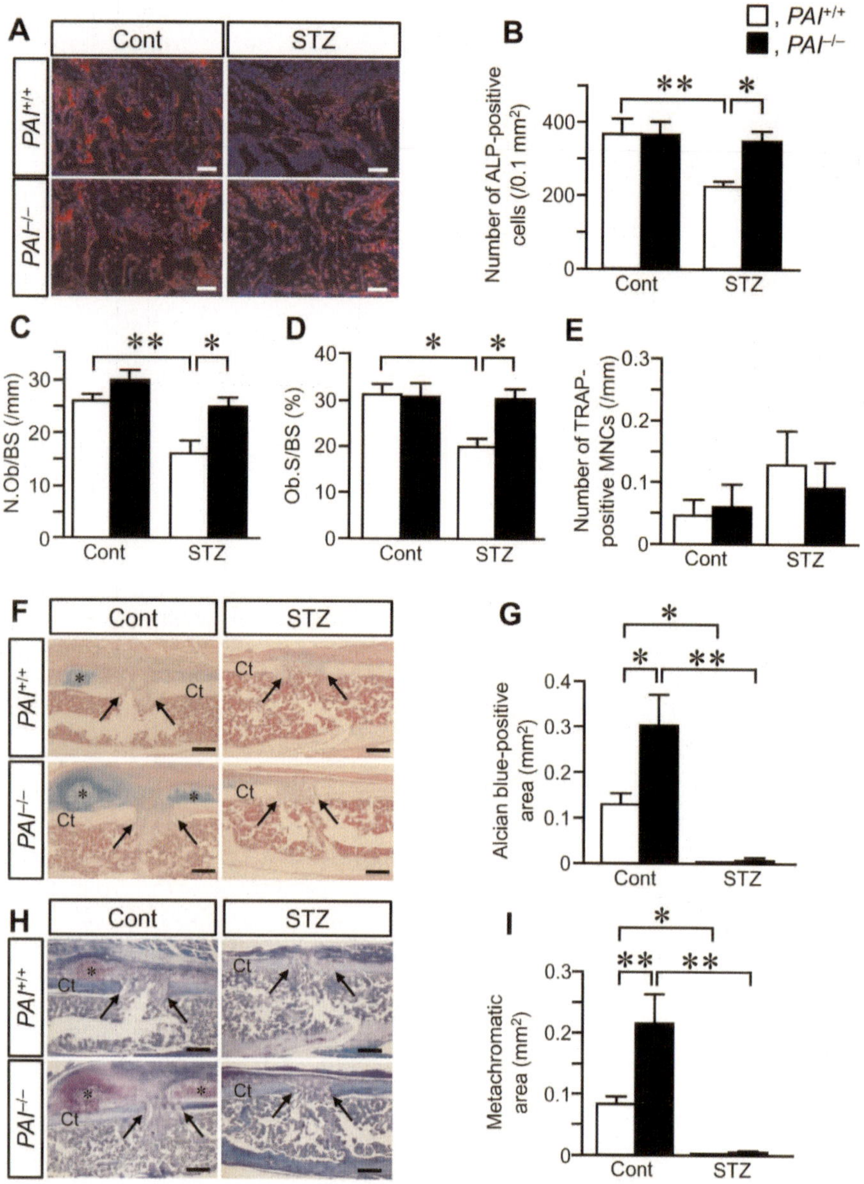

Figure 3. Histological analysis of the damaged site after a femoral bone defect. (A) Microphotographs of ALP-positive cells at the damaged site on day 7 after a femoral bone defect in female *PAI-1*$^{+/+}$ and *PAI-1*$^{-/-}$ mice with or without STZ treatment. (B) The number of ALP-positive cells per 0.1 mm^2 of the microscopic field in the damaged site on day 7 after a femoral bone defect in female *PAI-1*$^{+/+}$ and *PAI-1*$^{-/-}$ mice with or without STZ treatment. (C) The number of ALP-positive osteoblast-like cells per 1 mm of bone surface (N.Ob/BS) at the damaged site on day 7 in female *PAI-1*$^{+/+}$ and *PAI-1*$^{-/-}$ mice with or without STZ treatment. (D) Osteoblast surface per bone surface (Ob.S/BS) at the damaged site on day 7 in female *PAI-1*$^{+/+}$ and *PAI-1*$^{-/-}$ mice with or without STZ treatment. (E) The number of TRAP-positive multinucleated cells (MNCs) per 1 mm of bone surface at the damaged site on day 7 in female *PAI-1*$^{+/+}$ and *PAI-1*$^{-/-}$ mice with or without STZ treatment. (F) Microphotographs of Alcian blue-stained sections at the damaged site on day 7 after a femoral bone defect in female *PAI-1*$^{+/+}$ and *PAI-1*$^{-/-}$ mice with or without STZ treatment. The sections were counterstained with nuclear fast red. Asterisks indicate the Alcian blue-positive region. (G) Quantification of the Alcian blue-positive area at the damaged site on day 7 in female *PAI-1*$^{+/+}$ and *PAI-1*$^{-/-}$ mice with or without STZ treatment. (H) Microphotographs of toluidine blue-stained sections at the damaged site on day 7 after a femoral bone defect in female *PAI-1*$^{+/+}$ and *PAI-1*$^{-/-}$ mice with or without STZ treatment. Asterisks indicate the metachromatic region. (I) Quantification of the area of the metachromatic region in the sections stained with toluidine blue at the damaged site on day 7 in female *PAI-1*$^{+/+}$ and *PAI-1*$^{-/-}$ mice with or without STZ treatment. The results are from experiments performed on 5-6 mice in each group (A, F, H). Scale bars indicate 50 (A) and 300 μm (F, H). The arrows indicate the edge of the damaged site in the inner cortex (F, H). Data represent the mean ± SEM of 5-6 mice (B-E, G, I). *$p<0.05$, **$p<0.01$. Cont, control. Ct, cortical bone.

Bone repair after a femoral bone defect

The damaged site on the femur was progressively and similarly repaired in *PAI-1*$^{+/+}$ and *PAI-1*$^{-/-}$ mice without STZ treatment until day 7, as assessed by qCT (Fig. 2A, B). Conversely, the damaged site significantly remained on day 7 in *PAI-1*$^{+/+}$ mice with STZ treatment (Fig. 2A, B). This delay in bone repair was blunted in *PAI-1*$^{-/-}$ mice with STZ treatment.

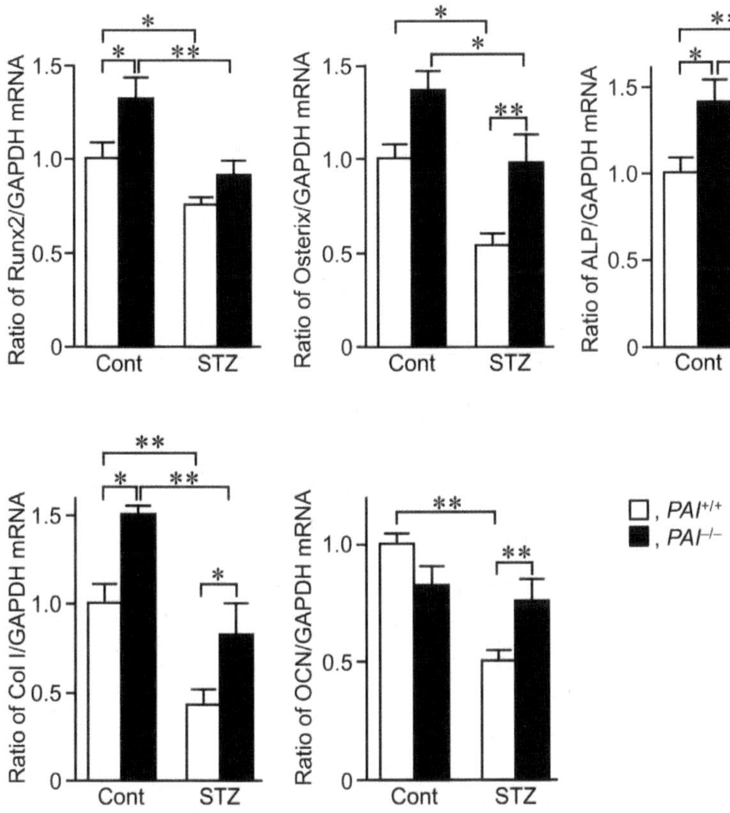

Figure 4. Effects of PAI-1 deficiency on osteogenic differentiation during bone repair in female mice. The levels of Runx2, Osterix, ALP, type I collagen (Col I), and osteocalcin (OCN) mRNA at the damaged site on day 7 after a femoral bone defect in female *PAI-1*$^{+/+}$ and *PAI-1*$^{-/-}$ mice with or without STZ treatment. Data are expressed relative to GAPDH mRNA values, and are expressed as the mean ± SEM. *$p<0.05$, **$p<0.01$ (n = 5–7 in each group). Cont, control.

Histological analysis of the damaged site after a femoral bone defect

The number of ALP-positive cells at the damaged site on day 7 was similar in both *PAI-1*$^{+/+}$ and *PAI-1*$^{-/-}$ mice without STZ treatment (Fig. 3A, B). STZ treatment significantly reduced the number of ALP-positive cells at the damaged site in female *PAI-1*$^{+/+}$ mice (Fig. 3A, B). However, consistent with the decreased bone repair observed in the diabetic state, PAI-1 deficiency significantly blunted the reduction in the number of ALP-positive cells at the damaged site in diabetic *PAI-1*$^{-/-}$ mice (Fig. 3A, B). N.Ob/BS and Ob.S/BS at the damaged site were similar on day 7 in *PAI-1*$^{+/+}$ and *PAI-1*$^{-/-}$ mice without STZ treatment (Fig. 3C, D). Although STZ treatment significantly reduced the N.Ob/BS and Ob.S/BS at the damaged site in female *PAI-1*$^{+/+}$ mice, PAI-1 deficiency significantly blunted the reductions in N.Ob/BS and Ob.S/BS induced by the diabetic state (Fig. 3C, D). Conversely, the number of TRAP-positive multinucleated cells per bone surface was not significantly different between *PAI-1*$^{+/+}$ and *PAI-1*$^{-/-}$ mice on day 7 regardless of STZ treatment (Fig. 3E).

PAI-1 deficiency significantly increased the formation of the cartilage matrix at the damaged site on day 7 after a femoral bone defect in sections stained with Alcian blue and toluidine blue (Fig. 3F–I). STZ treatment significantly reduced the formation of cartilage matrix in *PAI-1*$^{+/+}$ and *PAI-1*$^{-/-}$ mice. PAI-1 deficiency did not affect the formation of cartilage matrix suppressed by STZ (Fig. 3F–I).

Analysis of osteogenic, bone resorption, osteoclast, chondrogenic, and adipogenic marker gene expression in bone tissues at the damaged site

Next, we examined the levels of osteogenic marker mRNA in the bone tissues at the damaged site after a femoral bone defect in female *PAI-1*$^{+/+}$ and *PAI-1*$^{-/-}$ mice. The levels of Runx2, ALP, and type I collagen mRNA were significantly increased in *PAI-1*$^{-/-}$ mice, compared to those in *PAI-1*$^{+/+}$ mice without STZ treatment (Fig. 4). The levels of Osterix and osteocalcin mRNA were similar in *PAI-1*$^{+/+}$ and *PAI-1*$^{-/-}$ mice without STZ treatment on day 7 (Fig. 4). STZ treatment significantly reduced the levels of Runx2, Osterix, ALP, type I collagen, and osteocalcin mRNA in *PAI-1*$^{+/+}$ mice, and PAI-1 deficiency significantly blunted the levels of Osterix, ALP, type I collagen, and osteocalcin mRNA that were suppressed by STZ treatment. (Fig. 4).

We examined the levels of bone resorption markers in bone tissues at the damaged site after a femoral bone defect in female mice. The levels of TRAP, receptor activator of nuclear factor κB ligand (RANKL), and osteoprotegerin (OPG) mRNA as well as the ratio of RANKL/OPG were similar in *PAI-1*$^{+/+}$ and *PAI-1*$^{-/-}$ mice without STZ treatment on day 7 (Fig. 5A–D). STZ treatment significantly reduced the levels of RANKL mRNA in *PAI-1*$^{+/+}$ and *PAI-1*$^{-/-}$ mice (Fig. 5B), although it did not affect the levels of TRAP mRNA (Fig. 5A). STZ treatment seemed to reduce the levels of OPG mRNA and the ratio of RANKL/OPG in *PAI-1*$^{+/+}$ mice, although the differences were not statistically significant

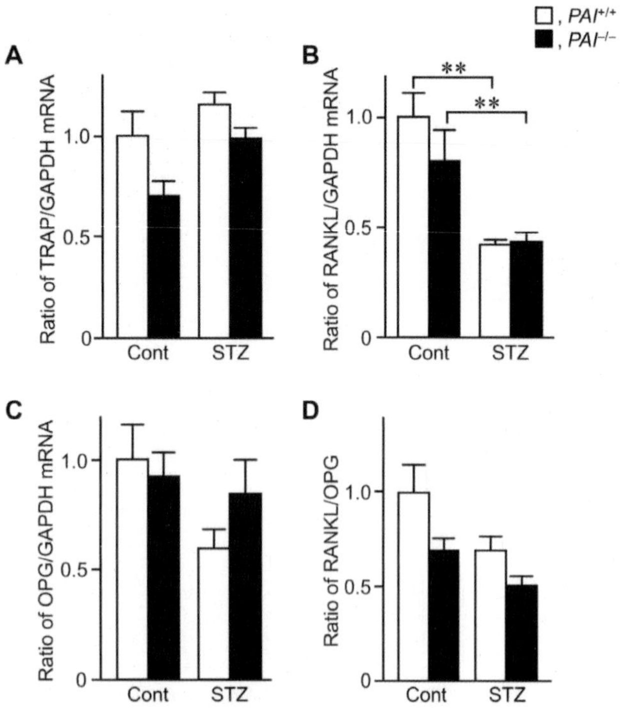

Figure 5. Effects of PAI-1 deficiency on bone resorption markers during bone repair in female mice. (A–C) The levels of TRAP, RANKL, and osteoprotegerin (OPG) mRNA at the damaged site on day 7 after a femoral bone defect in female *PAI-1*$^{+/+}$ and *PAI-1*$^{-/-}$ mice with or without STZ treatment. Data are expressed relative to GAPDH mRNA values, and are expressed as mean ± SEM. (D) The ratio of RANKL/OPG mRNA at the damaged site on day 7 after a femoral bone defect in female *PAI-1*$^{+/+}$ and *PAI-1*$^{-/-}$ mice with or without STZ treatment. **$p<0.01$ (n = 5–7 in each group). Cont, control.

(Fig. 5C, D). PAI-1 deficiency did not affect the levels of RANKL mRNA suppressed by STZ treatment (Fig. 5B).

Finally, we examined the levels of chondrogenic and adipogenic markers in bone tissues at the damaged site after a femoral bone defect in female *PAI-1*$^{+/+}$ and *PAI-1*$^{-/-}$ mice. As shown in Fig. 6A, PAI-1 deficiency significantly enhanced the levels of type II collagen and aggrecan mRNA in bone tissues at the damaged site after a femoral bone defect, although it did not affect the levels of type X collagen mRNA. STZ treatment significantly reduced the levels of chondrogenic markers in *PAI-1*$^{+/+}$ mice, and PAI-1 deficiency did not affect the levels of chondrogenic markers suppressed by STZ treatment (Fig. 6A). In contrast, PAI-1 deficiency decreased the levels of peroxisome proliferator-activated receptor γ (PPAR-γ) mRNA, but not adipocyte protein-2 (aP-2) mRNA at the damaged site after a femoral bone defect (Fig. 6B). STZ treatment enhanced the levels of aP-2 mRNA, but not PPAR-γ mRNA in *PAI-1*$^{+/+}$ mice. PAI-1 deficiency did not affect the levels of adipogenic marker genes in mice with STZ treatment (Fig. 6B).

Discussion

PAI-1, as a pivotal component of fibrinolytic system, belongs to the serine protease inhibitor (serpin) superfamily [25]. It is synthesized in several tissues, including bone, and is the principal inhibitor of plasminogen activators (PA) [26]. The fibrinolytic system participates in a wide variety of functions in mammals beyond its proteolytic effect on thrombi. Several studies have suggested the involvement of the PA/PAI-1 system in bone metabolism [27,28]. Our recent study using plasminogen-deficient mice showed that plasminogen deficiency decreases cartilage formation and osteoblastogenesis at the damaged site of femur after bone defect [23]. These findings imply that the tissue fibrinolytic system is involved in the bone repair process.

PAI-1 deficiency protects from increased bone turnover and trabecular bone loss in pathological states, such as estrogen deficiency [22]. Moreover, we recently demonstrated that PAI-1 deficiency protects against diabetic bone loss in female mice [20]. These observations suggest a specific role for PAI-1 in the regulation of trabecular bone turnover and osteoblastic bone formation, especially in some specific pathological conditions. The present study showed that diabetic wild-type mice displayed an obvious delay in bone repair, compared to non-diabetic wild-type mice from qCT analysis, which was compatible with previous evidence on fracture repair [16]. Moreover, PAI-1 deficiency rescued the impaired bone repair caused by the diabetic state, indicating that PAI-1 is involved in the delayed bone repair induced by the diabetic state in female mice. Our previous study suggested that the diabetic state increases PAI-1 expression in the liver, resulting in elevation of circulating PAI-1 levels in female mice [20]. The increased levels of circulating PAI-1 induced by the diabetic state might be responsible for the impaired bone repair, and the enhancement of the PA/plasminogen system induced by inactivation of PAI-1 might compensate the bone repair process suppressed by the diabetic state. These findings are consistent with our previous findings that plasminogen deficiency impairs bone repair [23]. Further studies will be necessary to clarify the mechanisms, by which PAI-1 impairs bone repair.

We previously revealed that the induction of diabetes decreases bone mineral density (BMD) and bone strength index and suppresses the expression of osteogenic genes in female wild-type mice, but not in PAI-1-deficient mice [20]. In the present study, we revealed that PAI-1 deficiency blunted the decrease in the number of ALP-positive osteoblastic cells induced by the diabetic state. Moreover, the levels of osteogenic genes, such as Osterix, ALP, type I collagen, and osteocalcin, were decreased at the damaged site of femur in female diabetic wild-type mice. These effects seemed to be reversed by PAI-1 deletion. In addition, our previous study revealed that active PAI-1 treatment reduces the levels of Runx2, Osterix, and ALP mRNA as well as ALP activity and mineralization in primary osteoblasts obtained from female wild-type mice [20]. These findings suggest that PAI-1 deficiency alleviates the impairment of bone repair associated with the diabetic state partly by protecting against diabetes-impaired osteoblastogenesis at the damaged site.

PAI-1 might impair osteoblast function by directly affecting osteoblasts in the diabetic state in female mice during bone repair. Accumulating evidence suggests that the diabetic state impairs stem cell function and negatively regulates tissue repair [6,11,29]. Extrinsic signaling from the surrounding ECM plays a pivotal role in converting mesenchymal stem cells into commitment osteogenic lineage, then terminally differentiating into osteoblasts [30]. PAI-1 inhibits the function of PA, hence suppresses activations of pro-matrix metalloproteinases (MMPs), which finally interfere with ECM remodeling, in pathological conditions. Previous studies revealed that MMPs activity is increased in the fibrotic liver and asthmatic lung in PAI-1-deficient mice [31,32]. Moreover, Krause *et al.* showed that the decrease in the levels of active MMP-9 in diabetic mice was restored by systemic treatment with a PAI-1 inhibitor, suggesting that the increase in PAI-1 levels induced by the diabetic state suppresses the activation of pro-MMPs [33]. Based on this knowledge, we can speculate that the protective

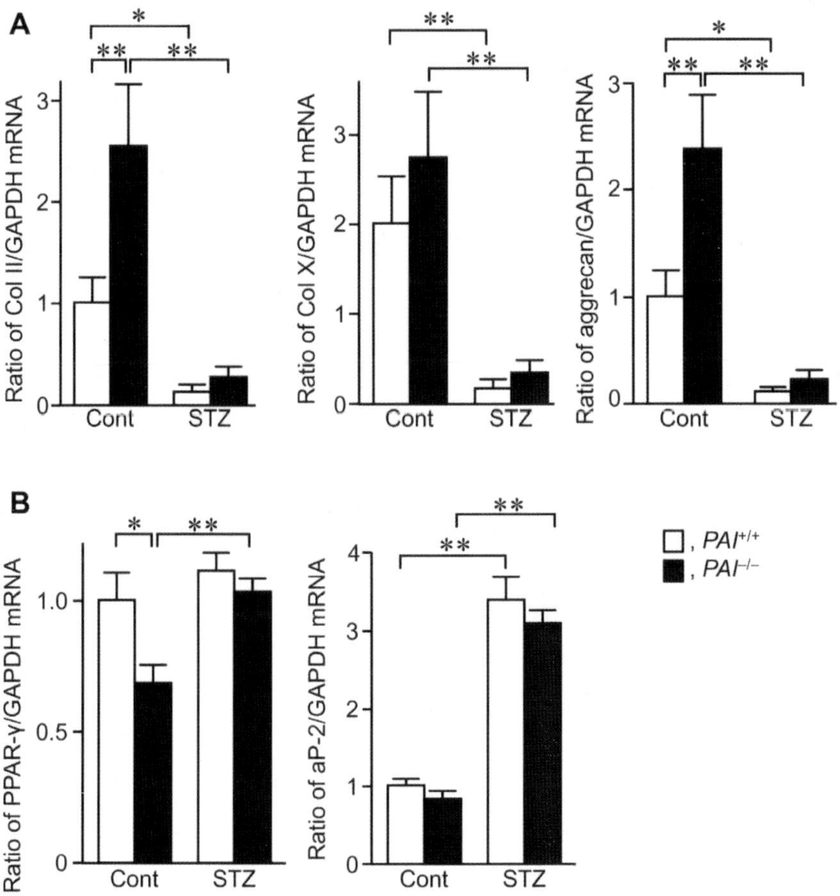

Figure 6. Effects of PAI-1 deficiency on chondrogenic or adipogenic differentiation during bone repair in female mice. (A) The levels of type II collagen (Col II), type X collagen (Col X), and aggrecan mRNA at the damaged site on day 7 after a femoral bone defect in female *PAI-1*$^{+/+}$ and *PAI-1*$^{-/-}$ mice with or without STZ treatment. Data are expressed relative to GAPDH mRNA values, and are expressed as mean ± SEM. **p*<0.05, ***p*<0.01 (n = 5–7 in each group). (B) The levels of PPAR-γ and aP-2 mRNA at the damaged site on day 7 after a femoral bone defect in female *PAI-1*$^{+/+}$ and *PAI-1*$^{-/-}$ mice with or without STZ treatment. Data are expressed relative to GAPDH mRNA values, and are expressed as mean ± SEM. **p*<0.05, ***p*<0.01 (n = 5–7 in each group). Cont, control.

effects of PAI-1 deficiency on the delayed bone repair induced by the diabetic state could be explained by the activation of MMPs, which modify the surrounding ECM microenvironments, consequently promoting mesenchymal stem cell differentiation into osteoblasts. Moreover, decreased growth factors such as insulin-like growth factor-I and fibroblast growth factor-2 are related to diminished bone formation during bone repair in diabetes [16]. The details of mechanism, by which PAI-1 is involved in the impaired bone repair process in the diabetic state, remain incompletely understood.

In the present study, PAI-1 deficiency significantly elevated the levels of Runx2, ALP, and type I collagen mRNA at the damaged site after a femoral bone defect in female mice without STZ treatment. Moreover, PAI-1 deficiency blunted the reduction in the number of ALP-positive cells induced by STZ treatment at the damaged site in mice. Our previous study showed that PAI-1 suppressed the levels of Runx2, ALP, and type I collagen mRNA in primary osteoblasts from mouse calvaria [20]. These findings suggest that PAI-1 suppresses osteoblast differentiation in both physiological and pathological states.

The fracture healing process can be divided into 3 stages: acute inflammation, repair, and remodeling. In the repair phase, the fracture site is repaired through the process of endochondral ossification, i.e., the formation of cartilage and the replacement of the cartilage by bone accompanied with the invasion of blood vessels [34]. Rundle *et al.* suggested that PAI-1 deficiency does not adversely affect the overall fracture healing process, but significantly enlarges the fracture callus in the non-diabetic state [35]. Our study showed that PAI-1 deficiency does not accelerate the bone repair process in female mice without diabetes, but it increases the cartilage matrix and the levels of chondrogenic marker mRNA such as type II collagen and aggrecan at the damaged site in female mice without diabetes. These results are consistent with the previous report by Rundle *et al.* [35]. However, their study showed that remodeling of the fracture callus was accelerated in PAI-1-deficient mice than in wild-type mice [35]. These data suggest enhancement of the tissue fibrinolytic system by PAI-1 deficiency that stimulates fracture healing through facilitation of ECM remodeling. The present study showed that PAI-1 deficiency rescued the impaired bone repair caused by the diabetic state. Taken together, PAI-1 might be involved in ECM remodeling during fracture healing in the diabetic state. Diabetes impairs cartilage formation during fracture healing through decreased chondrocyte differentiation and proliferation [17]. However, the diabetic state reduced the cartilage matrix and the levels of these chondrocyte markers in both wild-type and PAI-1-deficient mice in the present study, suggesting that PAI-1 deficiency could not compensate for the suppression of chondrogenesis induced by the diabetic state.

Mesenchymal stem cells have the ability to differentiate into chondrogenic and adipogenic lineage cells. Several studies revealed that an altered mesenchymal stem cell lineage selection toward adipocytes rather than osteoblasts is related to the mechanism of diabetic bone loss [6]. Bone marrow adiposity is observed in aged and type 1 diabetic bone tissues, which may be associated with a decrease in BMD [36]. Meanwhile, PAI-1 deficiency blunted the change in the levels of adipogenic genes that were increased with diabetes in tibia from female mice [20], suggesting that PAI-1 deficiency restores bone formation by promoting the differentiation of mesenchymal stem cells into osteoblasts instead of adipocytes. However, the present study revealed that the diabetic state did not induce PPAR-γ at the damaged site in wild-type female mice. Moreover, the levels of aP-2 mRNA were similar between diabetic wild-type and PAI-1-deficient mice, although the levels of aP-2 mRNA, known as an adipokine associated with the adipocyte phenotype, were increased in diabetic mice. These findings suggest that an altered mesenchymal stem cell lineage selection toward adipocytes rather than osteoblasts is not important for the bone repair process impaired by the diabetic state, compared to that in diabetic bone loss, because PPAR-γ is considered a key transcriptional factor that regulates adipogenesis [19,20,36].

In conclusion, our study showed that PAI-1 deficiency attenuates diabetic impaired bone repair in female mice partly through a reverse of the reduction in the number of osteoblasts induced by diabetic state, suggesting that PAI-1 is involved in the impaired bone repair induced by type I diabetes in female mice. Diabetic patients exhibit reduced BMD, an increase risk of fracture, and impairment in the fracture healing process. Our observations therefore provide a novel promising approach to ameliorate fracture healing impairment and promote bone regeneration in patients with diabetes.

Author Contributions

Conceived and designed the experiments: LM NK HK. Performed the experiments: LM NK YT K. Okumoto K. Okada MY OM. Analyzed the data: LM NK HK. Wrote the paper: LM HK.

References

1. Janghorbani M, Van Dam RM, Willett WC, Hu FB (2007) Systematic review of type 1 and type 2 diabetes mellitus and risk of fracture. Am J Epidemiol 166: 495–505.
2. Vestergaard P (2007) Discrepancies in bone mineral density and fracture risk in patients with type 1 and type 2 diabetes—a meta-analysis. Osteoporos Int 18: 427–444.
3. Hofbauer LC, Brueck CC, Singh SK, Dobnig H (2007) Osteoporosis in patients with diabetes mellitus. J Bone Miner Res 22: 1317–1328.
4. Merlotti D, Gennari L, Dotta F, Lauro D, Nuti R (2010) Mechanisms of impaired bone strength in type 1 and 2 diabetes. Nutr Metab Cardiovasc Dis 20: 683–690.
5. Wongdee K, Charoenphandhu N (2011) Osteoporosis in diabetes mellitus: Possible cellular and molecular mechanisms. World J Diabetes 2: 41–48.
6. McCabe LR (2007) Understanding the pathology and mechanisms of type I diabetic bone loss. J Cell Biochem 102: 1343–1357.
7. Shin L, Peterson DA (2012) Impaired therapeutic capacity of autologous stem cells in a model of type 2 diabetes. Stem Cells Transl Med 1: 125–135.
8. Liao YF, Chen LL, Zeng TS, Li YM, Fan Y, et al. (2010) Number of circulating endothelial progenitor cells as a marker of vascular endothelial function for type 2 diabetes. Vasc Med 15: 279–285.
9. Shoji T, Koyama H, Morioka T, Tanaka S, Kizu A, et al. (2006) Receptor for advanced glycation end products is involved in impaired angiogenic response in diabetes. Diabetes 55: 2245–2255.
10. Lerman OZ, Galiano RD, Armour M, Levine JP, Gurtner GC (2003) Cellular dysfunction in the diabetic fibroblast: impairment in migration, vascular endothelial growth factor production, and response to hypoxia. Am J Pathol 162: 303–312.
11. Fadini GP, Albiero M, Vigili de Kreutzenberg S, Boscaro E, Cappellari R, et al. (2013) Diabetes impairs stem cell and proangiogenic cell mobilization in humans. Diabetes Care 36: 943–949.
12. Simpson CM, Calori GM, Giannoudis PV (2012) Diabetes and fracture healing: the skeletal effects of diabetic drugs. Expert Opin Drug Saf 11: 215–220.
13. Kayal RA, Alblowi J, McKenzie E, Krothapalli N, Silkman L, et al. (2009) Diabetes causes the accelerated loss of cartilage during fracture repair which is reversed by insulin treatment. Bone 44: 357–363.
14. Kayal RA, Tsatsas D, Bauer MA, Allen B, Al-Sebaei MO, et al. (2007) Diminished bone formation during diabetic fracture healing is related to the premature resorption of cartilage associated with increased osteoclast activity. J Bone Miner Res 22: 560–568.
15. Kayal RA, Siqueira M, Alblowi J, McLean J, Krothapalli N, et al. (2010) TNF-alpha mediates diabetes-enhanced chondrocyte apoptosis during fracture healing and stimulates chondrocyte apoptosis through FOXO1. J Bone Miner Res 25: 1604–1615.
16. Retzepi M, Donos N (2010) The effect of diabetes mellitus on osseous healing. Clin Oral Implants Res 21: 673–681.
17. Gandhi A, Beam HA, O'Connor JP, Parsons JR, Lin SS (2005) The effects of local insulin delivery on diabetic fracture healing. Bone 37: 482–490.
18. Mathieu P, Lemieux I, Despres JP (2010) Obesity, inflammation, and cardiovascular risk. Clin Pharmacol Ther 87: 407–416.
19. Ma LJ, Mao SL, Taylor KL, Kanjanabuch T, Guan Y, et al. (2004) Prevention of obesity and insulin resistance in mice lacking plasminogen activator inhibitor 1. Diabetes 53: 336–346.
20. Tamura Y, Kawao N, Okada K, Yano M, Okumoto K, et al. (2013) Plasminogen activator inhibitor-1 is involved in streptozotocin-induced bone loss in female mice. Diabetes 62: 3170–3179.
21. Declerck PJ, Gils A (2013) Three decades of research on plasminogen activator inhibitor-1: a multifaceted serpin. Semin Thromb Hemost 39: 356–364.
22. Daci E, Verstuyf A, Moermans K, Bouillon R, Carmeliet G (2000) Mice lacking the plasminogen activator inhibitor 1 are protected from trabecular bone loss induced by estrogen deficiency. J Bone Miner Res 15: 1510–1516.
23. Kawao N, Tamura Y, Okumoto K, Yano M, Okada K, et al. (2013) Plasminogen plays a crucial role in bone repair. J Bone Miner Res 28: 1561–1574.
24. Dempster DW, Compston JE, Drezner MK, Glorieux FH, Kanis JA, et al. (2013) Standardized nomenclature, symbols, and units for bone histomorphometry: a 2012 update of the report of the ASBMR Histomorphometry Nomenclature Committee. J Bone Miner Res 28: 2–17.
25. Pannekoek H, Veerman H, Lambers H, Diergaarde P, Verweij CL, et al. (1986) Endothelial plasminogen activator inhibitor (PAI): a new member of the Serpin gene family. EMBO J 5: 2539–2544.
26. Sprengers ED, Kluft C (1987) Plasminogen activator inhibitors. Blood 69: 381–387.
27. Allan EH, Martin TJ (1995) The plasminogen activator inhibitor system in bone cell function. Clin Orthop Relat Res: 54–63.
28. Daci E, Udagawa N, Martin TJ, Bouillon R, Carmeliet G (1999) The role of the plasminogen system in bone resorption in vitro. J Bone Miner Res 14: 946–952.
29. Lu H, Kraut D, Gerstenfeld LC, Graves DT (2003) Diabetes interferes with the bone formation by affecting the expression of transcription factors that regulate osteoblast differentiation. Endocrinology 144: 346–352.
30. Stevens MM, George JH (2005) Exploring and engineering the cell surface interface. Science 310: 1135–1138.
31. Wang H, Zhang Y, Heuckeroth RO (2007) PAI-1 deficiency reduces liver fibrosis after bile duct ligation in mice through activation of tPA. FEBS Lett 581: 3098–3104.
32. Oh CK, Ariue B, Alban RF, Shaw B, Cho SH (2002) PAI-1 promotes extracellular matrix deposition in the airways of a murine asthma model. Biochem Biophys Res Commun 294: 1155–1160.
33. Krause MP, Moradi J, Nissar AA, Riddell MC, Hawke TJ (2011) Inhibition of plasminogen activator inhibitor-1 restores skeletal muscle regeneration in untreated type 1 diabetic mice. Diabetes 60: 1964–1972.
34. Claes L, Recknagel S, Ignatius A (2012) Fracture healing under healthy and inflammatory conditions. Nat Rev Rheumatol 8: 133–143.
35. Rundle CH, Wang X, Wergedal JE, Mohan S, Lau KH (2008) Fracture healing in mice deficient in plasminogen activator inhibitor-1. Calcif Tissue Int 83: 276–284.
36. Rosen CJ, Ackert-Bicknell C, Rodriguez JP, Pino AM (2009) Marrow fat and the bone microenvironment: developmental, functional, and pathological implications. Crit Rev Eukaryot Gene Expr 19: 109–124.

Abandoned Acid? Understanding Adherence to Bisphosphonate Medications for the Prevention of Osteoporosis among Older Women: A Qualitative Longitudinal Study

Charlotte Salter[1]*, Lisa McDaid[1], Debi Bhattacharya[2], Richard Holland[1], Tarnya Marshall[3], Amanda Howe[1]

1 Norwich Medical School, Faculty of Medicine & Health Science, University of East Anglia, Norwich, Norfolk, United Kingdom, **2** School of Chemistry and Pharmacy, University of East Anglia, Norwich, Norfolk. United Kingdom, **3** Rheumatology Department, Norfolk & Norwich University Foundation Trust Hospital. Norwich, Norfolk. United Kingdom

Abstract

Background: There is significant morbidity and mortality caused by the complications of osteoporosis, for which ageing is the greatest epidemiological risk factor. Preventive medications to delay osteoporosis are available, but little is known about motivators to adhere to these in the context of a symptomless condition with evidence based on screening results.

Aim: To describe key perceptions that influence older women's adherence and persistence with prescribed medication when identified to be at a higher than average risk of fracture.

Design of Study: A longitudinal qualitative study embedded within a multi-centre trial exploring the effectiveness of screening for prevention of fractures.

Setting: Primary care, Norfolk. United Kingdom

Methods: Thirty older women aged 70–85 years of age who were offered preventive medication for osteoporosis and agreed to undertake two interviews at 6 and 24 months post-first prescription.

Results: There were no overall predictors of adherence which varied markedly over time. Participants' perceptions and motivations to persist with medication were influenced by six core themes: understanding adherence and non-adherence, motivations and self-care, appraising and prioritising risk, anticipating and managing side effects, problems of understanding, and decision making around medication. Those engaged with supportive professionals could better tolerate and overcome barriers such as side-effects.

Conclusions: Many issues are raised following screening in a cohort of women who have not previously sought advice about their bone health. Adherence to preventive medication for osteoporosis is complex and multifaceted. Individual participant understanding, choice, risk and perceived need all interact to produce unpredictable patterns of usage and acceptability. There are clear implications for practice and health professionals should not assume adherence in any older women prescribed medication for the prevention of osteoporosis. The beliefs and motivations of participants and their healthcare providers regarding the need to establish acceptable medication regimes is key to promoting and sustaining adherence.

Editor: Christy Elizabeth Newman, The University of New South Wales, Australia

Funding: Funding came from Research for Patient Benefit Programme National Institute for Health Research PG-PB-0807-14068. The funder had no role in study design, data collection and analysis, decision to publish, or preparation of the manuscript.

Competing Interests: The authors have declared that no competing interests exist.

* E-mail: c.salter@uea.ac.uk

Introduction

There is significant morbidity and mortality caused by the complications of osteoporosis, for which ageing is the greatest epidemiological risk factor. While other risks such as immobility, persistent low body weight, early menopause and corticosteroid use may lead to early onset of osteoporosis, around 40% of women aged 70 will have osteoporosis, and as many as 90% will have a significantly increased risk of fracturing a bone in a fall or accident [1], [2]. This has led to a major research focus on the prevention of osteoporosis which has established that osteoporotic fractures can be significantly reduced by a combination of pharmacological (bisphosphonates with calcium and vitamin D supplements) and behavioural interventions (dietary intake, smoking cessation, and weight bearing exercise).

More recent initiatives include the development of treatment algorithms and encouragement for primary care practitioners to identify patients who may be at 'risk' of fracturing and may benefit from preventive options [3],[4]. However, as the National Institute for Clinical Excellence (NICE) acknowledge, *"identifying who will benefit from preventative treatment is imprecise"* [5]. No population screening programme currently exists for osteoporosis risk, and individuals are identified clinically on a case by case basis. Predictive risk of fracture compared to the norm for age and sex can now be calculated using clinical risk factors in conjunction with bone mineral density (BMD) measurements using Dual energy X-ray Absorbtiometry (DXA) scans [6], [7], creating new opportunities to identify individuals yet to sustain a fracture.

For screening to be effective, participants identified as high risk must be receptive to the intervention. Achieving long-term adherence to prescribed medications is more complex than just providing sufficient information or an acceptable medication regimen. The literature suggests adherence is highly variable in osteoporosis prevention with age and co-morbidity explaining relatively little of the variability [8], [9]. Attempts to reduce complexity in dosing regimens do not necessarily improve adherence [10], [11]. Patients are recommended to take their bisphosphonates first thing in the morning before eating or drinking and with a glass of water. There is a requirement for them to remain upright for 30 minutes to avoid irritation to the oesophagus. Calcium supplements are frequently provided in the form of chewy tablets. Patients may understand the potential for osteoporosis to have a negative effect on their lives, and express strong motivation to protect their health, but this does not always align with taking medications [12], [13]. This therefore makes the motivations and decision making of older women around uptake of preventive medication of primary importance to the public health impact of any potential screening programme as well as to the individual patient.

It is also known that patterns of adherence to osteoporosis medications vary over time [14], [15]. However, a survey of patients and physicians showed that poor adherence reflected patient scepticism about the risks and values of treatment, rather than a lack of factual knowledge. A qualitative synthesis of studies on lay experience of medicine taking found widespread caution about taking medication with many participants 'testing' prescribed medicines for efficacy and adverse side effects [14]. Our pilot study found as many as 50% of women at 'high risk' of fracture in the 70–85 age group were not receiving treatment four months later [16]. We therefore undertook this study to explore the factors that influence older women's adherence to prescribed prophylactic medication when assessed to have higher than average risk of fracture following screening. This paper describes the perceptions and motivations to which participants attributed their willingness and ability to adhere to osteoporosis prevention regimes, and considers implications for practice.

Methods

Participants and procedure

The Adherence To Osteoporosis Medication (ATOM Study) was established as a longitudinal qualitative study embedded within the Medical Research Council funded UK multi-centre randomised control trial on Screening for Osteoporosis in Older Women for the Prevention of Fractures (SCOOP). SCOOP [17] aims to explore the effectiveness of screening women aged 70–85 for the prevention of fractures using a risk-prediction algorithm. The qualitative study took place in Norfolk, United Kingdom.

Ethics Statement

We secured approval from North West National Health Service Research Ethics Committee (Ref: 07/H1010/70). Written informed consent was obtained from participants. Two participants with mild cognitive impairment were supported in the consenting and interview process by their husbands.

The research comprised a longitudinal design with two in-depth interviews conducted 18 months apart, the first at around 6 months post-randomisation. The sample was drawn from those found to be at 'higher than average' risk of a subsequent fracture and whose prescribing data showed they had started medications for the prevention of osteoporosis. Participants were purposively sampled from demographic and adherence data already collected by the SCOOP trial (see Table 1). As the focus of our study was to explore why older women were adherent, we constructed our sample to include more women self-reporting they were adherent when contacted by phone than reporting they were non-adherent to their osteoporosis medication.

For the purpose of this study 'adherent' included both women stating they were taking bisphosphonate medication as instructed, and those stating they were intentionally or unintentionally missing doses but no more than 1 in 5 (i.e. 80% adherence or more). Non-adherent' included all those who had discontinued bisphosphonate medication, or were taking them <80% of the time, but who might still be taking prescribed supplements (calcium and vitamin D).

The interviews

Interviews took place at participants' homes and lasted an average of 74 minutes. They were based on a topic guide developed to explore women's understanding of osteoporosis, responses to screening results, current usage of preventive medicine, motivators and detractors from taking medication and follow up with healthcare professionals. Interview recordings were transcribed verbatim and anonymised. Familiarisation, data management, coding and categorisation were carried out by the interdisciplinary research team including CS, LM and AH. Iteration between both data sets and the research literature helped inform the analysis at the explanatory level. The principles of Framework Analysis [18] were used to order, chart and search the data both manually and supported by relevant software (NVivo 9 Software, MSWord and Framework). Illustrative quotations are selected to elucidate the study findings. Extracts are labelled using participant number, age at interview and summary adherence status to both bisphosphonates and calcium supplements.

Results

Ninety women in the 'higher than average' risk group recruited to the Norwich arm of the SCOOP Trial indicated they would be willing to take part in the qualitative sub-study. From these we recruited a sample of 30 (33%) women, age range 73–85 years (Table 1). Five participants were unable to participate in the follow-up interview due to death or withdrawal from the study.

Understanding adherence and non-adherence

All 30 participants were prescribed bisphosphonates and all except one commenced their first course. Of the 10 participants shown in Table 2 who reported being non-adherent at Phase 1 Interviews, nine made this decision without discussion with their

Table 1. Sample characteristics using pre-collected trial data.

Sample Characteristic	Category	Number (%)
Self-reported adherence status given on phone at recruitment	Adherent	19 (63)
	Non-adherent	11 (37)
Age	70–74	9 (30)
	75–79	10 (33)
	80+	11 (37)
GP practice	Urban	14 (47)
	Rural	16 (53)
Social class	I	3 (10)
	II	6 (20)
	IIIN	6 (20)
	IIIM	10 (33)
	IV	5 (17)
	V	0

general pracitioner. All bar one said they had done this within a month of collecting their first prescription. The combination of bisphosphonate and calcium: vitamin D supplements was reported to be taken by 12 participants.

Of the 25 participants who took part in Phase 2 Interviews, thirteen had remained adherent to bisphosphonate medication and one previously non-adherent participant reported she had started taking her medication as prescribed. Eleven were non-adherent including three women that had given up their bisphosphonate medicine between interviews. Thus, a significant proportion of our sample were taking *no medication* for the prevention of fracture and osteoporosis at 18 months (44%). Even within the 'adherent' group, many women admitted deficits in their adherence; sometimes this was deliberate, to avoid inconvenience, sometimes it was because they forgot one day, but took it the next.

We found no obvious pattern or factors linking with adherence. Responses to screening, acceptance of risk status, existing medical history, previous experience of falls, fractures and family history did not appear to predict womens' adherence status.

Some participants complained about the complexity of the regimen, many had experienced side effects, some said their general practitioner had stopped the medication, and some had misunderstood the reasons for taking them long-term. However, many adherent women reported similar issues. Few cited 'forgetting' as a key cause of non-adherence. Almost all respondents declared a willingness to 'in principle' do what their general practitioner advised, but some non-adherent women cited medical permission or support for their choice to stop:

> He was quite happy, he said alright just stop. He said we've had no broken bones in your family, he said you'll probably be quite alright. (Participant 12, age 84 – became Non-Adherent to Bisphosphonates by Phase 2. Refused Calcium)

Personal scepticism about the value of the treatments did not seem to link clearly with non-adherence. For example, the following participant was adherent to her medications, but demonstrated very little belief that she needed them at her age:

> I thought well yes I am 80, so I probably have anyway (thinning bones) and I also thought it is a bit *late* to start treating me now I honestly did. That was my sort of attitude but the letter said 'go and see your doctor', so I went and saw my doctor and he gave me those. (Participant 24, age 80

Table 2. Summary of Patterns of Adherence.

	Bisphosphonates	Calcium Supplements	Bisphosphonates & Calcium Supplements
	N (%)	N (%)	N (%)
Phase 1			
Adherent	20 (67)	15 (50)	12 (40)
Non-adherent	10 (33)	10 (33)	13 (43)
Not prescribed	-	5 (17)	5 (17)
Total	30 (100)	30 (100)	30 (100)
Phase 2			
Adherent	14 (56)	12 (48)	9 (36)
Non-adherent	11 (44)	9 (36)	12 (48)
Not prescribed	-	4 (16)	4 (16)
Total	25 (100)	25 (100)	25 (100)

- Adherent to both Bisphosphonates & Calcium Phase 1, subsequently withdrew)

By contrast Participant 22 was non-adherent. She felt anyone could break a bone in the next 10 years and would have expected to fracture by now if she was really at risk. She described how her own mother had fallen and broken her hip yet appeared to remain personally unconcerned:

> When they said well look 'a higher risk of breaking a bone over the next 10 years' and I thought well *I'm over 80 so it's not surprising* (laughs). (Participant 22, age 84 – Continually Non-Adherent to both Bisphosphonates & Calcium)

Motivations, self-care and adherence

All the respondents regardless of adherence status seemed to have accepted the need for better self-care and an altered lifestyle in order to prevent fractures. Many believed they had been doing this all their lives through a good diet, plenty of physical activity and exercise:

> Because I've always taken calcium you know. I've always had a lot of cheese, a lot of yoghurt and I drink a certain amount of milk I have calcium and I have a lot of vegetables. (Participant 10, age 73 - Continually adherent bisphosphonates. Calcium not prescribed)

> I take a cod liver oil pill every day, winter and summer. I'm sure that's a help. (Participant 09, age 85 - Continually non-adherent bisphosphonates & calcium)

In addition, many participants had adjusted their daily routines to enhance their capacity to take their regimens as prescribed. Weekly doses were linked with memorable events, and chores such as ironing utilised to fulfil the half hour required in remaining upright:

> So I try and get up early, take it with this load of water and find something to do standing up, whether it's ironing for an hour which I did this week (laughs) or going round the garden seeing what's in flower. You have just got to find something to do which takes your mind off it. (Participant 06, age 80 – Continually Adherent to Bisphosphonates. Non-adherent to Calcium)

> Market day is a Wednesday and I always used to go down to buy plants every Wednesday. I always used to think I can't go down and get any plants, so I always remember Wednesday. That was my day. (Participant 30, age 75 – Continually Non-Adherent to Bisphosphonates. Took Calcium supplements at Phase 2)

Carers played a role in aiding adherence for two participants with cognitive impairments by bringing the medication to them and altering the routine to ensure no food or cup of tea at the same time:

> He'd put it on his computer to remind me (and) he puts them in front of me and lets me get on with it. (Participant 17, age 75 – Continually Adherent Bisphosphonates. Calcium not prescribed).

Autonomy was also a powerful motivator, characterised by the need to be independent and responsible in order to be able to care for self and others:

> Well it is just the independence. I don't want to be a nuisance to the family at all if I can help it, and if I haven't done something that might have helped I'd feel a bit guilty. If you can do anything to prevent that happening it does help a little bit. (Participant 03, age 83 – Continually Adherent Bisphosphonates. Calcium not prescribed)

> I like to protect myself as much as possible for my husband, well for me (too) for me I mean obviously. (Participant 18, age 80 – Non-Adherent Bisphosphonates by Phase 2. Non-adherent to Calcium)

Appraising and prioritising risk

Phase 1 interviews specifically asked participants about their reaction to their recent risk assessment. Risk perceptions at this phase were mostly expressed in 'sense making' comments regarding the context of ageing. There was added complexity for participants who had been given a risk status of 'higher than average' but had no visible signs or experience of symptoms:

> *Not in a million years.* I thought oh they'll come back and say oh you're fine. And they wrote back and said I wasn't. Yes I thought I couldn't believe it because I've always had a balanced diet. (Participant 29, age 75 – Continually Adherent to both Bisphosphonates & Calcium)

Many of those who had initially questioned their risk status and expressed negative reactions had adjusted to their status and cited measures taken to be self-protective such as not climbing ladders and prioritising a calcium rich diet:

> Oh yeah it's made me *more* careful since I had that density scan and had the letter to say that um (pause) you know on average, if I fell over I would more easily break a bone than you know than normal. So that was a *good* thing because it has made me more (careful) and as you notice, I've got no rugs. (Participant 24, age 80 - Adherent to both Bisphosphonates & Calcium Phase 1, subsequently withdrew)

We explored the data for links between positive self-caring attitudes (as exemplified by women in the first interviews giving examples of longstanding commitment to weight bearing exercise and good nutrition) and active embracing of pharmacological options for preventing fractures. We also looked for an interrelationship between women's 'accepting' versus 'questioning' of their risk assessment and adherence to prescribed medication, including their reported participation in the decision making process and recourse to other support and information. Neither state appeared to be linked with long-term adherence with equal numbers of women remaining adherent to their medication who were 'questioning' (n = 7) as 'accepting' (n = 7). Furthermore, there was no link to adherence from either an initial strong emotive reaction or passive acceptance. For example, the following initially adherent participant had moved from a state of shock to positive acceptance, and yet gave up on her medication within a year:

> Well in a way when I got over the shock I thought well I know something more about my body. (Participant 07, age 74 - Became Non- Adherent to Bisphosphonates by Phase 2. Adherent to Calcium)

However, the long-term and hidden changes of bones which 'thin' or 'crumble' seemed a lower priority than other illnesses. Participants' recall of medication reviews mirrored this, with most women reporting that their osteoporosis medications was rarely reviewed or mentioned in consultations.

Anticipating and managing side effects

Eighteen women experienced side effects from mild to very severe. These ranged from unsettled stomach problems to violent nausea, vomiting bile, and burning:

> They're *horrible* they really were. Well I mean honestly I got a really sore stomach and then on Monday my stomach was really bad and honestly it just felt full of air and I'd touch it and it was sore. (Participant 24, age 80 - Adherent to both Bisphosphonates & Calcium Phase 1, subsequently withdrew)

While severe side effects were linked to non-adherence, there was no simple relationship between side effects and persisting with medication, some trying up to 3 different medications. In fact, the anticipation of side effects seemed to be enough to put off some participants, with three in particular reporting that they were put off by the possible side effects described in the medicines information leaflet. Even the name 'alendronic acid' was cause for concern for some:

> Because it says *acid* (laughs). It isn't a natural thing. I just don't like the idea of taking an acid and not lying down. (Participant 13, age 75 – became adherent by Phase 2. Adherent to Calcium)

The need for support concerning side effects was also highlighted by a number of non-adherent women who anticipated side effects that might aggravate existing problems:

> To me it seemed more important that I, you know, (avoid) this reflux than breaking my hip because I thought I can be *careful*. (Participant 23, age 81 – tried one Bisphosphonate tablet only. Non-starter Calcium)

> The tablets that he gave me when I read the side effects it was like a *horror film* really. And I thought well I'm better off chancing, sort of breaking a bone, than all the horrible things it said on there about (how) you could get these stomach ulcers and all things like that. And I do suffer sort of with heartburn and things like that. You have to sort of keep upright for so long after taking the tablets. I thought well I'm better off as I am than more things wrong really. (Participant 21, age 75 – non-starter Bisphosphonates and Calcium)

Problems of understanding

A number of problems of understanding were evident in the interviews regarding osteoporosis risk, prevention and management in older women. Although there was fear and concern about developing osteoporosis, there was also a perception that falling and fracturing were normal in old age. Others debated the magnitude of risk, especially when compared to problems such as diabetes and heart disease. Some women questioned why the Dual energy X-ray Absorbtiometry screening had not been repeated to monitor the effectiveness of the medication. Nine patients adherent at Phase 1 mentioned this specifically, and 3 of these had become non-adherent by Phase 2:

> I really would like to have another scan to see how my body is now, if it's any worse or still the same or whatever. I'd like to do that but apparently they don't, they like to leave it a certain amount of years don't they? I've read that. (Participant 24, age 80 - Adherent to both Bisphosphonates & Calcium Phase 1, subsequently withdrew)

> I mean if you're going through all that performance, well it was for me with the lack of being able to swallow, but if you think you are doing that to no avail, you think well what's the point. (Participant 25, age 77 - became Non-adherent to Bisphosphonates & Calcium Phase 2)

A number of women in both groups expressed significant confusion about the nature and importance of the risk portrayed by the positive screening result. There was also confusion between falls and fractures, with some participants talking about their fracture risk in terms of instability rather than fragility:

> As I say, I would have thought somebody with osteoporosis would have fallen over and broken their bones. (Participant 07, age 74 - Non adherent to Bisphosphonates by Phase 2. Adherent to Calcium)

> I was surprised because I felt that I'd not had a lot of falls or tottery or anything. I thought people that were at higher risk were inclined to fall. (Participant 01, age 75 - Continually Adherent to Bisphosphonates. Took Calcium intermittently)

> So I thought well that (bisphosphonate medication) will prevent me falling cos the main reason was if my bones got stronger I could do more in the garden and things like that and get on the steps more often. I can't anyway cos I get dizzy (but) that was my thoughts. (Participant 30, age 75 - Continually Non adherent to Bisphosphonates. Took Calcium at Phase 2)

Confusion about the effectiveness of the medication was common and participants frequently reflected on 'not knowing' if they were getting any benefit from taking the medication or not. Participant 16 was fully adherent with no side effects, but felt it was 'discouraging not knowing if it works', as did others:

> I suppose the fact of never having broken anything coupled with the fact there's no signal in your body is there? There's nothing that tells you that there is anything wrong, so you

don't feel that there's anything wrong. (Participant 08, age 75 – Continually Adherence Bisphosphonates and Calcium)

Decision making around medication

Overall we found clear if unpredictable narratives around medication choice, with key factors being the initial result, side effects and subsequent health service intervention of medication prescription. Decisions were reviewed in a number of situations and personal costs weighed up against perceived benefits of taking the medication. Participant 09 described how she made the decision in the light of her own understanding of her needs and the relative benefit of taking the medication. She made her final decision in consultation with her doctor:

There is no bone disease or any sign of it in our family but I said I would take it and see what happened. It didn't suit me and I said I'm not taking them anymore and he (doctor) agreed. He said 'it's no good taking them if they upset you because your diabetes is more important'. (Participant 09, age 85 – became non adherent by Phase 2 to Bisphosphonates and Calcium)

Many of those non-adherent to bisphosphonate medication at Phase 2 had not asked for, or been offered, a change of medication (n = 10). However, five women still adherent to their medications and experiencing side effects had been back to their doctor at least once for an alternative prescription by Phase 2 (Table 3).

Although most participants cited encouragement by doctors, pharmacists, family, friends and the media, only three participants specifically mentioned any sort of formal follow-up (one at a diabetic review, one with a pharmacist and one with a nurse). Many felt specific follow-up would have given them more confidence:

I mean I'm all for taking it if I know what it's doing and if it's doing you good, but there's no follow up on these things. I have to go and get my blood pressure taken every six months. I feel like they know what's going on cos they have changed the different strengths at different times you know depending on how my blood pressure is. But you don't get any follow up with this.... I think they need to have more follow up on this. I'm taking it because it's doing me what it's supposed to be doing, but it's the not knowing and it's the not having the follow up to see whether you need to be taking it or not. (Participant 11, age 77 – Continually Adherent Bisphosphonates. Calcium not prescribed)

Table 3. Summary of Bisphosphonate medication changes and adherence for participants that experienced side effects at Phase 2 (n = 18).

	Adherent	Non-adherent
No change	2 (11)	10 (56)
Changed once	4 (22)	0
Changed twice	1 (6)	1 (6)
Total	**7 (39)**	**11 (61)**

One participant explicitly changed her mind and became adherent by Phase 2 having previously rejected the medication because of her doctor's insistence:

I didn't used to take that but then once I had this polymyalgia and I had to take the steroids. As I walked out of the doctors' room she said 'now look you must take that acid tablet because if not your bones will just crumble'. So whether I like it or not I'm taking it. (Participant 13, age 75 – became adherent by Phase 2. Adherent to Calcium)

In summary, many participants saw the medication as an adjunct to their own efforts to remain healthy and ward off the impacts of ageing. Additional convenience of medication dosing, a less off-putting name, and ways to reduce side effects would be likely to positively influence people's decisions to remain adherent to these medications.

Discussion

The data overall show a group of resilient older women doing their best to make sense of a particular set of health opportunities in their lives, and keen to manage the impacts of ageing and minimise increasing frailty and dependence. There was evidence that those who had engaged with professionals to establish and maintain regimens could tolerate and overcome barriers to adherence which had defeated others. The variation of adherence over time suggests that health professionals should not assume adherence in any older women who has relevant medication on their repeat medication list, and that the uncertainty of risk and desire not to worry participants must not confuse messages that these drugs can have a real positive health gain.

To our knowledge, no previous studies have undertaken longitudinal in depth interviews to identify factors which influence adherence to osteoporosis regimens in women who have been identified at high risk of fracture. Thus, the strength of this study is the repeat in depth interviews with older women that enabled follow up and discussion of change overtime. The limitations include potential sample bias: women who are keen to help research are potentially more motivated to self-care and take an active part in their own health.

However the context of this work is multifaceted and reflects the issues that arise following screening in a cohort of women who have not previously sought advice about their bone health. Overtime many medications that are routinely prescribed become objects embedded within everyday life and invested with particular meanings, values and identities [19]. However, our findings underline the fact that medications are complex social phenomena that may take time to embed and become routinized and acceptable to patients and healthcare professionals alike [20]. Medications, particularly medication prescribed prophylactically, have many levels of meaning [21]. Bisphosphonate medication for the prevention of osteoporosis and fracture is currently framed by a more complex social context where understanding, choice, risk and perceived need all interact to produce unpredictable patterns of usage and acceptability [22].

This study did not record consultation data or the perspective of general practitioners on their interactions around decision making on bisphosphonates. In depth sociolinguistic research has highlighted that patients talk and deploy different discourses and narratives depending on both the context and on the interactional resources available to them [23], [24], [25], [26]. Although most patients and their health care providers are likely to be keen to ensure that they utilise the outputs of modern medical advances, this is in the context of the increasing biomedicalisation of life, especially as people in developed countries are living longer [27]. Whether this is framed as a sophisticated commercial exploitation of societal fears of frailty and death, or as an unpredicted consequence of applying multiple disease related guidelines without considering the overall impact, there are consequences for individuals in making choices about their health-related practices each day. For example, recent authors have pointed out the likelihood of older people routinely being in receipt of multiple medications, even if they have not yet developed any specific disease [28], [29]. The cumulative costs of screenings, follow-ups, treatments and personal sequelae in terms of time, side effects, and perceived vulnerability or risk all need to be set against the potential benefits. The impacts of knowing that they are deemed to be at risk can move people from a narrative of their self as a healthy empowered person to one who is frail and in need of help, which can also have unexpected consequences [27].

Within this complex context, each patient and their doctor or nurse has to make individual decisions as to whether a risk factor should be prioritised or treated once detected. General practitioners are probably the medical professionals who are most aware of the extent to which the uptake of any new test or treatment is dependent on the beliefs, understanding, needs and expectations of the individual in front of them. It is a tenet of their discipline and training that any new health issue needs to be debated in the context of the person's whole life context, while maximising health gain and minimising adverse consequences of any intervention. It is the skill of a general practitioner to enable patients to make considered judgements in the face of these multiple choices. However, both the literature and our interviews suggest that preventive health measures often pose a challenge in time limited appointments, which may have influenced the decision made in some clinical encounters [30], [31], [32]. Furthermore, the fact that this was a research study may also have influenced overall uptake and follow-up in clinical practice. More research is needed on the effectiveness and efficacy of secondary prevention and the role of healthcare providers in this field.

Acknowledgments

We would like to acknowledge the staff and researchers of the Screening for Osteoporosis in Older women for the Prevention of fracture Trial from which this study grew, and the patients who were willing to undertake both studies. We also wish to thank our patient and public involvement leads from the NHS Norfolk 'PPIRes' panel, for their excellent guidance and input.

Disclaimer

This paper outlines independent research funded by the National Institute for Health Research (NIHR) under its Research for Patient Benefit Programme (RfPB) RfPB PB-PG-0807-14068. The views expressed are those of the authors and not necessarily those of the NHS, the NIHR or the Department of Health. The funders had no role in study design, data collection and analysis, decision to publish, or preparation of the manuscript.

Author Contributions

Conceived and designed the experiments: CS RH TM AH. Performed the experiments: CS LM. Analyzed the data: CS LM AH. Contributed reagents/materials/analysis tools: CS LM DB RH TM AH. Wrote the paper: CS LM DB RH TM AH.

References

1. Kanis JA (2002) Diagnosis of osteoporosis and assessment of fracture risk. Lancet 359: 1929–1936.
2. WHO (2003) Prevention and Management of osteoporosis. Geneva: WHO.
3. Verdijk NA, Romeijnders AC, Ruskus JJ, Van Der Sluijs C, Pop VJ (2009) Validation of the Dutch guidelines for dual X-ray absorptiometry measurement. The British Journal of General Practice 59: 256–260.
4. (SIGN) SIGN (2003) Management of osteoporosis risk.
5. NICE (2012) Osteoporosis: Assessing the risk of fragility fracture London: NICE.
6. WHO Fracture Risk Assessment Tool.
7. Kanis J, Glüer CC (2000) An update on the diagnosis and assessment of osteoporosis with densitometry. Osteoporosis International 11: 192–202.
8. Marshall IJ WC, McKevitt C (2012) Lay perspectives on hypertension and drug adherence: systematic review of qualitative research British Medical Journal 345.
9. Solomon DH AJ, Katz JN, Finklestein JS, Arnold M, Polinski JM, et al. (2005) Compliance with osteoporosis medications Arch Intern Med 165: 2414–2419.
10. Recker RR GR, MacCosbe PE (2005) Effect of dosing frequency on bisphosphonate medication adherence in a large longitudinal cohort of women Mayo Clin Proc 80: 856–861.
11. Rossini M BG, Di Munno O, Giannini S, Minisula S, Sinigaglia L, et al (2006) Determinants of adherence to osteoporosis treatment in clinical practice Osteoporosis International 17: 941-921.
12. (IOF) IOF (2005) The adherence gap: Why osteoporosis patients don't continue with treatment Nyon: IOF.
13. Pound P BN, Morgan M, Yardley L, Pope C, Daker-White G, et al. (2005) Resisting medicines: A synthesis of qualitative studies of medicine taking. Social Science & Medicine 61: 133–155.
14. Brookhart MA AJ, Katz JN, Finklestein JS, Arnold M, Polinski JM, et al. (2007) Gaps in treatment among users of osteoporosis medications: the dynamics of noncompliance Am J Med 120: 251–260.
15. Pickney CS AJ (2005) Correlation between patient recall of bone densitometry results and subsequent treatment adherence Osteoporosis International 16: 1156–1160.
16. L. S A Pragmatic Randomised Clinical Trail of the Effectiveness and Cost Effectiveness of Targeted Population Screening for Low Bone Mineral Density in the Prevention of next of Femur Fractures: ISRCTN 11021925.
17. Shepstone L FR, Lenaghan E, Harvey I, Cooper C, Gittoes N, et al. (2012) A pragmatic randomised controlled trial of the effectiveness and cost-effectiveness of screening older women for the prevention of fractures: Rationale, design and methods for the SCOOP study Osteoporosis International 23: 2507–2515.
18. Ritchie J LJ (2003) Qualitative research practice: A guide for social science students and researchers. London: Sage Publications.
19. Hodgetts D, Chamberlain K, Gabe J, Dew K, Radley A, et al. (2011) Emplacement and everyday use of medications in domestic dwellings. Health & Place 17: 353–360.
20. Cohen D, McCubbin M, Collin J, Pérodeau G (2001) Medications as social phenomena. Health: 5: 441–469.
21. Shoemaker SJ, Ramalho de Oliveira D, Alves M, Ekstrand M (2011) The medication experience: Preliminary evidence of its value for patient education and counseling on chronic medications. Patient education and counseling 83: 443–450.
22. Brown P, Calnan M (2012) Braving a faceless new world? Conceptualizing trust in the pharmaceutical industry and its products. Health: 16: 57–75.
23. Murdoch J, Salter C, Cross J, Smith J, Poland F (2013) Resisting medications: moral discourses and performances in illness narratives. Sociology of Health & Illness 35: 449–464.
24. Salter C, Holland R, Harvey I, Henwood K (2007) "I haven't even phoned my doctor yet." The advice giving role of the pharmacist during consultations for medication review with patients aged 80 or more: qualitative discourse analysis. BMJ 334: 1101.
25. Britten N, Stevenson F, Gafaranga J, Barry C, Bradley C (2004) The expression of aversion to medicines in general practice consultations. Social science & medicine 59: 1495–1503.
26. Murdoch J, Salter, C., Cross, J., & Poland, F. Misunderstandings, communicative expectations and resources in illness narratives: Insights from beyond interview transcripts.
27. Salter CI HA, Howe A, McDaid L, Lenaghan E, Blacklock J, et al (2011) Risk, significance and biomedicalisation of a new population: Older women's experience of osteoporosis screening Social Science & Medicine 73: 808–815.
28. Moynihan R DJ, Henry D (2012) Preventing overdiagnosis: How to stop harming the healthy British Medical Journal 244.
29. Moynihan R HI, Henry D (2002) Selling sickness: The pharmaceutical industry and disease mongering. British Medical Journal 324: 886–891.
30. Mirand AL BG, Kuo CL, Mahoney MC. (2003) Explaining the de-prioritization of primary prevention: Physicians' perceptions of their role in the delivery of primary care. BMC Public Health 3: 1–15.
31. Williams SJ CM (2008) Perspectives on prevention: The views of general practitioners. Sociol Health Ill 16: 372.393.
32. Poole KES CJ (2006) Osteoporosis and its management. BMJ 333.

9

Smoking and Body Fat Mass in Relation to Bone Mineral Density and Hip Fracture: The Hordaland Health Study

Jannike Øyen[1,2]*, Clara Gram Gjesdal[1,3], Ottar Kjell Nygård[3,4], Stein Atle Lie[5], Haakon E. Meyer[6,7], Ellen Margrete Apalset[1,2], Per Magne Ueland[3,8], Eva Ringdal Pedersen[3], Øivind Midttun[9], Stein Emil Vollset[2], Grethe S. Tell[2]

1 Department of Rheumatology, Haukeland University Hospital, Bergen, Norway, **2** Department of Global Public Health and Primary Care, University of Bergen, Bergen, Norway, **3** Department of Clinical Science, University of Bergen, Bergen, Norway, **4** Department of Heart Disease, Haukeland University Hospital, Bergen, Norway, **5** Department of Clinical Dentistry, University of Bergen, Bergen, Norway, **6** Section for Preventive Medicine and Epidemiology, University of Oslo, Oslo, Norway, **7** Norwegian Institute of Public Health, Division of Epidemiology, Oslo, Norway, **8** Laboratory of Clinical Biochemistry, Haukeland University Hospital, Bergen, Norway, **9** Bevital AS, Bergen, Norway

Abstract

Lower bone mineral density (BMD) in smokers may be attributable to lower body weight or fat mass, rather than to a direct effect of smoking. We analyzed the effects of smoking exposure, assessed by plasma cotinine, and body fat on BMD and the risk of subsequent hip fracture. In the community-based Hordaland Health Study (HUSK), 3003 participants 46–49 years and 2091 subjects 71–74 years were included. Cotinine was measured in plasma and information on health behaviors was obtained from self-administered questionnaires. BMD and total body soft tissue composition were measured by dual X-ray absorptiometry. Information on hip fracture was obtained from computerized records containing discharge diagnoses for hospitalizations between baseline examinations 1997–2000 through December 31st, 2009. In the whole cohort, moderate and heavy smokers had stronger positive associations between fat mass and BMD compared to never smokers (differences in regression coefficient (95% CI) per % change in fat mass = 1.38 (0.24, 2.52) and 1.29 (0.17, 2.4), respectively). In moderate and heavy smokers there was a nonlinear association between BMD and fat mass with a stronger positive association at low compared to high levels of fat mass (Davies segmented test, $p<0.001$). In elderly women and men, heavy smokers had an increased risk of hip fracture compared to never smokers (hazard ratio = 3.31, 95% CI: 2.05, 5.35; $p<0.001$). In heavy smokers there was a tendency of a lower risk of hip fracture with higher percentage of fat mass. The deleterious effect of smoking on bone health is stronger in lean smokers than in smokers with high fat mass.

Editor: Guoying Wang, Johns Hopkins Bloomberg School of Public Health, United States of America

Funding: This work was supported by the Western Norway Regional Health Authority and The Hordaland Health Study was partially funded by the Research Council of Norway. The funders had no role in study design, data collection and analysis, decision to publish, or preparation of the manuscript.

Competing Interests: The authors have declared that no competing interests exist.

* E-mail: jannike.oyen@igs.uib.no

Introduction

Cigarette smoking is associated with low bone mineral density (BMD) [1,2] and increased risk of fracture [1–4] in both women and men. The mechanisms behind the negative effects of smoking on bone are not completely known, but it is partly related to the influence from smoking on sex hormones in both genders [5]. A direct adverse effect of smoking on skeletal remodeling and bone cells has also been suggested [6], and in an animal model impaired bone formation was seen during nicotine exposure [7]. Further, smoking may decrease calcium absorption [8] and parathyroid hormone concentration [9].

Low body weight and low body mass index (BMI) are associated with low BMD [10], but the association between low BMI and fracture risk seems to be site specific. In some previous studies low BMI was associated with hip [11–13] and lower extremities fractures [12], while in a meta-analysis low BMI was associated with increased risk of all types of fractures [14]. In recently published studies the results are conflicting [15,16]. Low fat mass has been associated with increased risk of vertebral fractures in men [17] and hip fractures in women [11]. Accordingly, fat mass has been found to be positively associated with BMD in both women and men in some [18–20], but not all [21,22] studies. In a recently published meta-analysis including 44 studies, only four reported negative associations between fat mass and BMD in any participant subgroups [23]. Biochemical interactions between adipose tissue and bone are complex and linked by a multitude of pathways involving cytokines, adiponectin, insulin, and leptin, and hormones like insulin and estrogen [24].

On average, smokers have lower weight and lower fat mass than non-smokers [25]. In a Danish study on perimenopausal women a significant interaction was found between low fat mass ($<$13.3 kg) and current smoking on femoral neck BMD, demonstrating that among women with high fat mass ($>$19.0 kg) smoking did not affect BMD [25]. A Norwegian study described a 3-fold increased risk of hip fracture in lean (BMI$\leq$20 kg/m^2) female smokers compared to lean non-smokers, but no increased risk in smokers with BMI above the population mean ($>$25 kg/m^2) [3]. In men a 2-fold increased risk of hip fracture was found in smokers compared to non-smokers independently of BMI [3].

Studies of the association between smoking, BMD and fracture risk have mostly been based on self-reported smoking [1,2] with its inherent limitations. Cotinine is the main metabolite of nicotine and a sensitive marker of recent active and passive tobacco exposure. While nicotine has a half-life of only 2–3 hours, cotinine has a half-life of 11–37 hours [26].

To our knowledge, plasma cotinine-based classification of smoking habits has not been studied as a predictor of risk of hip fractures, and the effect of smoking exposure and fat mass on BMD and hip fracture risk has not been reported. We hypothesized that there is a higher risk of low BMD and hip fracture in lean smokers than in smokers with high fat mass. We also wanted to investigate the interaction between fat mass and smoking in relation to BMD and hip fracture.

The independent impact of fat mass and lean mass on BMD has been previously studied in this population [20]. The aim of the present study was to explore whether the deleterious effect of smoking on BMD and hip fracture risk was the same regardless of body composition/the proportion of fat mass.

Methods

Ethics statements

The study was approved by the Regional Committee for Medical Research Ethics review, REC West. Each participant signed an informed consent form.

Study population

Men and women, residing in Bergen (Norway) and three neighboring municipalities, born 1925–1927 and 1950–1951 were invited for the main Hordaland Health Study (HUSK) where the baseline examination was done during 1998–2000. Those invited had participated in a previous study (The Hordaland Homocysteine Study) during 1992–93 [27]. Altogether 77% met for the main study and they received an invitation for densitometry measurements. A total of 5408 (73.8%) met for this substudy. Inclusion criteria for the present study were participants with valid total body and femoral BMD scans and plasma cotinine measurements. Thirty subjects were excluded because of invalid BMD scans or bilateral hip prostheses. Total body soft tissue composition was invalid in 183 subjects (motion or metal artifacts). Thirty-nine persons were excluded because of non-white ethnicity. Lastly, plasma cotinine measurements were missing in 62 subjects. Thus, 5094 participants (1821 women and 1182 men aged 46–49 years and 1126 women and 965 men aged 71–74 years) comprise the cohort of the current study. Follow-up time was from inclusion until first hip fracture, while the observations were censored at death or on December 31st, 2009. As only eight participants in the youngest age group were diagnosed with a hip fracture during the follow-up period, only the oldest age group was included in the hip fracture analyses. During the follow-up period, 218 women and 309 men died without having suffered a hip fracture.

Bone mineral density and body composition

BMD and total body soft tissue composition was measured by dual X-ray absorptiometry (DXA) on a stationary fan beam densitometry (Expert-XL; Lunar Company Inc, Madison, Wis) by four trained technicians. The left hip was scanned except when there was a history of hip prosthesis or fracture. The results were based on measurements of femoral neck BMD as this measurement site is recommended as the reference standard for description of osteoporosis [28]. Fat mass (%) was calculated as fat mass (kg) in percent of total body weight (kg). Daily scanning of the manufacturer-supplied spine phantom showed no instrumentation drift and a coefficient of variation of <0.9% during the whole study period.

Hip fractures

Information on hip fracture was attained from computerized records containing discharge diagnoses for all hospitalizations occurring between HUSK baseline examinations through December 31st, 2009 at the six hospitals in Hordaland County. Mean follow-up time was 9.8 years. Hip fracture was defined as the first fracture of the proximal femur occurring during the observation period. Only hip fractures confirmed by a concurrent code of an adequate surgical procedure were included in order to validate the fracture registration; all hospital discharges with an identified hip fracture diagnosis were searched for adequate surgical treatment. Further description of the classification codes is previously described [29]. Information on time of death was attained from the Norwegian Population Register.

Other measurements

Height and weight were measured with light clothing. BMI was calculated as weight in kilograms divided by the square of height in meters. Self-administered questionnaires provided information on smoking, physical activity and hormone replacement therapy, which were missing in 13, 160 and 743 participants, respectively. Smoking habits were categorized as current, former or never-smokers. The number of cigarettes smoked daily was also collected. Leisure time physical activity was categorized as no or light regular activity (<1 hour/week), regular (1–2 hours/week) and hard regular activity (≥3 hours/week). Use of estrogen supplements was categorized as current or no use. Information on dietary intake was collected using a validated 169-item food frequency questionnaire (FFQ). FFQ was missing in 482 subject, and eight participants with energy intake extremes (<2.5 or >97.5 percentiles) were excluded.

Determination of cotinine and categorization of smoking

Non-fasting blood samples were collected and plasma was stored at −80 degrees Celsius. Plasma cotinine concentration was measured by liquid chromatography-tandem mass spectrometry at the laboratory Bevital A/S (Bergen, Norway) [30]. Never smoking was defined as plasma cotinine levels less than 85 nmol/L [31] and no report of previous smoking. Former smoking was defined as self-reported previous smoking and plasma cotinine levels less than 85 nmol/L. Moderate smoking was defined as plasma cotinine levels between 85 and 1199 nmol/L and heavy smoking as 1200 nmol/L or higher. A plasma cotinine level of 1200 nmol/L corresponded to a self-reported consumption of about 15 cigarettes per day among our study participants.

Statistical analyses

Categorical variables are expressed as numbers and percentages and continuous variables as means with standard deviations (SD). The hip fracture incidence rate per 10,000 person-years was calculated by summarizing the follow-up time (years) for the study population (person-years), and dividing the numbers of hip fractures on person-years. Linear representation of the categorical variables was used to test for trend. General linear regression models (GLM) with femoral neck BMD (g/cm^2) as the dependent variable and fat mass (%) as independent variable were used for each category of smoking habits. GLM was used to investigate a possible interaction between fat mass (%) or BMI and smoking on BMD. BMD was expressed in terms of g/cm^2 to give the direct strength of the relation between BMD and fat mass or BMI in each smoking category. To get more comprehensible regression coefficients, fat mass and BMI were divided by 1000 before the analyses. To test for nonlinearity in the slopes for the association between fat mass (%) and BMD for each of the different smoking categories, we used the Davies segmented test [32]. To graphically express the dose-response associations between fat mass (%) and BMD according to smoking categories, we used a generalized additive logistic regression model (GAM) with a smoothing spline term with adjustment for sex and age group.

Cox proportional hazards regression models were used to estimate associations between smoking categories in combination with fat mass (%) or BMI and subsequent hip fracture in the oldest subjects. These analyses were conducted with and without adjustments for physical activity and BMD. To study the dose-response associations between fat mass (%) and the risk of hip fracture according to smoking categories, a Cox model using a spline covariate smoothing with adjustment for sex was used. Two-tailed p-values <0.05 were considered statistically significant. The analyses were performed using SPSS for Windows (IBM SPSS Statistics 19). The generalized additive models were computed with the R (http://cran.r-project.org) package "gam" [33] and the Cox spline smoothed curves were constructed using the R package "survival".

Results

Study population

Characteristics of the female and male participants are shown in Tables 1 and 2, respectively. In women of both age groups, BMI (kg/m^2), fat mass (%), fat mass (kg), lean mass (kg), and BMD (g/cm^2) were significantly lower in heavy smokers than in moderate-, former-, and never smokers (Table 1). A similar trend was found among the oldest men (Table 2). In the youngest men, lean mass and BMD were significantly lower in heavy smokers compared with the other smoking categories. Among the youngest women and men, heavy smokers were less physically active than moderate-, former-, and never smokers. No significant differences between the smoking groups were found for total energy intake and use of estrogen supplementation in elderly women. During follow-up, 100 women and 52 men in the oldest age group suffered a hip fracture. The hip fracture incidence rates per 10,000 person-years were 83.5 for women and 54.2 for men. Among the oldest women, a higher proportion of heavy smokers suffered a hip fracture compared to moderate and never smokers.

Smoking, fat mass and bone mineral density

For all participants, BMD and fat mass were positively associated in all smoking categories, with the strongest association among moderate and heavy smokers (Table 3). Significant differences in the association (regression coefficients) between fat mass and BMD between the different smoking categories were found. Both heavy and moderate smokers had significantly stronger associations between fat mass and BMD compared to never smokers ($p=0.018$ and $p=0.024$, respectively) after adjustment for sex and age group (Table 3). The explained variance was 0.287 (28.7%) and an overall test of the model gave a significant fit ($F(9,5073)=226.5$, $p<0.001$). After additional adjustment for physical activity, the association was significant among heavy smokers only ($p=0.034$) (Table 3). The same tendency was observed after stratifying on sex and age groups, although the results were borderline significant (e.g. the oldest heavy smoking women: differences in regression coefficient = 4.64 per % change in fat mass, 95% confidence interval (CI): −0.07, 9.29; $p=0.050$).

Davies segmented test showed that for heavy and moderate smokers there was a nonlinear association, with a steeper positive association between BMD and fat mass at low compared to high values of fat mass, and a significant breakpoint at fat mass of 18.4% in heavy smokers, and at 21.1% in moderate smokers ($p<0.001$).

The non-linear dose-response associations (functional form) between BMD and fat mass are shown in figure 1. The curves show that BMD increased with increasing levels of fat mass, with the steepest increases among heavy and moderate smokers with low fat mass.

The associations were somewhat stronger for BMI as compared to fat mass (Table S1, Table 3).

Smoking, fat mass and hip fracture

For elderly women and men combined, heavy smokers had an increased risk of hip fracture compared to never smokers (hazard ratio = 3.31, 95% CI: 2.05, 5.35; $p<0.001$) after adjustment for sex and fat mass. Fat mass was not significantly related to risk of hip fracture in any of the smoking categories after adjustment for sex. However, there was a tendency towards heavy smokers having the strongest fracture risk reduction with increasing fat mass (Table 4). There were no significant differences between the associations for the different smoking categories (Table 4). Adjustment for physical activity and BMD did not materially change the results (Table 4). Similar results were found when BMI was used in the analyses instead of fat mass (Table S2).

The association (functional form) between fat mass and the risk of hip fracture is shown in figure 2, and reveals a non-linear dose-response relation. There was a tendency towards decreasing risk of hip fracture with increasing levels of fat mass for each of the smoking categories, with the steepest decrease among heavy smokers with low fat mass.

Discussion

In this study the positive association between fat mass and BMD was stronger among moderate and heavy smokers compared to never smokers, and the relation was stronger in smokers with low compared to high fat mass or BMI. In elderly women and men, an increased risk of hip fracture was associated with heavy smoking. Fat mass was not significantly related to risk of hip fracture in any of the smoking categories, but the tendency was that heavy smokers had higher risk of fractures at lower levels of fat mass, and that this risk decreased markedly with increasing fat mass.

Strengths of this study are the large number of participants of both genders, the population based cohort design, and the long follow-up time of more than 10 years for hip fractures. However, smoking status, BMD and fat mass were measured only at baseline; we therefore have no information on potential changes in these or in other factors during follow-up. All BMD and body composition measurements were performed on the same DXA machine. We measured cotinine, which have been reported to correlate better than self-reports with various effects of smoking [34]. A total number of 185 participants who reported no current smoking had plasma cotinine levels above 85 nmol/L. Misclassification might be related to under-reporting and/or passive smoking. Data on smokeless tobacco use was not collected, thus some of the participants with high cotinine levels might have been snuffers and not cigarette smokers. On the other hand, during 1998–2000, snuffing was very rare among adults and elderly in Norway, and we do not consider this to be of importance in the interpretation of our findings. In support of the latter, our results did not materially change when we used self-reported current

Table 1. Characteristics of the female study participants by baseline age group and smoking categories.

	Women 46–49 years old						*Women 71–74 years old*					
	All		**Smoking categories[b]**			**P for**	**All**		**Smoking categories[b]**			**P for**
	subjects[c]	**Never**	**Former**	**Moderate**	**Heavy**	**trend[d]**	**subjects[c]**	**Never**	**Former**	**Moderate**	**Heavy**	**trend[d]**
Number of participants	1821	728	423	341	329		1126	677	275	108	66	
	(100)	(40.0)	(23.2)	(18.7)	(18.1)		(100)	(60.1)	(24.4)	(9.6)	(5.9)	
Body mass index (kg/m²)	24.8	25.2	25.1	24.9	23.6	<0.001	26.2	26.3	27.1	25.0	23.0	<0.001
	(4.0)	(4.3)	(3.9)	(3.9)	(3.5)		(4.2)	(3.9)	(4.6)	(4.3)	(3.4)	
Total fat mass (kg)	24.5	25.4	25.1	24.7	21.5	<0.001	27.0	27.3	29.1	24.0	20.2	<0.001
	(9.7)	(10.1)	(9.7)	(9.8)	(8.2)		(9.6)	(9.1)	(10.4)	(9.3)	(8.0)	
Total lean mass (kg)	40.3	40.5	40.5	40.5	39.6	0.006	37.6	37.8	38.0	37.0	35.1	<0.001
	(4.5)	(4.6)	(4.2)	(4.9)	(4.4)		(4.3)	(4.0)	(4.4)	(4.7)	(4.5)	
Fat mass (%)	36.6	37.3	37.1	36.8	34.2	<0.001	40.6	40.9	42.2	38.0	35.3	<0.001
	(7.8)	(7.8)	(7.6)	(7.6)	(7.8)		(8.2)	(7.7)	(8.1)	(9.1)	(8.7)	
Fat mass <15%	6	1	0	0	5		8	2	1	3	2	
	(0.3)	(0.1)			(1.5)		(0.7)	(0.3)	(0.4)	(2.8)	(3.0)	
Fat mass >40%	577	263	138	108	68	<0.001	635	396	173	46	20	<0.001
	(31.7)	(36.1)	(32.6)	(31.7)	(20.7)		(56.4)	(58.5)	(62.9)	(42.6)	(30.3)	
Total energy (kJ/day)	7947.0	7827.8	8042.5	8140.2	7879.3	0.381	6575.9	6561.3	6573.4	6625.2	6666.5	0.701
	(2340.0)	(2193.7)	(2191.4)	(2642.8)	(2489.6)		(2221.1)	(2183.5)	(2188.9)	(2427.0)	(2470.3)	
No regular physical activity	655	241	140	116	158	<0.001	443	273	94	51	25	0.987
	(36.4)	(33.6)	(33.3)	(34.6)	(48.2)		(43.1)	(44.5)	(36.4)	(51.5)	(43.1)	
Estrogen supplementation	342	96	99	77	70	<0.001	125	72	29	15	9	0.406
	(25.1)	(17.9)	(30.6)	(30.9)	(27.5)		(14.9)	(14.6)	(13.6)	(17.6)	(18.8)	
Femoral neck BMD (g/cm²)	0.96	0.98	0.96	0.95	0.93	<0.001	0.76	0.77	0.77	0.74	0.73	0.002
	(0.12)	(0.13)	(0.12)	(0.12)	(0.13)		(0.11)	(0.11)	(0.12)	(0.12)	(0.13)	
Hip fracture during follow-up[e]	4	1	2	-	1	0.858	100	51	22	9	18	<0.001
	(0.2)	(0.1)	(0.5)		(0.3)		(8.9)	(7.5)	(8.0)	(8.3)	(27.3)	

The Hordaland Health Study[a].
Abbreviations: BMD, bone mineral density; BMI, body mass index.
[a]Values are given as mean (standard deviation (SD)) for continuous variables and number (%) for categorical variables.
[b]Never smoking, plasma cotinine levels <85 nmol/L and no self-reported previous smoking; former smoking, self-reported previous smoking and plasma cotinine levels <85 nmol/L; moderate smoking, plasma cotinine levels between 85 and 1199 nmol/L; heavy smoking, plasma cotinine levels ≥1200 nmol/L.
[c]Number of participants with data on femoral neck BMD, body soft tissue composition and plasma cotinine.
[d]*P*-value for trend across smoking categories.
[e]Hip fractures from inclusion in 1997–99 until December 31st, 2009.
Total numbers may vary between variables due to varying numbers of missing data.

smoking status instead of plasma cotinine in the analyses. Alcohol abuse is a potential confounding factor, but here were no major differences in reported alcohol intake within the different smoking categories, and adjustment for alcohol intake did not alter the results (data not shown). In addition, diabetes could also be a confounding factor since persons with diabetes usually have higher fat mass [35]. However, 166 HUSK participants reported diabetes and/or use of anti-diabetic medication, and 100 of these had fat mass above 30% (51 above 40%). Exclusion of these participants or including diabetes as a covariate did not alter the results.

Percent fat mass was positively related to BMD in all smoking categories in our study. In the meta-analysis by Ho-Pam et al [23], studies in which negative correlations between fat mass and BMD were found included few subjects (n<100) and the negative correlation coefficients reported were overall weaker than the (positive) correlations found in other studies. The significant association between fat mass and BMD may reflect a role of nutrition and sex hormones in bone building and bone tissue maintenance [23]. We found a stronger relation between fat mass and BMD in smokers than non-smokers and in smokers with low compared to high fat mass. This suggests that among smokers, the relative impact of fat tissue as an endocrine organ may be more important among those with little fat mass.

It has been suggested that lower BMD in smokers may be attributable to lower body weight rather than to a direct effect of smoking [36]. However, our results do not support that lower BMI is the predominant explanation as both moderate and heavy smokers with low fat mass had lower BMD compared to never

Table 2. Characteristics of the male study participants by baseline age group and smoking categories.

	Men 46–49 years old						*Men 71–74 years old*					
	All		**Smoking categories[b]**			**P for**	**All**		**Smoking categories[b]**			**P for**
	subjects[c]	**Never**	**Former**	**Moderate**	**Heavy**	**trend[d]**	**subjects[c]**	**Never**	**Former**	**Moderate**	**Heavy**	**trend[d]**
Number of participants	1182	404	349	188	241		965	245	555	87	78	
	(100)	(34.2)	(29.5)	(15.9)	(20.4)		(100)	(25.4)	(57.5)	(9.0)	(8.1)	
Body mass index (kg/m^2)	26.2	25.9	26.8	26.4	25.6	0.379	26.0	25.8	26.3	25.7	24.3	0.002
	(3.3)	(3.2)	(3.4)	(3.3)	(3.3)		(3.1)	(3.0)	(3.0)	(3.5)	(3.3)	
Total fat mass (kg)	20.6	19.6	22.5	20.8	19.4	0.690	21.2	19.9	22.4	20.4	17.8	0.202
	(9.0)	(8.4)	(9.7)	(8.4)	(8.9)		(8.5)	(7.9)	(8.5)	(8.6)	(7.9)	
Total lean mass (kg)	59.9	60.0	60.9	60.2	58.4	0.003	55.0	55.4	55.3	53.9	53.6	0.005
	(6.2)	(6.1)	(6.2)	(6.2)	(6.0)		(5.8)	(5.7)	(5.8)	(5.5)	(6.0)	
Fat mass (%)	24.7	23.9	26.1	24.9	23.9	0.981	27.0	25.7	28.1	26.6	23.9	0.315
	(7.4)	(7.2)	(7.3)	(7.1)	(7.8)		(7.4)	(7.3)	(7.2)	(7.1)	(7.7)	
Fat mass <15%	107	43	19	14	31		55	19	20	5	11	
	(9.1)	(10.6)	(5.4)	(7.4)	(12.9)		(5.7)	(7.8)	(3.6)	(5.7)	(14.1)	
Fat mass >40%	31	9	14	3	5	0.360	34	7	24	3	0	0.119
	(2.6)	(2.2)	(4.0)	(1.6)	(2.1)		(3.5)	(2.9)	(4.3)	(3.4)		
Total energy (kJ/day)	10547.4	10415.7	10509.4	10409.1	10953.5	0.073	8605.6	8775.5	8510.1	8531.2	8858.3	0.878
	(2870.6)	(2632.0)	(2799.1)	(2985.2)	(3252.8)		(2471.1)	(2467.6)	(2502.8)	(2528.9)	(2157.0)	
No regular physical activity	445	131	126	75	113	<0.001	273	58	156	40	19	0.059
	(38.0)	(32.7)	(36.3)	(40.3)	(47.7)		(29.3)	(24.3)	(29.2)	(47.6)	(25.3)	
Femoral neck BMD (g/cm^2)	0.99	1.00	1.00	0.97	0.95	<0.001	0.90	0.93	0.90	0.86	0.86	<0.001
	(0.13)	(0.13)	(0.14)	(0.13)	(0.12)		(0.14)	(0.15)	(0.14)	(0.12)	(0.14)	
Hip fracture during follow-up[e]	4	2	2	-	-	0.231	52	10	29	6	7	0.079
	(0.3)	(0.5)	(0.6)				(5.4)	(4.1)	(5.2)	(6.9)	(9.0)	

The Hordaland Health Study[a]
Abbreviations: BMD, bone mineral density; BMI, body mass index.
[a]Values are given as mean (standard deviation (SD)) for continuous variables and number (%) for categorical variables.
[b]Never smoking, plasma cotinine levels <85 nmol/L and no self-reported previous smoking; former smoking, self-reported previous smoking and plasma cotinine levels <85 nmol/L; moderate smoking, plasma cotinine levels between 85 and 1199 nmol/L; heavy smoking, plasma cotinine levels ≥1200 nmol/L.
[c]Number of participants with data on femoral neck BMD, body soft tissue composition and plasma cotinine.
[d]*P*-value for trend across smoking categories.
[e]Hip fractures from inclusion in 1997–99 until December 31st, 2009.
Total numbers may vary between variables due to varying numbers of missing data.

smokers with low fat mass. This is in accordance with a meta-analysis demonstrating a negative effect of smoking on BMD independent of differences in weight between smokers and non-smokers [2]. On the other hand, we found that smokers with low fat mass had significantly lower BMD than smokers with high fat mass. Thus, the negative effect of smoking on BMD seems to be especially deleterious among lean people.

To our knowledge, there are no published studies using cotinine to investigate the interaction with fat mass on BMD and subsequent hip fracture. However, urinary cotinine was investigated in relation to BMD in a study of pre- and postmenopausal Korean females, and a significant dose-related effect of smoking on BMD was observed [37]. In addition, serum cotinine in relation to bone mineral content (BMC) was investigated in a large cohort study in the USA and high serum cotinine levels were found to be a significant risk factor for low BMC in both women and men [38]. However, the interaction between smoking and fat mass was not examined in these studies. We found lower BMD in both moderate and heavy smokers with low fat mass compared to never smokers with low fat mass. Our

Table 3. Linear associations between fat mass (%) and femoral neck BMD (g/cm^2) for each category of smoking for all participants (n = 5094) in the Hordaland Health Study.

	Adjusted for sex and age						Adjusted for sex, age and physical activity					
	Regression coefficients			**Differences in regression coefficients**			**Regression coefficients**			**Differences in regression coefficients**		
Smoking categories[a]	B	95% CI	P value	B	95% CI	P value	B	95% CI	P value	B	95% CI	P value
Heavy	3.43	2.40, 4.47	<0.001	1.38	0.24, 2.52	0.018	3.60	2.54, 4.65	<0.001	1.26	0.10, 2.41	0.034
Moderate	3.35	2.33, 4.36	<0.001	1.29	0.17, 2.41	0.024	3.32	2.28, 4.36	<0.001	0.98	−0.17, 2.12	0.093
Former	1.30	0.59, 2.01	<0.001	-0.75	−1.60, 0.10	0.082	1.58	0.86, 2.31	<0.001	−0.76	−1.62, 0.10	0.084
Never	2.05	1.44, 2.67	<0.001	0 (ref.)	(-,-)	-	2.34	1.71, 2.98	<0.001	0 (ref.)	(-,-)	-

General linear regression models showing the regression coefficient between fat mass and BMD for each smoking category, and the differences in regression coefficients per % change in fat mass for each category, with never smokers as the reference group.
Abbreviations: BMD, bone mineral density (g/cm^2); B, Beta; CI, confidence interval.
[a]Never smoking, plasma cotinine levels less than 85 nmol/L and no self-reported previous smoking; former smoking, self-reported previous smoking and plasma cotinine level >85 nmol/L; moderate smoking, plasma cotinine levels between 85 and 1199 nmol/L; heavy smoking, plasma cotinine levels ≥1200 nmol/L.

results are similar with findings from a Danish study on 2015 perimenopausal women where a significant interaction was found between self-reported current smoking and fat mass in the lowest tertile (<13.3 kg) on femoral neck BMD, but not among those in the highest tertile of fat mass (>19.0 kg) [25]. Two studies demonstrated a higher risk of low BMD in current smokers compared with non-smokers in both genders, after adjustment for BMI [1,39]. In addition, a dose-dependent effect of cigarette smoking (cigarettes/day, years smoked) on BMD has been demonstrated in both genders; larger exposure was associated with lower BMD [2,40].

We observed an increased risk of hip fracture in elderly heavy smokers compared to never smokers. The association did not change materially after adjustment for physical activity and BMD,

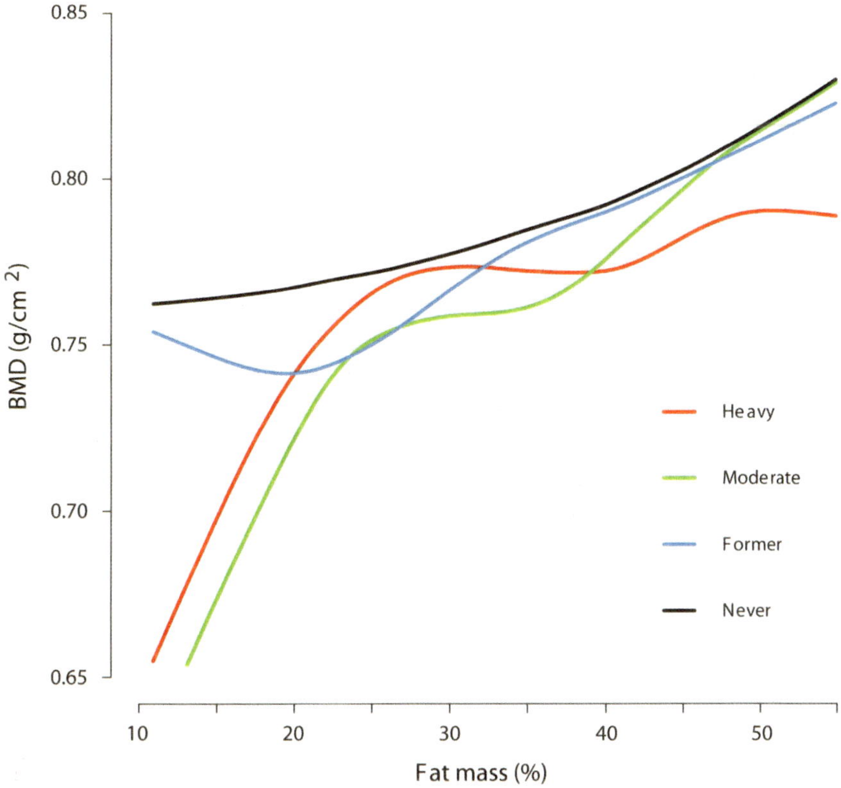

Figure 1. Dose-response curves between fat mass (%) and femoral neck bone mineral density (BMD, g/cm^2) for different smoking categories by generalized additive model (GAM). All participants (n = 5094) are included in the models, which are adjusted for sex and age group (The Hordaland Health Study). Never smoking is defined as plasma cotinine levels <85 nmol/L and no self-reported previous smoking; former smoking, self-reported previous smoking and plasma cotinine levels <85 nmol/L; moderate smoking, plasma cotinine levels between 85 and 1199 nmol/L; heavy smoking, plasma cotinine levels ≥1200 nmol/L.

Table 4. Associations between fat mass (%) and risk of hip fracture according to smoking status in elderly women and men (n = 2091) in the Hordaland Health Study.

	Adjusted for sex						**Adjusted for sex, physical activity and BMD**					
	HR for hip fracture by fat mass			**Differences in HR**			**HR for hip fracture by fat mass**			**Differences in HR**		
Smoking categories[a]	HR	95% CI	P value	HR	95% CI	P value	HR	95% CI	P value	HR	95% CI	P value
Heavy	0.67	0.42, 1.07	0.091	0.78	0.44, 1.37	0.391	0.80	0.62, 1.03	0.082	0.87	0.61, 1,24	0.424
Moderate	0.79	0.47, 1.32	0.368	0.92	0.50, 1.69	0.791	0.87	0,69, 1.11	0.259	0.95	0.68, 1.31	0.738
Former	1.05	0.73, 1.50	0.798	1.23	0.77, 1.96	0.394	0.92	0.65, 1.30	0.643	0.95	0.62, 1.45	0.811
Never	0.85	0.62, 1.19	0.348	1.00	(-,-)	-	0.88	0.62, 1,24	0.452	1.00	(-,-)	-

Cox proportional hazards regression models showing hazard ratio between fat mass and hip fracture within each smoking category, and differences in HRs between each smoking category compared to never smokers.
Abbreviations: HR, hazard ratio; CI, confidence interval.
[a]Never smoking, plasma cotinine levels <85 nmol/L and no self-reported previous smoking; former smoking, previous self-reported smoking and plasma cotinine levels <85 nmol/L; moderate smoking, plasma cotinine levels between 85 and 1199 nmol/L; heavy smoking, plasma cotinine levels ≥1200 nmol/L.

which suggests that increased fracture risk among heavy smokers may be independent of BMD. However, we did not find any significant interaction between fat mass or BMI and the different smoking categories on the risk of hip fracture which may be due to the relative small number of hip fractures. In a large Norwegian study a relative risk of 1.5 (95% CI: 1.0, 2.4) for suffering a hip fracture was found in female self-reported smokers with BMI below the population mean (25 kg/m^2), compared to lean non-smokers, increasing to a 3-fold RR when cut-off for BMI was set at 20 kg/m^2 [3]. On the other hand, a population-based case-control study from Sweden showed an increased risk of hip fracture in female smokers compared to never smokers (odds ratio = 1.66, 95% CI: 1.41, 1.95), but with similar results after dividing the group according to BMI above and below the median [41]. Hemenway et al [42], did not find any significant association between cigarettes smoked per day and risk of hip fracture among

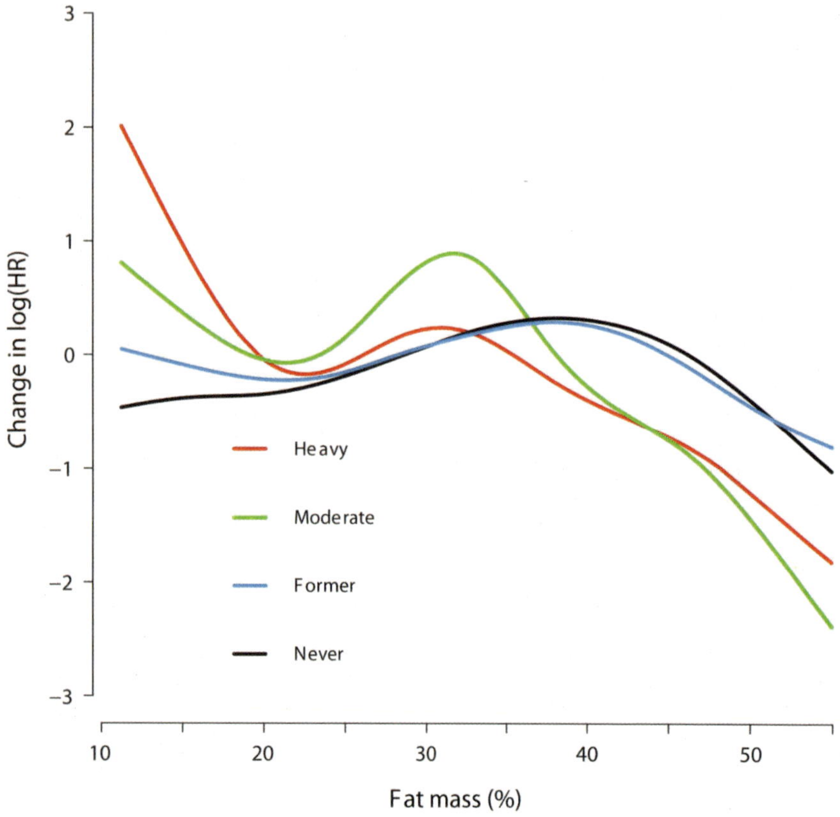

Figure 2. Dose-response curves between fat mass (%) and risk of hip fracture according to smoking status in elderly women and men (n = 2091) by generalized additive Cox modeling. The curves are adjusted for sex (The Hordaland Health Study). Never smoking is defined as plasma cotinine levels <85 nmol/L and no self-reported previous smoking; former smoking, previous self-reported smoking and plasma cotinine levels <85 nmol/L; moderate smoking, plasma cotinine levels between 85 and 1199 nmol/L; heavy smoking, plasma cotinine levels ≥1200 nmol/L.

women, nor any interaction with body weight. Forsen et al [3], found an increased risk of hip fractures in male smokers independently of BMI. In some other studies on male smokers the results are conflicting regarding impact of BMI or weight on risk of fracture [43,44].

We did not find any significant differences in the association between fat mass and the risk of low BMD or hip fracture in former smokers compared to never smokers. In some previous studies with adjustment for BMI, smoking cessation was found to both decrease the risk of low BMD [2,40] and hip fracture [44] as well as to increase the risk of hip fracture [45]. The number of years smoked and time since quitting may be important [2]. In the study by Hollenback et al [40], previous smokers with short time since smoking cessation had lower hip BMD than never smokers and long-term quitters, while current smokers had the lowest BMD. In a large Norwegian study of women and men under 75 years, the risk of hip fracture was higher in former smokers, even among those who had quit smoking more than 5 years before, compared to never smokers [45].

The mechanisms behind the negative effects of smoking on bone are not completely known. In women, positive associations between tobacco smoking, premature menopause [25], low estrogen levels [5] and low BMD have been found. In addition, a more rapid bone loss after menopause in smokers than non-smokers has been observed [46]. It has been estimated that smoking increases the lifetime risk of sustaining a hip fracture by 31% in women and 40% in men [2], and bone loss has been reported to be more rapid among male than female smokers [47]. The apparently higher risk among men may be due to a higher total consumption of cigarettes among male smokers, or a protective effect of hormone replacement therapy among women [2]. However, in the current study the prevalence of hip fracture was higher among female than male smokers. Smoking has also been shown to reduce testosterone levels in men [48]. A adverse effect of smoking on skeletal remodeling and bone cells has been observed [6]. Further, smoking may affect other hormones, minerals and enzymes involved in bone regulation resulting in reduced calcium absorption [8] and parathyroid hormone concentration [9]. Increased oxidative stress and inflammation are also observed in smokers [49].

Generally, and as we observed, smokers have lower BMI and lower fat mass than non-smokers [25]. It has been suggested that smoking has an appetite-suppressing effect, thereby leading to lower energy intake. However, we and others [50] did not find any significant differences in the total energy intake between smokers and non-smokers. A modestly increased rate of energy metabolism in smokers compared to non-smokers due to release of hormones as e.g. adrenaline from the central nervous system has been suggested [51].

The biochemical pathways linking adipose tissue to bone are complex [24]. For example, in women a decreased rate of bone loss might be explained by the production of extragonadal estrogen in adipose tissue after menopause. Thus, postmenopausal women with low fat mass have lower estrogen production and therefore a higher risk of osteoporosis [24]. In elderly men, androgen deficiency caused by hypogonadism may contribute to bone loss, but androgen deficiency is not related to fat mass [52]. However, low estradiol levels in elderly men may also cause faster bone loss [16].

Our findings indicate that the positive relation between fat mass and BMD was stronger among moderate and heavy smokers compared to never smokers, and the deleterious effect was stronger in smokers with low compared to high fat mass. Thus, physicians should be particularly attentive to lean smokers concerning the risk of osteoporosis. An uplifting finding in our study as well as in other studies [2] is that it seems that smoking cessation may slow down or partially reverse the accelerated bone loss caused by years of smoking. There is no convincing evidence that fat mass *per se* protects against osteoporosis or hip fractures. For a deeper understanding, further research should aim at investigating through which pathways fat tissue may exert a protective effect on bone exposed to toxic substances.

Supporting Information

Table S1 Linear associations between BMI (kg/cm^2) and femoral neck BMD (g/cm^2) for each category of smoking for all participants (n = 5094) in the Hordaland Health Study. General linear regression models showing the regression coefficient between BMI and BMD for each smoking category, and the differences in regression coefficients per unit change in BMI for each category, with never smokers as the reference group.

Table S2 Associations between BMI (kg/cm^2) and risk of hip fracture according to smoking status in elderly women and men (n = 2091) in the Hordaland Health Study. Cox proportional hazards regression models showing hazard ratio between BMI and hip fracture within each smoking category, and differences in HRs between each smoking category compared to never smokers.

Author Contributions

Conceived and designed the experiments: JØ CGG GST OKN PMU SEV. Performed the experiments: CGG GST OKN PMU SEV. Analyzed the data: JØ SAL SEV. Contributed reagents/materials/analysis tools: PMU CGG EMA ØM. Wrote the paper: JØ GST CGG. Critical revision of the manuscript: CGG GST OKN SAL PMU SEV EMA HEM ERP ØM. Data interpretation: JØ CGG GST OKN SAL PMU SEV EMA HEM ERP ØM.

References

1. Law MR, Hackshaw AK (1997) A meta-analysis of cigarette smoking, bone mineral density and risk of hip fracture: recognition of a major effect. BMJ 315: 841–846.
2. Ward KD, Klesges RC (2001) A meta-analysis of the effects of cigarette smoking on bone mineral density. Calcif Tissue Int 68: 259–270.
3. Forsen L, Bjorndal A, Bjartveit K, Edna TH, Holmen J, et al. (1994) Interaction between current smoking, leanness, and physical inactivity in the prediction of hip fracture. J Bone Miner Res 9: 1671–1678.
4. Jutberger H, Lorentzon M, Barrett-Connor E, Johansson H, Kanis JA, et al. (2010) Smoking predicts incident fractures in elderly men: Mr OS Sweden. J Bone Miner Res 25: 1010–1016.
5. Tanko LB, Christiansen C (2004) An update on the antiestrogenic effect of smoking: a literature review with implications for researchers and practitioners. Menopause 11: 104–109.
6. Walker LM, Preston MR, Magnay JL, Thomas PB, El Haj AJ (2001) Nicotinic regulation of c-fos and osteopontin expression in human-derived osteoblast-like cells and human trabecular bone organ culture. Bone 28: 603–608.
7. Riebel GD, Boden SD, Whitesides TE, Hutton WC (1995) The effect of nicotine on incorporation of cancellous bone graft in an animal model. Spine (Phila Pa 1976) 20: 2198–2202.
8. Krall EA, Dawson-Hughes B (1999) Smoking increases bone loss and decreases intestinal calcium absorption. J Bone Miner Res 14: 215–220.
9. Landin-Wilhelmsen K, Wilhelmsen L, Lappas G, Rosen T, Lindstedt G, et al. (1995) Serum intact parathyroid hormone in a random population sample of men and women: relationship to anthropometry, life-style factors, blood pressure, and vitamin D. Calcif Tissue Int 56: 104–108.
10. Felson DT, Zhang Y, Hannan MT, Anderson JJ (1993) Effects of weight and body mass index on bone mineral density in men and women: the Framingham study. J Bone Miner Res 8: 567–573.

11. Ensrud KE, Lipschutz RC, Cauley JA, Seeley D, Nevitt MC, et al. (1997) Body size and hip fracture risk in older women: a prospective study. Study of Osteoporotic Fractures Research Group. Am J Med 103: 274–280.
12. Joakimsen RM, Fonnebo V, Magnus JH, Tollan A, Sogaard AJ (1998) The Tromso Study: body height, body mass index and fractures. Osteoporos Int 8: 436–442.
13. Meyer HE, Tverdal A, Falch JA (1993) Risk factors for hip fracture in middle-aged Norwegian women and men. Am J Epidemiol 137: 1203–1211.
14. De Laet C, Kanis JA, Oden A, Johanson H, Johnell O, et al. (2005) Body mass index as a predictor of fracture risk: a meta-analysis. Osteoporos Int 16: 1330–1338.
15. Compston JE, Watts NB, Chapurlat R, Cooper C, Boonen S, et al. (2011) Obesity is not protective against fracture in postmenopausal women: GLOW. Am J Med 124: 1043–1050.
16. Prieto-Alhambra D, Premaor MO, Fina Aviles F, Hermosilla E, Martinez-Laguna D, et al. (2012) The association between fracture and obesity is site-dependent: a population-based study in postmenopausal women. J Bone Miner Res 27: 294–300.
17. Lau EM, Chan YH, Chan M, Woo J, Griffith J, Chan HH, Leung PC (2000) Vertebral deformity in chinese men: prevalence, risk factors, bone mineral density, and body composition measurements. Calcif Tissue Int 66: 47–52.
18. Edelstein SL, Barrett-Connor E (1993) Relation between body size and bone mineral density in elderly men and women. Am J Epidemiol 138: 160–169.
19. Reid IR, Ames R, Evans MC, Sharpe S, Gamble G, et al. (1992) Determinants of total body and regional bone mineral density in normal postmenopausal women—a key role for fat mass. J Clin Endocrinol Metab 75: 45–51.
20. Gjesdal CG, Halse JI, Eide GE, Brun JG, Tell GS (2008) Impact of lean mass and fat mass on bone mineral density: The Hordaland Health Study. Maturitas 59: 191–200.
21. Hsu YH, Venners SA, Terwedow HA, Feng Y, Niu T, et al. (2006) Li Z, Laird N, Brain JD, Cummings SR, Bouxsein ML, Rosen CJ, Xu X. Relation of body composition, fat mass, and serum lipids to osteoporotic fractures and bone mineral density in Chinese men and women. Am J Clin Nutr 83: 146–154.
22. Zhao LJ, Liu YJ, Liu PY, Hamilton J, Recker RR, et al. (2007) Relationship of obesity with osteoporosis. J Clin Endocrinol Metab 92: 1640–1646.
23. Ho-Pham LT, Nguyen UD, Nguyen TV (2014) Association Between Lean Mass, Fat Mass, and Bone Mineral Density: A Meta-analysis. J Clin Endocrinol Metab 99:30–38
24. Reid IR (2010) Fat and bone. Arch Biochem Biophys 503: 20–27.
25. Hermann AP, Brot C, Gram J, Kolthoff N, Mosekilde L (2000) Premenopausal smoking and bone density in 2015 perimenopausal women. J Bone Miner Res 15: 780–787.
26. Benowitz NL (1999) Nicotine addiction. Prim Care 26: 611–631.
27. Nygard O, Vollset SE, Refsum H, Stensvold I, Tverdal A, et al. (1995) Total plasma homocysteine and cardiovascular risk profile. The Hordaland Homocysteine Study. JAMA 274: 1526–1533.
28. Kanis JA, McCloskey EV, Johansson H, Oden A, Melton LJ, 3rd, et al. (2008) A reference standard for the description of osteoporosis. Bone 42: 467–475.
29. Gjesdal CG, Vollset SE, Ueland PM, Refsum H, Meyer HE, et al. (2008) Plasma homocysteine, folate, and vitamin B 12 and the risk of hip fracture: the hordaland homocysteine study. J Bone Miner Res 22: 747–756.
30. Midttun O, Hustad S, Ueland PM (2009) Quantitative profiling of biomarkers related to B-vitamin status, tryptophan metabolism and inflammation in human plasma by liquid chromatography/tandem mass spectrometry. Rapid Commun Mass Spectrom 23: 1371–1379.
31. Gorber SC, Schofield-Hurwitz S, Hardt J, Levasseur G, Tremblay M (2009) The accuracy of self-reported smoking: a systematic review of the relationship between self-reported and cotinine-assessed smoking status. Nicotine Tob Res 11: 12–24.
32. Davies RB (1987) Hypothesis testing when a nuisance parameter is present only under the alternative. Biometrika.
33. Hastie TJ, Tibshirani RJ (1990) Generalized additive models. London: Chapman & Hall.
34. Perez-Stable EJ, Benowitz NL, Marin G (1995) Is serum cotinine a better measure of cigarette smoking than self-report? Prev Med 24: 171–179.
35. Yaturu S (2009) Diabetes and skeletal health. J Diabetes 1: 246–254.
36. Jensen GF (1986) Osteoporosis of the slender smoker revisited by epidemiologic approach. Eur J Clin Invest 16: 239–242.
37. Myong JP, Kim HR, Choi SE, Koo JW (2012) Dose-related effect of urinary cotinine levels on bone mineral density among Korean females. Osteoporos Int 24: 1339–1346.
38. Benson BW, Shulman JD (2005) Inclusion of tobacco exposure as a predictive factor for decreased bone mineral content. Nicotine Tob Res 7: 719–724.
39. Egger P, Duggleby S, Hobbs R, Fall C, Cooper C (1996) Cigarette smoking and bone mineral density in the elderly. J Epidemiol Community Health 50: 47–50.
40. Hollenbach KA, Barrett-Connor E, Edelstein SL, Holbrook T (1993) Cigarette smoking and bone mineral density in older men and women. Am J Public Health 83: 1265–1270.
41. Baron JA, Farahmand BY, Weiderpass E, Michaelsson K, Alberts A, et al. (2001) Cigarette smoking, alcohol consumption, and risk of hip fracture in women. Arch Intern Med 161: 983–988.
42. Hemenway D, Colditz GA, Willett WC, Stampfer MJ, Speizer FE (1988) Fractures and lifestyle: effect of cigarette smoking, alcohol intake, and relative weight on the risk of hip and forearm fractures in middle-aged women. Am J Public Health 78: 1554–1558.
43. Kanis J, Johnell O, Gullberg B, Allander E, Elffors L, et al. (1999) Risk factors for hip fracture in men from southern Europe: the MEDOS study. Mediterranean Osteoporosis Study. Osteoporos Int 9: 45–54.
44. Hoidrup S, Prescott E, Sorensen TI, Gottschau A, Lauritzen JB, et al (2000) Tobacco smoking and risk of hip fracture in men and women. Int J Epidemiol 29: 253–259.
45. Forsen L, Bjartveit K, Bjorndal A, Edna TH, Meyer HE, et al. (1998) Ex-smokers and risk of hip fracture. Am J Public Health 88: 1481–1483.
46. Sowers MR, Clark MK, Hollis B, Wallace RB, Jannausch M (1992) Radial bone mineral density in pre- and perimenopausal women: a prospective study of rates and risk factors for loss. J Bone Miner Res 7: 647–657.
47. Hannan MT, Felson DT, Dawson-Hughes B, Tucker KL, Cupples LA, et al (2000) Risk factors for longitudinal bone loss in elderly men and women: the Framingham Osteoporosis Study. J Bone Miner Res 15: 710–720.
48. Baron JA, La Vecchia C, Levi F (1990) The antiestrogenic effect of cigarette smoking in women. Am J Obstet Gynecol 162: 502–514.
49. Yanbaeva DG, Dentener MA, Creutzberg EC, Wesseling G, Wouters EF (2007) Systemic effects of smoking. Chest 131: 1557–1566.
50. Perkins KA (1992) Effects of tobacco smoking on caloric intake. Br J Addict 87: 193–205.
51. Perkins KA (1992) Metabolic effects of cigarette smoking. J Appl Physiol 72: 401–409.
52. Seeman E (2002) Pathogenesis of bone fragility in women and men. Lancet 359: 1841–1850.

10

Molecular Mechanism of Thiazolidinedione-Mediated Inhibitory Effects on Osteoclastogenesis

Dongfeng Zhao[1,2], Zhenqi Shi[2], Amy H. Warriner[3], Ping Qiao[2], Huixian Hong[2], Yongjun Wang[1]*, Xu Feng[2]*

1 Longhua Hospital, Shanghai University of Traditional Chinese Medicine, Shanghai, People's Republic of China, **2** Department of Pathology, University of Alabama at Birmingham, Birmingham, Alabama, United States of America, **3** Department of Medicine, University of Alabama at Birmingham, Birmingham, Alabama, United States of America

Abstract

Thiazolidinediones are synthetic peroxisome proliferator-activated receptor γ agonists used to treat type 2 diabetes mellitus. Clinical evidence indicates that thiazolidinediones increase fracture risks in type 2 diabetes mellitus patients, but the mechanism by which thiazolidinediones augment fracture risks is not fully understood. Several groups recently demonstrated that thiazolidinediones stimulate osteoclast formation, thus proposing that thiazolidinediones induce bone loss in part by prompting osteoclastogenesis. However, numerous other studies showed that thiazolidinediones inhibit osteoclast formation. Moreover, the molecular mechanism by which thiazolidinediones modulate osteoclastogenesis is not fully understood. Here we independently address the role of thiazolidinediones in osteoclastogenesis *in vitro* and furthermore investigate the molecular mechanism underlying the *in vitro* effects of thiazolidinediones on osteoclastogenesis. Our *in vitro* data indicate that thiazolidinediones dose-dependently inhibit osteoclastogenesis from bone marrow macrophages, but the inhibitory effect is considerably reduced when bone marrow macrophages are pretreated with RANKL. *In vitro* mechanistic studies reveal that thiazolidinediones inhibit osteoclastogenesis not by impairing RANKL-induced activation of the NF-κB, JNK, p38 and ERK pathways in bone marrow macrophages. Nonetheless, thiazolidinediones inhibit osteoclastogenesis by suppressing RANKL-induced expression of NFATc1 and c-Fos, two key transcriptional regulators of osteoclastogenesis, in bone marrow macrophages. In addition, thiazolidinediones inhibit the RANKL-induced expression of osteoclast genes encoding matrix metalloproteinase 9, cathepsin K, tartrate-resistant acid phosphatase and carbonic anhydrase II in bone marrow macrophages. However, the ability of thiazolidinediones to inhibit the expression of NFATc1, c-Fos and the four osteoclast genes is notably weakened in RANKL-pretreated bone marrow macrophages. These *in vitro* studies have not only independently demonstrated that thiazolidinediones exert inhibitory effects on osteoclastogenesis but have also revealed crucial new insights into the molecular mechanism by which thiazolidinediones inhibit osteoclastogenesis.

Editor: Jean-Marc Vanacker, Institut de Génomique Fonctionnelle de Lyon, France

Funding: Research reported in this publication was supported by the National Institute of Arthritis and Musculoskeletal and Skin Diseases, part of the National Institutes of Health, under Award Number AR47830. This work was also supported by grants from the National Basic Research Program of China (2010CB530400), the Key Program of Natural Science Foundation of China (30930111), and the Program for Changjiang Scholars and Innovative Research Team in University (PCSIRT, IRT1270). The funders had no role in study design, data collection and analysis, decision to publish, or preparation of the manuscript.

Competing Interests: The authors have declared that no competing interests exist.

* Email: yjwang88@hotmail.com (YW); xufeng@uab.edu (XF)

Introduction

Types 2 diabetes mellitus (T2DM) accounts for 90–95% of all diabetes cases and causes significant economic and societal burdens globally [1,2]. Thiazolidinediones (TZDs) represent one class of drugs used to treat T2DM and they promote insulin sensitivity to enhance glucose consumption [3,4]. TZDs are highly effective oral mediators that exert their anti-hyperglycemic function through targeting peroxisome proliferator-activated receptor γ (PPARγ) [5,6], a master regulator of glucose metabolism [7,8]. In addition, PPARγ also regulates various other biological processes including adipogenesis, lipid metabolism, macrophage biology and inflammation [9–14].

However, clinical evidence has established that TZD treatments increase the risk of fracture in patients with T2DM [15–17]. Available data indicate that TZDs modulate bone remodeling through various bone cells including osteoblasts, osteocytes and osteoclasts [18]. It has been shown that TZDs induce preferential differentiation of mesenchymal stem cells into adipocytes instead of osteoblasts by activating PPARγ [19], leading to bone loss and structural deterioration [20,21]. Moreover, TZDs also negatively affect bone formation by inducing the apoptosis of osteocytes and increasing expression of sclerostin [22,23]. On the other hand, while a number of groups have also investigated the effects of TZDs on osteoclastogenesis [24–32], these studies generated controversial findings. Among these studies, seven demonstrated that TZDs exert inhibitory effects on osteoclastogenesis [24–30]; in contrast, two investigations showed that these PPARγ agonists promote osteoclast formation in an PPARγ-dependent manner [31,32].

Osteoclasts, the multinucleated bone-resorbing cells, not only play a crucial role in skeletal development and adult bone remodeling but are also implicated in the pathogenesis of various bone disorders [33,34]. Osteoclasts differentiate from mononuclear cells of the monocyte/macrophage lineage upon stimulation by the monocyte/macrophage colony stimulating factors (M-CSF) and the receptor activator of NF-κB ligand (RANKL) [35]. Whereas M-CSF mainly stimulates proliferation and survival of bone marrow macrophages (BMMs, namely, osteoclast precursors), RANKL primarily drives osteoclast differentiation. RANKL binds to its receptor RANK, a member of the TNF receptor superfamily, to activate numerous signaling pathways (NF-κB, JNK, ERK, p38 and Akt) [35,36]. RANKL also up-regulates the expression of nuclear factor of activated T-cells c1 (NFATc1), which plays an essential role in osteoclastogenesis [37]. c-Fos is another factor crucially involved in osteoclastogenesis [38]. RANKL increases the expression of c-Fos which cooperates with NFATc1 to regulate gene expression during osteoclastogenesis [37]. Thus, these RANKL-activated signaling pathways promote osteoclastogenesis in part by regulating the expression of genes including those encoding matrix metalloproteinase 9 (MMP9), cathepsin K (Ctsk), tartrate-resistant acid phosphatase (TRAP) and carbonic anhydrase II (Car2) [39,40].

RANKL promotes osteoclastogenesis in part by committing BMMs into the osteoclast lineage [41]. Moreover, we and others have previously revealed that RANKL-mediated osteoclast lineage commitment of BMMs determines the effects of numerous factors on osteoclastogenesis. Lipopolysaccharide (LPS), a common bacteria-derived product implicated in the periodontal bone loss, inhibits osteoclastogenesis from freshly isolated BMMs but stimulates osteoclast formation from RANKL-pretreated BMMs [42,43]. Furthermore, whereas interferon-γ (IFN-γ), a potent anti-osteoclastogenic factor, strongly inhibits osteoclastogenesis from fresh BMMs, the suppressive effect is significantly reduced when osteoclast precursors are pre-exposed to RANKL [44,45]. IL-1 and TNF-α, two proinflammatory cytokines, are unable to promote osteoclastogenesis without RANKL. However, they can do so in the presence of low levels of RANKL or with RANKL pretreatment [46–49].

In this work, given the controversy on the role of TZDs in osteoclastogenesis, first we independently and thoroughly carried out a series of *in vitro* assays to further investigate the effects of TZDs on osteoclastogenesis. In particular, we performed the assays with rosiglitazone and pioglitazone, which are two common forms of TZDs used to treat T2DM, in parallel to obtain more convincing data. Moreover, given that RANKL-mediated osteoclast lineage commitment of BMMs has been shown to determine the effects of LPS, IFN-γ, IL-1 and TNF-α on osteoclastogenesis, we also examined whether RANKL-mediated osteoclast lineage commitment alters the effect of TZDs on osteoclastogenesis. Finally, we carried out mechanistic studies to gain insights into the molecular mechanism by which TZDs modulate osteoclastogenesis.

Materials and Methods

Chemicals, biological reagents and mice

Rosiglitazone (R2408), pioglitazone hydrochloride (E6910) and dimethyl sulfoxide (DMSO) (D2438) were purchased from Sigma-Aldrich (St. Louis, MO). Stock solutions (2×10^4 μM) of rosiglitazone and pioglitazone were prepared in DMSO monthly and stored at 4°C. Recombinant purified glutathione S-transferase-RANKL was purified as described previously [50]. Mouse M-CSF was prepared from an M-CSF-producing cell line as previously described [51]. Recombinant mouse TNF-α (410-TRNC-050) was purchased from R&D system (Minneapolis, MN). The following antibodies were purchased from Cell Signaling Technology, Inc. (Beverly, MA): antibodies against IκBα (#9242), phosphor-IκBα (#2859s), p44/42ERK (#9102), phospho-44/42ERK (#9101s), JNK (#9252), phospho-JNK (#9251s), p38 (#9212), phospho-p38 (#9211s), and lamin A/C (#2032s). Antibodies against NFATc1 (sc-7294), RANK (sc-7624) and c-Fos (sc-253) were purchased from Santa Cruz Biotechnology (Santa Cruz, CA). Catalog numbers for the chemicals and biological reagents are provided in parentheses. C57BL/6 mice were purchased from Harlan Industries (Indianapolis, IN), and were maintained in the animal facility at University of Alabama at Birmingham (UAB). The study was approved by UAB institutional animal care and use committee (IACUC) (animal protocol number: 130407854). The experiments involving mice were performed in accordance with the Instructions and Regulations of UAB IACUC.

In vitro osteoclastogenesis assays

BMMs were isolated from long bones of 4-to-6-week-old male and female C57BL/6 mice. To generate osteoclasts, 5×10^4 cells were plated per well in 24-well tissue culture plates and treated with different doses of M-CSF and RANKL as indicated in individual experiments. Osteoclasts were stained for TRAP activity with a leukocyte acid phosphatase commercial kit (Sigma, 387-A). The images of osteoclastogenesis assays were obtained using Olympus IX70 Fluorescence Microscope (Shinjuku, Japan).

In vitro bone resorption assays

BMMs, 5×10^4 cells per/well, were seeded on bovine cortical bone slices in 24-well tissue culture plates. Cells were treated under conditions indicated in individual experiments to promote osteoclastogenesis and bone resorption for up to 10 days. Then, bone slices were harvested, and cells were removed from bone slices with 0.25 M ammonium hydroxide and mechanical agitation. Bone slices were subjected to scanning electron microscopy (SEM) using a Philips 515 SEM (Materials Engineering Department, UAB). Bone resorption surfaces were quantified by measuring the percentage of the pits area in 5 random areas using the ImageJ analysis software obtained from National Institutes of Health.

Western blot assays

For the assays performed to assess the activation of IκBα/NF-κB, ERK, JNK, p38 pathways, BMMs were washed twice with ice cold PBS and then lysed with the lysis buffer from Cell Signaling Technology (#9803s), supplemented with protease inhibitor (#8340) and phosphatase inhibitor cocktail 1 (#2850) and 2 (#5726) from Sigma-Aldrich. For NFATc1, RANK and c-Fos expression assays, BMMs were washed twice with ice cold PBS and then lysed with the lysis buffer from Cell Signaling Technology (#9803), supplemented with protease inhibitor (#8340). Cytoplasmic and nuclear extracts were prepared using the NE-PER Nuclear and Cytoplasmic Extraction Reagents (Catalog No: 78833) from Thermo Scientific (Rockford, IL). Lysates were then subjected to Western blot analysis as described in our previous study [47] except that the primary antibodies against NFATc1, RANK and c-Fos were incubated in 5% nonfat dry milk solution (TBS containing 0.1% Tween 20). Membranes were washed extensively, and an ECL detection assay was performed using a Super Signal West Dura kit from Pierce. Densitometric analysis of Western blot bands was performed using FluiorChem 8900 imager from Alpha Innotech (Santa Clara, CA).

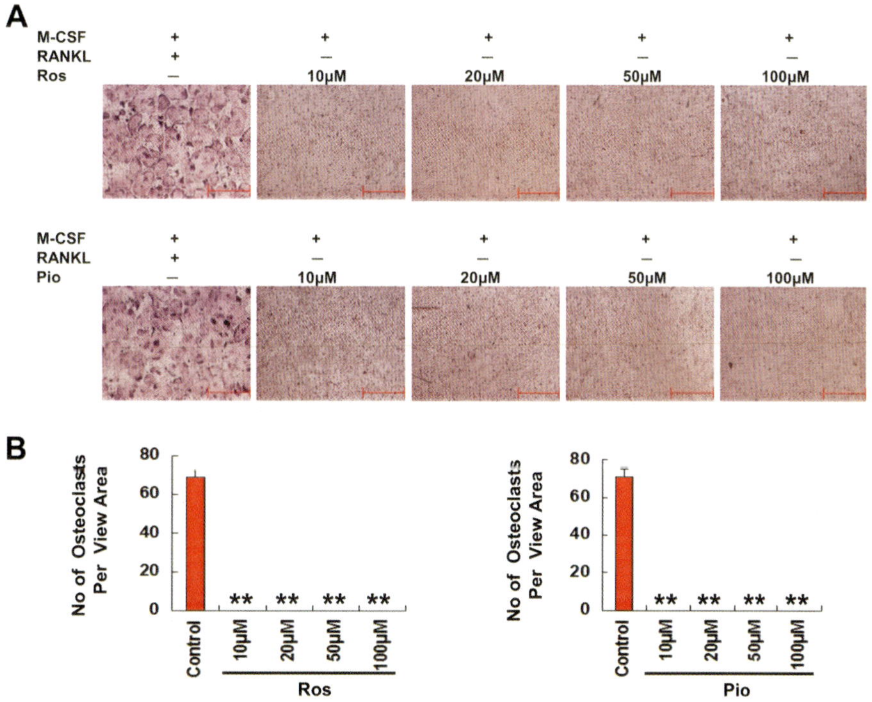

Figure 1. Rosiglitazone and pioglitazone do not induce osteoclastogenesis in the absence of RANKL. (A) BMMs were treated with M-CSF (44 ng/ml) and RANKL (100 ng/ml) as control, or M-CSF (44 ng/ml) plus different doses (10 μM, 20 μM, 50 μM and 100 μM) of rosiglitazone (Ros) or pioglitazone (Pio) for 4 days. The cultures were stained for TRAP activity. All assays were performed in triplicate and repeated 3 times. One representative view from each condition is shown. (B) Quantification of the osteoclastogenesis assays in A for Ros (left panel) and Pio (right panel). The number of multinucleated TRAP-positive cells (>3nuclei) per representative view area (40× magnification) was obtained. Bars show averages of three replicates ±S.D. TZD-treated cultures were compared with control cultures. **: $P<0.001$.

Semi-quantitative RT-PCR analysis

Total RNA was isolated from BMMs using TRIzol reagent from Invitrogen (Carlsbad, CA). Reverse transcription was performed using the Superscript III RT-PCR system (Invitrogen) according to standard protocol. In brief, 2 μg of total RNA was reverse-transcribed to cDNA with oligo (dT) in a 20 μl volume at 50°C for 60 min. The reverse transcription reaction was then followed by enzyme inactivation and RNA H digestion. PCR amplification of the MMP9, Ctsk, TRAP, Car2, and GAPDH genes was carried out as in our previous [47]. 25 μl of PCR products was loaded and separated on 2% agarose gel for electrophoretic analysis. The images of PCR product bands were obtained using FluorChem 8900 imager from Alpha Innotech Corporation (San Leandro, CA).

Statistical analysis

Bone resorption data are expressed as mean ± S.D. of the percentage of resorbed bone surface and osteoclastogenesis assay data are expressed as mean ± S.D. of the number of TRAP-positive cells/view area at 40× magnification. Statistical analyses were carried out using ANOVA with Bonferroni adjustment or Student's *t*-test. *p* values less than 0.05 are considered significant.

Results

TZDs dose-dependently inhibit osteoclastogenesis

Given the controversy on the effect of TZDs on osteoclastogenesis, in this study we seek to perform a series of experiments to fully and independently investigate the role of TZDs in osteoclast biology. It has been established that M-CSF and RANKL are two essential and sufficient factors for osteoclastogenesis [35]. While M-CSF functions to stimulate proliferation and survival of osteoclast precursors, RANKL is the key factor driving osteoclast differentiation. Therefore, our initial set of experiments aims to address whether TZDs can replace RANKL in promoting osteoclastogenesis in the presence of M-CSF. BMMs were treated with M-CSF and RANKL as positive control, or with M-CSF plus different doses of rosiglitazone or pioglitazone in tissue culture plates to promote osteoclastogenesis (Figure 1). While RANKL treatment led to the formation of osteoclasts, rosiglitazone and pioglitazone failed to induce osteoclastogenesis, indicating that TZDs cannot replace RANKL in promoting osteoclastogenesis.

Previously, we showed that whereas TNF-α or IL-1 cannot stimulate osteoclastogenesis in the presence of M-CSF, they can do so with low/permissive levels (10 ng.ml) of RANKL or RANKL pretreatment [47,52]. Therefore, we performed assays to determine whether TZDs can induce osteoclastogenesis with low levels of RANKL or RANKL pretreatment. As shown in Figure 2A–2B, TNF-α (5 ng/ml) induced the formation of numerous osteoclasts in the presence of 10 ng/ml RANKL. However, rosiglitazone and pioglitazone at concentrations as high as 100 μM were unable to promote osteoclastogenesis in the presence of 10 ng/ml RANKL. Similarly, TNF-α (5 ng/ml) promoted osteoclastogenesis from BMMs pretreated with 100 ng/ml RANKL for 24 hours (Figure 2C–2D), rosiglitazone and pioglitazone at concentrations as high as 100 μM failed to do so from RANKL-pretreated BMMs. These data indicate that TZDs are unable to promote osteoclastogenesis with low levels of RANKL or RANKL pretreatment.

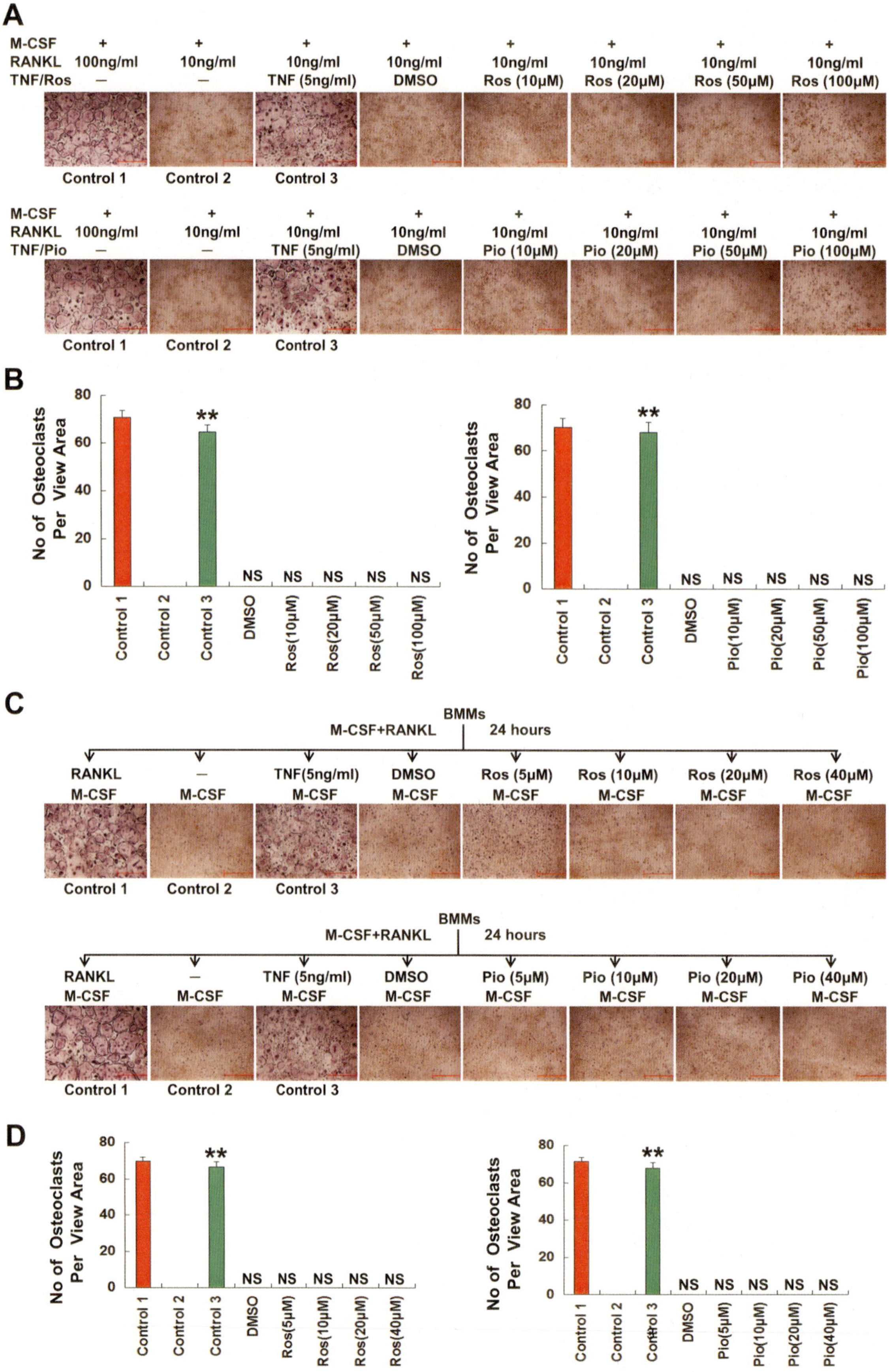
A
M-CSF + + + + + + + +
RANKL 100ng/ml 10ng/ml 10ng/ml 10ng/ml 10ng/ml 10ng/ml 10ng/ml 10ng/ml
TNF/Ros — — TNF (5ng/ml) DMSO Ros (10μM) Ros (20μM) Ros (50μM) Ros (100μM)
Control 1 Control 2 Control 3
M-CSF + + + + + + + +
RANKL 100ng/ml 10ng/ml 10ng/ml 10ng/ml 10ng/ml 10ng/ml 10ng/ml 10ng/ml
TNF/Pio — — TNF (5ng/ml) DMSO Pio (10μM) Pio (20μM) Pio (50μM) Pio (100μM)
Control 1 Control 2 Control 3
B
No of Osteoclasts Per View Area
80
60
40
20
0
**
NS NS NS NS NS
Control 1 Control 2 Control 3 DMSO Ros(10μM) Ros(20μM) Ros(50μM) Ros(100μM)
Control 1 Control 2 Control 3 DMSO Pio(10μM) Pio(20μM) Pio(50μM) Pio(100μM)
C
BMMs
M-CSF+RANKL 24 hours
RANKL — TNF(5ng/ml) DMSO Ros (5μM) Ros (10μM) Ros (20μM) Ros (40μM)
M-CSF M-CSF M-CSF M-CSF M-CSF M-CSF M-CSF M-CSF
Control 1 Control 2 Control 3
BMMs
M-CSF+RANKL 24 hours
RANKL — TNF (5ng/ml) DMSO Pio (5μM) Pio (10μM) Pio (20μM) Pio (40μM)
M-CSF M-CSF M-CSF M-CSF M-CSF M-CSF M-CSF M-CSF
Control 1 Control 2 Control 3
D
No of Osteoclasts Per View Area
80
60
40
20
0
**
NS NS NS NS NS
Control 1 Control 2 Control 3 DMSO Ros(5μM) Ros(10μM) Ros(20μM) Ros(40μM)
Control 1 Control 2 Control 3 DMSO Pio(5μM) Pio(10μM) Pio(20μM) Pio(40μM)

Figure 2. Rosiglitazone and pioglitazone do not induce osteoclastogenesis with low levels of RANKL or RANKL pretreatment. (A) BMMs were treated with M-CSF (44 ng/ml) and RANKL (100 ng/ml) as control 1, M-CSF (44 ng/ml) and RANKL (10 ng/ml) as control 2, M-CSF (44 ng/ml) and RANKL (10 ng/ml) plus TNF-α (TNF, 5 ng/ml) as control 3, M-CSF (44 ng/ml) and RANKL (10 ng/ml) plus DMSO or different doses (5 μM, 10 μM, 20 μM or 40 μM) of rosiglitazone (Ros) or pioglitazone (Pio) for 4 days and then stained for TRAP activity. The assays were performed in triplicate and repeated 3 times. One representative view from each condition is shown. (B) Quantification of the osteoclastogenesis assays in A for Ros (left panel) and Pio (right panel). The number of multinucleated TRAP-positive cells (>3nuclei) per representative view area (40×magnification) was obtained. Bars show averages of three replicates ±S.D. Control 3, DMSO, or TZD-treated cultures were compared with control 2. **: P<0.001. NS: not significant. (C) BMMs were treated with M-CSF (44 ng/ml) and RANKL (100 ng/ml) for 24 hours and then were continued with M-CSF (44 ng/ml) and RANKL (100 ng/ml) as control 1, M-CSF (44 ng/ml) alone as control 2, M-CSF (44 ng/ml) and TNF (5 ng/ml) as control 3, M-CSF (44 ng/ml) and DMSO, or M-CSF (44 ng/ml) plus different doses (5 μM, 10 μM, 20 μM or 40 μM) of Ros or Pio for additional 3 days. The cultures were stained for TRAP activity. The experiments were performed in triplicate and repeated 3 times. One representative view from each condition is shown. (D) Quantification of the osteoclastogenesis assays in A for Ros (left panel) and Pio (right panel). The number of multinucleated TRAP-positive cells (> 3nuclei) per representative view area (40×magnification) was obtained. Bars show averages of three replicates ±S.D. Control 3, DMSO, or TZD-treated cultures were compared with control 2. **: P<0.001. NS: not significant.

Having shown that TZDs are incapable of inducing osteoclastogenesis in the absence of RANKL, in the presence of low levels of RANKL, or with RANKL pretreatment, we further investigated their effects on osteoclastogenesis with optimal levels (100 ng/ml) of RANKL. We found that both rosiglitazone and pioglitazone dose-dependently inhibited RANKL-mediated osteoclastogenesis with complete inhibition of osteoclastogenesis at 40 µM (Figure 3). Bone surfaces represent the physiological substratum for osteoclastogenesis. To further investigate the effect of TZDs on osteoclastogenesis in a more physiologically relevant manner, we repeated the assays on bone slices. The data reveal that both rosiglitazone and pioglitazone treatment led to a significant reduction in bone resorption at 20 µM and complete absence of bone resorption at 40 µM (Figure 4), further indicating that TZDs inhibit RANKL-induced osteoclastogenesis.

TZDs do not affect RANKL-induced activation of the NF-κB and MAPK pathways in BMMs

To elucidate the molecular mechanism by which TZDs inhibit osteoclastogenesis, we first examine whether TZDs exert an effect on known RANK signaling pathways (NF-κB, JNK, ERK and p38) involved in osteoclastogenesis. BMMs were treated with M-CSF and RANKL only, or M-CSF and RANKL plus vehicle

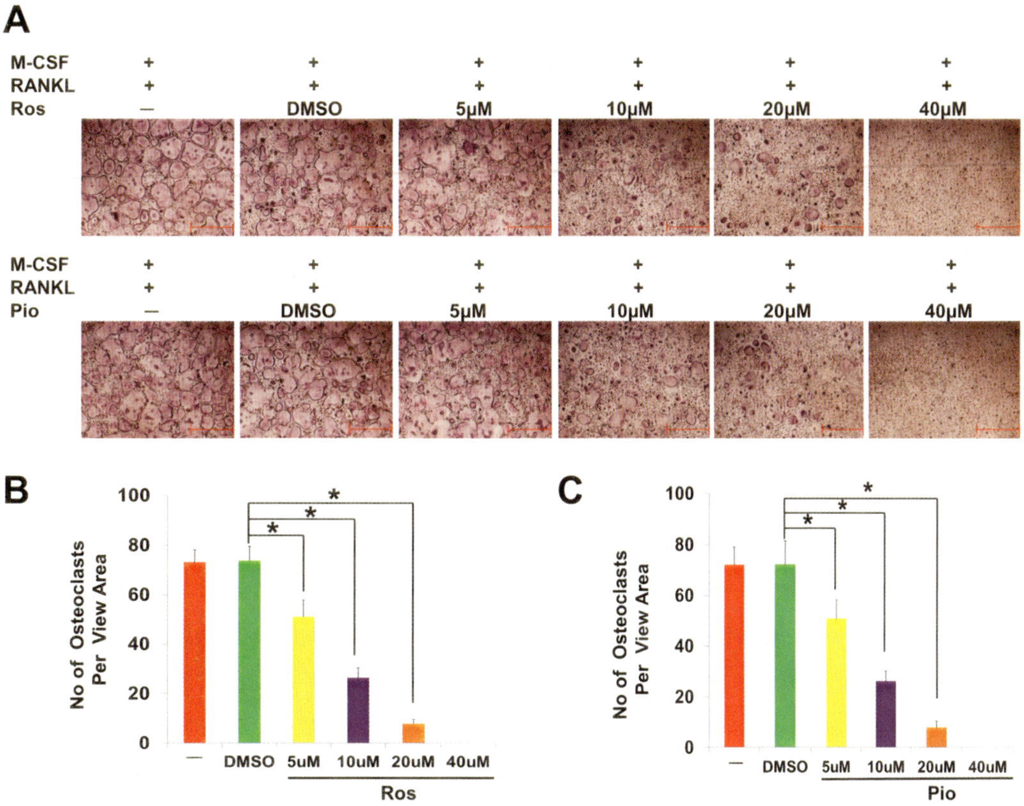

Figure 3. Rosiglitazone and pioglitazone inhibit RANKL-mediated osteoclastogenesis in tissue culture plates. (A) BMMs were treated with M-CSF (44 ng/ml) and RANKL (100 ng/ml), or M-CSF (44 ng/ml) and RANKL (100 ng/ml) plus vehicle (DMSO) or different doses (5 μM, 10 μM, 20 μM or 40 μM) of rosiglitazone (Ros) or pioglitazone (Pio) for 4 days. The cultures were then stained for TRAP activity. All assays were performed in triplicate and repeated 3 times. One representative view from each condition is shown. (B) Quantification of osteoclastogenesis assays for Ros in A. (C) Quantification of osteoclastogenesis assays for Pio in A. The number of multinucleated TRAP-positive cells (>3nuclei) per representative view area at 40× magnification was obtained. Bars show averages of three replicates ±S.D. *P<0.05.

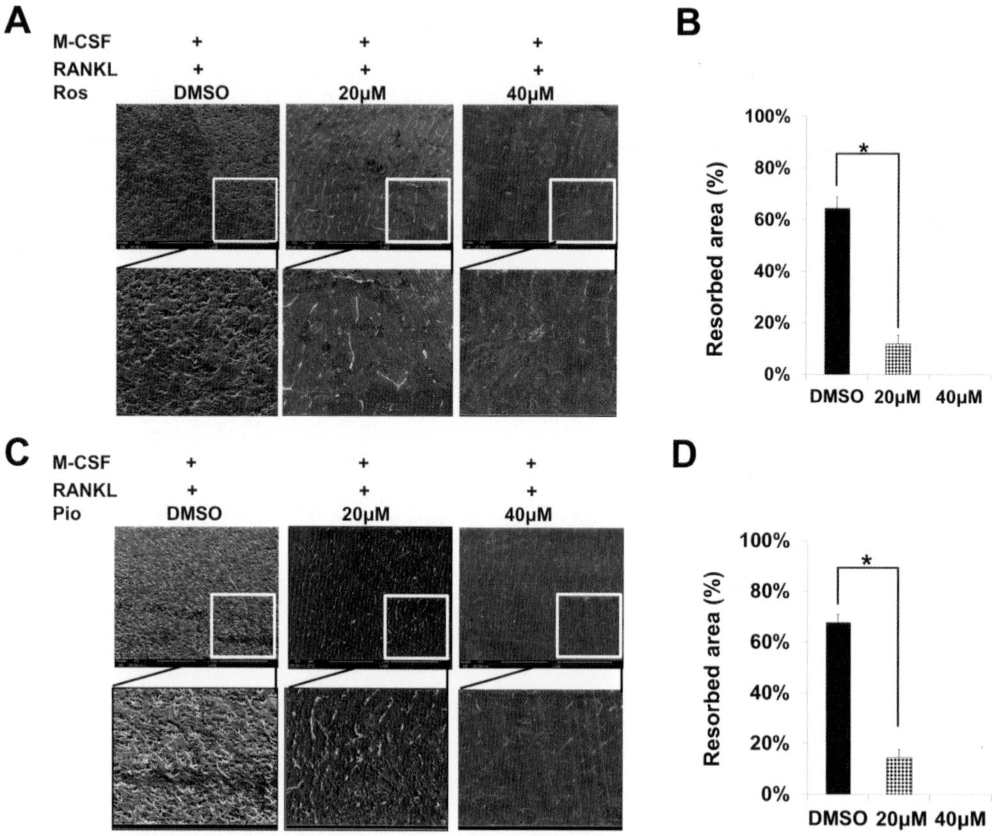

Figure 4. Rosiglitazone and pioglitazone significantly inhibit the formation of functional osteoclasts on bone slices. (A) BMMs were seeded on bone slices and treated with M-CSF (44 ng/ml) and RANKL (100 ng/ml) plus vehicle (DMSO), 20 μM or 40 μM of rosiglitazone (Ros) for 10 days. Bone resorption pits were visualized by SEM. One representative view from each condition is shown. (B) Quantification of resorbed bone area for Ros in A. Bars show percentage averages of resorbed bone area ±S.D. *P<0.05. (C) The same assays in A were carried out with pioglitazone (Pio). (D) Quantification of resorbed bone area for Pio in C. Bars show percentage averages of resorbed bone area ±S.D. *P<0.05.

(DMSO), rosiglitazone or pioglitazone for 5 or 10 minutes. Activation of NF-κB, JNK, ERK and p38 pathways was determined using Western bot analysis as the levels of phosphorylated form of IκB, JNK, ERK and p38, respectively (Figure 5). RANKL treatment led to increased phosphorylation of IκB, JNK, ERK and p38 at 5 minute (lane 2) and 10 minutes (lane 6) compared to those without RANKL treatment (lane 1), replicating previous findings that RANKL activates NF-κB, JNK, ERK and p38 pathways in osteoclast precursors. However, phosphorylation of IκB, JNK, ERK and p38 were not considerably affected by DMSO (lanes 3 and 7), rosiglitazone (lanes 4 and 8) or pioglitazone (lanes 5 and 9). These findings indicate that rosiglitazone and pioglitazone do not exert considerable effects on the activation of the NF-κB, JNK, ERK or p38 pathways in osteoclast precursors.

TZDs repress RANKL-induced expression of NFATc1, c-Fos and osteoclast genes

NFATc1 and c-Fos are two important transcriptional regulators of osteoclastogenesis [37,38]. To address whether TZDs exert an effect on NFATc1 and c-Fos expression, BMMs were treated with 40 μM rosiglitazone or pioglitazone for 1 or 2 days for Western blot analysis of NFATc1 and c-Fos expression. We found that both rosiglitazone and pioglitazone significantly suppressed RANKL-induced expression of NFATc1 (lane 2 vs. lanes 3 and 4; also lane 6 vs. lanes 7 and 8, top panel, Figure 6A) and c-Fos (lane 2 vs. lanes 3 and 4; also lane 6 vs. lanes 7 and 8, bottom panel, Figure 6A) in BMMs. Notably, RANKL not only induces NFATc1 expression but also activates NFATc1 by promoting its nuclear translocation in osteoclast precursors [37]. Thus, we further examined whether TZDs affect NFATc1 nuclear translocation in osteoclast precursors. BMMs were treated with 40 μM rosiglitazone or pioglitazone for 2 days and then cytoplasmic and nuclear extracts were prepared for Western blot analysis of NFATc1 levels in these subcellular fractions. We found that TZDs do not exert considerable effects on RANKL-induced nuclear translocation of NFATc1 (Figure 6B). These results indicate that TZDs inhibit osteoclastogenesis in part by suppressing RANKL-induced expression of the two key transcriptional regulators of osteoclastogenesis, NFATc1 and c-Fos.

Moreover, osteoclastogenesis involves differential regulation of the expression of numerous genes [39,40]. Particularly, RANKL considerably up-regulates the expression of genes encoding MMP9, Car2, Ctsk, and TRAP [39,40]. Thus, we next investigated whether TZDs affect the expression of these four representative osteoclast genes. As shown in Figure 6C, RANKL activated the expression of MMP9, Ctsk, TRAP and Car2 genes in BMMs at 24, 48 or 96 hours (lanes 2, 7 and 12). Rosiglitazone or pioglitazone markedly suppressed RANKL-induced expression of MMP9, Ctsk, TRAP and Car2 genes in BMMs at 24 (lanes 4–5), 48 (lanes 9–10), and 96 hours (lanes 14–15). The results indicated that TZDS significantly suppress RANKL-mediated expression of

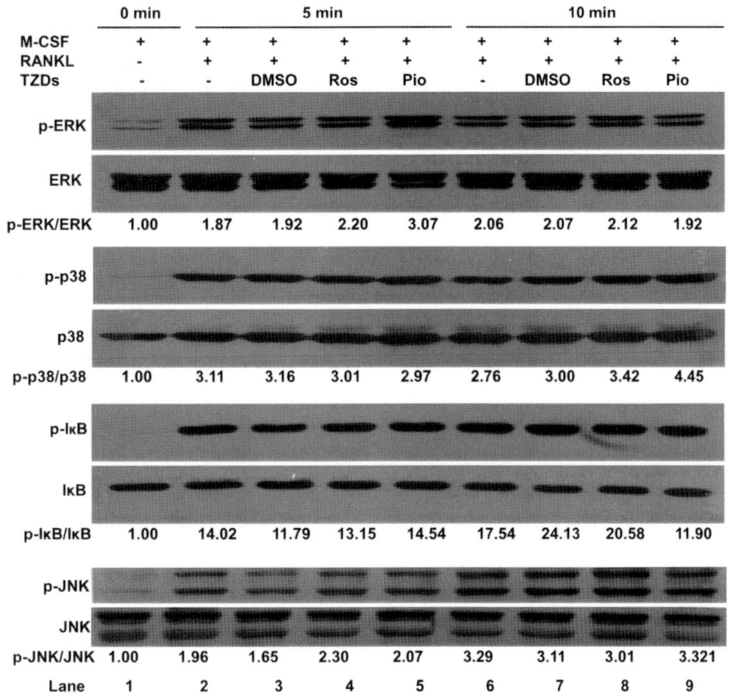

Figure 5. Rosiglitazone and pioglitazone exert no effects on RANKL-induced activation of the NF-κB, JNK, ERK and p38 pathways in BMMs. BMMs were cultured with M-CSF (44 ng/ml) to 20–30% confluence on 60-mm tissue culture dishes, and then treated with M-CSF (44 ng/ml) alone, M-CSF (44 ng/ml) and RANKL (100 ng/ml), M-CSF (44 ng/ml) and RANKL (100 ng/ml) plus vehicle (DMSO), 40 μM rosiglitazone (Ros) or pioglitazone (Pio) for 5 or 10 minutes (min). Activation of ERK, p38, NF-κB and JNK pathways was assessed as the level of the phosphorylated form of ERK, p38, IκB and JNK using Western analysis with antibodies against phospho-ERK, phospho-p38, phospho-IκB, and phospho-JNK, respectively. The blots were stripped and re-probed with antibodies against ERK, p38 and IκB for the expression levels of total proteins. Separate blots were probed with the antibody against JNK for the expression levels of the total JNK. Ratios of the phosphorylated form to the total protein for these signaling proteins were obtained by dividing the densitometric reading of the phosphorylated form with that of the total protein, and then the value calculated for 0 min was set as 1.00. All assays were repeated three times. One representative set of experiments is shown.

NFATc1, MMP9, Ctsk, TRAP and Car2 genes during osteoclastogenesis.

Given that previous studies demonstrated that TZDs inhibit osteoclastogenesis by decreasing the expression of RANK in bone marrow cells and RAW264.7 cells [29,30], we independently examined the effect of rosiglitazone or pioglitazone on RANK expression in BMMs. Towards this end, we treated BMMs with 40 μM rosiglitazone or pioglitazone for 1 or 2 days for Western blot analysis of RANK expression. In contrast, our data indicate that these two TZDs do not significantly affect the expression of RANK (lane 2 vs. lanes 3 and 4; also lane 6 vs. lanes 7 and 8, Figure 6D). Therefore, we conclude that TZDs directly inhibit RANKL-induced expression of NFATc1, c-Fos and osteoclast genes, not indirectly through the suppression of RANK expression.

The inhibitory effect of TZDs on osteoclastogenesis is significantly reduced in RANKL-pretreated BMMs

We and others previously established that RANKL-mediated osteoclast lineage commitment dictates the effects of various factor including LPS, IFN-γ, IL-1 and TNF-α on osteoclastogenesis [42–49]. To determine whether RANKL-mediated osteoclast lineage commitment also modulates the action of TZDs in osteoclastogenesis, rosiglitazone or pioglitazone was added at the beginning of the osteoclastogenic assays, or 24 and 48 hours after the start of the assays. The data revealed that BMMs pretreated with RANKL for as short as 24 hours formed much more osteoclasts compared to BMMs without RANKL pretreatment in the presence of rosiglitazone (Figures 7A–7B) or pioglitazone (Figures 7C–7D). Notably, rosiglitazone or pioglitazone completely abolished osteoclastogenesis from fresh BMMs at the concentration of 40 μM, replicating our assays above (Figure 3). However, numerous osteoclasts formed from RANKL-pretreated BMMs in the presence of these TZDs at 40 μM. These findings indicate that RANKL-mediated osteoclast lineage commitment decreases the effects of TZDs on osteoclastogenesis.

To further substantiate this notion, we carried out additional assays to investigate whether RANKL-mediated osteoclast lineage commitment affects the role of TZDs in osteoclastogenesis on bone slices since bone surfaces represent the physiological substratum for osteoclastogenesis and assays with bone slices are more physiologically relevant. Similar to our assays above in Figure 4, no bone resorption pits were found on bone slices with fresh BMMs cultured in the presence of 40 μM rosiglitazone (top row, Figure 8A) or 40 μM pioglitazone (top row, Figure 8C). But, bone slices with RANKL-pretreated BMMs in the presence of 40 μM rosiglitazone (middle and bottom rows, Figure 8A) or 40 μM pioglitazone (middle and bottom rows, Figure 8C) exhibited numerous resorption pits. Quantification of the bone resorption assays indicates that RANKL pretreatment significantly reduced TZD-mediated inhibitory effects on osteoclastogenesis on bone slices (Figures 8B and 8D). These findings further demonstrate that RANKL-mediated osteoclast lineage commitment diminishes the inhibitory effects of TZDs on osteoclastogenesis.

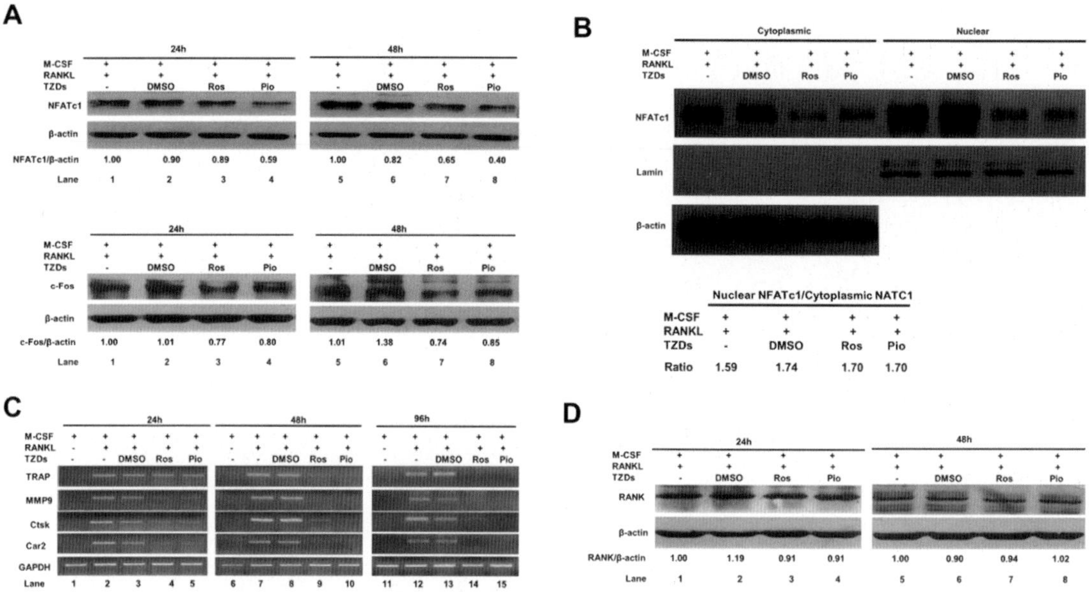

Figure 6. Rosiglitazone and pioglitazone repress RANKL-induced expression of NFATc1, c-Fos, TRAP, MMP9, Ctsk and Car2 genes but exert no effects on RANK expression. (A) BMMs were treated with M-CSF (44 ng/ml) and RANKL (100 ng/ml), M-CSF (44 ng/ml) and RANKL (100 ng/ml) plus DMSO or 40 μM rosiglitazone (Ros) or pioglitazone (Pio) for 24 hours (h), 48 h prior to lysis for Western blot assays with antibodies against NFATc1 (top panel) or c-Fos (bottom panel). The blots were stripped and then re-probed with β-actin antibody for loading control. Ratios of NFATc1/c-Fos to β-actin were obtained by dividing the densitometric reading of NFATc1/c-Fos with that of β-actin, and then the value calculated for the assay treated with M-CSF (44 ng/ml) and RANKL (100 ng/ml) was set as 1.00. The assays were repeated three times. One representative set of experiments is shown. (B) BMMs were treated with M-CSF (44 ng/ml) and RANKL (100 ng/ml), M-CSF (44 ng/ml) and RANKL (100 ng/ml) plus DMSO or 40 μM Ros or Pio for 48 h, and then cytoplasmic and nuclear extracts were prepared from the cells for Western analysis of NFATc1 expression. Lamin A/C was used to determine the quality of the cytoplasmic and nuclear extracts and also used as loading control for nuclear extract samples. β-actin was used as loading control for cytoplasmic extract samples. Densitometric values of cytoplasmic NFATc1 were normalized by β-actin densitometric values, whereas densitometric values of nuclear NFATc1 were normalized by those of lamin A/C. Ratios of nuclear NFATc1 to cytoplasmic NFATc1 were obtained by dividing normalized densitometric values of nuclear NFATc1 with normalized densitometric values of cytoplasmic NFATc1. The assays were repeated two times and one set of data is shown. (C) BMMs were treated with M-CSF (44 ng/ml), M-CSF (44 ng/ml) and RANKL (100 ng/ml), M-CSF (44 ng/ml) and RANKL (100 ng/ml) plus DMSO, or 40 μM Ros/Pio for 24 h, 48 h and 96 h prior to isolation of total RNAs for semi-quantitative RT-PCR analysis. The assays were repeated three times. One representative set of experiments is shown. (D) BMMs were treated with M-CSF (44 ng/ml) and RANKL (100 ng/ml), M-CSF (44 ng/ml) and RANKL (100 ng/ml) plus DMSO or 40 μM Ros/Pio for 24 h, 48 h prior to lysis for Western blot assays with an antibody against RANK. The blots were stripped and then re-probed with β-actin antibody for loading control. Ratios of RANK to β-actin were obtained by dividing the densitometric reading of RANK with that of β-actin, and then the value calculated for the assay treated with M-CSF (44 ng/ml) and RANKL (100 ng/ml) was set as 1.00. All assays were repeated three times. One representative set of experiments is shown.

The inhibitory effect of TZDs on the expression of NFATc1, c-Fos and osteoclast genes is significantly impaired in RANKL-pretreated BMMs

To delineate the molecular mechanism by which RANKL-mediated osteoclast lineage commitment modulates the action of TZDs in osteoclastogenesis, we examined the effect of TZDs on the expression of NFATc1 and c-Fos in RANKL-pretreated BMMs. Similar to our above assays in Figure 6A, rosiglitazone and pioglitazone dramatically suppressed RANKL-induced expression of NFATc1 (top panel, lane 2 vs. lanes 3 and 4, Figure 9A) and c-Fos (bottom panel, lane 2 vs. lanes 3 and 4, Figure 9A) in fresh BMMs, the inhibitory effect of these two TZDs on NFATc1 (top panel, lane 6 vs. lanes 7 and 8, Figure 9A) and c-Fos (bottom panel, lane 6 vs. lanes 7 and 8, Figure 9A) was almost abrogated when BMMs were pretreated with RANKL. Finally, we also assessed the effects of TZDs on RANKL-mediated expression of the four osteoclast genes in RANKL-pretreated BMMs. Similarly, rosiglitazone or pioglitazone significantly inhibited RANKL-induced expression of MMP9, Ctsk, TRAP and Car2 genes in fresh BMMs (left panel, lane 2 vs. lane 3 and 4, Figure 9B). In contrast, once BMMs were treated with RANKL, the capacity of these two TZDs to suppress RANKL-induced expression of these osteoclast genes was considerably reduced (right panel, lane 6 vs. lanes 7 and 8, Figure 9B). Taken together, these results indicate that RANKL pretreatment reduces the inhibitory effect of TZDs on osteoclastogenesis in part by rendering NFATc1, c-Fos and osteoclast genes refractory to the action of TZDs.

Discussion

Effects of TZDs on osteoclastogenesis were initially investigated almost 15 years ago by Okazaki and coworkers who carried out their study using mouse whole bone marrow cultures and demonstrated that rosiglitazone, pioglitazone and troglitazone all inhibited osteoclastogenesis in the whole bone marrow culture system [24]. Although whole bone marrow cultures contain different cell types including bone marrow stromal cells, TZDs are likely to exert inhibitory effects on osteoclastogenesis directly by targeting osteoclast precursors rather than indirectly by modulating the production of RANKL and/or OPG by bone marrow stromal cells since these investigators showed that troglitazone did not affect the expression of RANKL or OPG in bone marrow stromal cells [24]. Subsequently, two groups demonstrated that rosiglitazone suppressed RANKL-induced osteoclast formation

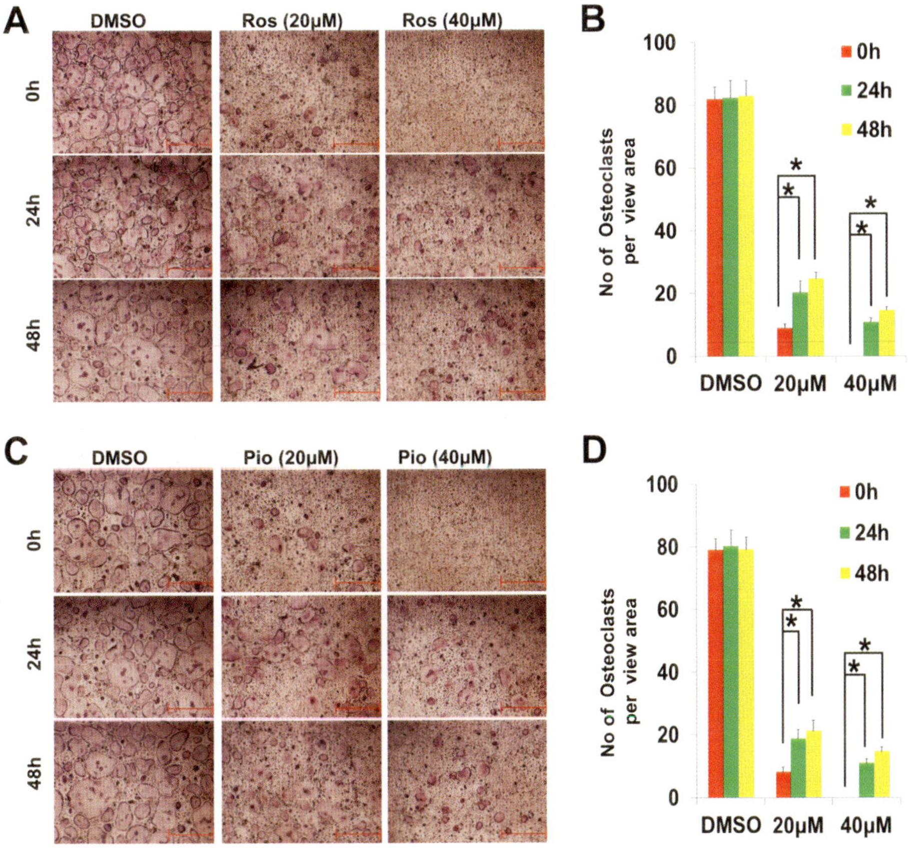

Figure 7. The inhibitory effects of rosiglitazone and pioglitazone on osteoclastogenesis are significantly decreased in RANKL-pretreated BMMs. (A) BMMs were cultured with M-CSF (220 ng/ml) until 30–40% confluence. Then, BMMs were treated with M-CSF (44 ng/ml) and RNAKL (100 ng/ml) for 4 days to stimulate osteoclastogenesis. Vehicle (DMSO), 20 μM or 40 μM of rosiglitazone (Ros) was added at the beginning of the assays (0 hour – 0 h) or 24 h and 48 h after the start of the assays. The cultures were stained for TRAP activity. All assays were performed in triplicate and repeated 3 times and one representative view from each condition is shown. (B) Quantification of the osteoclastogenesis assays in A. The number of multinucleated TRAP-positive cells (>3nuclei) per representative view area at 40× magnification was obtained. Bars show averages of three replicates ±S.D. *$P<0.05$. (C) The same set of assays in A was performed with pioglitazone (Pio). (D) The osteoclastogenesis assays in C were quantified as described in B. *$P<0.05$.

from primary bone marrow macrophages [30] and MOCP-5 cells [27], a mouse osteoclast precursor cell line [53]. Pioglitazone was shown to inhibit RANKL-induced osteoclastogenesis from mouse macrophage-like cell line RAW264.7 cells [29]. Moreover, it was also demonstrated that rosiglitazone and pioglitazone block TNF-α-induced osteoclast differentiation from RAW264.7 cells [28]. These findings indicate that TZDs exert inhibitory effects on murine osteoclastogenesis and they do so directly by targeting osteoclast precursors. Finally, two studies demonstrated that ciglitazone inhibits RANKL- and TNF-α-induced differentiation of human peripheral monocytes into osteoclasts [25,26]. Collectively, these seven independent investigations provide several lines of evidence supporting a notion that TZDs exert inhibitory effects on osteoclastogenesis.

Intriguingly, in 2007 Wan and coworkers demonstrated that rosiglitazone enhances RANKL-induced osteoclastogenesis in an PPARγ-dependent manner, proposing a concept that TZDs induce bone loss in patients with T2DM in part by promoting osteoclastogenesis [31]. Furthermore, a recent study has also shown that rosiglitazone exerts a stimulatory effect on osteoclastogenesis in vitro [32]. The stimulatory role of TZDs in osteoclastogenesis has been highlighted in several recent review papers [54,55], further promoting the view that TZDs induce bone loss in T2DM patients in part by enhancing osteoclast formation.

Several factors prompted us to carry out this study to further address the role of TZDs in osteoclastogenesis. First, the role of TZDs in osteoclastogenesis remains highly contentious and this controversy raises a concern about the notion that TZDs induce bone loss in T2DM patients in part by enhancing osteoclastogenesis [54,55]. We feel that a precise understanding of the role of TZDs in osteoclast formation is a prerequisite for further delineating the mechanism by which TZDs increase fracture risks; Secondly, a better understanding of the role of TZDs in osteoclastogenesis can assist in elucidating the precise role of PPARγ in osteoclastogenesis, which will facilitate future efforts to develop better PPARγ agonists; Thirdly, this study was also promoted by our recent studies revealing that RANKL-mediated osteoclast lineage commitment dictates the effect of various factors such as LPS, IFN-γ, IL-1 and TNF-α on osteoclastogenesis [42–49]. For example, early investigations on the role of LPS in osteoclastogenesis also generated conflicting results; while the majority of studies showed that LPS stimulates osteoclast formation, a few demonstrated that LPS exerts an inhibitory effect on the process. We later found that LPS inhibits osteoclast formation from normal BMMs but enhances osteoclastogenesis

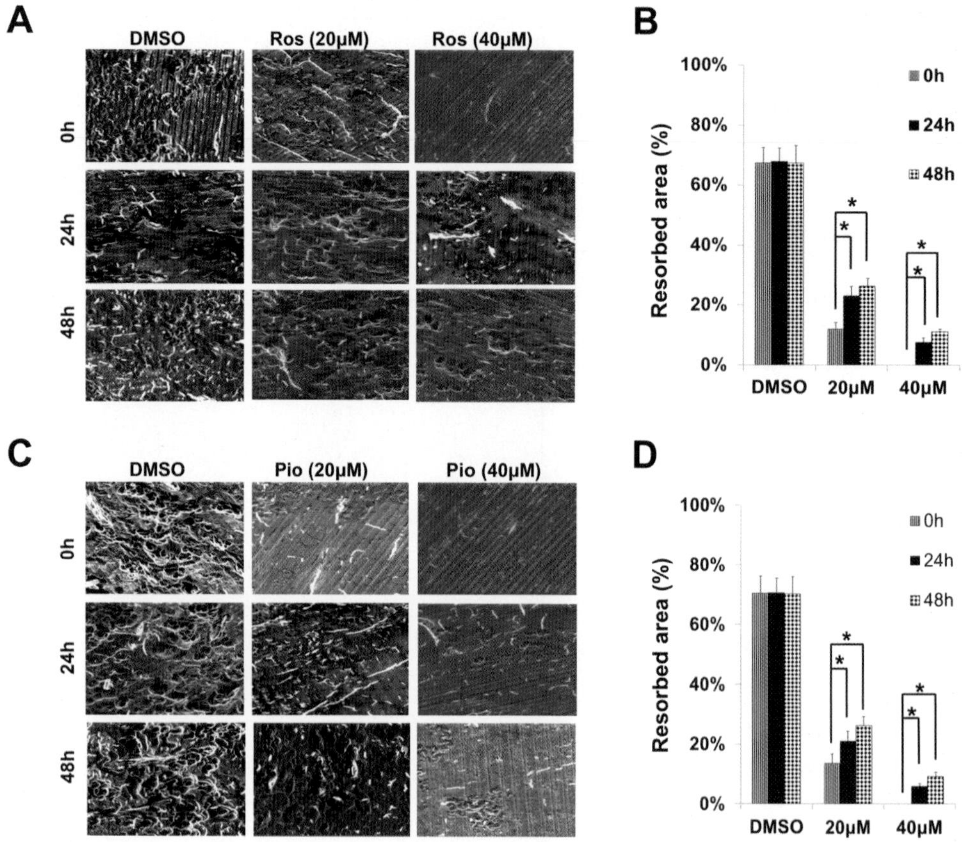

Figure 8. The inhibitory effects of rosiglitazone and pioglitazone on the formation of functional osteoclasts on bone slices are significantly decreased in RANKL-pretreated BMMs. (A) BMMs were seeded on bone slices and treated with M-CSF (44 ng/ml) and RNAKL (100 ng/ml) for 10 days. Vehicle (DMSO), 20 μM or 40 μM of rosiglitazone (Ros) was added at the beginning of the assays (0 hour – 0 h), or 24 h and 48 h after the start of the assays. Bone resorption pits were visualized by SEM and one representative view from each condition is shown. All assays were performed in duplicates and were repeated 2 times. (B) Quantification of bone resorption assays for rosiglitazone in A. 5 view areas on each bone slice were randomly chosen. Bars show mean percentage of resorbed bone area ±S.D. *$P<0.05$. (C) The same set of assays in A was performed with pioglitazone (Pio). (D) The bone resorption assays in C were quantified as described in B. *$P<0.05$.

when BMMs are pretreated with RANKL [42]; this led to a realization that the conflicting data on the role of LPS in osteoclastogenesis might result from cells with different states of lineage commitment used by different groups. So, our initial hypothesis was that RANKL-mediated osteoclast lineage commitment also modulates the effect of TZDs on osteoclastogenesis; specifically, TZDs inhibit osteoclastogenesis from normal BMMs but enhances osteoclastogenesis from RANKL-pretreated BMMs. Finally, a need for further studies to address the controversy is also raised by other investigators [18].

In light of the controversy, we carried out a series of *in vitro* osteoclastogenesis assays in this study to independently and thoroughly investigate the effect of TZDs on osteoclastogenesis using primary BMMs (namely, authentic osteoclast precursors) and two TZDs (rosiglitazone and pioglitazone). More importantly, we also validated key osteoclastogenesis data obtained from tissue culture plates by performing bone resorption assays to assess the formation of functional osteoclasts on bone slices, which represent the physiological substratum for osteoclastogenesis. We found that both rosiglitazone and pioglitazone dose-dependently inhibit osteoclastogenesis *in vitro* from normal BMMs (namely, primary BMMs which were freshly isolated and not subjected to treatments with RANKL or any other factors), replicating the findings from these seven previous studies [24–30]. To test our hypothesis that TZDs inhibit osteoclastogenesis from normal BMMs but enhances osteoclastogenesis from RANKL-pretreated BMMs, we further determined whether rosiglitazone and pioglitazone can promote osteoclastogenesis with low levels of RANKL or from RANKL-pretreated BMMs. Unexpectedly, we found that neither rosiglitazone nor pioglitazone was able to mediate osteoclastogenesis in the presence of low levels of RANKL or from RANKL-pretreated BMMs. Nonetheless, we found that the inhibitory effect of both rosiglitazone and pioglitazone is significantly reduced in RANKL-pretreated BMMs compared to normal BMMs. Thus, our data indicate that rosiglitazone and pioglitazone are unable to enhance osteoclastogenesis under any circumstances and this finding is inconsistent with those from two previous studies [31,32].

Obviously, the inhibitory effect of TZDs on osteoclastogenesis is counterintuitive given that clinical data indicate that TZD treatments cause bone loss and increase fracture risks in T2DM patients. So, how can our findings explain the clinical observation? To address this issue, we would like to highlight following important observations: a) TZDs inhibit osteoblast differentiation and bone formation [19–21]; b) TZDs induce bone loss in ovariectomized rats but not in intact rats [56]; c) TZD-induced bone loss is more pronounced in postmenopausal women [57], who have increased levels of RANKL expression on bone marrow cells compared to premenopausal counterparts [58]. Based on these observations and our current findings, we propose the following hypothesis to explain how TZDs induce bone loss and

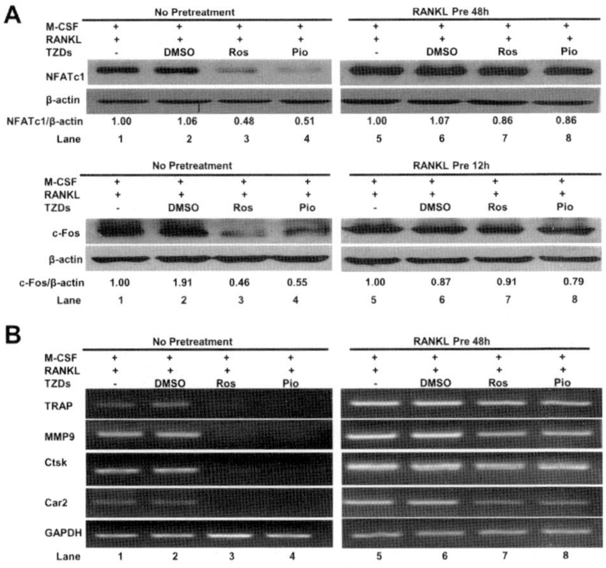

Figure 9. The inhibitory effects of rosiglitazone and pioglitazone on the expression of NFATc1, c-Fos, TRAP, MMP9, Ctsk and Car2 genes are significantly impaired in RANKL-pretreated BMMs. (A) Fresh BMMs (No Pretreatment) or BMMs pretreated with M-CSF (44 ng/ml) and RANKL (100 ng/ml) for 48 h (RANKL Pre 48 h) were treated with M-CSF (44 ng/ml) and RANKL (100 ng/ml), M-CSF (44 ng/ml) and RANKL (100 ng/ml) plus DMSO, 40 μM rosiglitazone (Ros) or pioglitazone (Pio) for 48 hours (h). Cells were then lysed for Western blot analysis of NFATc1 expression. For c-Fos assays, BMMs were pretreated with RANKL for 12 h before culturing with two TZDs for additional 12 h prior to Western blot analysis. The blots were stripped and then re-probed with β-actin antibody for loading control. Ratios of NFATc1/c-Fos to β-actin were obtained by dividing the densitometric reading of NFATc1/c-Fos with that of β-actin, and then the value calculated for the assay treated with M-CSF (44 ng/ml) and RANKL (100 ng/ml) was set as 1.00. The assays were repeated 3 times and the same results were obtained. One typical set of assays is shown. (B) The same set of cultures in A for NFATc1 was repeated for semi-quantitative RT-PCR analysis of the expression of TRAP, MMP9, Ctsk and Car2 genes using GAPDH gene as control. The assays were repeated 3 times and the same results were obtained. One set of assays is shown.

increase fracture risks in postmenopausal T2DM patients: in premenopausal T2DM patients, TZDs inhibit both osteoblast differentiation (bone formation) and osteoclast differentiation (bone resorption) probably to similar extents, thus resulting in no significant net change in bone mass. However, the onset of menopause leads to increases in RANKL levels, which augment the commitment of BMMs into the osteoclast lineage. As a consequence, the inhibitory effect of TZDs on osteoclast differentiation (bone resorption) is reduced based on our current finding while the extent of TZDs-mediated inhibition on osteoblast differentiation (bone formation) remains the same; this therefore leads to bone loss and increases in fracture risks in postmenopausal T2DM patients. Future studies should be carried out to test this hypothesis using ovariectomized mouse and/or rat models.

We extended our study to investigate the molecular mechanism by which TZDs suppress osteoclastogenesis. Our data indicate that rosiglitazone and pioglitazone inhibit osteoclastogenesis not through impairing RANKL-induced activation of the NF-κB, JNK, p38 and ERK pathways in BMMs. However, both rosiglitazone and pioglitazone inhibit RANKL-induced expression of NFATc1 and c-Fos, two key transcriptional regulators of osteoclastogenesis [37,38], and four osteoclast genes (TRAP, Ctsk, MMP9 and Car2). This observation is consistent with previous studies showing that rosiglitazone inhibits osteoclastogenesis from MOCP-5 osteoclast precursor cell line by down-regulating TRAP expression [27] and that rosiglitazone and pioglitazone block TNF-α-induced osteoclastogenesis by suppressing NFATc1 expression [28]. Interestingly, two groups demonstrated that RANK expression was down-regulated by rosiglitazone in BMMs [30] and by pioglitazone in RAW264.7 cells [29], suggesting that these TZDs may inhibit osteoclastogenesis by down-regulating RANK expression. It is noted that Wan et al previously showed that rosiglitazone not only enhances osteoclastogenesis but also mechanistically does so by up-regulating the expression of NFATc1 and the four osteoclast genes [31]. Their findings completely conflicts with ours in this study in that rosiglitazone and pioglitazone inhibits osteoclastogenesis in part by down-regulating the expression of NFATc1, c-Fos and the four osteoclast genes, and even in RANKL-pretreated BMMs rosiglitazone and pioglitazone were unable to up-regulate the expression of NFATc1 and the four osteoclast genes.

Our study has also raised several crucial issues which need to be further addressed to gain a complete understanding of the role and mechanisms of TZDs in osteoclast biology. The first question is whether TZDs mediate the inhibitory effects on osteoclastogenesis through PPARγ. Although TZDs were established as agonists of PPARγ, these synthetic compounds may also bind to other intracellular molecules. So, future studies are needed to address whether TZDs inhibit osteoclastogenesis in PPARγ-dependent or -independent manner. Secondly, if TZDs inhibit osteoclastogenesis in PPARγ-dependent fashion, a question arises regarding the molecular mechanism by which TZDs suppress osteoclastogenesis. Elucidation of the molecular mechanism underlying the inhibitory role of TZDs in osteoclastogenesis may guide the future development of new and better PPARγ agonists for therapy. Thirdly, it is noted that Wan et al investigated the role of PPARγ in osteoclastogenesis *in vivo* using a mouse model in which PPARγ is deleted in endothelial cells and multiple hematopoietic lineages [31]. If future *in vitro* studies demonstrate that TZDs inhibit osteoclastogenesis in PPARγ-dependent fashion, new animal models in which PPARγ is selectively deleted in osteoclast precursors (namely, hematopoietic cells of the monocyte/macrophage lineage) should be developed to better address the role of PPARγ in osteoclastogenesis *in vivo*.

In summary, the findings from this study combined with those from seven previous studies collectively support the notion that TZDs inhibit osteoclastogenesis. Moreover, our study also reveals new insights into the molecular mechanism by which TZDs inhibit osteoclastogenesis. These findings are significant since the precise understanding of the role of TZDs on osteoclastogenesis *in vitro* is required for designing proper animal model studies to delineate the mechanisms by which TZDs induce bone loss *in vivo*. Furthermore, our findings in this study highlight the importance of further investigation of the role of PPARγ in osteoclastogenesis *in vitro* and *in vivo*. These future studies will not only provide a better understanding of the role and mechanisms of TZDs and PPARγ in osteoclast biology but, more importantly, also facilitate development of better PPARγ agonists with no or fewer side effects for T2DM patients.

Acknowledgments

We thank Joel Jules, Erin M. McCoy and Huaping Chen in the Department of Pathology, and Yan Li in the Department of Nutritional Sciences at UAB for their expert technical assistance and Robin D. Foley in the Department of Materials Science & Engineering at UAB for her assistance in performing SEM and data analysis. Disclaimer: The content is solely the responsibility of the authors and does not necessarily represent the official views of the National Institutes of Health.

Author Contributions

Conceived and designed the experiments: XF YW AHW. Performed the experiments: DZ ZS HH PQ. Analyzed the data: DZ ZS HH PQ. Wrote the paper: DZ YW AHW XF.

References

1. Shaw JE, Sicree RA, Zimmet PZ (2010) Global estimates of the prevalence of diabetes for 2010 and 2030. Diabetes Res Clin Pract 87: 4–14.
2. Zhang P, Zhang X, Brown J, Vistisen D, Sicree R, et al. (2010) Global healthcare expenditure on diabetes for 2010 and 2030. Diabetes Res Clin Pract 87: 293–301.
3. Krishnaswami A, Ravi-Kumar S, Lewis JM (2010) Thiazolidinediones: a 2010 perspective. Perm J 14: 64–72.
4. Krentz AJ, Bailey CJ (2005) Oral antidiabetic agents: current role in type 2 diabetes mellitus. Drugs 65: 385–411.
5. Reginato MJ, Lazar MA (1999) Mechanisms by which Thiazolidinediones Enhance Insulin Action. Trends Endocrinol Metab 10: 9–13.
6. Tontonoz P, Spiegelman BM (2008) Fat and beyond: the diverse biology of PPARgamma. Annual review of biochemistry 77: 289–312.
7. Kim HI, Ahn YH (2004) Role of peroxisome proliferator-activated receptor-gamma in the glucose-sensing apparatus of liver and beta-cells. Diabetes 53 Suppl 1: S60–65.
8. Barroso I, Gurnell M, Crowley VE, Agostini M, Schwabe JW, et al. (1999) Dominant negative mutations in human PPARgamma associated with severe insulin resistance, diabetes mellitus and hypertension. Nature 402: 880–883.
9. Tontonoz P, Hu E, Spiegelman BM (1994) Stimulation of adipogenesis in fibroblasts by PPAR gamma 2, a lipid-activated transcription factor. Cell 79: 1147–1156.
10. Tontonoz P, Nagy L, Alvarez JG, Thomazy VA, Evans RM (1998) PPARgamma promotes monocyte/macrophage differentiation and uptake of oxidized LDL. Cell 93: 241–252.
11. Chawla A, Boisvert WA, Lee CH, Laffitte BA, Barak Y, et al. (2001) A PPAR gamma-LXR-ABCA1 pathway in macrophages is involved in cholesterol efflux and atherogenesis. Mol Cell 7: 161–171.
12. Jiang C, Ting AT, Seed B (1998) PPAR-gamma agonists inhibit production of monocyte inflammatory cytokines. Nature 391: 82–86.
13. Ricote M, Li AC, Willson TM, Kelly CJ, Glass CK (1998) The peroxisome proliferator-activated receptor-gamma is a negative regulator of macrophage activation. Nature 391: 79–82.
14. Lehrke M, Lazar MA (2005) The many faces of PPARgamma. Cell 123: 993–999.
15. Moseley KF (2012) Type 2 diabetes and bone fractures. Curr Opin Endocrinol Diabetes Obes 19: 128–135.
16. Betteridge DJ (2011) Thiazolidinediones and fracture risk in patients with Type 2 diabetes. Diabet Med 28: 759–771.
17. Bazelier MT, de Vries F, Vestergaard P, Herings RM, Gallagher AM, et al. (2013) Risk of fracture with thiazolidinediones: an individual patient data meta-analysis. Front Endocrinol (Lausanne) 4: 11.
18. Mabilleau G, Chappard D, Basle MF (2011) Cellular and molecular effects of thiazolidinediones on bone cells: a review. Int J Biochem Mol Biol 2: 240–246.
19. Lecka-Czernik B, Moerman EJ, Grant DF, Lehmann JM, Manolagas SC, et al. (2002) Divergent effects of selective peroxisome proliferator-activated receptor-gamma 2 ligands on adipocyte versus osteoblast differentiation. Endocrinology 143: 2376–2384.
20. Ali AA, Weinstein RS, Stewart SA, Parfitt AM, Manolagas SC, et al. (2005) Rosiglitazone causes bone loss in mice by suppressing osteoblast differentiation and bone formation. Endocrinology 146: 1226–1235.
21. Rzonca SO, Suva LJ, Gaddy D, Montague DC, Lecka-Czernik B (2004) Bone is a target for the antidiabetic compound rosiglitazone. Endocrinology 145: 401–406.
22. Soroceanu MA, Miao D, Bai XY, Su H, Goltzman D, et al. (2004) Rosiglitazone impacts negatively on bone by promoting osteoblast/osteocyte apoptosis. J Endocrinol 183: 203–216.
23. Mabilleau G, Mieczkowska A, Edmonds ME (2010) Thiazolidinediones induce osteocyte apoptosis and increase sclerostin expression. Diabet Med 27: 925–932.
24. Okazaki R, Toriumi M, Fukumoto S, Miyamoto M, Fujita T, et al. (1999) Thiazolidinediones inhibit osteoclast-like cell formation and bone resorption in vitro. Endocrinology 140: 5060–5065.
25. Chan BY, Gartland A, Wilson PJ, Buckley KA, Dillon JP, et al. (2007) PPAR agonists modulate human osteoclast formation and activity in vitro. Bone 40: 149–159.
26. Hounoki H, Sugiyama E, Mohamed SG, Shinoda K, Taki H, et al. (2008) Activation of peroxisome proliferator-activated receptor gamma inhibits TNF-alpha-mediated osteoclast differentiation in human peripheral monocytes in part via suppression of monocyte chemoattractant protein-1 expression. Bone 42: 765–774.
27. Hassumi MY, Silva-Filho VJ, Campos-Junior JC, Vieira SM, Cunha FQ, et al. (2009) PPAR-gamma agonist rosiglitazone prevents inflammatory periodontal bone loss by inhibiting osteoclastogenesis. International immunopharmacology 9: 1150–1158.
28. Yang CR, Lai CC (2010) Thiazolidinediones inhibit TNF-alpha-mediated osteoclast differentiation of RAW264.7 macrophages and mouse bone marrow cells through downregulation of NFATc1. Shock 33: 662–667.
29. Jiang M, Lu S, Wu L, Liu J, Cheng P, et al. (2010) [Effect of pioglitazone on receptor activator of nuclear factor-kappa B expression in osteoclast from RAW264.7 cells]. Zhonghua Yi Xue Za Zhi 90: 2282–2285.
30. Cho ES, Kim MK, Son YO, Lee KS, Park SM, et al. (2012) The effects of rosiglitazone on osteoblastic differentiation, osteoclast formation and bone resorption. Mol Cells 33: 173–181.
31. Wan Y, Chong LW, Evans RM (2007) PPAR-gamma regulates osteoclastogenesis in mice. Nature medicine 13: 1496–1503.
32. Wu H, Li L, Ma Y, Chen Y, Zhao J, et al. (2013) Regulation of selective PPARgamma modulators in the differentiation of osteoclasts. J Cell Biochem 114: 1969–1977.
33. Teitelbaum SL (2007) Osteoclasts: what do they do and how do they do it? Am J Pathol 170: 427–435.
34. Feng X, McDonald JM (2011) Disorders of bone remodeling. Annu Rev Pathol 6: 121–145.
35. Boyle WJ, Simonet WS, Lacey DL (2003) Osteoclast differentiation and activation. Nature 423: 337–342.
36. Feng X (2005) Regulatory roles and molecular signaling of TNF family members in osteoclasts. Gene 350: 1–13.
37. Takayanagi H, Kim S, Koga T, Nishina H, Isshiki M, et al. (2002) Induction and activation of the transcription factor NFATc1 (NFAT2) integrate RANKL signaling in terminal differentiation of osteoclasts. Dev Cell 3: 889–901.
38. Grigoriadis AE, Wang ZQ, Cecchini MG, Hofstetter W, Felix R, et al. (1994) c-Fos: a key regulator of osteoclast-macrophage lineage determination and bone remodeling. Science 266: 443–448.
39. Cappellen D, Luong-Nguyen NH, Bongiovanni S, Grenet O, Wanke C, et al. (2002) Transcriptional program of mouse osteoclast differentiation governed by the macrophage colony-stimulating factor and the ligand for the receptor activator of NFkappa B. J Biol Chem 277: 21971–21982.
40. Rho J, Altmann CR, Socci ND, Merkov L, Kim N, et al. (2002) Gene expression profiling of osteoclast differentiation by combined suppression subtractive hybridization (SSH) and cDNA microarray analysis. DNA Cell Biol 21: 541–549.
41. Xu D, Wang S, Liu W, Liu J, Feng X (2006) A novel receptor activator of NF-kappaB (RANK) cytoplasmic motif plays an essential role in osteoclastogenesis by committing macrophages to the osteoclast lineage. The Journal of biological chemistry 281: 4678–4690.
42. Liu J, Wang S, Zhang P, Said-Al-Naief N, Michalek SM, et al. (2009) Molecular mechanism of the bifunctional role of lipopolysaccharide in osteoclastogenesis. The Journal of biological chemistry 284: 12512–12523.
43. Zou W, Bar-Shavit Z (2002) Dual modulation of osteoclast differentiation by lipopolysaccharide. Journal of bone and mineral research : the official journal of the American Society for Bone and Mineral Research 17: 1211–1218.
44. Huang W, O'Keefe RJ, Schwarz EM (2003) Exposure to receptor-activator of NFkappaB ligand renders pre-osteoclasts resistant to IFN-gamma by inducing terminal differentiation. Arthritis Res Ther 5: R49–59.
45. Cheng J, Liu J, Shi Z, Jules J, Xu D, et al. (2012) Molecular mechanisms of the biphasic effects of interferon-gamma on osteoclastogenesis. J Interferon Cytokine Res 32: 34–45.
46. Lam J, Takeshita S, Barker JE, Kanagawa O, Ross FP, et al. (2000) TNF-alpha induces osteoclastogenesis by direct stimulation of macrophages exposed to permissive levels of RANK ligand. The Journal of clinical investigation 106: 1481–1488.
47. Jules J, Shi Z, Liu J, Xu D, Wang S, et al. (2010) Receptor activator of NF-{kappa}B (RANK) cytoplasmic IVVY535–538 motif plays an essential role in tumor necrosis factor-{alpha} (TNF)-mediated osteoclastogenesis. The Journal of biological chemistry 285: 37427–37435.
48. Jules J, Zhang P, Ashley JW, Wei S, Shi Z, et al. (2012) Molecular basis of requirement of receptor activator of nuclear factor kappaB signaling for interleukin 1-mediated osteoclastogenesis. J Biol Chem 287: 15728–15738.
49. Wei S, Kitaura H, Zhou P, Ross FP, Teitelbaum SL (2005) IL-1 mediates TNF-induced osteoclastogenesis. The Journal of clinical investigation 115: 282–290.
50. McHugh KP, Hodivala-Dilke K, Zheng MH, Namba N, Lam J, et al. (2000) Mice lacking beta3 integrins are osteosclerotic because of dysfunctional osteoclasts. The Journal of clinical investigation 105: 433–440.
51. Takeshita S, Kaji K, Kudo A (2000) Identification and characterization of the new osteoclast progenitor with macrophage phenotypes being able to differentiate into mature osteoclasts. J Bone Miner Res 15: 1477–1488.
52. Jules J, Zhang P, Ashley JW, Wei S, Shi Z, et al. (2012) Molecular basis of requirement of receptor activator of nuclear factor kappaB signaling for interleukin 1-mediated osteoclastogenesis. The Journal of biological chemistry 287: 15728–15738.

53. Chen W, Li YP (1998) Generation of mouse osteoclastogenic cell lines immortalized with SV40 large T antigen. J Bone Miner Res 13: 1112–1123.
54. Wan Y (2010) PPARgamma in bone homeostasis. Trends Endocrinol Metab 21: 722–728.
55. Ahmadian M, Suh JM, Hah N, Liddle C, Atkins AR, et al. (2013) PPARgamma signaling and metabolism: the good, the bad and the future. Nat Med 19: 557–566.
56. Sottile V, Seuwen K, Kneissel M (2004) Enhanced marrow adipogenesis and bone resorption in estrogen-deprived rats treated with the PPARgamma agonist BRL49653 (rosiglitazone). Calcified tissue international 75: 329–337.
57. Grey A, Bolland M, Gamble G, Wattie D, Horne A, et al. (2007) The peroxisome proliferator-activated receptor-gamma agonist rosiglitazone decreases bone formation and bone mineral density in healthy postmenopausal women: a randomized, controlled trial. The Journal of clinical endocrinology and metabolism 92: 1305–1310.
58. Eghbali-Fatourechi G, Khosla S, Sanyal A, Boyle WJ, Lacey DL, et al. (2003) Role of RANK ligand in mediating increased bone resorption in early postmenopausal women. The Journal of clinical investigation 111: 1221–1230.

Parkinson's Disease and Risk of Fracture: A Meta-Analysis of Prospective Cohort Studies

Li Tan[9], Ying Wang[9], Lingling Zhou, Yun Shi, Fan Zhang, Li Liu, Shaofa Nie*

Department of Epidemiology and Biostatistics, School of Public Health, Tongji Medical College, Huazhong University of Science and Technology, Wuhan, P. R. China

Abstract

Backgrounds/Objective: Parkinson's disease (PD) is the second most common neurodegenerative disease among the elderly population. However, epidemiological evidence on the relationship of PD with risk of fracture has not been systematically assessed. Therefore, we performed this meta-analysis of prospective studies to explore the association between PD and risk of fracture.

Methods: PubMed, Embase, Web of Science and Cochrane Library up to February 26, 2014 were searched to identify eligible studies. Random-effects model was used to pool the results.

Results: Six studies that totally involved 69,387 participants were included for analysis. Overall, PD patients had an increased risk of fracture compared with control subjects (pooled hazard ratio = 2.66, 95% confidence interval: 2.10–3.36). No publication bias was observed across studies and the subgroup as well as sensitivity analysis suggested that the general results were robust.

Conclusion: The present study suggested that PD is associated with an increased risk of fracture. However, given the limited number and moderate quality of included studies, well-designed prospective cohort studies are required to confirm the findings from this meta-analysis.

Editor: Katriina Aalto-Setala, University of Tampere, Finland

Funding: The authors have no support or funding to report.

Competing Interests: The authors have declared that no competing interests exist.

* E-mail: sf_nie@mails.tjmu.edu.cn

[9] These authors contributed equally to this work.

Introduction

Parkinson's disease (PD) is the second most common neurodegenerative disease among the elderly population. It is characterized clinically by three motor symptoms including resting tremors, rigidity and bradykinesia [1,2], with an estimated prevalence of about 1% among people aged over 60 years old [3]. PD is still an incurable progressive neurological disease and seriously impairs the quality of life (QOL) [4]. Therefore, it is of great importance to improve QOL and functional capacity as well as reduce the risk of subsequent adverse results.

Previous studies have suggested that PD patients have an increased risk of falls and reduced bone mineral density (BMD) compared with healthy controls [5,6]. However, both falls and lower BMD are recognized determinants for the increased risk for fractures [7–9]. In recent years, there is growing evidence suggesting an increased risk for developing fractures in patients with PD [6,10–17]. Nevertheless, epidemiological evidence on the relationship of PD with fracture risk has not been systematically assessed. Since the strength of prospective studies is stronger than retrospective studies, we conducted a meta-analysis of prospective cohort studies to explore the effects of PD on incidence of fracture.

Methods and Materials

Search Strategy

We followed the Meta-Analysis of Observational Studies in Epidemiology guidelines [18] to conduct this meta-analysis. We undertook a systematic search on PubMed, EMBASE, Web of Science and the Cochrane library up to February 26, 2014 for relevant prospective cohort studies that reported the association between Parkinson disease and risk of fracture. We also scanned the reference lists of all retrieved articles to find if there were any additional literatures. The search terms used were '(Parkinson's disease OR Parkinson disease) AND Fracture'. There was no language restriction.

Study Selection Criteria

Studies were included if they met the following criteria: i.) had a prospective cohort design, ii.) evaluated the association between PD and at least one anatomical site of fracture, iii.) reported the relative risk (RR) or hazard ratio (HR) and its 95% confidence interval(CI), iv.) excluded participants with fractures at baseline. Studies that had retrospective design or did not report risk estimates or were conference abstract were excluded. Only the most recent study with the longest follow-up duration was included

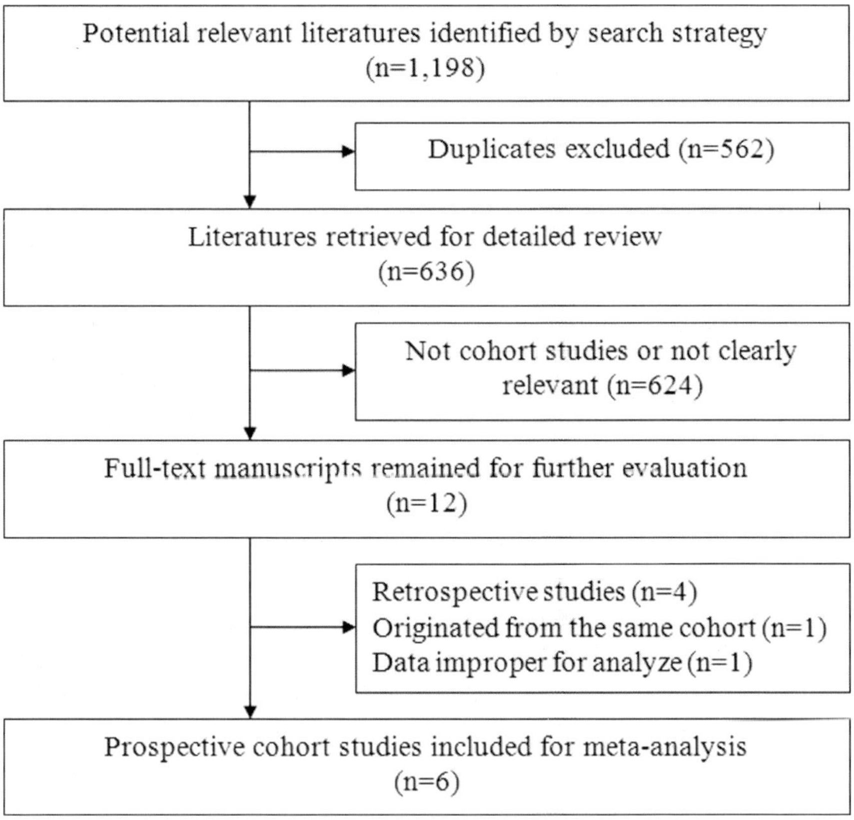

Figure 1. Selection flow of studies included in the meta-analysis. Two authors independently performed the literature search and selection to include prospective cohort studies regarding association between PD and risk of fracture, disagreement were resolved by discussion.

if publications were duplicated or originated from the same study population.

Data Extraction and Quality Assessment

Data extraction was performed by two independent reviewers, with any discrepancies resolved by discussion. We extracted the following data from the included studies: name of the first author, year of publication, study location, age of the study population, ratio of males to females, follow-up years, outcome assessment method, total number of fracture cases and study population, site of fracture and the corresponding risk estimates with 95%CI, and confounders that were adjusted for in the analysis.

We used a 9-star system based on the Newcastle-Ottawa Scale (NOS) [19] to assess the study quality. The maximum score of 9 points could be assigned to a study which had the highest methodological quality, with 4, 2, 3 scores respectively being assigned to selection of study groups, comparability of study groups, assessment of outcomes and adequacy of follow-up. Studies with scores of 0–3, 4–6, 7–9 were respectively deemed as low, moderate, and high quality.

Data Analysis

Data for any site of facture were included for main meta-analysis. However, for studies that only reported one specific site of fracture, the corresponding risk estimates with 95%CI were also included for analysis. In a study [6] which reported both hip fracture and non-spine, non-hip fracture in two separate analysis cohorts, only the HR regarding hip fracture was extracted for main analysis as hip fracture is the most devastating type of fracture [20]. We transformed HRs or RRs by taking their natural logarithms. Standard errors were calculated from ln (HR) or ln (RR) and corresponding CIs. Heterogeneity in results across studies was assessed using the Cochrane's Q test and I^2 statistic [21,22]. The heterogeneity was considered statistically significant when $P \leq 0.10$ and $I^2 > 50\%$. A random-effects model [23] was used to pool the results because this model takes into account both study sample size and between-study variation [24]. We also performed sensitivity analysis to explore the potential influence of each individual study on overall results. Subgroup analyses were carried out according to sex, study location, site of fracture, follow-up years, quality score and number of confounders for adjustment.

Publication bias was detected by using both Begg's test [25] and Egger's test [26]. Begg's test or Egger's test was considered to indicate significant statistical publication bias when P-value<0.05. All data analyses were conducted using STATA version 11.0 (Stata Corporation, College Station, TX).

Results

Literature Search

Figure 1 presents the study selection flow. A total of 1,198 articles were identified by the search strategy. After removing 562 duplicates, 636 articles were left for screening. After screening of titles or abstracts, 624 articles that were not clearly relevant or not cohort studies were excluded. After reading the full text of the remained 12 articles, 4 articles [13,15,17,27] were excluded as they were retrospective studies, 1 article [11] was excluded as we included another article reported the same study with a longer follow-up duration. 1 study [28] calculated the odds ratio (OR)

Table 1. Characteristics of epidemiological studies of parkinson's disease and risk of fracture included in the meta-analysis.

Studies	Study location	Ratio of Males to Females, %	Age, years	Total cases/ Total population	Follow-up years	Outcome Assessment	Site of fracture	Adjustment for Confounders
Taylor, 2004 [30]	U.S.	0:100	73.3 ± 4.9[1]	604/6,787	8.9	Self-report and confirmed by review of radiological reports	Hip	Age
Melton, 2006 [16]	U.S.	61:39	Median 71 (range 40–97)	100/392	13	Inpatient and outpatient records	Any/hip/spine/skull or face/pelvis/ribs/clavicle or scapula or sternum/ distal forearm/other arm or hands/other leg or feet	NA[2]
Schneider, 2008 [6]	U.S.	0:100	≧65	850/8,105	9(hip cohort); 8 (non-spine, non-hip cohort)	Self-reported, confirmed by expert review of radiology reports	Hip/Non-spine and non-hip	Age, walking speed, depression, self-reported health status, falls in past year, weight change, and total hip bone mineral density
Fink, 2008 [12]	U.S.	100:0	≧65	431/5,937	4.6	Self-report, confirmed by central review of radiographic reports	Non-spine	Age
Chen, 2012 [10]	Taiwan	49:51	68.6 ± 7.3[1]	201/4,334	8	Discharge diagnosis	Hip	Age, gender, state of co-morbid hypertension, diabetes, diabetic neuropathy, osteoporosis, and hyperlipidemia
Gregson, 2013 [29]	10 countries[3]	0:100	≧55	2,945/43,832	3	Self-report	Any	NA[2]

[1]It was mean age ± standard deviation.
[2]NA: Not available.
[3]Australia, Belgium, Canada, France, Germany, Italy, Netherlands, Spain, U.K., and U.S.

Table 2. Methodological quality of cohort studies included in the meta-analysis.

Studies	Selection				Comparability	Outcome			Total scores
	Representativeness of the exposed cohort	Selection of the unexposed cohort	Ascertainment of exposure	Outcome of interest not present at start of study	Control for important factor or additional factor[1]	Outcome assessment	Follow-up long enough for outcomes to occur	Adequacy of follow-up of cohorts	
Taylor, 2004 [30]	–	☆	☆	☆	☆☆	☆	☆	–	7
Melton, 2006 [16]	☆	☆	☆	☆	–	☆	☆	☆	7
Schneider, 2008 [6]	☆	☆	–	–	☆☆	☆	☆	☆	7
Fink, 2008 [12]	☆	☆	–	–	☆☆	☆	☆	–	6
Chen, 2012 [10]	☆	☆	☆	☆	☆☆	☆	☆	☆	9
Gregson, 2013 [29]	☆	☆	☆	–	–	–	☆	☆	5

[1]A maximum of 2 stars could be assigned to this item.

and its 95%CI based on an estimated number of people with PD using a crude PD prevalence from two studies. Because this kind of estimation failed to consider many potential confounding factors and thus the OR might not be accurate, thus we did not included this study. Finally, a total of 6 prospective cohort studies [6,10,12,16,29,30] were included for meta-analysis.

Study Characteristics

Table 1 summarizes the main characteristics of the studies for analysis. Of the 6 studies, 4 studies [6,12,16,30] were conducted in the United States, 1 study [10] was conducted in Taiwan, while 1 study [29] was a conducted in 10 countries including Australia, Belgium, Canada, France, Germany, Italy, Netherlands, Spain, U.K., and U.S. 3 studies [6,29,30] only consisted of females, 1 study [12] only consisted of males while 2 studies [10,16] involved both sex. The study population ranged from 392 to 43,832, with a total of 69,387 participants involved in. Adjusted HR was reported in 4 studies [6,10,12,30]. The follow-up years were 3, 4.6, 8, 8.9, 9, and 13 respectively for the 6 studies. For the outcome assessment, 4 studies [6,12,29,30] were based on self-report, while 1 [10] was ascertained by discharge diagnosis and 1 [16] was based on inpatient and outpatient records. Fractures were most frequently reported in the hip [6,10,16,30]. Table 2 presents the results of quality assessment based on NOS, 4 studies were in high quality (1 [10] scored 9 and 3 [6,16,30] scored 7, respectively) while the other 2 studies [12,29] were in moderate quality (scored 6 and 5 respectively).

Main Analysis

Figure 2 shows a forest plot presenting individual and overall results. No statistically significant heterogeneity was observed across studies ($P_{heterogeneity} = 0.159$, $I^2 = 37.1\%$). Overall, meta-analysis of the included studies by random-effects model suggested an increased risk of fracture in those with PD compared to those without PD (Overall HR = 2.66, 95% CI: 2.10–3.36).

Subgroup and Sensitivity Analysis

Table 3 shows the effects of PD on fracture risk in subgroup analysis. From the results, we observed a similar summary HR in men (HR = 2.55, 95%CI: 1.77–3.67) and in women (HR = 2.54, 95%CI: 1.67–3.86), and greater summary HR in studies with a follow-up duration of less than 6 years (HR = 3.46, 95%CI: 2.30–5.19) than that of more than 6 years (HR = 2.36, 95%CI: 1.92–2.90). Subgroup analysis on other strata generally had similar results with the overall result.

For the result of sensitivity analysis, the pooled HR was not substantially influenced by any of the individual studies when omitting one study each time and recalculated the overall results, with a range from 2.36(95% CI: 1.94–2.88) to 2.87(95% CI: 2.22–3.73). As two included studies [16,29] reported unadjusted HRs, we excluded them and re-pooled the result. However, the re-pooled HR was only slightly reduced and was similar to the general result (HR = 2.51, 95%CI: 1.92–3.27).

Publication Bias

The Begg's and Egger's test suggested no evidence of publication bias in studies of PD and fracture risk (all $P>0.05$).

Discussion

To our knowledge, this is the first meta-analysis of prospective cohort studies on PD and risk of fracture. Findings from the present analysis suggest that PD was associated with a 2.66-fold increased risk for fracture. Subgroup analysis and sensitivity

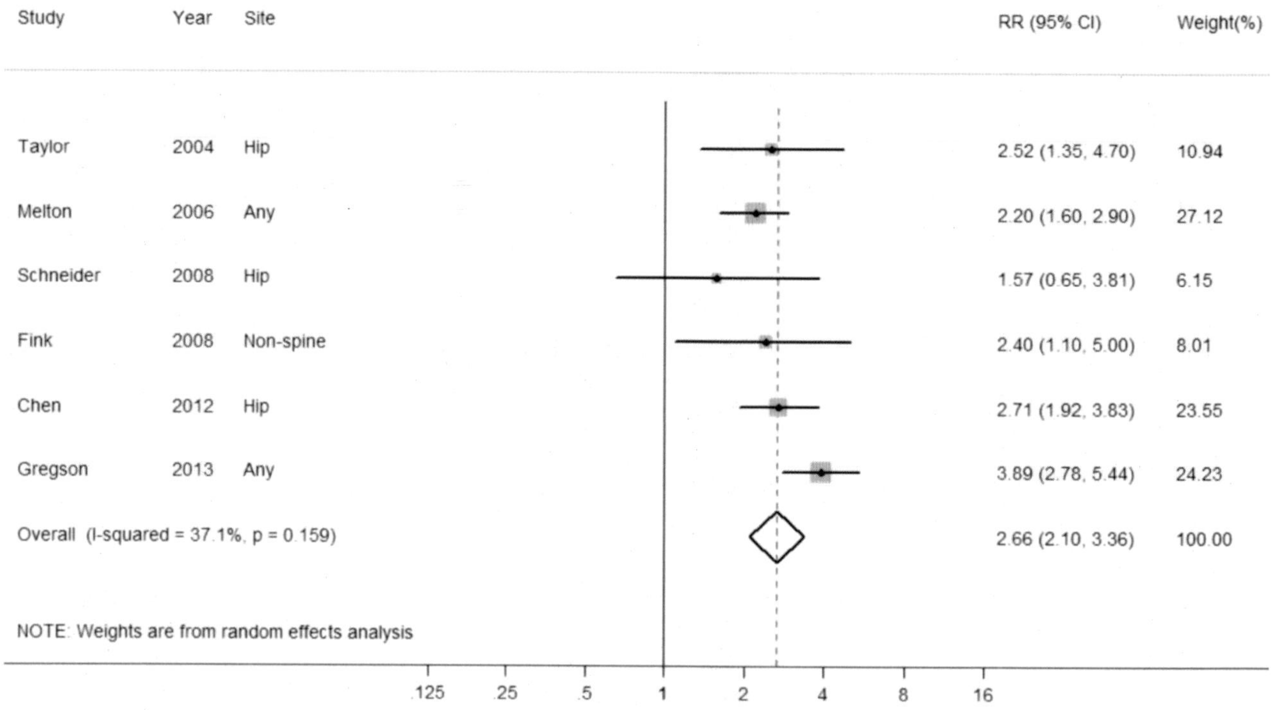

Figure 2. A forest plot of the association between PD and risk of fracture. Random-effects model was used to pool the overall hazard ratios (HRs) and 95% confidence intervals (CIs). The diamond represents the pooled HR and, the squares and the horizontal lines respectively represent the HR and 95% CI of each individual study.

Table 3. Summary risk estimates of the association between PD and risk of fracture[1].

Factors	**No. of studies**	**Summary adjusted HR (95%)**	**Heterogeneity I^2 (%)**
Sex			
Male	2	2.55(1.77, 3.67)	0
Female	4	2.54(1.67, 3.86)	62.2
Study location			
US/Europe	5	2.60(1.89, 3.57)	49.7
Asia	1	2.71(1.92, 3.83)	NA
Site of fracture			
Any	2	2.91(1.66, 5.09)	83.9
Hip	4	2.66(2.07, 3.42)	0
Non-spine	2	1.61(0.70, 3.73)	51.8
Follow-up years			
>6	4	2.36(1.92, 2.90)	0
<6	2	3.46(2.30, 5.19)	23.5
No. of factors for adjustment			
>5	4	2.75(1.98, 3.83)	53.6
<5	2	2.42(1.56, 3.74)	21.3
Quality scroe			
≥7	4	2.75(1.98, 3.83)	53.6
<7	2	2.42(1.56, 3.74)	21.3

[1]PD: Parkinson's disease.
[2]HR: Hazard ratio.

analysis suggested that the overall result of this analysis was robust and there was no publication bias.

The underlying mechanism involved in the association between PD and fracture is still not clear. However, two main concerns might be explainable for their association. First, falls are important risk factors for fractures and 90% of fractures in older people result from a fall [13]. It was estimated that the annual incidence of falls among PD patients was 68%, with the majority of the fallers fell again in the following year [31]. Moreover, as the disease progresses, the occurrence of falls increased in PD patients [5]. Second, PD patients have lower BMD than healthy controls [32] and thus may have higher risk of fracture. In addition, low BMD in PD patients may be related to various factors, including reduced mobility, vitamin D deficiency, vitamin K deficiency, dysautonomia, and altered estrogen or growth hormone levels [33]. As all these factors are common in PD patients, they may act synergistically to the increased risk of fracture [34].

Along with the improvement and development of living conditions and medical care services, people tend to live longer compared with several decades ago, the global average life expectancy at birth increased from 64 years in 1990 to 70 years in 2011 according to WHO [35]. The estimated number of PD patients is expected to increase considerably because of the burden of chronic diseases being closely related to the increase of life expectancy in the most populous nations [36]. Meanwhile, the number of falls increases as the number of elderly population increases in many nations throughout the world [37]. Although it is not clear to what an extent the incidence of fractures were attributed to PD, the potential PD-related fracture and its corresponding burden of disease should not be neglected. Therefore, the findings from this study call for sufficient attention and care for the PD patients so as to reduce the subsequent fracture risk.

Both men and women have potential risk of fractures. In our study, we observed a similar summary HR in men (HR = 2.55, 95%CI: 1.77–3.67) and in women (HR = 2.54, 95%CI: 1.67–3.86). However, previous studies [38,39] have suggested that postmenopausal women tend to have a higher fracture incidence than older men, which might be explained by the estrogen deficiency-related substantial decline in bone mass and changes in bone architecture [40]. The reason why men had similar pronounced risk might be related to the inconsistent conditions of individual studies, including age, site of fractures, progression stages of PD and ethnicity. Moreover, the stability of these findings is limited by the rare number of included studies.

Both severity and duration of PD are independent predictors of recurrent falls [41,42], which implies that longer duration and more severity of PD may be associated with increased risk of fracture. However, in our study we found that the magnitude of increased risk in studies with shorter duration of follow-up was stronger than that with longer length of follow-up period (HR: 3.46 vs. 2.36). Nevertheless, considering the limited number of included studies, this finding should be interpreted with caution and further studies are required to determine the potential period for high risk of fracture in PD patients.

The present study has several strengths. Only prospective cohort studies were included for analysis, thus precluding the possibility of recall and selection biases. Meanwhile, no publication bias was observed, which suggests that no statistically significant effect of potential unpublished papers existed.

There are still several potential limitations. Firstly, while 4 included studies [6,10,12,30] adjusted for several factors, 2 studies [16,29] only reported unadjusted HRs. However, studies that reported unadjusted HR either used age as the time scale or were ordered by age in their estimation models, and the subgroup analysis excluding this two studies did not alter the general result, Nevertheless, the possibility that the association between PD and risk of fracture could be attributed to other potential confounders (such as vitamin D intake, dysautonomia, and growth hormone levels) could not be excluded. Secondly, although no statistical heterogeneity was observed between studies, there was potential clinical heterogeneity and methodological heterogeneity. However, results from sensitivity analysis and subgroup analysis suggested that the general result of this meta-analysis was rather robust. Thirdly, the information on fractures was self-reported without any objective ascertainments in one study [29], there was a possibility that it may lead to misclassification of fracture status due to potential recall bias. Nevertheless, the validity and accuracy of self-reported information for fractures were supported by previous studies [43,44]. Finally, the length of follow-up varied among included studies, with 3 years in the shortest and 13 years in the longest; it is therefore difficult to determine the long-term impact of PD on fractures among the studies with insufficient follow-up duration.

Conclusion

In conclusion, this meta-analysis indicates that PD is associated with an increased risk of fracture. However, given the limited number and quality of included studies, further well-designed studies are warranted to confirm the findings from our study.

Author Contributions

Conceived and designed the experiments: SFN LT YW. Performed the experiments: LT YW LLZ. Analyzed the data: LT YW LLZ YS. Contributed reagents/materials/analysis tools: LT YW FZ LLZ. Wrote the paper: LT YW.

References

1. De Lau LM, Breteler MM (2006) Epidemiology of Parkinson's disease. Lancet Neurol 5: 525–535.
2. Gottlich M, Munte TF, Heldmann M, Kasten M, Hagenah J, et al. (2013) Altered resting state brain networks in Parkinson's disease. PLoS One 8: e77336.
3. Nussbaum RL, Ellis CE (2003) Alzheimer's disease and Parkinson's disease. N Engl J Med 348: 1356–1364.
4. Chen S, Zheng J (2012) Translational Neurodegeneration, a platform to share knowledge and experience in translational study of neurodegenerative diseases. Translational Neurodegeneration 1: 1–3.
5. Hiorth YH, Lode K, Larsen JP (2013) Frequencies of falls and associated features at different stages of Parkinson's disease. Eur J Neurol 20: 160–166.
6. Schneider JL, Fink HA, Ewing SK, Ensrud KE, Cummings SR (2008) The association of Parkinson's disease with bone mineral density and fracture in older women. Osteoporos Int 19: 1093–1097.
7. Edwards MH, Jameson K, Denison H, Harvey NC, Sayer AA, et al. (2013) Clinical risk factors, bone density and fall history in the prediction of incident fracture among men and women. Bone 52: 541–547.
8. Marshall D, Johnell O, Wedel H (1996) Meta-analysis of how well measures of bone mineral density predict occurrence of osteoporotic fractures. BMJ 312: 1254–1259.
9. Hartholt KA, Oudshoorn C, Zielinski SM, Burgers PT, Panneman MJ, et al. (2011) The epidemic of hip fractures: are we on the right track? PLoS One 6: e22227.
10. Chen YY, Cheng PY, Wu SL, Lai CH (2012) Parkinson's disease and risk of hip fracture: an 8-year follow-up study in Taiwan. Parkinsonism Relat Disord 18: 506–509.

11. Dennison EM, Compston JE, Flahive J, Siris ES, Gehlbach SH, et al. (2012) Effect of co-morbidities on fracture risk: findings from the Global Longitudinal Study of Osteoporosis in Women (GLOW). Bone 50: 1288–1293.
12. Fink HA, Kuskowski MA, Taylor BC, Schousboe JT, Orwoll ES, et al. (2008) Association of Parkinson's disease with accelerated bone loss, fractures and mortality in older men: the Osteoporotic Fractures in Men (MrOS) study. Osteoporos Int 19: 1277–1282.
13. Genever RW, Downes TW, Medcalf P (2005) Fracture rates in Parkinson's disease compared with age- and gender-matched controls: a retrospective cohort study. Age Ageing 34: 21–24.
14. Grisso JA, Kelsey JL, Strom BL, Chiu GY, Maislin G, et al. (1991) Risk factors for falls as a cause of hip fracture in women. The Northeast Hip Fracture Study Group. N Engl J Med 324: 1326–1331.
15. Johnell O, Melton LJ, 3rd, Atkinson EJ, O'Fallon WM, Kurland LT (1992) Fracture risk in patients with parkinsonism: a population-based study in Olmsted County, Minnesota. Age Ageing 21: 32–38.
16. Melton LJ, 3rd, Leibson CL, Achenbach SJ, Bower JH, Maraganore DM, et al. (2006) Fracture risk after the diagnosis of Parkinson's disease: Influence of concomitant dementia. Mov Disord 21: 1361–1367.
17. Pouwels S, Bazelier MT, de Boer A, Weber WE, Neef C, et al. (2013) Risk of fracture in patients with Parkinson's disease. Osteoporos Int 24: 2283–2290.
18. Stroup DF, Berlin JA, Morton SC, Olkin I, Williamson GD, et al. (2000) Meta-analysis of observational studies in epidemiology: a proposal for reporting. Meta-analysis Of Observational Studies in Epidemiology (MOOSE) group. JAMA 283: 2008–2012.
19. Wells G, Shea B, O'connell D, Peterson J, Welch V, et al. (2000) The Newcastle-Ottawa Scale (NOS) for assessing the quality of nonrandomised studies in meta-analyses.
20. Boonen S, Singer AJ (2008) Osteoporosis management: impact of fracture type on cost and quality of life in patients at risk for fracture I. Current Medical Research and Opinion 24: 1781–1788.
21. Higgins JP, Thompson SG (2002) Quantifying heterogeneity in a meta-analysis. Stat Med 21: 1539–1558.
22. Higgins JP, Thompson SG, Deeks JJ, Altman DG (2003) Measuring inconsistency in meta-analyses. BMJ 327: 557–560.
23. DerSimonian R, Laird N (1986) Meta-analysis in clinical trials. Control Clin Trials 7: 177–188.
24. Rosenthal L, Schisterman E (2010) Meta-analysis: drawing conclusions when study results vary. Methods Mol Biol 594: 427–434.
25. Begg CB, Mazumdar M (1994) Operating characteristics of a rank correlation test for publication bias. Biometrics 50: 1088–1101.
26. Egger M, Davey Smith G, Schneider M, Minder C (1997) Bias in meta-analysis detected by a simple, graphical test. BMJ 315: 629–634.
27. Bhattacharya RK, Dubinsky RM, Lai SM, Dubinsky H (2012) Is there an increased risk of hip fracture in Parkinson's disease? A nationwide inpatient sample. Mov Disord 27: 1440–1443.
28. Walker RW, Chaplin A, Hancock RL, Rutherford R, Gray WK (2013) Hip fractures in people with idiopathic Parkinson's disease: incidence and outcomes. Mov Disord 28: 334–340.
29. Gregson CL, Dennison EM, Compston JE, Adami S, Adachi JD, et al. (2013) Disease-specific perception of fracture risk and incident fracture rates: GLOW cohort study. Osteoporos Int.
30. Taylor BC, Schreiner PJ, Stone KL, Fink HA, Cummings SR, et al. (2004) Long-term prediction of incident hip fracture risk in elderly white women: study of osteoporotic fractures. J Am Geriatr Soc 52: 1479–1486.
31. Wood BH, Bilclough JA, Bowron A, Walker RW (2002) Incidence and prediction of falls in Parkinson's disease: a prospective multidisciplinary study. J Neurol Neurosurg Psychiatry 72: 721–725.
32. Zhao Y, Shen L, Ji HF (2013) Osteoporosis risk and bone mineral density levels in patients with Parkinson's disease: a meta-analysis. Bone 52: 498–505.
33. Fink HA, Kuskowski MA, Orwoll ES, Cauley JA, Ensrud KE (2005) Association between Parkinson's disease and low bone density and falls in older men: the osteoporotic fractures in men study. J Am Geriatr Soc 53: 1559–1564.
34. van den Bos F, Speelman AD, Samson M, Munneke M, Bloem BR, et al. (2013) Parkinson's disease and osteoporosis. Age Ageing 42: 156–162.
35. WHO World health statistics 2013. Available at: http://www.who.int/gho/publications/en/.
36. Dorsey ER, Constantinescu R, Thompson JP, Biglan KM, Holloway RG, et al. (2007) Projected number of people with Parkinson disease in the most populous nations, 2005 through 2030. Neurology 68: 384–386.
37. Ageing WHO, Unit LC (2008) WHO global report on falls prevention in older age: World Health Organization.
38. Cummings SR, Cawthon PM, Ensrud KE, Cauley JA, Fink HA, et al. (2006) BMD and risk of hip and nonvertebral fractures in older men: a prospective study and comparison with older women. J Bone Miner Res 21: 1550–1556.
39. Nguyen ND, Ahlborg HG, Center JR, Eisman JA, Nguyen TV (2007) Residual lifetime risk of fractures in women and men. J Bone Miner Res 22: 781–788.
40. Yang J, Hu X, Zhang Q, Cao H, Wang J, et al. (2012) Homocysteine level and risk of fracture: A meta-analysis and systematic review. Bone 51: 376–382.
41. Allen NE, Schwarzel AK, Canning CG (2013) Recurrent falls in Parkinson's disease: a systematic review. Parkinsons Dis 2013: 906274.
42. Wood BH, Bilclough JA, Bowron A, Walker RW (2002) Incidence and prediction of falls in Parkinson's disease: a prospective multidisciplinary study. J Neurol Neurosurg Psychiatry 72: 721–725.
43. Chen Z, Kooperberg C, Pettinger MB, Bassford T, Cauley JA, et al. (2004) Validity of self-report for fractures among a multiethnic cohort of postmenopausal women: results from the Women's Health Initiative observational study and clinical trials. Menopause 11: 264–274.
44. Hundrup YA, Hoidrup S, Obel EB, Rasmussen NK (2004) The validity of self-reported fractures among Danish female nurses: comparison with fractures registered in the Danish National Hospital Register. Scand J Public Health 32: 136–143.

Obesity and Risk of Hip Fracture in Adults: A Meta-Analysis of Prospective Cohort Studies

Xianye Tang[1], Gang Liu[1], Jian Kang[1], Yang Hou[1], Fungui Jiang[2], Wen Yuan[1]*, Jiangang Shi[1]*

1 Orthopaedic Department, Changzheng Hospital, Second Military Medical University, Shanghai, China, 2 Department of Orthopaedics, People's Hospital of Wujiang City, Wujiang, China

Abstract

Background: Many observational studies assessed the association between obesity and risk of hip fracture in adults, but reported controversial results. Our goal was to evaluate the association between obesity and risk of hip fracture in adults by conducting a meta-analysis of prospective cohort studies.

Methods: Three databases, PubMed, Embase and Web of Science, were searched through May 2012 to identify eligible cohort studies. Either a fixed- or a random-effects model was used to calculate the pooled relative risk (RR) with its 95% confidence interval (95%CI).

Results: Fifteen prospective cohort studies involving a total 3,126,313 participants were finally included into this meta-analysis. Overall, adults with obesity compared with the normal weight group had a significantly decreased risk of hip fracture (RR: 0.66, 95% CI 0.57 to 0.77, P<0.001). Meta-analyses by the adjusted status of RRs also suggested adults with obesity compared with the reference group had a significantly decreased risk of hip fracture (adjusted RR: 0.48, 95% CI 0.39 to 0.58, P<0.001; unadjusted RR: 0.66, 95% CI 0.56 to 0.78, P<0.001). Subgroup analyses by gender suggested individuals with obesity had a significantly decreased risk for developing hip fracture compared with the reference group in both men (RR 0.54, 95% CI 0.48 to 0.60, P<0.001) and women (RR 0.70, 95% CI 0.58 to 0.84, P<0.001). No evidence of publication bias was observed in this meta-analysis.

Conclusions: This meta-analysis of prospective cohort studies suggests that obesity significantly decreases the risk of hip fracture in adults, and obesity is probably a protective factor of hip fracture in adults.

Editor: Reury F.P. Bacurau, University of Sao Paulo, Brazil

Funding: The authors have no support or funding to report.

Competing Interests: The authors have declared that no competing interests exist.

* E-mail: fuguidoctor@yahoo.com (JS); wenyuancz19@yahoo.com (WY)

Introduction

Osteoporotic fractures are a major and increasing cause of morbidity, and they have caused a serious burden to health services in the world [1,2]. Hip fracture is a major part of osteoporotic fractures, and is associated with low independence, excess morbidity and high mortality [3,4]. With the increasing ageing population and the high prevalence of osteoporosis, hip fracture is causing more serious damage to the public health [1,5]. Thus, to decrease the prevalence of hip fracture, multifaceted interventions for preventing hip fracture are urgently needed [6–8]. To make more effective therapeutic or lifestyle interventions, we need have a better knowledge of both the risk factors and the protective factors of hip fracture [9–11]. Low body mass index (BMI) is a recognized risk factor for fracture, particularly for the hip fracture [7,12]. However, whether obesity is protective against fracture has recently been challenged, and the association between obesity and fracture is controversial [13,14]. As obesity has risen in adults (BMI >30 kg/m2), so has the number of studies examining the association between obesity and fracture risk [7,14]. Many epidemiologic were published to investigate the association between obesity and risk of hip fracture, but the magnitudes of the association varied among those studies [15–29]. Furthermore, whether obesity is an independent protective factor or merely a silent marker of hip fracture remains unclear [13,14]. An improved understanding of this issue may have important public health and clinical implications given more effective therapeutic or lifestyle interventions can be made [13,14]. Thus, to evaluate the association between obesity and risk of hip fracture in adults, we performed a meta-analysis of 15 prospective cohort studies [15–29]. We performed the meta-analysis by following the PRISMA in the systematic review and meta-analysis [30].

Methods

Search strategy

We conducted a literature search in PubMed and Embase databases through May 6, 2012 for relevant studies that tested the association between adult obesity and risk of hip fracture. The following key words were used the literature search: 1) obesity, body mass index, BMI, or overweight; 2) fracture, or fractures; and 3) cohort study, cohort studies, prospective study, or prospective studies or longitudinal study. There was no language restriction in

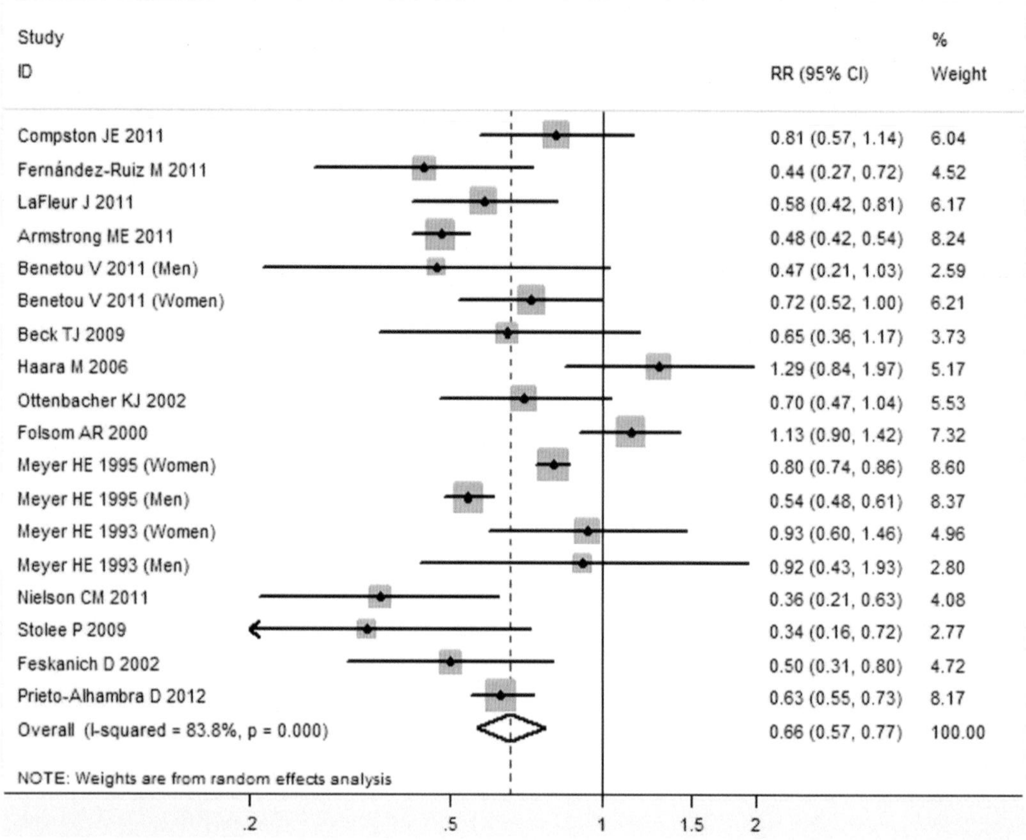

Figure 1. Forest plot showed an association between adult obesity and decreased risk of hip fracture (Meta-analysis of total included studies).

the literature search. In addition, we reviewed the reference lists of retrieved papers and recent reviews for additional studies.

Study selection

We first performed an initial screening of titles or abstracts. A second screening was based on full-text review. Studies were considered eligible if they met the following criteria: 1) the study design was a prospective cohort study; 2) the exposure of interest was obesity; 3) the outcome of interest was hip fracture; and 4) relative risk (RR) and the corresponding 95% confidence interval (95%CI) (or data to calculate them) were reported.

Data extraction and quality assessment

Two authors independently conducted the studies selection and data extraction, and any disagreements were resolved by discussion. The key exposure variable was the presence or absence of obesity at baseline. In most studies, people with normal weight served as the reference group. Outcome of interest in this study was hip fracture. Data extraction was then performed using a standardized data-collection form. We extracted any reported RRs, hazard ratios, or incidence density ratios of outcomes for patients with obesity compared with the reference group. We also extracted study characteristics for each trial, and data were recorded as follows: first author's last name, year of publication, country of origin, study period and duration of follow-up, characteristics of study population and age at baseline, number of participants with obesity, number of participants with normal weight, number of hip fracture events, ascertainments of obesity, and statistical adjustments for confounding factors. To clarify that all papers were based on different cohorts, we carefully checked the basic characteristics of included studies including the country of origin, study period, duration of follow-up, characteristics of study population and age at baseline. Quality assessment for cohort studies in this meta-analysis was assessed using the Newcastle Ottawa scale (NOS) as recommended by the Cochrane Non-Randomized Studies Methods Working Group [31]. Given the variability in quality of observational studies found on our initial literature search, we considered studies that met 5 or more of the NOS criteria as high quality.

Statistical analyses

RR with its 95%CI was used as a common measure of the association between obesity and risk of hip fracture across studies. Homogeneity of RRs across studies was tested by the I^2 statistic, which is a quantitative measure of inconsistency across studies [32]. The pooled RR were computed using either fixed-effects models [33] or, in the presence of heterogeneity (I^2 >50.0%), random-effects models [34]. To find the possible heterogeneity, we performed subgroup analyses by gender. We also used meta-regression to investigate if there is a difference in effect between men and women. Because characteristics of populations, and adjustments for confounding factors were not consistent between studies, we further conducted a sensitivity analysis to explore possible explanations for heterogeneity and to examine the influence of various exclusion criteria on the overall pooled RR. We investigated the influence of a single study on the overall risk

Table 1. Characteristics of 15 prospective cohort studies included into this meta-analysis.

study	Enrolment time	Setting	Number of participants	Definition	Follow up	Adjustment
Meyer HE 1993 [16]	1974–1978	Norway	52313	BMI ≥28.0 kg/m2	10 years	Age, height, physical activity, diabetes mellitus, and smoking
Meyer HE 1995 [19]	1963–1975	Norway	673848	Women BMI >29.3 kg/m2; Men BMI >27.5 kg/m2	16.4 years	None
Folsom AR 2000 [18]	1985–1986	USA	31702	BMI ≥30.2 kg/m2	11 to 12 years	Age, educational level, physical activity, alcohol intake, smoking status, vitamin use, et al.
Ottenbacher KJ 2002 [27]	1998–1999	USA	3050	BMI ≥30.0 kg/m2	7 years	None
Feskanich D 2002 [29]	1976	USA	61200	BMI ≥30.0 kg/m2	12 years	Age, smoking, postmenopausal hormone use, and intakes of calcium, vitamin use, et al.
Haara M 2005 [15]	1978–1980	Finland	3561	BMI ≥30.0 kg/m2	15 years	None
Beck TJ 2009 [24]	1991–2002	USA	4642	BMI ≥30.0 kg/m2	8.5 years	None
Stolee P 2009 [28]	2002–2006	Canada	40279	BMI ≥35.0 kg/m2	5 years	Age, smoking, height, et al.
Benetou V 2011 [20]	1992–2000	Europe	27982	BMI ≥30.0 kg/m2	8 years	Age at recruitment, educational level, smoking habits and history of diabetes mellitus at enrolment.
Armstrong ME 2011 [23]	1996–2001	UK	925345	BMI ≥30.0 kg/m2	6.2 years	None
LaFleur J 2011 [22]	1995–2005	USA	190847	BMI ≥30.0 kg/m2	29.1 months	None
Fernandez-Ruiz M 2011 [21]	1994–1995	Spain	5278	BMI ≥30.0 kg/m2	13 years	Age, gender, osteoporosis, circulatory disorders, et al.
Compston JE 2011 [17]	2006–2008	USA	60393	BMI ≥30.0 kg/m2	2 years	None
Nielson CM 2011 [25]	2000–2002	USA	5995	BMI ≥30.0 kg/m2	7 years	None
Prieto-Alhambra D 2012 [26]	2009	Spain	1,039,878	(BMI≥30 kg/m2	1 year	Age, smoking status, high alcohol intake, type 2 diabetes, and oral corticosteroid use.

(BMI, body mass index).

estimate by omitting 1 study in each turn. Potential publication bias was assessed by visual inspection of the Begg's funnel plots in which the logRRs was plotted against their stand errors (SEs) [35]. We also performed the Begg's rank correlation test and Egger's linear regression test to assess the publication bia [35,36]. All analyses were performed using STATA version 11.0 (StataCorp LP, College Station, Texas). A P value <0.05 was considered statistically significant, except where otherwise specified.

Results

Study characteristics

We initially retrieved 1326 unique citations from the PubMed and Embase databases. Of these, the majority were excluded after the first screening based on abstracts or titles, mainly because they were reviews, case-control studies, cross-sectional studies, or not relevant to our analysis. 23 full-text papers were preliminarily included into this study. After full-text review of those papers, 5 studies were excluded for lack of necessary dada and 3 studies were excluded because they used a retrospective cohort design. Finally, 15 studies with a total of 3,126,313 participants were included in our meta-analysis (Supply figure 1) [15–29]. The characteristics of the 15 prospective cohort studies are presented in Table 1. These studies were published between 1993 and 2011 [15–29]. Seven studies were conducted in the United States [17,18,22,24,25,27,29], 7 in Europe [15,16,19–21,23,26], and 1 in Canada [28]. The mean length of follow-up ranged from 1 to 16.4 years. Three studies reported the RRs by gender and the data were extracted as RR for men and RR for women, respectively. The sizes of the cohorts ranged from 3050 to 9,006 (total 3,126,313). Outcome assessments were from a variety of sources, including medical record, self-report, and hospital database. Seven studies reported adjusted RRs, and the mainly including age, diabetes, cholesterol, and smoking. According to the NOS system, thirteen studies were considered as high quality (meeting 5 or more of the NOS criteria) [16–19,21–26,28,29].

Adult obesity and risk of hip fracture

Overall, there was substantial heterogeneity observed among those studies ($I^2 = 83.8\%$). Figure 1 showed the results from the random-effects model combining the RRs for hip fracture (Figure 1). Individuals with obesity compared with the reference group had a significantly decreased risk for developing hip fracture (RR: 0.66, 95% CI 0.57 to 0.77, P<0.001) (Figure 1). Further exclusion of any single study did not materially alter the overall combined RR.

Subgroup analyses were firstly performed by the adjusted RRs or unadjusted RRs. Figure 2 showed the results from the random-effects model combining the adjusted RRs for hip fracture (Figure 2). Individuals with obesity compared with the reference group had a significantly decreased risk for developing hip fracture (adjusted RR: 0.48, 95% CI 0.39 to 0.58, P<0.001). Further exclusion of any single study also did not materially alter the overall combined RR. Figure 3 showed the results from the

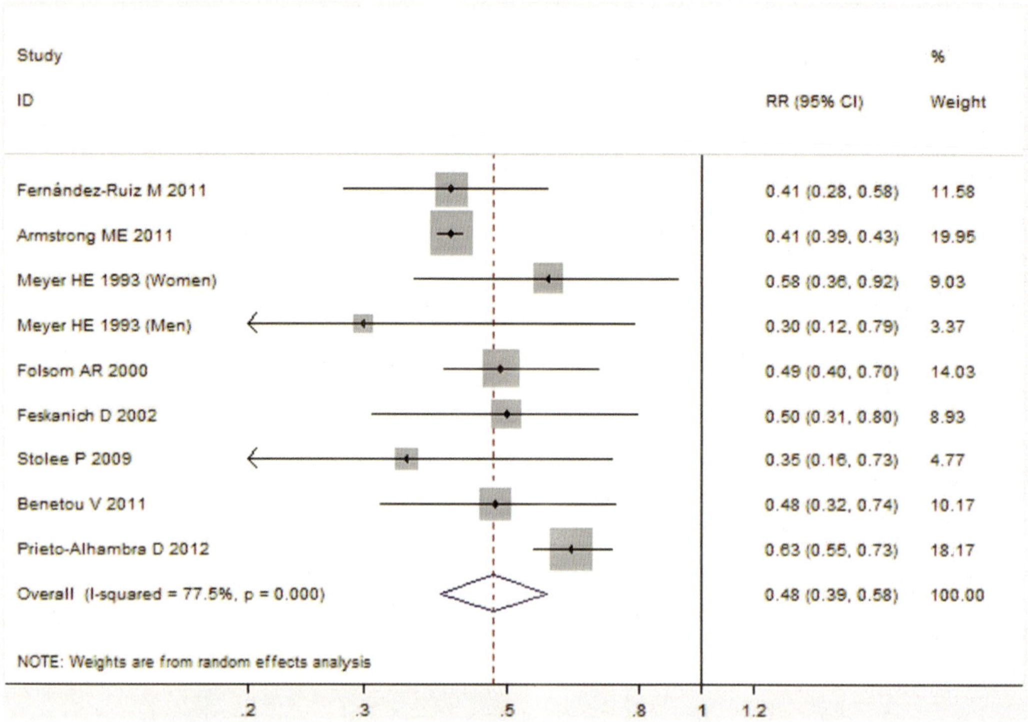

Figure 2. Forest plot showed an association between adult obesity and decreased risk of hip fracture (Analysis of adjusted RRs).

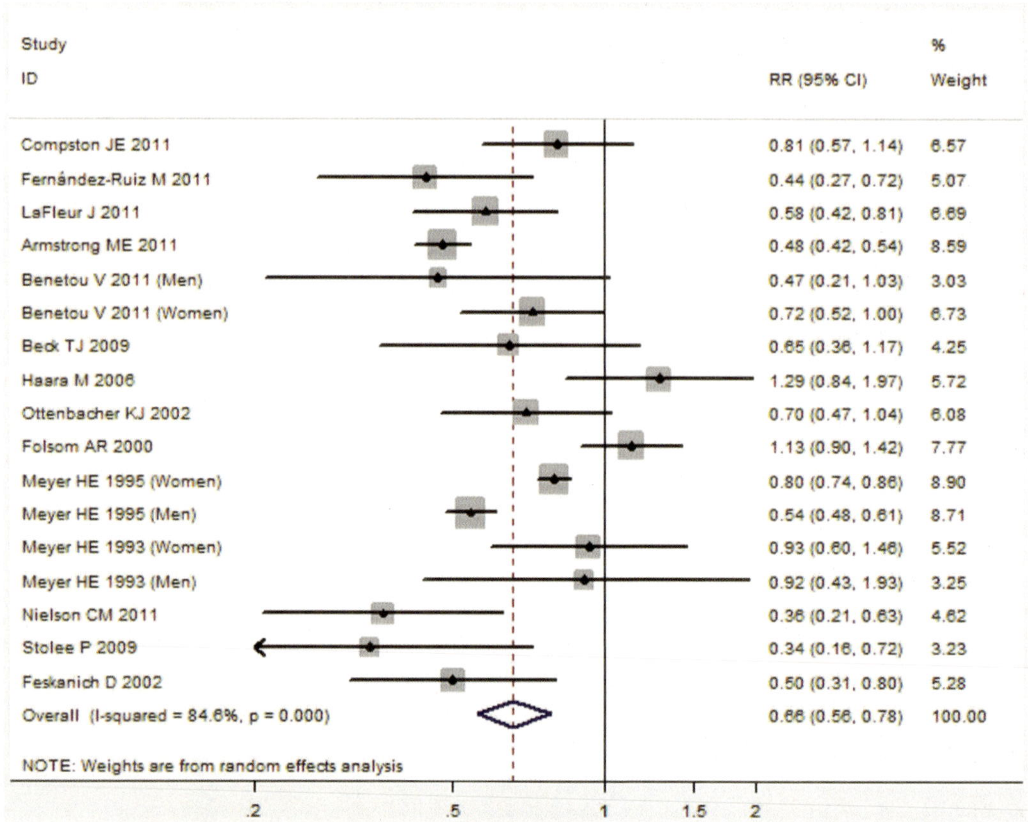

Figure 3. Forest plot showed an association between adult obesity and decreased risk of hip fracture (Analysis of unadjusted RRs).

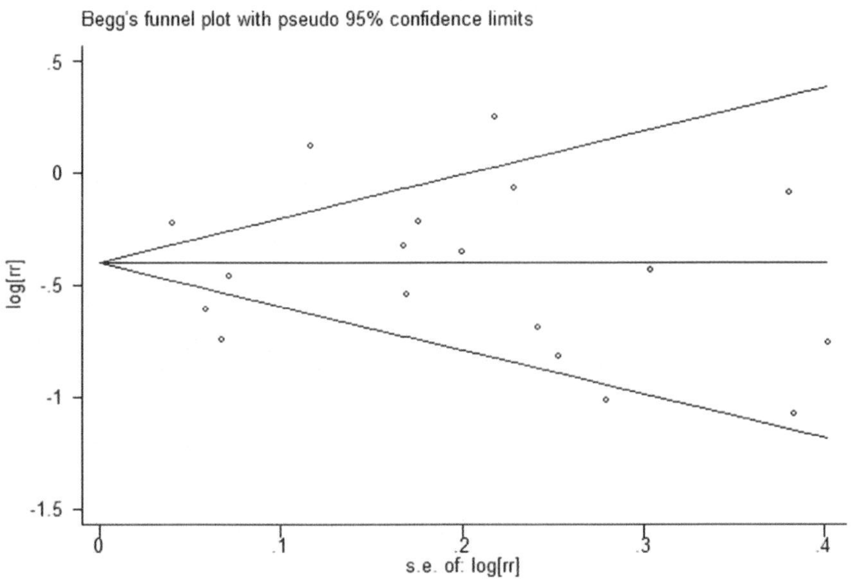

Figure 4. Begg's funnel plot did not identify substantial asymmetry in the meta-analysis of total 15 studies.

random-effects model combining the unadjusted RRs for hip fracture (Figure 3). Individuals with obesity compared with the reference group had a significantly decreased risk for developing hip fracture (unadjusted RR: 0.66, 95% CI 0.56 to 0.78, P<0.001). Further exclusion of any single study also did not materially alter the overall combined RR.

Subgroup analyses were then performed by gender. Individuals with obesity compared with the reference group had a significantly decreased risk for developing hip fracture in both men (RR 0.54, 95% CI 0.48 to 0.60, P<0.001) and women (RR 0.70, 95% CI 0.58 to 0.84, P<0.001). Further exclusion of any single study did not materially alter the overall pooled RRs above. Besides, meta-regression was performed to investigate if there was a difference in effect between men and women, but we found that there was no obvious difference in effect between men and women (P>0.05).

Risk of publication bias

Visual inspection of the Begg funnel plot did not identify substantial asymmetry (Figure 4). The Begg rank correlation test and Egger's linear regression test also indicated no evidence of publication bias (Begg's rank correlation test, P = 0.89; Egger's linear regression test, P = 0.73). Besides there was also no evidence of publication bias in the subgroup analyses (Table 2). Thus, there was no obvious risk of publication bias in this meta-analysis.

Discussion

There is rapidly growing interest in the association between obesity in adults and risk of hip fracture. Many observational studies have been published to evaluate the association between obesity in adults and risk of hip fracture, but controversial results are reported. To comprehensively evaluate the association between obesity in adults and risk of hip fracture, we conducted

Table 2. Summary of the results in the meta-analysis of adult obesity and risk of hip fracture.

Outcomes	No of studies	RR(95% CI)	P value	Pooled model	I^2	$P_{Egger\ test}$
Total population						
Total studies	18	0.66(0.57–0.77)	<0.001	Random	83.8%	0.732
Unadjusted RR	17	0.66(0.56–0.78)	<0.001	Random	84.6%	0.726
Adjusted RR	9	0.48(0.39–0.58)	<0.001	Random	77.5%	0.364
Women						
Total studies	10	0.70(0.58–0.84)	<0.001	Random	86.6%	0.845
Unadjusted RR	9	0.71(0.57–0.89)	<0.001	Random	87.6%	0.851
Adjusted RR	5	0.51(0.40–0.66)	<0.001	Random	88.4%	0.256
Men						
Total studies	4	0.54(0.48–0.60)	<0.001	Fixed	26.9%	0.912
Unadjusted RR	4	0.54(0.48–0.60)	<0.001	Fixed	26.9%	0.912
Adjusted RR	1	0.30(0.12–0.77	0.012	Fixed	NA	NA

(NA = not applicable).

a meta-analysis of 15 prospective cohort studies with a total 3,126,313 participants [15–29]. Our meta-analysis provides evidence that obesity in adults is significantly and independently associated with a decreased risk of hip fracture. Adults with obesity compared with the reference group had a significantly decreased risk for developing hip fracture (RR: 0.66, 95% CI 0.57 to 0.77, $P<0.001$; adjusted RR: 0.48, 95% CI 0.39 to 0.58, $P<0.001$; unadjusted RR: 0.66, 95% CI 0.56 to 0.78, $P<0.001$). Subgroup analyses by gender suggest with obesity compared with the reference group have a significantly decreased risk for developing hip fracture in both men (RR 0.54, 95%CI 0.48 to 0.60, $P<0.001$) and women (RR 0.70, 95% CI 0.58 to 0.84, $P<0.001$). Thus, our meta-analysis suggests that obesity in adults significantly decreases the risk of hip fracture, and obesity is probably a protective factor of hip fracture in adults.

Low bone mineral density (BMD) has been considered one of the major causes of the increased risk of fracture in those with low weight, while higher BMD in adults is posited to mitigate risk of fractures [10,37]. Body weight is directly associated with BMD, and a low BMI has been identified as an important risk factor for lower BMD and predicts greater bone loss in older age [13]. On the other hand, BMD is moderately positively correlated with BMI, many obese individuals have relatively higher BMD, and bone strength may increase in proportion to increases in total or fat mass. An increased strain on the bones imposed by higher body mass may lead to increased BMD and improved structural integrity of the bones. The higher BMD and bone mineral content in obesity are attributed to multiple factors. These include a greater mechanical loading on bone and the altered hormonal milieu and higher serum levels of adipokines associated with obesity, which play an important role in influencing bone mass in obesity [13]. Thus, obesity is an important protective factor for fractures by an effect mediated predominantly through high BMD [13]. Besides, obesity is also widely believed to be protective against fracture because of the effect of increased soft-tissue padding. Individuals who carry more fat mass may benefit from cushioning of their hip by gluteofemoral adipose tissue, which reduces impact forces when they fall and hence their chance of fracture [13].

To our knowledge, this is the first comprehensive systematic review and meta-analysis on the effect of obesity on the risk of hip fracture in adults. We carried out an extensive quality assessment, and investigated heterogeneity with sensitivity analyses and subgroup analyses. We compared the results of crude and adjusted data to try to determine if the observed risks were due to body mass index independently or were explained by confounding factors. We also performed subgroup analyses by gender, to explore if the gender specific effect existed. All those above could add the strength of evidence for the protective effect obesity on hip fracture in adults from our meta-analysis. Besides, we conclude that obesity is a protective factor of hip fracture in adults and it is similar in both sexes.

Obesity is growing concerns worldwide, and an estimated 1.5 billion people were obese in the year 2008 worldwide, and 34% of the population of the United States is obese [13,38,39]. Obesity has led to an increased risk for several comorbidities, including cardiovascular disease (CVD), diabetes, and certain cancers [40–42]. In addition, although weight reduction is recommended to reduce comorbidities related to obesity, it also induces bone loss and increases risk of fracture in older individuals [13,14]. Besides, a high BMD can be due to increased physical activity or obesity, and bone loss could result in an increased risk of fractures due to weight reduction [13]. Since obesity is a protective factor of hip fracture in adults and it is similar in both sexes, dietary and clinical interventions can be used to help attenuate bone loss with weight reduction during weight reduction, such as increasing a specific micro- or macronutrient and physical activity [13].

Limitations of this systematic review include the obvious inconsistency across studies, especially in the confounding factors and lengths of follow up. Some confounding factors might account for the observed association between obesity and risk of hip fracture, which were not adjusted for in some of those included studies. Among those studies adjusted for confounding factors, those factors varied greatly among different studies. Besides, the length of follow up also varied greatly among different studies, arranging from 1 to 16.4 years. In addition, we did not try to contact the authors of those included studies for relevant information where it was not available in published form, and there was also possibility of having missed studies in the literature search and selective presenting of results from those included studies, therefore a meta-analysis of individual patients data is urgently needed to further provide a more precise estimation on the effect of obesity on hip fracture. Finally, we pooled data based on the original studies' definitions of obesity. There was a problem of varying cut-offs of definitions of obesity between studies. All the inconsistency across studies could cause the obvious heterogeneity in this meta-analysis (Table 2).

In conclusion, this meta-analysis of prospective cohort studies suggests that obesity in adults significantly decreases the risk of hip fracture, and obesity is probably a protective factor of hip fracture in adults.

Author Contributions

Conceived and designed the experiments: XT GL WY JS. Performed the experiments: XT GL JS. Analyzed the data: JK YH FJ. Contributed reagents/materials/analysis tools: XT GL WY JS . Wrote the paper: XT GL WY JS.

References

1. Cummings SR, Melton LJ (2002) Epidemiology and outcomes of osteoporotic fractures. Lancet 359 (9319): 1761–7.
2. Delmas PD (2002) Treatment of postmenopausal osteoporosis. Lancet 359 (9322): 2018–26.
3. Mayhew PM, Thomas CD, Clement JG, Loveridge N, Beck TJ, et al. (2005) Relation between age, femoral neck cortical stability, and hip fracture risk. Lancet 366 (9480): 129–35.
4. Orwig DL, Chan J, Magaziner J (2006) Hip fracture and its consequences: differences between men and women. Orthop Clin North Am 37 (4): 611–22.
5. Hartholt KA, Oudshoorn C, Zielinski SM, Burgers PT, Panneman MJ, et al. (2011) The epidemic of hip fractures: are we on the right track? PLoS One 6 (7): e22227.
6. Bischoff-Ferrari HA, Willett WC, Orav EJ, Lips P, Meunier PJ, et al. (2012) A pooled analysis of vitamin D dose requirements for fracture prevention. N Engl J Med 367 (1): 40–9.
7. Nasser KM, Quinonez Obiols A, Silverman SL (2011) Identifying individuals at risk for fracture in Guatemala. PLoS One 6 (11): e28042.
8. Tang BM, Eslick GD, Nowson C, Smith C, Bensoussan A (2007) Use of calcium or calcium in combination with vitamin D supplementation to prevent fractures

and bone loss in people aged 50 years and older: a meta-analysis. Lancet 370 (9588): 657–66.
9. Chudyk AM, Ashe MC, Gorman E, Al Tunaiji HO, Crossley KM (2012) Risk of hip fracture with hip or knee osteoarthritis: a systematic review. Clin Rheumatol 31 (5): 749–57.
10. Johnell O, Kanis JA, Oden A, Johansson H, De Laet C, et al. (2005) Predictive value of BMD for hip and other fractures. J Bone Miner Res 20 (7): 1185–94.
11. Visschedijk J, Achterberg W, Van Balen R, Hertogh C (2010) Fear of falling after hip fracture: a systematic review of measurement instruments, prevalence, interventions, and related factors. J Am Geriatr Soc 58 (9): 1739–48.
12. Sienkiewicz E, Magkos F, Aronis KN, Brinkoetter M, Chamberland JP, et al. (2011) Long-term metreleptin treatment increases bone mineral density and content at the lumbar spine of lean hypoleptinemic women. Metabolism 60 (9): 1211–21.
13. Shapses SA, Sukumar D (2012) Bone metabolism in obesity and weight loss. Annu Rev Nutr 32 287–309.
14. Dimitri P, Bishop N, Walsh JS, Eastell R (2012) Obesity is a risk factor for fracture in children but is protective against fracture in adults: a paradox. Bone 50 (2): 457–66.
15. Haara M, Heliovaara M, Impivaara O, Arokoski JP, Manninen P, et al. (2006) Low metacarpal index predicts hip fracture: a prospective population study of 3,561 subjects with 15 years of follow-up. Acta Orthop 77 (1): 9–14.
16. Meyer HE, Tverdal A, Falch JA (1993) Risk factors for hip fracture in middle-aged Norwegian women and men. Am J Epidemiol 137 (11): 1203–11.
17. Compston JE, Watts NB, Chapurlat R, Cooper C, Boonen S, et al. (2011) Obesity is not protective against fracture in postmenopausal women: GLOW. Am J Med 124 (11): 1043–50.
18. Folsom AR, Kushi LH, Anderson KE, Mink PJ, Olson JE, et al. (2000) Associations of general and abdominal obesity with multiple health outcomes in older women: the Iowa Women's Health Study. Arch Intern Med 160 (14): 2117–28.
19. Meyer HE, Tverdal A, Falch JA (1995) Body height, body mass index, and fatal hip fractures: 16 years' follow-up of 674,000 Norwegian women and men. Epidemiology 6 (3): 299–305.
20. Benetou V, Orfanos P, Benetos IS, Pala V, Evangelista A, et al. (2011) Anthropometry, physical activity and hip fractures in the elderly. Injury 42 (2): 188–93.
21. Fernandez-Ruiz M, Guerra-Vales JM, Trincado R, Medrano MJ, Benito-Leon J, et al. (2011) Hip fracture in three elderly populations of central Spain: data from the NEDICES study. Intern Emerg Med.
22. LaFleur J, McAdam-Marx C, Alder SS, Sheng X, Asche CV, et al. (2011) Clinical risk factors for fracture among postmenopausal patients at risk for fracture: a historical cohort study using electronic medical record data. J Bone Miner Metab 29 (2): 193–200.
23. Armstrong ME, Spencer EA, Cairns BJ, Banks E, Pirie K, et al. (2011) Body mass index and physical activity in relation to the incidence of hip fracture in postmenopausal women. J Bone Miner Res 26 (6): 1330–8.
24. Beck TJ, Petit MA, Wu G, LeBoff MS, Cauley JA, et al. (2009) Does obesity really make the femur stronger? BMD, geometry, and fracture incidence in the women's health initiative-observational study. J Bone Miner Res 24 (8): 1369–79.
25. Nielson CM, Marshall LM, Adams AL, LeBlanc ES, Cawthon PM, et al. (2011) BMI and fracture risk in older men: the osteoporotic fractures in men study (MrOS). J Bone Miner Res 26 (3): 496–502.
26. Prieto-Alhambra D, Premaor MO, Fina Aviles F, Hermosilla E, Martinez-Laguna D, et al. (2012) The association between fracture and obesity is site-dependent: a population-based study in postmenopausal women. J Bone Miner Res 27 (2): 294–300.
27. Ottenbacher KJ, Ostir GV, Peek MK, Goodwin JS, Markides KS (2002) Diabetes mellitus as a risk factor for hip fracture in mexican american older adults. J Gerontol A Biol Sci Med Sci 57 (10): M648–53.
28. Stolee P, Poss J, Cook RJ, Byrne K, Hirdes JP (2009) Risk factors for hip fracture in older home care clients. J Gerontol A Biol Sci Med Sci 64 (3): 403–10.
29. Feskanich D, Willett W, Colditz G (2002) Walking and leisure-time activity and risk of hip fracture in postmenopausal women. JAMA 288 (18): 2300–6.
30. Moher D, Liberati A, Tetzlaff J, Altman DG; PRISMA Group (2009) Preferred reporting items for systematic reviews and meta-analyses: the PRISMA statement. PLoS Med 6 (7):e1000097.
31. Wells G, Shea B, O'connell D, Peterson J, Welch V, et al. (2012) The Newcastle-Ottawa Scale (NOS) for assessing the quality of nonrandomised studies in meta-analyses. Ottawa Health Research Institute Web site.
32. Higgins JP, Thompson SG, Deeks JJ, Altman DG (2003) Measuring inconsistency in meta-analyses. BMJ 327 (7414): 557–60.
33. Mantel N, Haenszel W (1959) Statistical aspects of the analysis of data from retrospective studies of disease. J Natl Cancer Inst 22 (4): 719–48.
34. DerSimonian R, Laird N (1986) Meta-analysis in clinical trials. Control Clin Trials 7 (3): 177–88.
35. Begg CB, Mazumdar M (1994) Operating characteristics of a rank correlation test for publication bias. Biometrics 50 (4): 1088–101.
36. Egger M, Davey Smith G, Schneider M, Minder C (1997) Bias in meta-analysis detected by a simple, graphical test. BMJ 315 (7109): 629–34.
37. Jamal SA, Hayden JA, Beyene J (2007) Low bone mineral density and fractures in long-term hemodialysis patients: a meta-analysis. Am J Kidney Dis 49 (5): 674–81.
38. Han JC, Lawlor DA, Kimm SY (2010) Childhood obesity. Lancet 375 (9727): 1737–48.
39. Plourde G, Prud'homme D (2012) Managing obesity in adults in primary care. CMAJ 184 (9): 1039–44.
40. Renehan AG, Tyson M, Egger M, Heller RF, Zwahlen M (2008) Body-mass index and incidence of cancer: a systematic review and meta-analysis of prospective observational studies. Lancet 371 (9612): 569–78.
41. Romero-Corral A, Montori VM, Somers VK, Korinek J, Thomas RJ, et al. (2006) Association of bodyweight with total mortality and with cardiovascular events in coronary artery disease: a systematic review of cohort studies. Lancet 368 (9536): 666–78.
42. Yoon KH, Lee JH, Kim JW, Cho JH, Choi YH, et al. (2006) Epidemic obesity and type 2 diabetes in Asia. Lancet 368 (9548): 1681–8.

13

Delayed Fracture Healing and Increased Callus Adiposity in a C57BL/6J Murine Model of Obesity-Associated Type 2 Diabetes Mellitus

Matthew L. Brown[1,2], Kiminori Yukata[1], Christopher W. Farnsworth[1,6], Ding-Geng Chen[1,3], Hani Awad[1,4,5], Matthew J. Hilton[1,4], Regis J. O'Keefe[1,4], Lianping Xing[1,6], Robert A. Mooney[1,6], Michael J. Zuscik[1,4]*

1 Center for Musculoskeletal Research, University of Rochester Medical Center, Rochester, New York, United States of America, **2** School of Medicine and Dentistry, University of Rochester Medical Center, Rochester, New York, United States of America, **3** Department of Biostatistics and Computational Biology, University of Rochester Medical Center, Rochester, New York, United States of America, **4** Department of Orthopaedics and Rehabilitation, University of Rochester Medical Center, Rochester, New York, United States of America, **5** Department of Biomechanical Engineering, University of Rochester, Rochester, New York, United States of America, **6** Department of Pathology and Laboratory Medicine, University of Rochester Medical Center, Rochester, New York, United States of America

Abstract

Introduction: Impaired healing and non-union of skeletal fractures is a major public health problem, with morbidity exacerbated in patients with diabetes mellitus (DM). DM is prevalent worldwide and affects approximately 25.8 million US adults, with >90% having obesity-related type 2 DM (T2DM). While fracture healing in type 1 DM (T1DM) has been studied using animal models, an investigation into delayed healing in an animal model of T2DM has not yet been performed.

Methods: Male C57BL/6J mice at 5 weeks of age were placed on either a control lean diet or an experimental high-fat diet (HFD) for 12 weeks. A mid-diaphyseal open tibia fracture was induced at 17 weeks of age and a spinal needle was used for intra-medullary fixation. Mice were sacrificed at days 7, 10, 14, 21, 28, and 35 for micro-computed tomography (μCT), histology-based histomorphometry and molecular analyses, and biomechanical testing.

Results: HFD-fed mice displayed increased body weight and impaired glucose tolerance, both characteristic of T2DM. Compared to control mice, HFD-fed mice with tibia fractures showed significantly ($p<0.001$) decreased woven bone at day 28 by histomorphometry and significantly ($p<0.01$) decreased callus bone volume at day 21 by μCT. Interestingly, fracture calluses contained markedly increased adiposity in HFD-fed mice at days 21, 28, and 35. HFD-fed mice also showed increased PPARγ immunohistochemical staining at day 14. Finally, calluses from HFD-fed mice at day 35 showed significantly ($p<0.01$) reduced torsional rigidity compared to controls.

Discussion: Our murine model of T2DM demonstrated delayed fracture healing and weakened biomechanical properties, and was distinctly characterized by increased callus adiposity. This suggests altered mesenchymal stem cell fate determination with a shift to the adipocyte lineage at the expense of the osteoblast lineage. The up-regulation of PPARγ in fracture calluses of HFD-fed mice is likely involved in the proposed fate switching.

Editor: Brenda Smith, Oklahoma State University, United States of America

Funding: This work was supported by NIH P50 AR054041 (R.J.O. & M.J.Z.), NIH R01 AR052011 (M.J.Z.), and an AOTrauma Clinical Priority Program Grant (R.A.M.). Trainee support (for M.L.B.) was provided by NIH CTSA TL1 RR024135, and support for Core Services was provided by NIH P30 AR061307. The content is solely the responsibility of the authors and does not necessarily represent the official views of the National Institutes of Health. The funders had no role in study design, data collection and analysis, decision to publish, or preparation or the manuscript.

Competing Interests: The authors have declared that no competing interests exist.

* E-mail: michael_zuscik@urmc.rochester.edu

Introduction

Delayed and failed fracture repair and bone healing are major public health issues in the United States. Musculoskeletal disease impairs the performance of normal daily activities, compromises the performance of other organ systems, and impairs psychological health and social function [1–7]. While all patients with bone injury are affected, morbidity is significantly exacerbated in patients with diabetes, which is recognized clinically to delay bone healing and contribute to increased incidence of fibrous non-union (i.e. failure to heal) [8,9].

Diabetes mellitus (DM) is one of the most common diseases in the United States. The Centers for Disease Control and Prevention (CDC) estimated that as of 2011, approximately 11.3% of the United States population ≥20 years of age were symptomatic diabetics, which includes a total of approximately 25.8 million people – 18.8 million diagnosed and 7.0 million undiagnosed [10]. With DM incidence doubling between 1990 and 2005, the CDC has declared it an epidemic in our society.

Despite this warning, the incidence of DM in the US in 2010 was approximately 1.9 million cases [10].

Two types of diabetes exist, each with a distinct etiology. In type 1 DM (T1DM) the loss of insulin-secreting pancreatic β cells causes an absolute insulin insufficiency, resulting from an autoimmune process that has a strong genetic component. The hyperglycemia that occurs in T1DM causes long-term damage to tissues and organs. Type 2 DM (T2DM) is more prevalent in the United States and accounts for >90% of all patients with diabetes [10]. Patients with T2DM, which was previously referred to as non-insulin dependent diabetes (NIDDM) or adult onset diabetes, have elevated blood glucose levels secondary to insulin insensitivity and relative insulin deficiency. Importantly, while T2DM also has a genetic component, it has been more widely associated with obesity and consumption of a high fat diet that is rich in unsaturated fats. Thus, lifestyle and dietary modifications provide an opportunity to mollify the incidence, prevalence and societal burden of T2DM overall.

Rodent models of fracture healing in diabetes have focused on T1DM, which was either caused by an autoimmune destruction of pancreatic β cells or was induced via administration of streptozotocin (STZ) to these cells. Fracture repair studies in these models of T1DM have led to the discovery of several tissue-level defects that alter the normal bone healing program. Normal bone healing involves recruitment and proliferation of stem cell populations at the injury site, chondrogenic commitment and cartilage differentiation, formation of woven bone and osteoclast-mediated remodeling of the callus [11,12] [11,12]. In T1DM, there is evidence for decreased progenitor cell proliferation [13–17], decreased callus cartilage content [13,14,17,18], premature cartilage resorption [13,18,19], decreased callus bone content [14–16,20,21], and biomechanically inferior repair [14–17,20]. Several groups have demonstrated that administration of sufficient systemic insulin to achieve tight glucose control rescued progenitor cell proliferation, callus bone content, and biomechanical strength [15,16,20]. Alternatively, intramedullary insulin delivery rescued the decreased cellular proliferation, cartilage percentage, bone percentage, and mechanical strength that characterize the fracture callus of diabetic rats [14].

Even though T2DM is a much more prevalent and growing disease condition compared to T1DM, the tissue and molecular events that impair fracture healing in T2DM have not been investigated. Here, for the first time, we examine tibia fracture healing in a high fat diet-fed mouse, a classic model of T2DM. Our results demonstrate that the metabolic dysregulation in this model is associated with defective fracture repair that is distinct from that seen in T1DM and is likely related to an aberrant increase in adipocytes in the fracture callus of mice with T2DM.

Materials and Methods

Animals

All animal experiments described in this report were reviewed and approved by the University Committee on Animal Resources (IACUC) at the University of Rochester Medical Center. Male C57BL/6J mice (Jackson Laboratories, Bar Harbor, ME, USA) were obtained at 5 weeks of age and housed 5 per microisolator cage in a vivarium housing room on a 12-hour light/dark cycle at the University of Rochester Medical Center. Upon arrival, mice were immediately provided *ad libitum* access to either a control lean diet with 10% total kcal from saturated fat or an experimental high fat diet with 60% total kcal from saturated fat (Catalog Nos. D12450B and D12492 respectively, Open Source Diets, Research Diets Inc., New Brunswick, NJ, USA). The high fat diet (HFD) has been shown to cause weight gain, insulin resistance, and hyperglycemia in this strain of mice [22,23]. Each mouse was weighed before fracture and again at sacrifice. Glucose tolerance testing (GTT) was performed on representative lean (n = 5) and HFD-fed (n = 5) mice preoperatively [24,25]. Briefly, mice were fasted for 6 hours, anesthetized with isoflurane (5%) and tail vein blood was sampled using a commercially available glucometer (One Touch Ultra; Lifescan, Inc., Milpitas, CA, USA). A glucose bolus (300 mg/kg) was then injected intraperitoneally. Additional glucose levels were obtained at 15, 30, 60, 90, and 120 minutes, with isoflurane again employed to ensure anesthetic plane for each blood draw. To quantify metabolic status, the net area under the curve (AUC) was calculated from the GTT curve of each mouse (GraphPad PRISM, version 4, GraphPad Software, La Jolla, CA, USA).

Tibia Fracture Model

Using a model previously established in our Center, we administered open tibia fractures to mice fed either a lean or HF diet [26]. The rationale for using this approach instead of the commonly employed Einhorn method (utilizing the Einhorn device to induce closed fractures via delivery of a blunt force that causes traumatic 3 point bending to initiate failure) is as follows: Our own work [27] as well as studies published by others [28,29] definitively establish that the HFD induces an osteoclast-dependent bone loss that leads to a weaker skeleton. If we had performed the trauma-induced fracture model developed by Einhorn, there would be a concern that mode of fracture and comminution might be distinct in the diabetic animals due to their skeletal fragility. To avoid this potential complication, and to make the fractures as reproducible as possible across experimental groups, we opted to perform the open tibial fracture osteotomy model, which is a surgical transection of the tibia (without injury to the fibula) that is carefully applied with a scalpel blade. Initial differences in bone strength or fragility do not influence the nature of the injury and insure that at the start of the healing process, the fracture is the same in both control and HFD-fed mice. Since our interest was to further understand the healing process post-fracture, this approach is the best available to factor out bone strength issues that exist pre-fracture. To administer the tibial fractures, mice were anesthetized via isoflurane inhalation (5% induction, 2.5% maintenance). Under sterile conditions, a 15-mm skin incision was made over the anterior aspect of the right lower leg. A 26G, five-eighths inch intradermal needle (BD Medical Systems, Franklin Lakes, NJ, USA) was inserted through the anteromedial tibial plateau to access the medullary canal. This was removed and a 26G Quincke-type spinal needle (BD Medical Systems, Franklin Lakes, NJ, USA) was inserted for trial fit and removed. The mid-diaphysis of the right tibia was identified and a #11 scalpel blade was gently scribed over the posterolateral cortex and slowly drawn back and forth over the developing furrow to complete the osteotomy while preventing comminution. The distal tibia was mobilized to confirm a complete osteotomy. The 26G spinal needle was reinserted to provide intramedullary fixation. The skin was closed using simple 5-0 nylon (Ethicon, Inc., Somerville, NJ, USA) interrupted sutures. Radiographs (Faxitron X-Ray Cabinet, Wheeling, IL, USA) were obtained postoperatively to evaluate the fracture and fixation. Banamine (2.5 mg/kg) or buprenorphine (0.5 mg/kg) was administered for analgesia.

Micro-Computed Tomography and Microvascular Analysis

Fractured tibiae were harvested at 7, 10, 14, 21, 28, and 35 days postoperatively by disarticulating the right lower-extremity at the knee and cutting the tibia just distal to origin of the fibula. High-resolution micro-computed tomography (vivaCT 40; Scanco Medical AG, Basserdorf, Switzerland) was used to render a three-dimensional image of the tibia. Bone and vascular volumes within the fracture callus were determined by routine methods that we employ regularly in our Center [26,30,31] and involves the expertise of our Molecular and Anatomic Imaging Core. Regarding assessment of bone values, samples were scanned using the following parameters: 55 kV energy setting, 300 millisecond integration time, 10.5 μM voxel size, 10 μM slice increment, and a threshold of 210. To analyze external callus bone volume, two contours were created for each slice; the first traced the perimeter of the external fracture callus and the second surrounded all cortical bone from the adjacent uninjured cortices. Subtraction included all mineralized tissues above the threshold between the two contour lines, which encompassed the entire fracture callus. Analysis of vascular volume within the external fracture callus was also performed for selected samples harvested at 10 and 14 days postoperatively. As previously described, lead chromate paint was perfused to visualize all vascular structures [32]. Briefly, mice were anesthetized and a thoracotomy was performed to permit catheterization of the left ventricle and an incision to the right atrium. Approximately 20 mL mixture of 0.9% NaCl and heparin (100 IU/mL) was slowly injected into the left ventricle followed by 20 mL of 10% neutral buffered formalin (NBF). Finally, 4 mL of lead chromate paint (Microfil MV-122 yellow; Flow Tech, Inc., Carver, MA, USA) was injected into the left ventricle and continued until the liver and footpads became yellow. After 30 min at room temperature (RT) carcasses were placed in 10% NBF for 24 hours. Right tibiae were harvested and placed into NBF for 3 days. Tissues were μCT scanned as described above to capture fracture callus bone volume as well as total vascular volume in the callus. Tissues were decalcified in 10% ethylenediaminetetraacetic acid (EDTA) for 3 weeks and then rescanned, which provided the total vascular volume.

Histology and Histomorphometry

Fractured tibiae harvested for μCT analysis were processed for histology as previously described [33]. Briefly, tibiae were disarticulated at the knee, denuded of soft tissue, cut distally and fixed at RT in 10% NBF for 72 hours. After three washes in phosphate buffered saline (PBS), fixed tibiae were decalcified in 10% EDTA for 7 to 14 days. Tissues were then processed using a Tissue-Tek VIP 6 tissue processor (Sakura Finetek USA, Inc., Torrance, CA, USA) and embedded in paraffin. Serial 3 μm thick sagittal sections were obtained from a 60 μm region spanning the center of the fracture callus. Three sections, each separated by approximately 10 to 15 μm, were stained with Alcian Blue Hematoxylin/Orange G (ABH/OG) and histomorphometric analysis was performed using a point counting method as described previously [34]. Briefly, blinded sections were analyzed using a standardized eyepiece grid under the 10x objective to determine the percent of total callus area composed of cartilage, woven bone, adipocytes, osteoblasts and stromal cells. Each crossing point on the grid was scored to either be cartilage, woven bone, adipocyte or stromal area. Cartilage was defined as tissue with positive Alcian Blue stain. Woven bone was counted whenever a trabecular structure was observed, regardless of staining. Adipocytes were defined as any tissue completely lacking stain and exhibiting a circular or elliptical shape characteristic of adipocytes. Osteoblasts, including stromal cells, were defined as the population that was directly residing bone surfaces that was not multinucleated. Stromal cells were considered to be all cellular tissues within the fracture callus that did not meet the above criteria for cartilage, woven bone or adipocytes or osteoblasts. Cortical bone and internal callus were not included in these analyses. The relative percentage of each tissue type, normalized to the entire callus area as well as the percent of bone perimeter occupied by an osteoblast population was calculated for each section.

Osteoclast Quantification

One section per sample was stained for tartrate-resistant acid phosphatase (TRAP). Briefly, after deparaffinization and rehydration with distilled water, sections were incubated at 37°C for 25 minutes in a solution of anhydrous sodium acetate (Sigma S-2889), L-(+) tartaric acid (Sigma T-6521), glacial acetic acid, fast red violet LB salt (Sigma F-3381), naphthol AS-MX phosphate (Sigma N-4875), ethylene glycol monoethyl ether (Sigma E-2632), and distilled water. Sections were rinsed in distilled water, counterstained with hematoxylin for 10 sec and then placed in ammonia water for 5 seconds. Quantification was completed using the 10x objective and Osteomeasure software (OsteoMetrics, Inc., Decatur, GA, USA) to contour bone perimeter (B.Pm.) within the anterior callus and identify osteoclasts (Oc.N.), which were defined as multi-nucleated, TRAP-positive cells seated on bone surfaces.

Immunohistochemical Staining

Immunohistochemistry was performed as described previously [35]. Briefly, an avidin-biotin peroxidase system (Vector Lab, Burlingame, CA, USA) was used to detect two primary antibodies; anti-perilipin rabbit monoclonal antibody (1:100: Cat. #9349: Cell Signaling Technology, Inc., Danvers, MA) and anti-PPARγ rabbit monoclonal antibody (1:100: Cat. #2435: Cell Signaling Technology, Inc., Danvers, MA). Reactions were then visualized with diaminobenzidine (DAB) as substrate (Vector Lab, Burlingame, CA, USA). The sections were counterstained with hematoxylin. All staining procedures were followed as instructed by the manufacturer.

Biomechanical Testing

Biomechanical properties of healed fractures were assessed at 14 and 35 days postoperatively as described previously [36]. Briefly, right tibiae were harvested, immediately flash-frozen in liquid nitrogen and then stored at −80°C. Prior to testing, samples were thawed over 30 minutes at RT and sent for μCT scanning. After μCT, polymethylmethacrylate (PMMA) bone cement (Endurance Cement; Depuy Orthopaedics, Inc., Warsaw, IN) was used to cement tibiae into square 6.35 mm^2 aluminum sleeves, taking care to align the long axis of each tibia with the sleeve's center of rotation. Samples were rehydrated and loaded into an EnduraTec TestBench TM System (200 Nmm torque cell; Bose Corporation, Minnetonka, MN, USA) and tested in torsion at a rate of 1°/s until failure. Torque data were plotted against rotational deformation and maximum torque at the point of failure was recorded for each sample. All samples were blinded throughout preparation and testing.

Statistical Analyses

Data presented are the mean and standard error for lean and HFD-fed mice, unless specified otherwise. Two-tailed, unpaired Student's t tests were calculated using Excel software (Microsoft Corporation, Redmond, WA, USA). Two-way ANOVA tests were calculated using GraphPad PRISM software, (GraphPad Software, La Jolla, CA, USA). Significance is indicated using asterisks; *$p<0.05$, **$p<0.01$, and ***$p<0.001$.

Results

Induction of obesity and glucose intolerance by HFD

To confirm that HFD-fed mice recapitulated key pathogenic features of human T2DM, we weighed all mice and performed glucose tolerance testing (GTT) on a representative group. After twelve weeks of *ad libitum* access to the assigned diet, the HFD-fed mice weighed significantly more than lean controls ($p<0.001$). Importantly, HFD-fed mice remained significantly heavier throughout the postoperative period compared to time-matched lean controls (Fig. 1A, $p<0.001$). GTT performed preoperatively showed that HFD-fed mice were unable to restore basal blood glucose levels 120 minutes after glucose bolus while lean-fed control mice restored blood glucose levels after 90 minutes, indicating that HFD-fed mice had impaired glucose handling, which is characteristic of human patients with T2DM (Fig. 1B) [24]. This was confirmed by calculating the net area under the curve (AUC) for each mouse. HFD-fed mice had a significantly larger net AUC preoperatively, indicating impaired glucose handling (Fig. 1C, $p<0.05$). Taken together, these results confirm that our HFD-fed mice recapitulate two important features of T2DM in human patients.

HFD does not impair neovascularization of the fracture callus

Human T2DM is characterized by numerous microvascular complications leading to retinopathy [37], renal dysfunction [38], and peripheral neuropathy [39]. Furthermore, in rodent models of fracture healing in the context of T1DM, reduced callus vascularization during healing has been documented [40,41]. Thus, we performed lead chromate perfusion-based vascular µCT at days 10 and 14 to investigate whether HFD-fed mice exhibited impaired neovascularization of the fracture callus. Serial µCT scanning was performed to capture bone and lead chromate volume prior to decalcification and a second scan after decalcification yielded lead chromate volume within vascular spaces. Representative three-dimensional reconstructions from µCT scans after decalcification show a qualitative trend towards decreased callus vascular volume in HFD-fed mice (Fig. 2A). Quantification confirmed this trend but significance was not achieved at either time point (Fig. 2B). This trend towards decreased callus vascularity in HFD-fed mice was not apparent after normalizing vascular volume to bone volume for each sample (Fig. 2C), indicating that apparent reduced vascularity in the calluses was likely associated with a net reduction in callus. This experiment confirms the positive correlation between vascular volume and bone volume but a definitive link between reduced fracture callus vascular volume and feeding of a HFD cannot be established from this experiment.

HFD-fed mice display decreased fracture callus bone content in late-stage healing

Fracture callus bone volume was determined via µCT studies performed at various time points during healing. Representative µCT reconstructions are presented for all time points (Fig. 3), with the correlated quantitation shows significantly decreased bone volume at day 21 and an apparent delay in achieving peak bone volume and in HFD-fed mice compared to lean-fed controls (Fig. 4). Alcian Blue Hematoxylin/Orange G-stained histologic sections (Fig. 5A) were used to perform histomorphometry-based study of the callus, revealing no differences in cartilage content between the groups at any timepoint (Fig. 5B), but confirming decreased bone content, with HFD-fed mice showing a significant decrease in woven bone area as a percentage of total callus area at day 28 (Fig. 5C). Interestingly, HFD-fed mice showed significantly decreased stromal area at day 35, which may be due to expansion of the adipocyte population with possible suppression of bone marrow stem cells and/or other progenitor or stromal cell populations (Fig. 5D). It should be noted that TRAP-staining to examine ratio of osteoclast number to bone perimeter was performed, indicating that the ratio of osteoclast number (Oc.N.) to bone perimeter (B.Pm.) was not different between lean- and HFD-fed mice at any time point (data not shown).

HFD-fed mice display increased fracture callus adiposity and decreased osteoblast-occupied bone surface area

Within the fracture callus, cells with spherical morphology and lacking intracellular organelles were observed. These presumptive adipocytes were markedly more abundant in fracture calluses of HFD-fed mice (Fig. 6B) than in those of lean diet controls (Fig. 6A). To confirm that these cells were adipocytes, immunohistochemical staining was performed using a monoclonal antibody for perilipin, a protein associated with the membranes of lipid vacuoles within

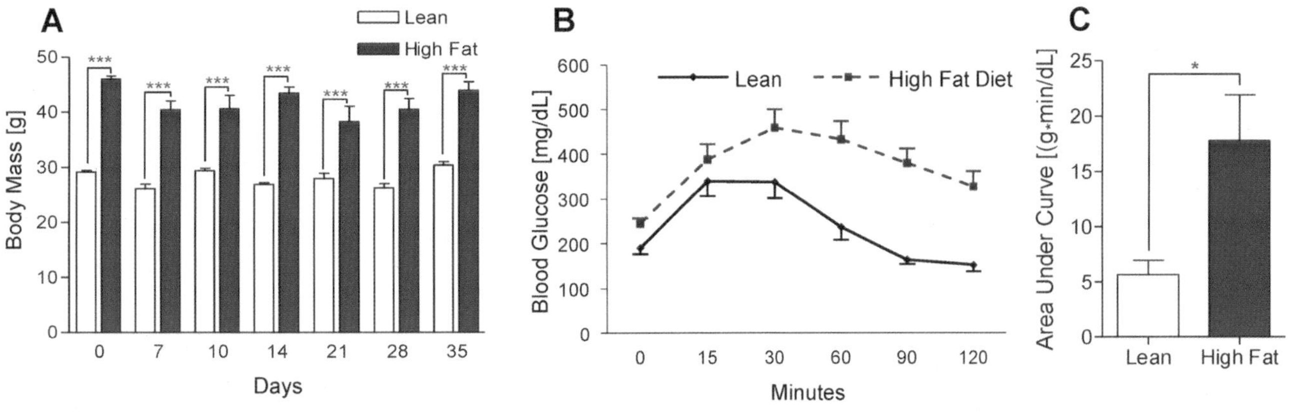

Figure 1. HFD-fed mice are obese and glucose intolerant. (**A**) Body weights of HFD-fed and control lean diet-fed mice at various time points after surgical fracture. Bars represent means ± SEM (n≥5). ***$p<0.001$ using a two-way, unpaired ANOVA with a Bonferroni post-test. (**B**) Glucose tolerance testing (GTT) was performed immediately prior to fracture on lean and HFD-fed mice. Plotted data points represent means ± SEM (n = 5). (**C**) Net area under the curve (AUC) was calculated for each mouse that underwent GTT (n = 5). *$p<0.05$ compared to respective lean diet controls using an unpaired, two-tailed Student's *t* test. Bars represent means ± SEM (n = 5).

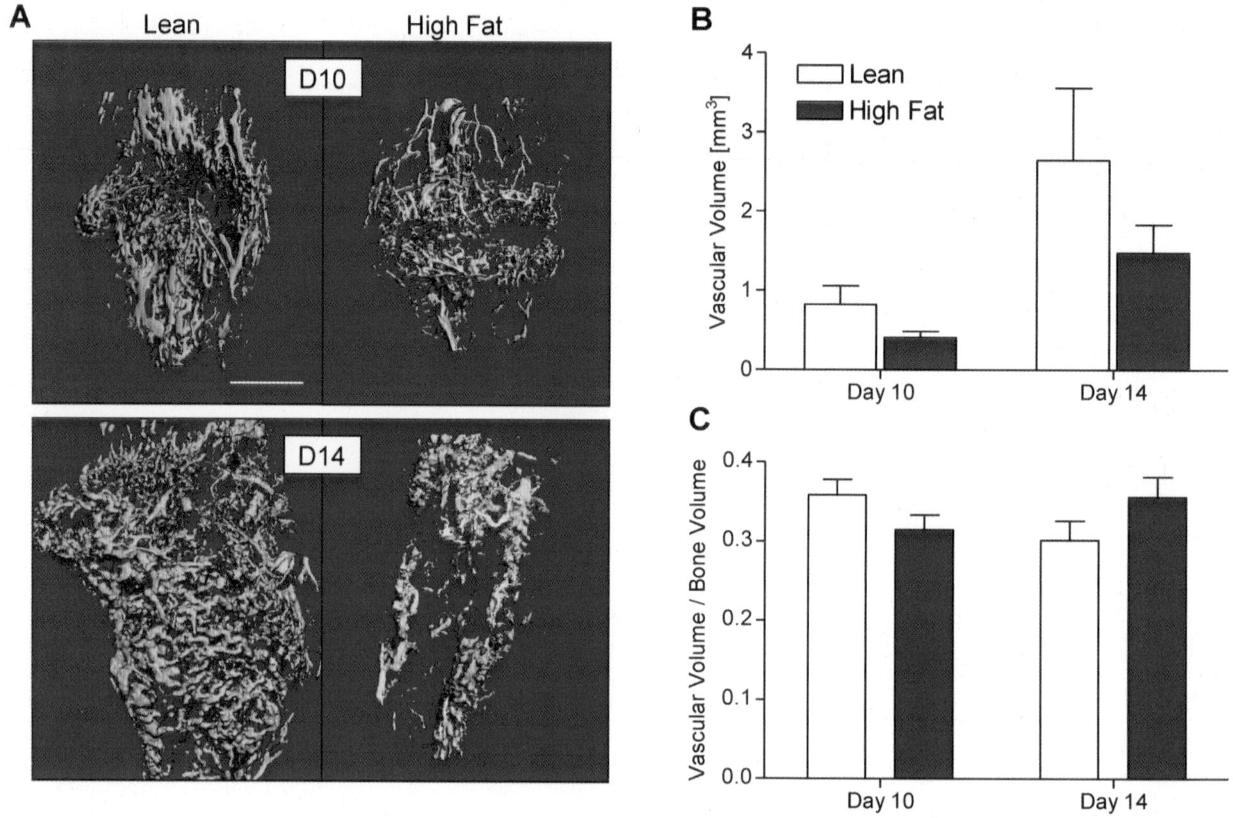

Figure 2. Callus neovascularization in lean- and HFD-fed mice is similar. μCT scans of fractured tibiae that were perfused with lead chromate paint after decalcification were performed in lean and HFD-fed mice at 10 and 14 days post-fracture. Representative three-dimensional reconstructions are presented in panel (**A**). Vascular volume (**B**) and vascular volume normalized to callus bone volume (**C**) was quantified from μCT data. Bars represent means ± SEM (n≥5). Scale bar (white line) = 1 mm.

adipocytes [42]. As shown in Fig. 6B, the ribbon-like lipid vacuole membranes within presumptive adipocytes specifically stained for perilipin, confirming that these are adipocytes. Conversely, the fracture calluses of lean diet control mice exhibited a paucity of perilipin-positive adipocytes (Fig. 6A). Correlated with this, histomorphometry revealed that adipose tissue area as a percentage of total callus area was significantly increased in HFD-fed mice at days 21, 28 and 35 (Fig. 6C). Interestingly, adipose tissue was minimal at early time points through day 14 in both HFD-fed and lean control mice. Increased adiposity was observed in the HFD-fed mice only at day 21 and the later time points. This change in adipocyte area was coincident with a significant decrease in percentage of bone surface occupied by osteoblast-like cells in HFD-fed mice, an effect that was significant at day 21 and 35 post-fracture, with a trend toward a decrease at day 28 (Fig. 6D). Taken together, these data establish that during the later stages of healing, HFD-fed mice have a concomitant increase in callus adiposity, and a decrease in woven bone content/osteoblast-occupied bone surface suggesting a single pathophysiological process may be responsible for both defects.

PPARγ expression is up-regulated in the callus of HFD-fed mice

Given the increase in the number of adipocytes in fracture callus from HFD-fed mice, we further examined the expression of peroxisome-proliferation activated receptor, subtype gamma (PPARγ), widely recognized as a master regulator of adipogenesis [43,44]. Since we observed callus adipocyte number to increase at time points from days 21 through 35 post-fracture (Fig. 6C), we chose to perform PPARγ immunohistochemistry at the previous time point (day 14), where PPARγ might be expected to be up-regulated to drive the commitment of progenitor populations toward adipocyte formation. While PPARγ expression was detectable in day 14 fracture callus from both lean- (Fig. 7A) and HFD-fed (Fig. 7B) mice, the HFD-fed group had increased PPARγ staining overall, particularly in cells adjacent to trabecular bone (Fig. 7B, red arrows), compared to lean diet controls (Fig. 7A, blue arrows).

Biomechanical strength during late-stage healing was decreased in HFD-fed mice

Torsional testing was performed on surgically fractured tibiae at days 14 and 35. HFD-fed mice had significantly weaker healed fractures at day 35 (Fig. 8), but no difference in maximum torque to failure was observed at day 14. This finding corresponds with our data that shows no differences in woven bone or adipocyte percentage between HFD-fed and lean control diet mice until day 21.

Discussion

Endochondral-based healing, which predominates in repair of long bones, requires the correct temporospatial coordination of a series of molecular and cellular events [45]. From a tissue architecture perspective, these events are organized into four overlapping phases: (1) inflammation, (2) soft (cartilaginous) callus

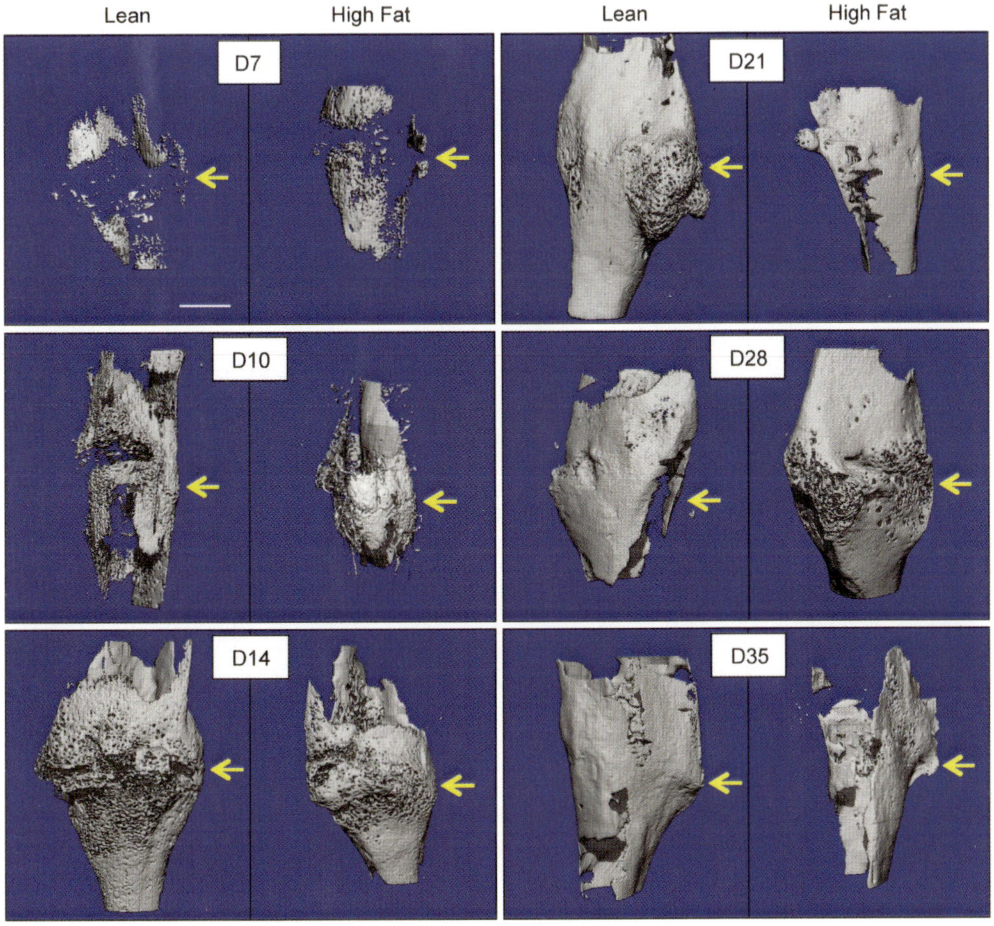

Figure 3. μCT imaging reveals a trend toward decreased bone volume in HFD-fed mice. μCT scans were performed on tibiae at 7, 10, 14, 21, 28, and 35 days post-fracture. Representative three-dimensional reconstructions, from groups of 5–7 tibiae, show bone volume within the external fracture callus. Scale bar (white line) = 1 mm. Fracture sites are denoted with yellow arrows.

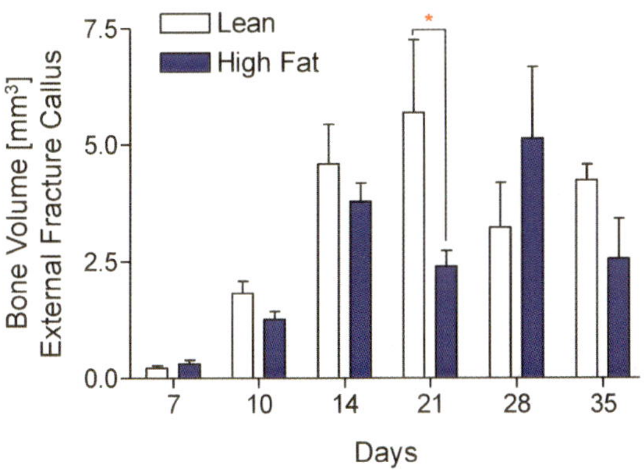

Figure 4. Quantitative analysis confirms decreased and delayed accrual of peak bone volume in fracture callus of HFD-fed mice. Using μCT scans that were used create the reconstructions shown Fig. 3, bone volume was quantified from lean- and HFD-fed mice at 7, 10, 14, 21, 28, and 35 days post-fracture. Bars represent means ± SEM (n≥5). $*p<0.05$ compared to time-matched lean diet controls using two-way, unpaired ANOVA with Bonferroni post-tests.

formation, (3) hard (woven bone) callus formation, and (4) woven bone remodeling. Mesenchymal cells (MSCs) and chondro-/osteo-progenitor populations that primarily reside in the periosteum are essential throughout fracture repair [45–49]. Angiogenesis and neovascularization are required as a conduit for MSC delivery during hard callus formation and to provide oxygen tension sufficient to induce MSCs to differentiate into osteoblasts [4,11,12,45,47]. From the perspective of the work presented in this report, it is interesting to note that osteoblastic progenitors [11] and preadipocytes [44] have both been identified as populations of progenitor cells whose source is perivascular. Overall, it is generally held that fracture healing is impaired when MSCs are dysfunctional, which can include a decreased progenitor pool, ineffective recruitment, aberrant fate determination, or impaired differentiation.

Patients with T1DM and T2DM sustain pathologic changes to normal skeletal homeostasis and repair. Osteopenia and osteoporosis, human disease states characterized by decreased bone mineral density and/or bone quality, are more prevalent in patients with either type of DM [50]. Furthermore, the constellation of pathologic changes that accumulate in patients with DM coalesce to impair skeletal repair, manifesting as an increased incidence of delayed healing or fracture non-union [8] and increased rates of pseudoarthrosis after surgical arthrodesis [51–53]. Work focused on understanding the impact of T1DM on

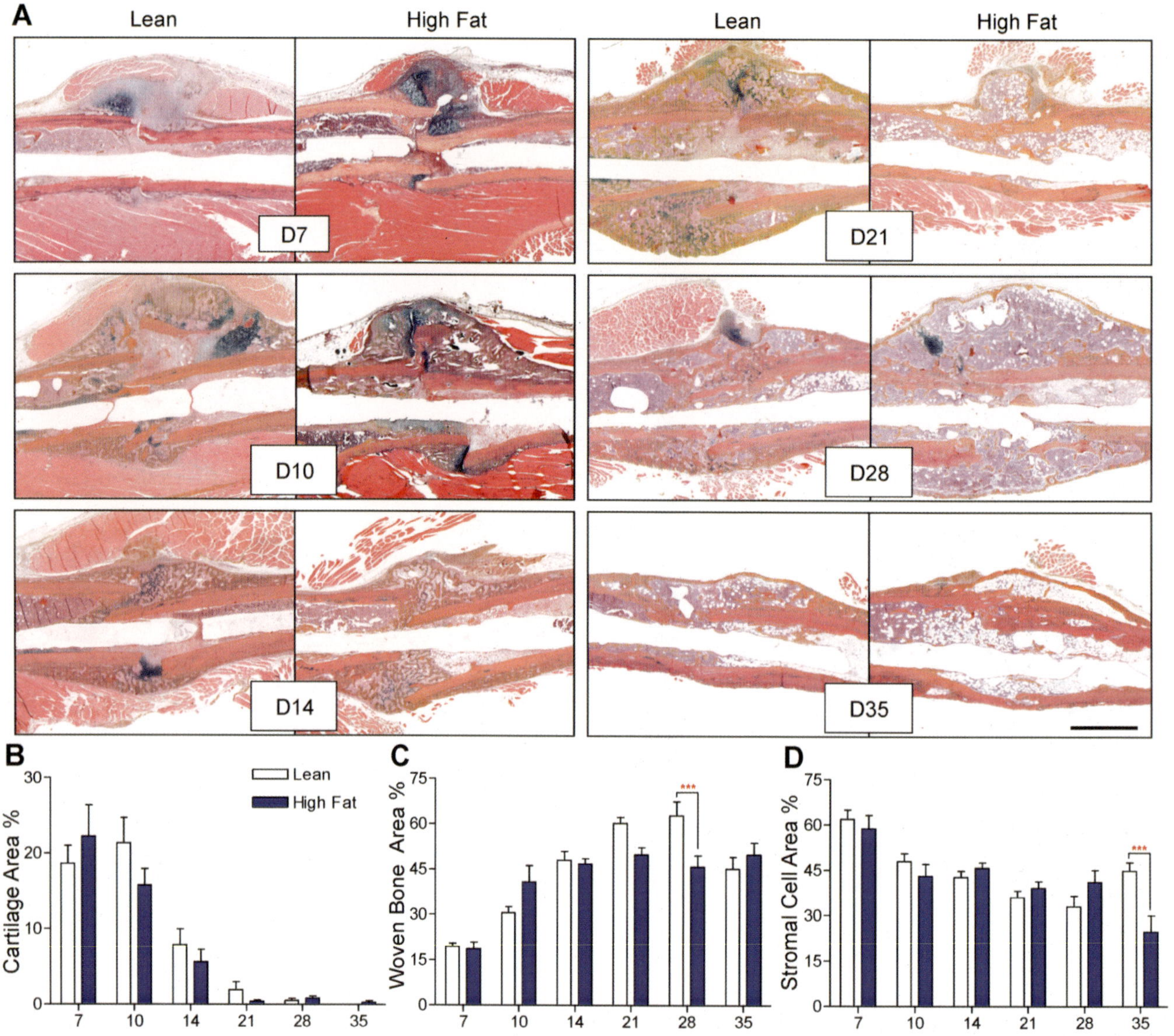

Figure 5. Woven bone content is decreased at later stages of fracture healing in HFD-fed mice. (**A**) Representative Alcian Blue Hematoxylin/Orange G stained histologic sections of fracture callus in lean- and HFD-fed mice at 7, 10, 14, 21, 28, and 35 days post-fracture. Quantification of cartilage (**B**), woven bone (**C**), and stromal cell areas (**D**), expressed as percentages of total callus area, were determined using a point-counting histomorphometric method. Bars represent means ± SEM (n≥5). ****p*<0.001 compared to time-matched controls using two-way, unpaired ANOVA with Bonferroni post-tests. The black size marker in the lower right panel = 1 mm.

skeletal repair has been published previously in rodent models of tibia and femur fracture following STZ-dependent pancreatic beta cell depletion. As mentioned, these studies have revealed that key defects include decreased progenitor cell proliferation [13–17], decreased callus cartilage content [13,14,17,18], premature cartilage resorption [13,18,19], reduced neovascularization of the callus [40,41], decreased callus bone content [14–16,20,21], and a biomechanically inferior repair at later time points [14–17,20]. Based on these clinical and animal data establishing an impairment of bone healing in DM, and because T2DM in particular is highly prevalent and a major health crises in the US and worldwide, we characterized the fracture healing process in mice induced to have obesity-related type 2 diabetes that was induced via consumption of a high fat Western diet. We hypothesized that the deleterious effect of T2DM on the bone healing process involves an alteration in one or more of the phases of healing.

Findings presented here establish that obesity-associated T2DM leads to defective fracture repair that is distinct from the defect seen in T1DM from the perspective of early callus tissue morphogenesis. The two most striking differences relate to neovascularization of the callus during early healing and induction of osteoclast formation and numbers during mid-late healing. Regarding the vascular phenotype, while a key defect in T1DM is reduced cartilage content [13,14,17,18] and a correlated impairment in callus neovascularization [40,41], T2DM did not significantly impair the cartilage phase of healing or the subsequent propagation of vascular tissue within the callus. Since it is established that chondrocyte-dependent production of VEGF is a critical signal for vascular ingrowth during bone repair [54], the reduced cartilage phenotype in T1DM is consistent with the

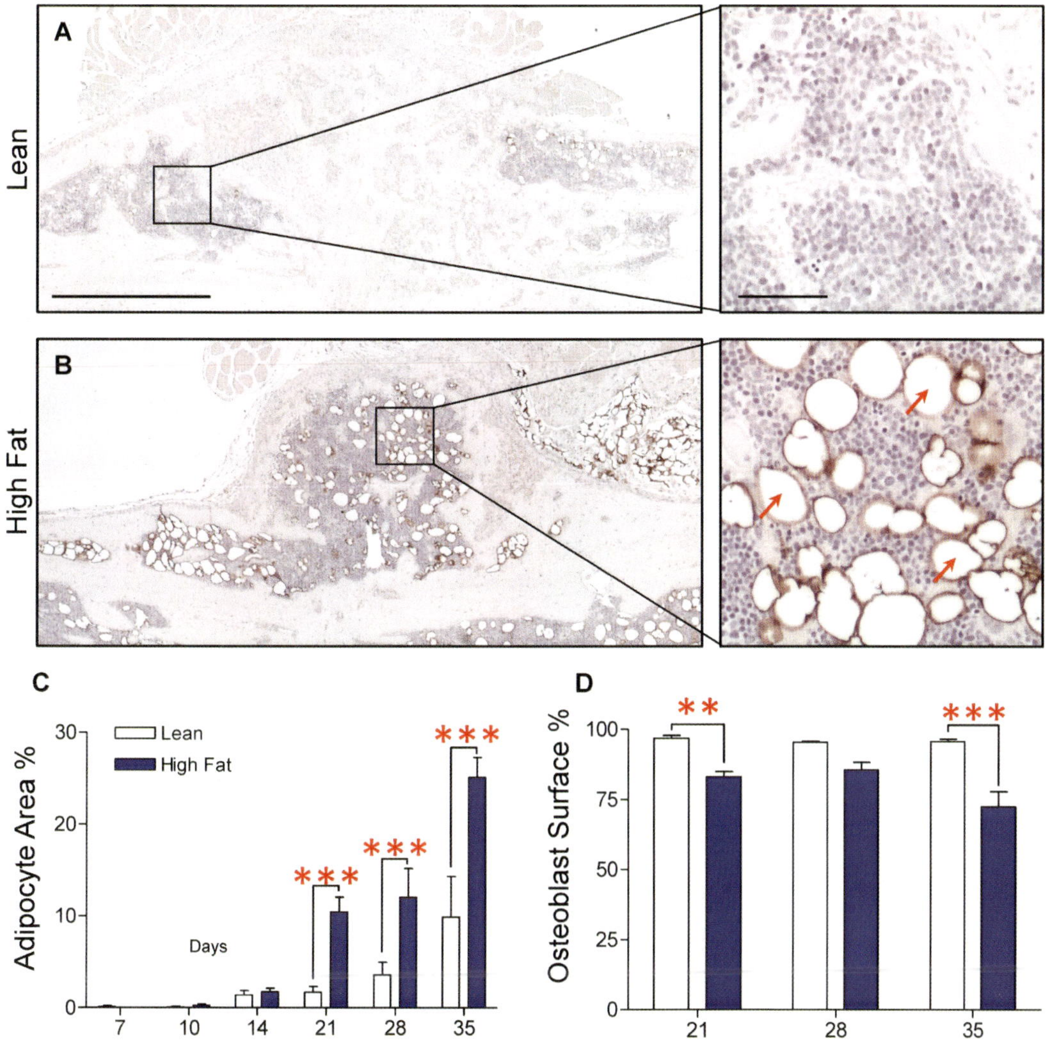

Figure 6. Adiposity is increased and osteoblast-occupied bone surface is decreased within the external fracture callus during late stage healing in HFD-fed mice. Immunohistochemical staining for perilipin was performed to confirm the presence of adipocytes within the fracture callus. Representative sections from day 21 post-fracture demonstrate an increased number of adipocytes within the fracture callus of the HFD-fed mouse (**B**) compared to the lean diet control (**A**). Higher magnifications of selected regions from lean and HFD-fed calluses illustrate specificity of perilipin staining, with several typical perilipin-positive adipocytes denoted with red arrows. (**C**) Adipocyte area as a percentage of total callus area and percent of osteoblast occupied bone surface were determined using histomorphometric methods in lean- and HFD-fed mice at the indicated time points. Bars represent the means $\pm$ SEM ($n \geq 5$). **$p<0.01$ and ***$p<0.001$ compared to time-matched controls using an unpaired, two-way ANOVA with Bonferroni post-test. The black size marker in the low magnification images (left panels of **A** and **B**) = 1 mm. The black size marker for the high magnification images (right panels of **A** and **B**) = 100 μm.

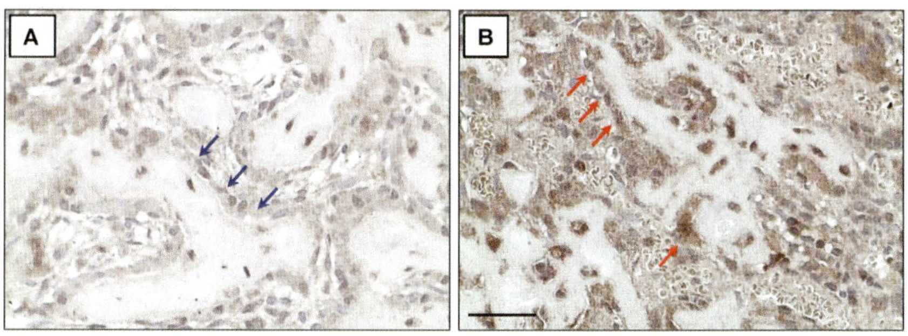

Figure 7. PPARγ expression is increased in fracture callus of HFD-fed mice. Sections were subjected to immunohistochemical staining for PPARγ and representative fracture calluses at day 14 show increased PPARγ expression in the fracture callus of HFD-fed mice (**B**) compared to lean controls (**A**), particularly in cells adjacent to trabecular bone elements (marked by blue arrows in callus from lean-fed mice and red arrows in callus from HFD-fed mice). The black size marker (panel **B**) = 20 μm.

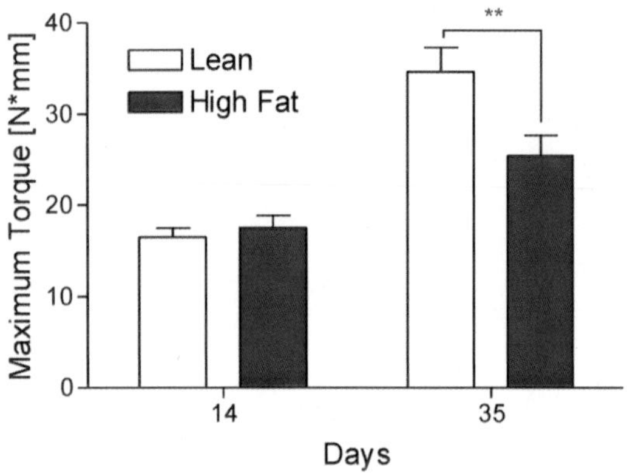

Figure 8. Healed tibiae from HFD-fed mice are biomechanically weaker. (**A**) Surgically fractured right tibiae from lean- and HFD-fed mice (n≥8) were subjected to biomechanical torsional testing at days 14 and 35 post-fracture, with a significant decrease in strength observed in the HFD-fed group at day 35. Bars represent the means ± SEM (n≥8). $^{**}p<0.01$ compared to time-matched controls using an unpaired, two-way ANOVA with Bonferroni post-tests.

decreased neovascularization observed in that model. Conversely, a normal cartilage phase in T2DM, which would presumable include appropriate expression of VEGF, may account for the absence of a vascular phenotype in this model. This tissue dynamic (i.e. chondrocyte hypertrophy leading to VEGF-dependent neovascularization) is likely unique to bone healing, and may explain why impaired vascularization in other situations, such as during dermal wound healing [55,56], is a phenotype shared by T1DM and T2DM. Regarding the osteoclast phenotype, it is established that in T1DM, increased levels of TNF-α lead to increased osteoclastogenesis and a higher number of osteoclasts [19,57], which may account for the accelerated resorption of the cartilage callus during mid-stage healing in this model. This phenotype is not observed in T2DM based on our assessment of osteoclast number, an analysis that revealed no differences between mice fed the normal versus the HFD. It may be that the complete loss of insulin in T1DM leads to molecular and tissue effects during healing that are more robust and/or distinct from the impact of the diet-induced insulin resistance (i.e. incomplete ablation of insulin sensitivity or insulin production) that occurs in T2DM. It has been shown that osteoclast numbers/function during skeletal homeostasis is enhanced in T2DM [28], and that this effect could lead to obesity-related bone loss [29], but results presented here suggest that in the stressed situation present during fracture repair, the osteoclast phenotype is unaffected. Understanding the molecular and tissue basis for this distinction is an important focus for ongoing study.

Further differences in bone repair between T1DM and T2DM are also seen in the post-cartilage phases of healing within the callus. While T1DM shows late stage healing defects that likely result from the initial soft callus defects (reduced cartilage/neovascularization), the central tissue defect we observed in T2DM is a significant increase in fracture callus adiposity in HFD-fed mice during the woven bone formation and remodeling phases that was coincident with a decrease in both the area of osteoblast-occupied bone surface and callus bone volume during mid to late healing. This ultimately led to a biomechanically weaker repair at day 35 post-fracture. Interestingly, adipocytes were not appreciably observed within the fracture callus until day 14, with calluses from both lean and HFD-fed mice up through this time point possessing a minimal and approximately equal number of adipocytes. After 14 days, a significant increase in adipose tissue content was observed in calluses from HFD-fed mice, coinciding with the period of maximal woven bone formation and subsequent remodeling driven by osteoblast formation and osteoblast-osteoclast coupling respectively. The simultaneous increase in adipose tissue and decrease in osteoblast-occupied surface area and woven bone content in HFD-fed mice compared to lean diet controls suggests a potential MSC fate switch, with a possible shift toward the adipocyte lineage at the expense of osteoblastic commitment. This idea that fate switching drives the phenotype is further supported by the observation of increased PPARγ expression within the fracture callus of HFD-fed mice, particularly in the population of cells lining bone trabeculae.

Mounting evidence for the mutual exclusivity of bone and adipose tissue formation suggests a reciprocal regulation of MSC fate with respect to adipogenesis and osteoblastogenesis [46,58–60]. PPARγ, one of 3 known subtypes of peroxisome-proliferation activated receptors (PPARs), which are transcription factors of the steroid/thyroid hormone receptor superfamily [61,62], has traditionally been regarded as the master regulator of adipogenesis and has been implicated as a key regulator that drives MSCs down either the adipocytic or osteoblastic lineage [43,63]. This idea has been most definitively demonstrated in animal studies of PPARγ signaling and its influence on skeletal biology. Akune et al. deleted the PPARγ gene in mice to characterize its role in the regulation of adipogenesis and osteoblastogenesis. Embryonic stem (ES) cells cultured from PPAR$\gamma^{-/-}$ embryos in medium lacking osteogenic stimulation demonstrated a complete absence of adipogenesis coupled with increased bone nodule formation [59]. Col1α1, osteocalcin, and Runx2 expression were significantly increased in PPAR$\gamma^{-/-}$ ES cells compared to WT ES cells, providing molecular evidence of fate switching in the cultures. These findings correlate with in vivo data from PPAR$\gamma^{+/-}$ mice demonstrating increased bone volume and expression of osteoblast markers in conjunction with decreased adipocyte volume and expression of adipocyte markers [59]. Furthermore, epidemiological data suggest that PPARγ agonists from the thiazolidinedione (TZD) family of drugs adversely affect skeletal homeostasis with multiple large, prospective clinical trials demonstrating an excess fracture risk among diabetic patients treated with TZDs [64–66]. The TZDs have been used extensively to treat patients with T2DM [64,67] and the excess fracture risk in patients exposed to TZDs is likely due to the development of osteoporosis. While these observations do not speak directly to fracture healing, they do support the idea that PPARγ likely plays an important role in the balance between the osteoblastic and adipogenic pathways [46,58–60]. Overall, these results suggest that PPARγ, either independently or in concert with other emerging candidate signaling regulators of adipogenesis, such as the non-canonical Wnt signaling pathway [68], plays a central role in balancing adipogenesis and osteoblastogenesis. This concept is consistent with the increased PPARγ expression and the increased adiposity/decreased osteoblast number and woven bone content in mid- to late-stage healing that we observed in T2DM.

Data presented in this report support the concept that adipogenesis and osteoblastogenesis are interrelated in the context of fracture repair. Normally, a balance between these fates exists during healing, with the osteoblast fate the dominant outcome. Osteoblastic commitment supports woven bone formation and the downstream production of osteoblast-produced factors known to regulate osteoclast formation (RANKL and osteoprotegerin) and callus remodeling. Based on our findings, we propose that the balance of progenitor cell differentiation is partially shifted toward the adipocyte lineage in HFD-fed mice. This results in an increase in adipocyte formation and an associated decrease in osteoblast commitment. Based on immunohistochemistry findings, we propose that increased PPARγ expression may contribute to this altered fate for progenitor cells leading to the healing defect seen in the HFD-fed population.

As mentioned, insulin has known anabolic effects on bone, with both systemic and local delivery improving fracture repair in T1DM animal models [13–15,19]. Furthermore, clinical reports suggest that better glycemic control, as measured by lower hemoglobin A1c percentage, results in fewer complications of diabetes mellitus [69]. Of specific relevance to the work presented here, rates of healing after transmetatarsal foot amputation were significantly lower in diabetic patients with poorly controlled disease (HbA1c ≥8%), compared to diabetic patients with better control (HbA1c <8%) [70]. Based on these observations and our current work, we suggest that a method to improving fracture repair in patients with T2DM, with the potential to normalize the balance between adipogenesis and osteoblastogenesis in the callus, would be to employ insulin therapy to control the diabetes during the healing process. While multiple and distinct mechanisms have been implicated in mediating diabetic complications in various target tissues, intensive insulin therapy has been shown to be effective in decreasing the frequency and severity of most diabetic complications. Other than insulin, it will require further investigation to identify novel therapeutic approaches, including strategies to inhibit adipogenesis in the fracture callus, to address impaired fracture repair in type 2 diabetes.

Acknowledgments

The authors would like to acknowledge the outstanding technical assistance of Michael Thullen, Sarah Mack and Robert Maynard, all in the Center for Musculoskeletal Research at the University of Rochester Medical Center.

Author Contributions

Conceived and designed the experiments: MLB KY HA RJO LX RAM MJZ. Performed the experiments: MLB KY CWF RAM. Analyzed the data: MLB KY CWF DGC MJH LX RAM MJZ. Contributed reagents/materials/analysis tools: HA MJH RJO LX RAM MJZ. Wrote the paper: MLB RAM MJZ.

References

1. Alarcon T, Gonzalez-Montalvo JI, Gotor P, Madero R, Otero A (2011) Activities of daily living after hip fracture: profile and rate of recovery during 2 years of follow-up. Osteoporos Int 22: 1609–1613.
2. Brenneman SK, Barrett-Connor E, Sajjan S, Markson LE, Siris ES (2006) Impact of recent fracture on health-related quality of life in postmenopausal women. J Bone Miner Res 21: 809–816.
3. Ding R, McCarthy ML, Houseknecht E, Ziegfeld S, Knight VM, et al. (2006) The health-related quality of life of children with an extremity fracture: a one-year follow-up study. J Pediatr Orthop 26: 157–163.
4. Giannoudis PV, Harwood PJ, Kontakis G, Allami M, Macdonald D, et al. (2009) Long-term quality of life in trauma patients following the full spectrum of tibial injury (fasciotomy, closed fracture, grade IIIB/IIIC open fracture and amputation). Injury 40: 213–219.
5. Lonnroos E, Kautiainen H, Sund R, Karppi P, Hartikainen S, et al. (2009) Utilization of inpatient care before and after hip fracture: a population-based study. Osteoporos Int 20: 879–886.
6. Olerud P, Ahrengart L, Soderqvist A, Saving J, Tidermark J (2010) Quality of life and functional outcome after a 2-part proximal humeral fracture: a prospective cohort study on 50 patients treated with a locking plate. J Shoulder Elbow Surg 19: 814–822.
7. Silverman SL, Shen W, Minshall ME, Xie S, Moses KH (2007) Prevalence of depressive symptoms in postmenopausal women with low bone mineral density and/or prevalent vertebral fracture: results from the Multiple Outcomes of Raloxifene Evaluation (MORE) study. J Rheumatol 34: 140–144.
8. Loder RT (1988) The influence of diabetes mellitus on the healing of closed fractures. ClinOrthopRelat Res: 210–216.
9. Khazai NB, Beck GR Jr, Umpierrez GE (2009) Diabetes and fractures: an overshadowed association. Curr Opin Endocrinol Diabetes Obes 16: 435–445.
10. Gregg EW, Li Y, Wang J, Burrows NR, Ali MK, et al. (2014) Changes in diabetes-related complications in the United States, 1990–2010. N Engl J Med 370: 1514–1523.
11. Einhorn TA (1998) The cell and molecular biology of fracture healing. ClinOrthop: S7–21.
12. Tsiridis E, Upadhyay N, Giannoudis P (2007) Molecular aspects of fracture healing: which are the important molecules? Injury 38 Suppl 1: S11–25.
13. Ogasawara A, Nakajima A, Nakajima F, Goto K, Yamazaki M (2008) Molecular basis for affected cartilage formation and bone union in fracture healing of the streptozotocin-induced diabetic rat. Bone 43: 832–839.
14. Gandhi A, Beam HA, O'Connor JP, Parsons JR, Lin SS (2005) The effects of local insulin delivery on diabetic fracture healing. Bone 37: 482–490.
15. Follak N, Kloting I, Merk H (2005) Influence of diabetic metabolic state on fracture healing in spontaneously diabetic rats. Diabetes Metab Res Rev 21: 288–296.
16. Follak N, Kloting L, Wolf E, Merk H (2004) Delayed remodeling in the early period of fracture healing in spontaneously diabetic BB/OK rats depending on the diabetic metabolic state. Histol Histopathol 19: 473–486.
17. Macey LR, Kana SM, Jingushi S, Terek RM, Borretos J, et al. (1989) Defects of early fracture-healing in experimental diabetes. J Bone Joint Surg Am 71: 722–733.
18. Kayal RA, Tsatsas D, Bauer MA, Allen B, Al-Sebaei MO, et al. (2007) Diminished bone formation during diabetic fracture healing is related to the premature resorption of cartilage associated with increased osteoclast activity. J Bone Miner Res 22: 560–568.
19. Kayal RA, Alblowi J, McKenzie E, Krothapalli N, Silkman L, et al. (2009) Diabetes causes the accelerated loss of cartilage during fracture repair which is reversed by insulin treatment. Bone 44: 357–363.
20. Beam HA, Parsons JR, Lin SS (2002) The effects of blood glucose control upon fracture healing in the BB Wistar rat with diabetes mellitus. Journal of Orthopaedic Research 20: 1210–1216.
21. Gandhi A, Doumas C, O'Connor JP, Parsons JR, Lin SS (2006) The effects of local platelet rich plasma delivery on diabetic fracture healing. Bone 38: 540–546.
22. Surwit RS, Kuhn CM, Cochrane C, McCubbin JA, Feinglos MN (1988) Diet-induced type II diabetes in C57BL/6J mice. Diabetes 37: 1163–1167.
23. Mooney RA, Sampson ER, Lerea J, Rosier RN, Zuscik MJ (2011) High-fat diet accelerates progression of osteoarthritis after meniscal/ligamentous injury. Arthritis Res Ther 13: R198.
24. Andrikopoulos S, Blair AR, Deluca N, Fam BC, Proietto J (2008) Evaluating the glucose tolerance test in mice. Am J Physiol Endocrinol Metab 295: E1323–1332.
25. Clementi AH, Gaudy AM, Zimmers TA, Koniaris LG, Mooney RA (2011) Deletion of interleukin-6 improves pyruvate tolerance without altering hepatic insulin signaling in the leptin receptor-deficient mouse. Metabolism 60: 1610–1619.
26. Kung MH, Yukata K, O'Keefe RJ, Zuscik MJ (2012) Aryl hydrocarbon receptor-mediated impairment of chondrogenesis and fracture healing by cigarette smoke and benzo(a)pyrene. J Cell Physiol 227: 1062–1070.
27. Inzana JA, Kung M, Shu L, Hamada D, Xing LP, et al. (2013) Immature mice are more susceptible to the detrimental effects of high fat diet on cancellous bone in the distal femur. Bone 57: 174–183.
28. Kawashima Y, Fritton JC, Yakar S, Epstein S, Schaffler MB, et al. (2009) Type 2 diabetic mice demonstrate slender long bones with increased fragility secondary to increased osteoclastogenesis. Bone 44: 648–655.
29. Cao JJ (2011) Effects of obesity on bone metabolism. J Orthop Surg Res 6: 30.
30. Dhillon RS, Schwarz EM (2011) Teriparatide Therapy as an Adjuvant for Tissue Engineering and Integration of Biomaterials. J Mater Res 4: 1117–1131.
31. Dhillon RS, Xie C, Tyler W, Calvi LM, Awad HA, et al. (2013) PTH-enhanced structural allograft healing is associated with decreased angiopoietin-2-mediated arteriogenesis, mast cell accumulation, and fibrosis. J Bone Miner Res 28: 586–597.
32. Zhang X, Xie C, Lin AS, Ito H, Awad H, et al. (2005) Periosteal progenitor cell fate in segmental cortical bone graft transplantations: implications for functional tissue engineering. Journal of Bone and Mineral Research 20: 2124–2137.
33. Zhang X, Schwarz EM, Young DA, Puzas JE, Rosier RN, et al. (2002) Cyclooxygenase-2 regulates mesenchymal cell differentiation into the osteoblast lineage and is critically involved in bone repair. JClinInvest 109: 1405–1415.
34. Naik AA, Xie C, Zuscik MJ, Kingsley P, Schwarz EM, et al. (2009) Reduced COX-2 expression in aged mice is associated with impaired fracture healing. Journal of Bone and Mineral Research 24: 251–264.
35. Mungo DV, Zhang X, O'Keefe RJ, Rosier RN, Puzas JE, et al. (2002) COX-1 and COX-2 expression in osteoid osteomas. J Orthop Res 20: 159–162.
36. Reynolds DG, Hock C, Shaikh S, Jacobson J, Zhang X, et al. (2007) Micro-computed tomography prediction of biomechanical strength in murine structural bone grafts. JBiomech 40: 3178–3186.

37. Jackson GR, Scott IU, Quillen DA, Walter LE, Gardner TW (2012) Inner retinal visual dysfunction is a sensitive marker of non-proliferative diabetic retinopathy. Br J Ophthalmol 96: 699–703.
38. Thomas MC, Groop PH, Tryggvason K (2012) Towards understanding the inherited susceptibility for nephropathy in diabetes. Curr Opin Nephrol Hypertens 21: 195–202.
39. Tesfaye S, Selvarajah D (2012) Advances in the epidemiology, pathogenesis and management of diabetic peripheral neuropathy. Diabetes Metab Res Rev 28 Suppl 1: 8–14.
40. Coords M, Breitbart E, Paglia D, Kappy N, Gandhi A, et al. (2011) The effects of low-intensity pulsed ultrasound upon diabetic fracture healing. J Orthop Res 29: 181–188.
41. Wang CY, Yang HB, Hsu HS, Chen LL, Tsai CC, et al. (2012) Mesenchymal stem cell-conditioned medium facilitates angiogenesis and fracture healing in diabetic rats. J Tissue Eng Regen Med 6: 559–569.
42. Greenberg AS, Egan JJ, Wek SA, Garty NB, Blanchette-Mackie EJ, et al. (1991) Perilipin, a major hormonally regulated adipocyte-specific phosphoprotein associated with the periphery of lipid storage droplets. J Biol Chem 266: 11341–11346.
43. Nuttall ME, Gimble JM (2004) Controlling the balance between osteoblastogenesis and adipogenesis and the consequent therapeutic implications. Curr Opin Pharmacol 4: 290–294.
44. Cristancho AG, Lazar MA (2011) Forming functional fat: a growing understanding of adipocyte differentiation. Nat Rev Mol Cell Biol 12: 722–734.
45. Schindeler A, McDonald MM, Bokko P, Little DG (2008) Bone remodeling during fracture repair: The cellular picture. Semin Cell Dev Biol 19: 459–466.
46. Owen M (1988) Marrow stromal stem cells. J Cell Sci Suppl 10: 63–76.
47. Gruber R, Koch H, Doll BA, Tegtmeier F, Einhorn TA, et al. (2006) Fracture healing in the elderly patient. ExpGerontol 41: 1080–1093.
48. Zuscik MJ, O'Keefe RJ (2009) Skeletal Healing. In: Rosen CJ, editor. Primer on the Metabolic Bone Diseases and Disorders of Mineral Metabolism: American Society of Bone and Mineral Research. pp. 61–65.
49. Zhang X, Naik A, Xie C, Reynolds D, Palmer J, et al. (2005) Periosteal stem cells are essential for bone revitalization and repair. JMusculoskeletNeuronalInteract 5: 360–362.
50. Montagnani A, Gonnelli S, Alessandri M, Nuti R (2011) Osteoporosis and risk of fracture in patients with diabetes: an update. Aging Clin Exp Res 23: 84–90.
51. Papa J, Myerson M, Girard P (1993) Salvage, with arthrodesis, in intractable diabetic neuropathic arthropathy of the foot and ankle. J Bone Joint Surg Am 75: 1056–1066.
52. Stuart MJ, Morrey BF (1990) Arthrodesis of the diabetic neuropathic ankle joint. Clin Orthop Relat Res: 209–211.
53. Perlman MH, Thordarson DB (1999) Ankle fusion in a high risk population: an assessment of nonunion risk factors. Foot Ankle Int 20: 491–496.
54. Athanasopoulos AN, Schneider D, Keiper T, Alt V, Pendurthi UR, et al. (2007) Vascular endothelial growth factor (VEGF)-induced up-regulation of CCN1 in osteoblasts mediates proangiogenic activities in endothelial cells and promotes fracture healing. Journal of Biological Chemistry 282: 26746–26753.
55. Lerman OZ, Galiano RD, Armour M, Levine JP, Gurtner GC (2003) Cellular dysfunction in the diabetic fibroblast: impairment in migration, vascular endothelial growth factor production, and response to hypoxia. Am J Pathol 162: 303–312.
56. Jazwa A, Kucharzewska P, Leja J, Zagorska A, Sierpniowska A, et al. (2010) Combined vascular endothelial growth factor-A and fibroblast growth factor 4 gene transfer improves wound healing in diabetic mice. Genet Vaccines Ther 8: 6.
57. Alblowi J, Kayal RA, Siqueira M, McKenzie E, Krothapalli N, et al. (2009) High levels of tumor necrosis factor-alpha contribute to accelerated loss of cartilage in diabetic fracture healing. Am J Pathol 175: 1574–1585.
58. Beresford JN, Bennett JH, Devlin C, Leboy PS, Owen ME (1992) Evidence for an inverse relationship between the differentiation of adipocytic and osteogenic cells in rat marrow stromal cell cultures. J Cell Sci 102 (Pt 2): 341–351.
59. Akune T, Ohba S, Kamekura S, Yamaguchi M, Chung UI, et al. (2004) PPARgamma insufficiency enhances osteogenesis through osteoblast formation from bone marrow progenitors. JClinInvest 113: 846–855.
60. Sen B, Styner M, Xie Z, Case N, Rubin CT, et al. (2009) Mechanical loading regulates NFATc1 and beta-catenin signaling through a GSK3beta control node. J Biol Chem 284: 34607–34617.
61. Green S, Wahli W (1994) Peroxisome proliferator-activated receptors: finding the orphan a home. Mol Cell Endocrinol 100: 149–153.
62. Lehrke M, Lazar MA (2005) The many faces of PPARgamma. Cell 123: 993–999.
63. McCauley LK (2010) c-Maf and you won't see fat. J Clin Invest 120: 3440–3442.
64. Meier C, Kraenzlin ME, Bodmer M, Jick SS, Jick H, et al. (2008) Use of thiazolidinediones and fracture risk. Arch Intern Med 168: 820–825.
65. Kahn SE, Haffner SM, Heise MA, Herman WH, Holman RR, et al. (2006) Glycemic durability of rosiglitazone, metformin, or glyburide monotherapy. N Engl J Med 355: 2427–2443.
66. Hampton T (2007) Diabetes drugs tied to fractures in women. JAMA 297: 1645.
67. Yki-Jarvinen H (2005) The PROactive study: some answers, many questions. Lancet 366: 1241–1242.
68. Kanazawa A, Tsukada S, Kamiyama M, Yanagimoto T, Nakajima M, et al. (2005) Wnt5b partially inhibits canonical Wnt/beta-catenin signaling pathway and promotes adipogenesis in 3T3-L1 preadipocytes. Biochem Biophys Res Commun 330: 505–510.
69. Wukich DK, Kline AJ (2008) The management of ankle fractures in patients with diabetes. J Bone Joint Surg Am 90: 1570–1578.
70. Younger AS, Awwad MA, Kalla TP, de Vries G (2009) Risk factors for failure of transmetatarsal amputation in diabetic patients: a cohort study. Foot Ankle Int 30: 1177–1182.

14

Microstructural Parameters of Bone Evaluated Using HR-pQCT Correlate with the DXA-Derived Cortical Index and the Trabecular Bone Score in a Cohort of Randomly Selected Premenopausal Women

Albrecht W. Popp[1]*, Helene Buffat[1], Ursula Eberli[2], Kurt Lippuner[1], Manuela Ernst[2], R. Geoff Richards[2], Vincent A. Stadelmann[2], Markus Windolf[2]

1 Department of Osteoporosis, Inselspital, Berne University Hospital and University of Berne, Berne, Switzerland, **2** AO Research Institute Davos, Davos, Switzerland

Abstract

Background: Areal bone mineral density is predictive for fracture risk. Microstructural bone parameters evaluated at the appendicular skeleton by high-resolution peripheral quantitative computed tomography (HR-pQCT) display differences between healthy patients and fracture patients. With the simple geometry of the cortex at the distal tibial diaphysis, a cortical index of the tibia combining material and mechanical properties correlated highly with bone strength ex vivo. The trabecular bone score derived from the scan of the lumbar spine by dual-energy X-ray absorptiometry (DXA) correlated ex vivo with the micro architectural parameters. It is unknown if these microstructural correlations could be made in healthy premenopausal women.

Methods: Randomly selected women between 20–40 years of age were examined by DXA and HR-pQCT at the standard regions of interest and at customized sub regions to focus on cortical and trabecular parameters of strength separately. For cortical strength, at the distal tibia the volumetric cortical index was calculated directly from HR-pQCT and the areal cortical index was derived from the DXA scan using a Canny threshold-based tool. For trabecular strength, the trabecular bone score was calculated based on the DXA scan of the lumbar spine and was compared with the corresponding parameters derived from the HR-pQCT measurements at radius and tibia.

Results: Seventy-two healthy women were included (average age 33.8 years, average BMI 23.2 kg/m^2). The areal cortical index correlated highly with the volumetric cortical index at the distal tibia (R = 0.798). The trabecular bone score correlated moderately with the microstructural parameters of the trabecular bone.

Conclusion: This study in randomly selected premenopausal women demonstrated that microstructural parameters of the bone evaluated by HR-pQCT correlated with the DXA derived parameters of skeletal regions containing predominantly cortical or cancellous bone. Whether these indexes are suitable for better predictions of the fracture risk deserves further investigation.

Editor: Dominique Heymann, Faculté de médecine de Nantes, France

Funding: This study was funded by the AO Research program. The funders had no role in study design, data collection and analysis, decision to publish, or preparation of the manuscript.

Competing Interests: The authors have declared that no competing interests exist.

* E-mail: albrecht.popp@insel.ch

Introduction

In addition to low bone mass, osteoporosis was characterized in the WHO Technical Report of 1994 [1] by the micro architectural deterioration of bone tissue. Predominantly driven by sex steroid hormone levels changing with aging, the structures of the long bones are altered by enhanced endosteal resorption and are only in part compensated by periosteal apposition [2]. This change translates into altered micro architecture of the trabecular and cortical bone in vivo as assessed by high resolution imaging techniques, such as high-resolution peripheral quantitative computed tomography (HR-pQCT) [3]. For the cortex, trabecularization of the cortical bone with aging has been suggested [4]. Accordingly, ex-vivo micrographs of the femoral cortex demonstrated increasing porosity and thinning of the cortex by coalescence of the intracortical pores [5].

Different studies have demonstrated the direct relationship between the mechanical properties of specific anatomical regions and their architecture ex vivo [6,7] and in silico [8–10]. Even if the differences in the areal bone mineral density (aBMD) measurements by dual-energy X-ray absorptiometry (DXA) at the standardized sites were inexistent or mild, these structural parameters could distinguish between individuals with or without prevalent low velocity fractures [11,12]. The standard regions of interest (ROI) used in the clinically applied HR-pQCT measurements at the distal radius and tibia were formerly focused on the trabecular bone [13], but meanwhile the quantification of the cortical bone derived indices, including the cortical porosity (Ct.Po) based on automated segmentation from HR-pQCT images, has been implemented [14].

A low aBMD is predictive of the individual fracture risk in postmenopausal women when measured at the hip, lumbar spine, or radius [15,16]. The best predictive ability was observed when the measurements were performed at the same skeletal sites that sustained a fracture later. Whereas the tibial epiphysis (T-EPI) consists predominantly of trabecular bone, the tibial diaphysis (T-DIA) is predominantly composed of cortical bone. The authors previously showed that, in a cohort of randomly selected postmenopausal women, aBMD measured by DXA at both tibial subregions was predictive for non-vertebral fracture risk [17]. T-scores were generally higher at the T-DIA than at the T-EPI suggesting that the T-DIA might be suitable for identifying other contributors of an individual's fracture risk, including parameters related to the shape and size.

Because of the growing share of cortex from distal to proximal the ratio of trabecular and cortical bone is highly variable at the tibial metaphysis [18]. A more proximal region of interest with thicker and more homogeneous cortices, such as the T-DIA, has a simple geometric structure, similar to a hollow cylinder. The combination of the aBMD at the T-DIA and the structural parameters derived from DXA scans and confirmed by HR-pQCT can improve the prediction of local bone strength ex vivo [19]. It is unknown whether this combination of material and structural competence can be confirmed by both of the techniques in a standardized procedure in vivo.

The trabecular bone score (TBS) is a DXA-derived parameter that focuses on the cancellous architecture. This score quantifies the gray-level texture out of the DXA scan of the lumbar spine [20]. TBS was shown not to correlate or to correlate weakly with the aBMD in postmenopausal women ranging from 0.2 to 0.58 [21–23]. In epidemiological studies, TBS was significantly lower in the women with incidental fractures compared to the controls [24]. Even improvements in the TBS could be observed in postmenopausal women under antiresorptive treatment in a randomized controlled trial [22]. While the correlation of this texture parameter to the parameters of microarchitecture, e.g., the degree of connectivity, the trabecular number and separation, was performed ex vivo by micro-computed tomography [25], little is known if these correlations can be confirmed by the HR-pQCT measurement of these parameters at the appendicular skeleton in vivo.

The aim of this study was to evaluate whether and to what extent the DXA-derived cortical and trabecular structural parameters correlate with the bone microstructural parameters assessed using HR-pQCT in premenopausal women.

Materials and Methods

Study participants

In December 2012, study invitations were mailed to a total of 485 women selected from commercially available address listings categorized by sex, age, and the region of Davos, Switzerland. Mobile, non-institutionalized, not pregnant (confirmed by a negative pregnancy test) randomly selected women between 20–40 years old were eligible. The exclusion criteria were a known bone disease or immobilization (relative or absolute immobilization was defined as unable to stand or walk at least one hour per day). In total, 72 women were included in this study, sixty-nine of these women were white. The left upper and lower extremities were examined or the nonfractured contralateral extremity in cases of prior fracture on the left side (Fig. 1). All of the measurements occurred at the AO Research Institute Davos, Switzerland.

Ethical Statement

The study was approved by the local ethics committee for medical sciences (Ethics Committee of the Canton of Zurich, Switzerland, registration number 2012-0464). All of the participants provided prior written informed consent and were monetarily compensated for their efforts.

DXA Measurements

DXA densitometer measurements (Hologic Discovery C^{TM}, Hologic, Bedford, MA, USA) were performed with a mobile device provided by the Department of Osteoporosis, University Hospital Berne, Switzerland. aBMD was measured at the lumbar spine (L1-4; LS), the femoral neck (FN) and total hip (TH), the distal radius (Rad 1/3), and at the two customized subregions of the distal tibia (T-EPI, T-DIA). The detailed standardized procedures for the tibial BMD measurements by DXA were previously published [26]. The ROI is defined as the 120 mm height and 129 mm width area that starts 10 mm above the top of the ankle joint space. T-EPI corresponds to the distal 40 mm of the ROI, and T-DIA corresponds to the proximal 40 mm of the ROI (Fig. 2). aBMD is expressed in grams of hydroxyapatite (HA) per square centimeter of the projected area. The obtained aBMD values of the femoral neck were expressed as the standard deviation (SD) of the mean value of the young healthy population (T-scores) derived from the National Health and Nutrition Examination Survey in the United States of America (NHANES III) [27]. The scans were performed according to the manufacturer's guidelines, and the analyses were conducted according to the recommendations of the International Society of Clinical Densitometry. Spine phantom scanning was routinely performed on a daily basis for quality control. A least significant change at the 95% confidence level of 0.020 g/cm^2 for the aBMD at the total hip was achieved as the reproducibility index for the technician involved.

DXA-Derived Parameters of Cortical and Trabecular Bone

Assuming a hollow cylindrical shape of the T-DIA, the DXA-derived cortical thickness (Ct.Th) was calculated using the DICOM images of the DXA scan at the distal tibia. DXA grayscale images were imported into Matlab^{TM} programming environment (MATLAB^{TM}, MathWorks Inc., Natick, MA, USA). The region of interest was automatically extracted for all data sets. Image data was segmented using an edge detection filter based on the algorithm proposed by Canny [28]. Canny threshold was kept constant at 0.05 resulting in a binary image showing the inner and outer borders of the cortex. A Butterworth filter was applied for smoothing the edges (Fig. 3). Cortex diameter (DIA) was defined as mean pixel distance between the outermost edges. Ct.Th was calculated as mean distance between outer and inner edges of the medial cortex projection, because the individual variation of Ct.Th is wider at the medial cortex than at the lateral cortex, i.e., the cortex closer to the fibula (own observation, unpublished data). Values were transformed to millimeter by isometric scaling (2.0 pixels/mm). Estimating the bony cross section as ideal tube the polar moment of inertia (pMOI) was computed according to formula I.

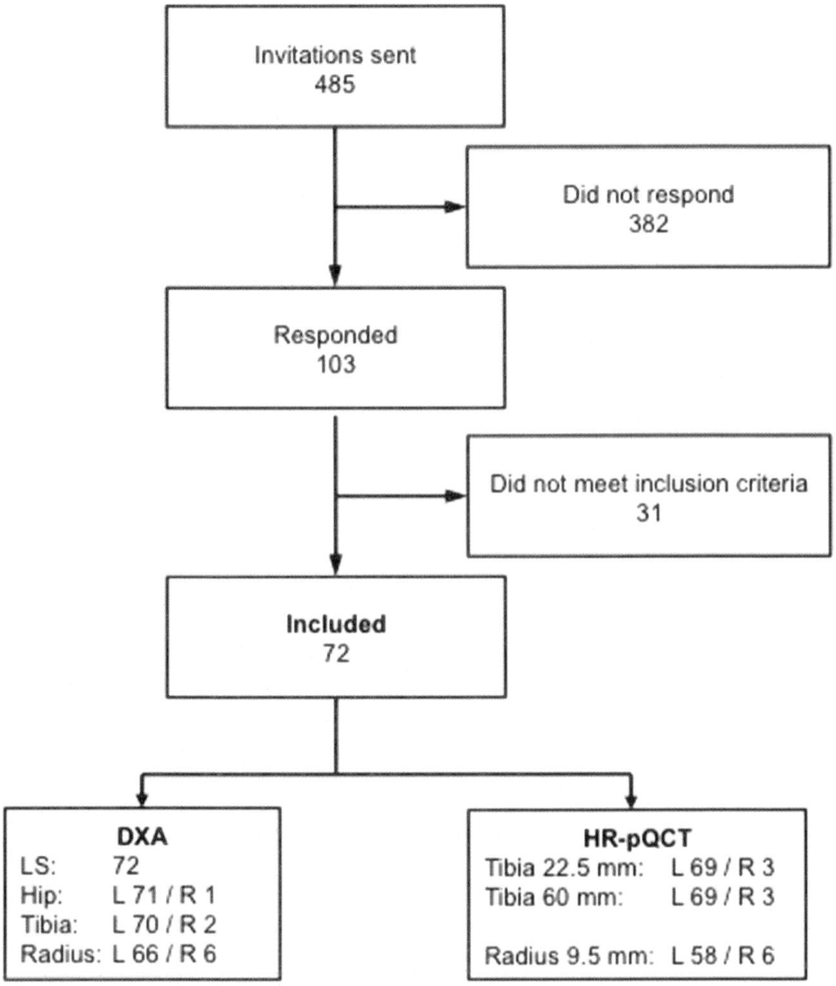

Figure 1. Consort flow diagram.

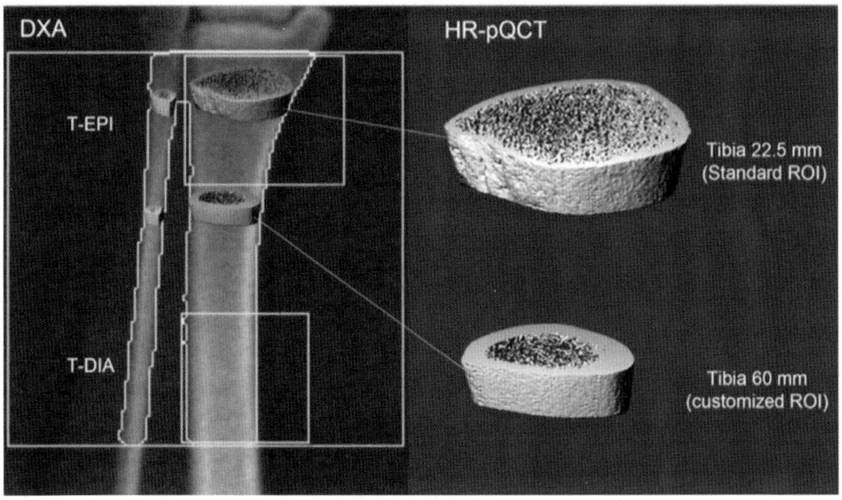

Figure 2. Regions of interest at the left distal tibia by DXA (left) and the volumes of interest as 3D reconstructions by HR-pQCT (right).

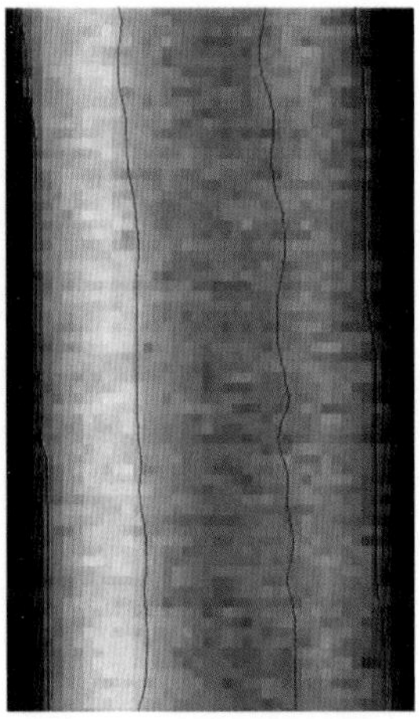

Figure 3. ROI of a representative DXA data set of the tibial diaphysis. The cortex edges as derived from image filtering are depicted as blue (outer diameter) and red lines (intramedullary channel).

$$pMOI = \frac{\pi}{4}\left[\left(\frac{DIA}{2}\right)^4 - \left(\frac{DIA}{2} - Ct.Th\right)^4\right] \quad (I)$$

A new parameter was introduced as cortical index for diaphyseal bone strength (CI), defined as product of a material (aBMD) and a structural component (pMOI). Because this CI is calculated from the two-dimensional DXA data, it is called the areal CI (aCI) in formula II.

$$aCI = aBMD * pMOI \quad (II)$$

TBS was evaluated in the identical ROI as those used for the LS BMD. The dimensionless TBS values were calculated as the mean of the individual measurements for vertebrae L1-L4 from the DXA using TBS iNsight® Software (version 1.8.2; Med-Imaps, Bordeaux, France).

HR-pQCT Measurements

HR-pQCT (XtremeCT, Scanco Medical AG, Brüttisellen, Switzerland) measurements were performed by immobilizing the left forearm and the left distal tibia in a carbon fiber shell and scanning as previously described [29–31]. In addition to the standard ROI at the radius (radius 9.5 mm) and at the tibia (tibia 22.5 mm), a third customized ROI was scanned starting at the distal tibia 60 mm above the endplate (tibia 60 mm) to increase the amount of cortex measured (Fig. 2). A stack of 110 parallel CT slices was acquired at the distal starting points of all of the sites in the proximal direction using 60 kVp and a 126 mm field of view reconstructed across an image matrix size of 1536×1536, with a voxel size of 82 μm. These provided a 3D image of 9.02 mm in the axial direction. The attenuation data were converted to the equivalent hydroxyapatite (HA) densities. The manufacturer's phantom was scanned daily for quality control.

The bone morphological parameters were evaluated using the standard protocols provided by the manufacturer. The parameters of interest were the total volumetric bone mineral density (vBMD), the bone volume fraction (BV/TV), the trabecular bone density (Tb. BMD), the trabecular thickness (Tb.Th), the trabecular number (Tb.N), the trabecular separation (Tb.Sp), the inhomogeneity of the trabecular network, defined as Tb.1/N.SD, and connectivity density of the trabecular network (Conn.D), the cortical bone density (Ct.BMD) and the cortical thickness (Ct.Th). The cortical porosity (Ct.Po) and the polar moment of inertia (pMOI), as a structural index of resistance to torsion, were calculated using an automated image processing chain [14,32]. As an analogue to the calculation from DXA, the vBMD at both ROI of the tibia multiplied by the pMOI leads to the volumetric cortical index (vCI) as a potential parameter of cortical strength. Scans with severe movement artifacts, such as a blurry trabecular area or skewed or discontinued cortical faces, were excluded. Based on the categories (1 = best, 5 = worst), seven forearm scans of grade 3 and higher were excluded [33]. Additionally, a single forearm measurement by HR-pQCT was lost for technical reasons.

Table 1. Baseline characteristics.

n = 72	mean	SD
Age (years)	33.8	5.5
Height (cm)	167.6	6.2
Weight (kg)	65.2	12.1
BMI (kg/m2)	23.2	4.1
Calcium intake (mg per day)	816.0	402
	n	%
Nulliparas	42	58.3
Smoker total	19	26.4
former	10	13.9
current	9	12.5
Family history for osteoporosis	22	30.6
BMI $<$ 18.5 kg/m^2	3	4.2
Ever glucocorticoid use	6	8.3

Table 2. Areal BMD and the structural derivates by DXA.

DXA		mean	SD
aBMD			
FN	g/cm^2	0.853	0.119
TH	g/cm^2	0.952	0.116
LS	g/cm^2	1.039	0.138
Rad 1/3	g/cm^2	0.712	0.046
T-DIA	g/cm^2	1.362	0.108
T-EPI	g/cm^2	0.750	0.096
Structural derivates			
Ct.Th (T-DIA)	mm	3.8	0.58
pMOI (T-DIA)	mm^4	1.9298	0.64
aCI	g*cm^2	2.62	0.856
TBS	-	1.399	0.087

Table 3. Volumetric BMD and the structural parameters by HR-pQCT.

HR-pQCT		radius 9.5 mm		tibia 22.5 mm		tibia 60 mm	
	Unit	*mean*	*SD*	*mean*	*SD*	*mean*	*SD*
total vBMD	mgHA/cm^3	307.6	53.3	303.2	50.1	550.3	79.3
BV/TV	%	13.7	2.8	14.1	2.9	7.6	2.6
Cortical parameters							
Ct.BMD	mgHA/cm^3	846.2	44.7	874.8	33.2	997.9	20.9
Ct.Th	mm	0.760	0.151	1.229	0.221	2.521	0.267
pMOI	mm^4	7694	2228	41104	11140	20031	4967
Ct.Po	%	2.8	1.0	4.3	1.2	1.2	0.5
vCI	gHA*cm	0.234	0.072	1.231	0.352	1.079	0.222
Trabecular parameters							
Tb.BMD	mgHA/cm^3	164.4	34.2	169.7	34.5	91.2	31.2
Tb.N	1/mm	1.944	0.246	1.912	0.312	1.476	0.424
Tb.Th	mm	0.070	0.009	0.074	0.011	0.052	0.011
Tb.Sp	mm	0.453	0.073	0.464	0.094	0.690	0.247
Inhomogeneity	mm	0.187	0.038	0.209	0.053	0.373	0.177
Conn.D	mm^{-3}	3.300	0.816	3.39	1.01	1.020	0.570

Statistical Analysis

The analyses were conducted with PASW statistical software (version 21.0; SPSS™, Chicago, IL). The two-sided p values <0.05 were considered to indicate statistical significance. The descriptive data were presented as the mean $\pm$ standard deviation (SD). After checking the variables of interest for normality (Kolmogorov-Smirnov test), the correlations between the structural parameters were expressed as R Pearson's coefficient. To compare correlations, Fisher's transformation was applied.

Results

Baseline Characteristics

Seventy-two healthy premenopausal women were included in the study. The anthropometric baseline characteristics are shown

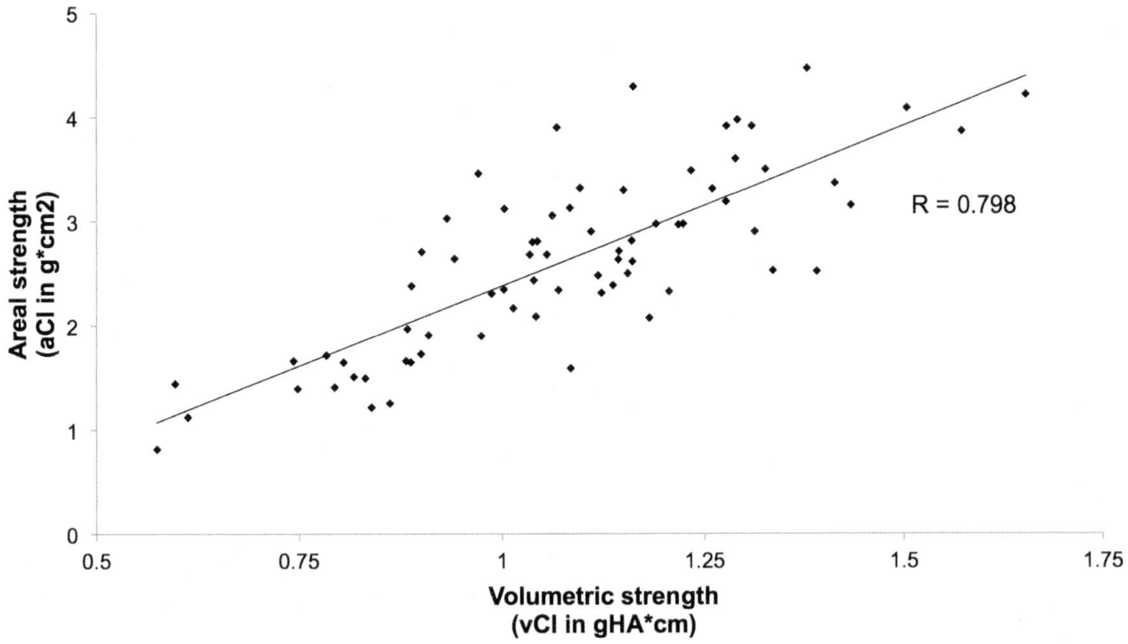

Figure 4. Correlation between the aCI (DXA) and the vCI (HR-pQCT) at the distal tibia.

Table 4. Correlations between the parameters derived from DXA and HR-pQCT.

HR-pQCT radius tibia 22.5 mm tibia 60 mm	DXA aBMD FN	aBMD TH	aBMD LS	aBMD Rad 1/3	aBMD T-DIA	aBMD T-EPI	Ct.Th T-DIA	pMOI T-DIA	aCI T-DIA	TBS
total vBMD	**0.501 0.532** *0.295*	**0.586 0.603 0.307**	**0.334** *0.275* 0.020	**0.521 0.496 0.429**	**0.459 0.570 0.601**	**0.564 0.748 0.467**	*0.259* **0.586 0.566**	**−0.440 −0.333 −0.600**	*−0.337* −0.177 **−0.433**	0.242 *0.254* 0.029
BV/TV	**0.544 0.659 0.594**	**0.707 0.736 0.644**	**0.608 0.631 0.680**	**0.363 0.407** 0.227	**0.457 0.558 0.442**	**0.736 0.889 0.664**	**0.374 0.521** *0.247*	−0.117 0.075 0.169	0.015 0.220 *0.290*	**0.494 0.508 0.572**
Ct.BMD	*0.300* 0.196 −0.101	*0.288* 0.210 −0.113	0.045 −0.117 *−0.293*	**0.465 0.377** *0.257*	0.241 0.183 0.073	0.209 0.184 −0.068	0.065 0.119 −0.007	**−0.492 −0.436 −0.525**	**−0.417 −0.370 −0.494**	0.008 −0.017 *−0.295*
Ct.Th	**0.441 0.399 0.382**	**0.506 0.492 0.440**	*0.288* 0.163 0.186	**0.525 0.446 0.471**	**0.422 0.542 0.791**	**0.506 0.650 0.665**	0.230 **0.612 0.755**	**−0.326** *−0.285* *−0.242*	−0.212 −0.134 −0.029	0.154 0.185 0.167
pMOI	0.115 0.205 0.149	*0.295* **0.302** *0.234*	**0.479 0.514 0.412**	−0.003 −0.030 −0.063	0.135 0.118 0.073	**0.448 0.368 0.466**	0.245 0.105 −0.002	**0.704 0.829 0.892**	**0.748 0.821 0.897**	*0.276* **0.351 0.315**
vCI	**0.411 0.542 0.452**	**0.640 0.680 0.564**	**0.684 0.708 0.588**	**0.324** *0.284* *0.267*	**0.408 0.477 0.585**	**0.764 0.820 0.714**	**0.384 0.461 0.450**	**0.417 0.599 0.645**	**0.542 0.729 0.798**	**0.408 0.512 0.447**
Ct.Po	0.016 0.135 0.271	0.109 0.200 0.259	0.289 **0.415** *0.298*	−0.166 −0.122 −0.024	0.128 0.208 *0.301*	0.236 **0.308** *0.300*	0.110 *0.252* **0.308**	0.171 **0.338** 0.131	0.196 **0.392** 0.208	0.227 0.155 *0.247*
Tb.BMD	**0.544 0.659 0.593**	**0.707 0.735 0.643**	**0.608 0.630 0.681**	**0.363 0.408** 0.227	**0.458 0.559 0.442**	**0.737 0.889 0.665**	**0.373 0.522** *0.248*	−0.118 0.073 0.167	0.014 0.221 *0.288*	**0.493 0.508 0.570**
Tb.N	**0.467 0.525 0.604**	**0.532 0.565 0.611**	**0.517 0.645 0.565**	*0.307 0.268* *0.274*	**0.400 0.420 0.552**	**0.589 0.627 0.636**	0.230 *0.260* **0.321**	−0.058 *0.253* 0.189	0.056 **0.358 0.330**	**0.432 0.527 0.497**
Tb.Th	**0.432 0.353** 0.115	**0.624 0.411** 0.167	**0.455** 0.136 *0.287*	*0.296 0.280* −0.082	**0.363** *0.293* −0.098	**0.608 0.533** 0.167	**0.389 0.437** −0.035	−0.152 −0.195 −0.002	−0.046 −0.011 −0.015	**0.373** 0.109 0.188
Tb.Sp	**−0.452 −0.517 −0.546**	**−0.551 −0.570 −0.582**	**−0.528 −0.672 −0.592**	**−0.322** *−0.280* *−0.301*	**−0.415 −0.422 −0.526**	**−0.614 −0.656 −0.610**	*−0.272 −0.287* *−0.295*	0.079 *−0.257* −0.208	−−0.040 **−0.360 −0.337**	**−0.428 −0.572 −0.570**
Inhomogeneity	**−0.475 −0.482 −0.571**	**−0.531 −0.503 −0.584**	**−0.487 −0.634 −0.536**	*−0.306 −0.233* **−0.355**	*−0.394 −0.322* **−0.550**	**−0.547 −0.563 −0.595**	−0.222 −0.183 **−0.306**	0.071 *−0.264* −0.100	−0.043 **−0.344** *−0.243*	**−0.408 −0.498 −0.510**
Conn.D	**0.425 0.432 0.466**	**0.496 0.464 0.473**	**0.499 0.596 0.575**	0.188 0.142 0.092	**0.377 0.346** *0.279*	**0.558 0.497 0.449**	0.228 0.155 0.040	0.061 **0.310 0.376**	0.172 **0.397 0.450**	**0.416 0.461 0.428**

$p<0.05$ (italic); **p<0.01 (bold).**

in Table 1. The mean age was 33.8 years; the mean height and BMI were 167.6 cm and 23.2 kg/m^2, respectively. Forty-two women were nulliparas, and 9 of 72 women were current smokers. The mean calcium intake was 816 mg per day. Thirty-eight females had prevalent fractures, mainly in the forearms (18), phalanges (14) and ankle (6). Twenty-two women or 30.6 % reported a potentially positive family history for osteoporosis, i.e. any self-reported major osteoporotic fracture (clinical spine, forearm, hip or shoulder fracture) among first-/second-grade relatives. As shown in Table 2, the femoral neck BMD was 0.853 g/cm^2, corresponding to a mean NHANES T-score of 0.04 ($\pm$1.08) SD. All of the areal and volumetric density parameters at all of the ROI were normally distributed (Tables 2 and 3). While the magnitude of extent of the vBMD was similar at the standard ROI of the radius 9.5 mm and the tibia 22.5 mm, the one at the tibia 60 mm was higher because of the higher portion of the cortical compartment. The Ct.Po was lower at the tibia 60 mm compared to the tibia 22.5 mm (1.2$\pm$0.5 % vs. 4.3$\pm$1.2 %).

Correlation Analysis Between the Cortical Parameters

For the cortex at the distal tibia, a significant correlation ($R = 0.74$, $p<0.01$, Table 4) was found between the CI measured at the tibia 22.5 mm by DXA and HR-pQCT, indicating that the bone strengths assessed by both techniques were predictive of each other. The correlation coefficient was even higher at the tibia 60 mm (Fig. 4), where the portion of cortical bone is more substantial, but without reaching statistical significance ($p = 0.3$).

Correlation Analysis Between the DXA-derived and HR-pQCT Parameters of the Trabecular Bone

The TBS of L1-4 correlated significantly ($p<0.01$) with the following parameters at the radius 9.5 mm and the tibia 22.5 mm: positively with the Tb.BMD, BV/TV, Tb.N, Conn.D, and negatively with the TbSp, inhomogeneity (Table 4). Correlations between the TBS and the Tb.Th, the total vBMD, the Ct.BMD, the Ct.Th or the Ct.Po were absent or inconsistent between the different skeletal sites. Among these healthy women, the TBS correlated with the aBMD at the lumbar spine and femoral neck ($R = 0.660$ and 0.532).

Discussion

The CI and TBS represent DXA derived parameters of the cortical and cancellous bone. This study showed for the first time that the corresponding structural parameters of the bone evaluated by HR-pQCT correlate with these DXA derived parameters in a cohort of randomly selected premenopausal women. In clinical practice, the aBMD is the only bone-specific parameter currently used to assess the fracture risk. By integrating the cortical and cancellous bone of a defined skeletal area, DXA scans provide bone mass of the projected area as expressed as the aBMD. If specific skeletal sites revealed a substantial amount of cortical or cancellous bone, these structural parameters could be quantified. The distal tibial diaphysis offers simple geometry similar to a hollow cylinder and a high percentage of cortical bone. Ex vivo material and structural characteristics of the bone at the T-DIA were previously shown to be predictive of the bone strength assessed by biomechanical testing [19]. As shown in the present study, the determination of the pMOI on a DXA scan of the tibia allowed for calculation of the CI by integrating the potential bone material (BMD) and the mechanical properties (pMOI). This index correlated highly with the index obtained by applying HR-pQCT. The correlation between those cortical parameters is stepwise, increasing from the radius 9 mm to the tibia 22.5 mm to the tibia 60 mm, which may reflect that a higher cortex portion better predicts its quantity, even if it is enhanced by considering two subregions of the same tibia. Interestingly, the cortical porosity at the distal tibia decreases the more proximal it is measured, which might reflect less transition from trabecular to cortical bone in the tibial diaphysis. Further studies are needed to confirm if this standardized quantification of the cortex in individuals at risk is predictive for the incidences of fractures.

By focusing on the cancellous bone contained in the lumbar spine, this ROI is predestinated for the assessment of the trabecular structure. TBS is a texture parameter that evaluates the pixel gray-level variations in DXA images of the lumbar spine. Ex vivo, these variations reflect the altered micro architecture of the trabecular bone such as the Conn.D, Tb.Sp or Tb.N assessed by high-resolution micro computed tomography [20,25]. In our cohort of healthy young women, the TBS correlated highly with these parameters of the microstructures, although the resolution of HR-pQCT is lower compared to that used ex vivo. Similar correlations were described recently in a pooled cohort of pre- and postmenopausal Chinese American and white women with exception that the strongest association has been found between TBS and vBMD [34]. In postmenopausal women with osteoporosis, the TBS did not correlate or correlated weakly with the aBMD of the lumbar spine [22]. In contrast to that, R was highly significant between aBMD at the LS and TBS in this study in healthy controls indicating that normal bone mass and not altered, homogeneous texture correlate highly with each other.

This study has some limitations. All of the measurements were performed in healthy premenopausal women and will not necessarily translate into findings of other cohorts, e.g., postmenopausal women or men. The sample might be selective (e.g., the subjects were from rural mountain areas; the regional calcium rich dietary habits of the subjects may have had an effect). For both of the bone structures, only one skeletal region was considered, and the findings may differ when applying a similar methodology to other sites of the skeleton. Whether the CI reflects more than regional bone strength is speculative. The strengths of the study included the number of randomly selected healthy women and the consistency of the study results of the hip aBMD to the data obtained by the NHANES III, which demonstrates the balance of the sample.

In this cohort of randomly selected healthy women, microstructural parameters of bone assessed by the 3D technique were predictable through information deducted from regular 2D DXA scans. This approach may add information to improve the prediction of individual fracture risks in a clinical setting.

Author Contributions

Conceived and designed the experiments: AP MW. Performed the experiments: HB VS UE ME AP. Analyzed the data: HB UE ME MW VS AP. Contributed reagents/materials/analysis tools: RGR MW VS KL. Wrote the paper: AP MW HB. Revised the manuscript content: MW RGR VS KL AP. Takes responsibility for the integrity of the data analysis: MW AP.

References

1. WHO Study Group - no authors listed (1994) Assessment of fracture risk and its application to screening for postmenopausal osteoporosis. Report of a WHO Study Group. World Health Organ Tech Rep Ser 843: 1–129.

2. Seeman E (2003) Invited Review: Pathogenesis of osteoporosis. J Appl Physiol 95: 2142–2151.

3. Khosla S, Riggs BL, Atkinson EJ, Oberg AL, McDaniel LJ, et al. (2006) Effects of sex and age on bone microstructure at the ultradistal radius: a population-based noninvasive in vivo assessment. J Bone Miner Res 21: 124–131.
4. Seeman E, Delmas PD (2006) Bone quality—the material and structural basis of bone strength and fragility. N Engl J Med 354: 2250–2261.
5. Zebaze RM, Ghasem-Zadeh A, Bohte A, Iuliano-Burns S, Mirams M, et al. (2010) Intracortical remodelling and porosity in the distal radius and post-mortem femurs of women: a cross-sectional study. Lancet 375: 1729–1736.
6. Cordey J, Schneider M, Belendez C, Ziegler WJ, Rahn BA, et al. (1992) Effect of bone size, not density, on the stiffness of the proximal part of normal and osteoporotic human femora. J Bone Miner Res 7 Suppl 2: S437–444.
7. Holzer G, von Skrbensky G, Holzer LA, Pichl W (2009) Hip fractures and the contribution of cortical versus trabecular bone to femoral neck strength. J Bone Miner Res 24: 468–474.
8. Hernandez CJ, Gupta A, Keaveny TM (2006) A biomechanical analysis of the effects of resorption cavities on cancellous bone strength. J Bone Miner Res 21: 1248–1255.
9. Liu XS, Zhang XH, Sekhon KK, Adams MF, McMahon DJ, et al. (2010) High-resolution peripheral quantitative computed tomography can assess microstructural and mechanical properties of human distal tibial bone. J Bone Miner Res 25: 746–756.
10. Nishiyama KK, Macdonald HM, Hanley DA, Boyd SK (2012) Women with previous fragility fractures can be classified based on bone microarchitecture and finite element analysis measured with HR-pQCT. Osteoporos Int.
11. Stein EM, Liu XS, Nickolas TL, Cohen A, Thomas V, et al. (2010) Abnormal microarchitecture and reduced stiffness at the radius and tibia in postmenopausal women with fractures. J Bone Miner Res 25: 2572–2581.
12. Vico L, Zouch M, Amirouche A, Frere D, Laroche N, et al. (2008) High-resolution pQCT analysis at the distal radius and tibia discriminates patients with recent wrist and femoral neck fractures. J Bone Miner Res 23: 1741–1750.
13. Laib A, Ruegsegger P (1999) Calibration of trabecular bone structure measurements of in vivo three-dimensional peripheral quantitative computed tomography with 28-microm-resolution microcomputed tomography. Bone 24: 35–39.
14. Burghardt AJ, Buie HR, Laib A, Majumdar S, Boyd SK (2010) Reproducibility of direct quantitative measures of cortical bone microarchitecture of the distal radius and tibia by HR-pQCT. Bone 47: 519–528.
15. Black DM, Cummings SR, Genant HK, Nevitt MC, Palermo L, et al. (1992) Axial and appendicular bone density predict fractures in older women. J Bone Miner Res 7: 633–638.
16. Marshall D, Johnell O, Wedel H (1996) Meta-analysis of how well measures of bone mineral density predict occurrence of osteoporotic fractures. BMJ 312: 1254–1259.
17. Popp AW, Senn C, Franta O, Krieg MA, Perrelet R, et al. (2009) Tibial or hip BMD predict clinical fracture risk equally well: results from a prospective study in 700 elderly Swiss women. Osteoporos Int 20: 1393–1399.
18. Sode M, Burghardt AJ, Kazakia GJ, Link TM, Majumdar S (2010) Regional variations of gender-specific and age-related differences in trabecular bone structure of the distal radius and tibia. Bone 46: 1652–1660.
19. Popp AW, Windolf M, Senn C, Tami A, Richards RG, et al. (2012) Prediction of bone strength at the distal tibia by HR-pQCT and DXA. Bone 50: 296–300.
20. Pothuaud L, Carceller P, Hans D (2008) Correlations between grey-level variations in 2D projection images (TBS) and 3D microarchitecture: applications in the study of human trabecular bone microarchitecture. Bone 42: 775–787.
21. Hans D, Goertzen AL, Krieg MA, Leslie WD (2011) Bone microarchitecture assessed by TBS predicts osteoporotic fractures independent of bone density: the Manitoba study. J Bone Miner Res 26: 2762–2769.
22. Popp AW, Guler S, Lamy O, Senn C, Buffat H, et al. (2013) Effects of zoledronate versus placebo on spine bone mineral density and microarchitecture assessed by the trabecular bone score in postmenopausal women with osteoporosis: A three-year study. J Bone Miner Res 28: 449–454.
23. Silva BC, Boutroy S, Zhang C, McMahon DJ, Zhou B, et al. (2013) Trabecular bone score (TBS)--a novel method to evaluate bone microarchitectural texture in patients with primary hyperparathyroidism. J Clin Endocrinol Metab 98: 1963–1970.
24. Boutroy S, Hans D, Sornay-Rendu E, Vilayphiou N, Winzenrieth R, et al. (2012) Trabecular bone score improves fracture risk prediction in non-osteoporotic women: the OFELY study. Osteoporos Int.
25. Hans D, Barthe N, Boutroy S, Pothuaud L, Winzenrieth R, et al. (2011) Correlations between trabecular bone score, measured using anteroposterior dual-energy X-ray absorptiometry acquisition, and 3-dimensional parameters of bone microarchitecture: an experimental study on human cadaver vertebrae. J Clin Densitom 14: 302–312.
26. Casez JP, Troendle A, Lippuner K, Jaeger P (1994) Bone mineral density at distal tibia using dual-energy X-ray absorptiometry in normal women and in patients with vertebral osteoporosis or primary hyperparathyroidism. J Bone Miner Res 9: 1851–1857.
27. Looker AC, Wahner HW, Dunn WL, Calvo MS, Harris TB, et al. (1998) Updated data on proximal femur bone mineral levels of US adults. Osteoporos Int 8: 468–489.
28. Canny J (1986) A computational approach to edge detection. IEEE Trans Pattern Anal Mach Intell 8: 679–698.
29. Boutroy S, Bouxsein ML, Munoz F, Delmas PD (2005) In vivo assessment of trabecular bone microarchitecture by high-resolution peripheral quantitative computed tomography. J Clin Endocrinol Metab 90: 6508–6515.
30. Cohen A, Liu XS, Stein EM, McMahon DJ, Rogers HF, et al. (2009) Bone microarchitecture and stiffness in premenopausal women with idiopathic osteoporosis. J Clin Endocrinol Metab 94: 4351–4360.
31. Sornay-Rendu E, Boutroy S, Munoz F, Delmas PD (2007) Alterations of cortical and trabecular architecture are associated with fractures in postmenopausal women, partially independent of decreased BMD measured by DXA: the OFELY study. J Bone Miner Res 22: 425–433.
32. Nishiyama KK, Macdonald HM, Buie HR, Hanley DA, Boyd SK (2010) Postmenopausal women with osteopenia have higher cortical porosity and thinner cortices at the distal radius and tibia than women with normal aBMD: an in vivo HR-pQCT study. J Bone Miner Res 25: 882–890.
33. Sode M, Burghardt AJ, Pialat JB, Link TM, Majumdar S (2011) Quantitative characterization of subject motion in HR-pQCT images of the distal radius and tibia. Bone 48: 1291–1297.
34. Silva BC, Walker MD, Abraham A, Boutroy S, Zhang C, et al. (2013) Trabecular Bone Score Is Associated With Volumetric Bone Density and Microarchitecture as Assessed by Central QCT and HRpQCT in Chinese American and White Women. J Clin Densitom 16: 554–561.

15

Characteristics of Bone Turnover in the Long Bone Metaphysis Fractured Patients with Normal or Low Bone Mineral Density (BMD)

Christoph Wölfl[1], Daniela Schweppenhäuser[1], Thorsten Gühring[1], Caner Takur[1], Bernd Höner[2], Ulrich Kneser[3], Paul Alfred Grützner[1], Leila Kolios[3]*

1 Department for Traumatology and Orthopaedic Surgery, BG Traumacenter Ludwigshafen, Ludwigshafen, Germany, **2** SRH Hochschule Heidelberg, Dpt. Of Social Sciences and Law, Heidelberg, Germany, **3** Department for Plastic-, Reconstructive and Handsurgery, Burn Care Centre, Department of Plastic Surgery of Heidelberg University, BG Traumacenter Ludwigshafen, Ludwigshafen, Germany

Abstract

The incidence of osteoporotic fractures increases as our population ages. Until now, the exact biochemical processes that occur during the healing of metaphyseal fractures remain unclear. Diagnostic instruments that allow a dynamic insight into the fracture healing process are as yet unavailable. In the present matched pair analysis, we study the time course of the osteoanabolic markers bone specific alkaline phosphatase (BAP) and transforming growth factor β1 (TGFβ1), as well as the osteocatabolic markers crosslinked C-telopeptide of type-I-collagen (β-CTX) and serum band 5 tartrate-resistant acid phosphatase (TRAP5b), during the healing of fractures that have a low level of bone mineral density (BMD) compared with fractures that have a normal BMD. Between March 2007 and February 2009, 30 patients aged older than 50 years who suffered a metaphyseal fracture were included in our study. BMDs were verified by dual energy Xray absorptiometry (DXEA) scans. The levels of BTMs were examined over an 8-week period. Osteoanabolic BAP levels in those with low levels of BMD were significantly different from the BAP levels in those with normal BMD. BAP levels in the former group increased constantly, whereas the latter group showed an initial strong decrease in BAP followed by slowly rising values. Osteocatabolic β-CTX increased in the bone of the normal BMD group constantly, whereas these levels decreased significantly in the bone of the group with low BMD from the first week. TRAP5b was significantly reduced in the low level BMD group. With this work, we conduct first insights into the molecular biology of the fracture healing process in patients with low levels of BMD that explains the mechanism of its fracture healing. The results may be one reason for the reduced healing qualities in bones with low BMD.

Editor: João Costa-Rodrigues, Faculdade de Medicina Dentária, Universidade do Porto, Portugal

Funding: No external funding was used. The study was done by the cooperation partners as listed in the authors section. The funding was done by the BG Klinik Ludiwgshafen Research Center. Besides the authors no one had a role in the study design, the data collection and analysis, decision to publish, or preparation of the manuscript.

Competing Interests: The authors have declared that no competing interests exist.

* E-mail: lkolios@bgu-ludwigshafen.de

Introduction

Bone formation markers reflect the enzymatic activity of bone building cells, mostly osteoblasts, which are excess products from the bone formation process that are released during the breakdown of matrix components [1]. Serum osteocalcin (OC), bone specific alkaline phosphatase (BAP), transforming growth factor β1 (TGFβ1) and the N-terminal propeptide of type-I-collagen (Col1a1) represent the most sensitive bone formation markers. Bone resorption markers are products from the deposition of bone tissue, such as the crosslinked C-(CTX) and N-(NTX) telopeptides of type-I-collagen, or indicate the activity of bone catabolic cells, such as osteoclasts. The serum band 5 tartrate-resistant acid phosphatase (TRAP 5b) as one example is a safe and sensitive marker for detecting the high turnover typical in osteoporosis [2]. In the osteoporotic (non fractured) bone, the microarchitecture deteriorates as a result of altered bone turnover and is characterized by typical changes of these BTMs.

Typically, osteoporosis is a silent disease until the first fracture occurs. After an osteoporotic fracture, callus- and bone remodeling is required [3,4]. Bone formation and resorption rates increase to repair the bone defect, and the accelerated bone metabolism can be detected using elevated serum levels of BTMs [5–11]. The elevation in BTMs may result from increased bone remodeling activity at the fracture sites or reflect accelerated bone resorption close to the fracture [12–15]. However, until now, the exact metabolism processes at play during the healing of fractured bone that has a low level of bone mineral density has not been elucidated. Diagnostic instruments that allow a dynamic insight into the fracture healing process and that may be used in collecting decision criteria for treatment of fractures and for monitoring the healing course are as yet unavailable [16].

There are only a few studies examining the characteristics of BTM levels during the healing of osteoporotic fractures [16,17], and there is no matched pair-analysis comparing the early (up to 8 weeks after fracture) time course of BTM levels during the fracture healing of bones with a low level of bone mineral density versus normal BMD bone. In the present matched-pair study, we analyse the time course of the osteoanabolic markers BAP and TGFβ1 (transforming growth factor β1), as well as the osteocatabolic markers β-CTX and TRAP5b, during the fracture healing process of bone with a low level of bone mineral density compared with fractures of bones with normal bone mineral density.

Materials and Methods

Between March 2009 and February 2011, patients older than 50 years who suffered a metaphyseal fracture (distal radius, proximal humerus and proximal femur fracture) that required surgical stabilization and who agreed to take part in this special protocol were included in this study. All patients underwent state of the art operative treatment. Exclusion criteria were polytrauma, significant soft tissue injury, highly open fracture, >24 h mechanical ventilation after surgery, dialysis, long-term therapy with immunosuppressants, collagenosis, chronic inflammatory bowel disease, hematological disorders and malignancies.

In all patients, radiographs of the fracture region and the lumbar spine were performed with anterior-posterior and lateral views. Radiographs of the lumbar spine were used to exclude the possibility of morphological changes of the vertebrae that may lead to false values in the DEXA scans for bone density measurement. To monitor the clinical course of fracture healing, radiographs of the fracture site were obtained at 4 and 8 weeks and one year after osteosynthetic stabilization.

Out of this collective, 15 matched pairs were created according to the matching criteria presented in Table 1. Among these matched pairs were 7 pairs with fractures of the distal radius, 3 pairs with proximal humeral fractures and 5 pairs with proximal femoral fractures (including femoral neck and intertrochanteric fractures). The patients' baseline demographic data showed no significant differences (Table 2).

The study was designed as an epidemiologic case-control study. After receiving results from the DEXA measurements, patients were matched in a low bone mineral density group and a normal bone mineral density group. Further matching criteria were age (+/−5 years), sex (male, female), fracture localization (proximal humerus, distal radius, proximal femur), fracture type (according to AO-classification; A-, B- or C-type fractures) and operation method (plate, intramedular nail). Thus, we received a collective of 15 matched pairs, or 30 patients in total (Table 1), out of a total of 78 patients who met the inclusion criteria. All appropriate patients were included; there were no patients selectively included to match with previously included patients. We did not subdivide groups further because all patients were older than 50 years and represented the collective of patients at risk for osteoporosis and osteoporotic fractures.

The healing of fractures was assessed clinically and radiologically during the usual follow-up examinations that are planned at the fourth and eighth week after surgery, as well as one year later. The fracture consolidation was scored by 2 members of our departments (1 orthopedic surgeon, 1 radiologist) who did not participate in the study and who were blind to the group assignments. Fracture consolidation was scored by the Lane-Sandhu Score (Table 3). In cases where there were post-surgical complications, patients were seen more frequently in the osteoporotic fracture care center in the outpatient clinic of our department.

The bone mineral density (BMD) was examined within one week after surgery by a standardized protocol at the lumbar spine and both femoral necks except for the patients with fractures of the hip (in which case, the injured side was not examined) by DEXA (Lunar iDPX, GE Medical Systems Germany, Solingen, Germany), based on Encore TM Version II.X software. Using normative data for young adult white people, the BMD was categorized as normal or low, as defined by the World Health Organization[17]. Participants with a T-score ≤2.5 SD were categorized as having osteoporosis.

A laboratory analysis was performed the morning after injury with the patient in a fasting state. In addition to the typical routine laboratory values, the bone formation markers BAP (bone specific alkaline phosphatase) and TGFβ1 (transforming growth factor β1), as well as the osteocatabolic markers β-CTX (crosslinked C-(CTX) telopeptide of type-I-collagen) and TRAP5b (serum band 5 tartrate-resistant acid phosphatase), were examined. Quantitative measurements were obtained using the chemiluminescence immunoassay "Access Ostase assay 37300" (Beckman Coulter, Brea, USA) and the electrochemiluminescence immunoassay ECLIA (Roche, Basel, Switzerland). Laboratory tests were repeated at the first, fourth and eighth postoperative week, as well as one year postoperatively.

Statistics were performed using the software SPSS 11.0.0 (IBM Germany, Munich, Germany) and Microsoft Excel 2003/2007 (Microsoft Corp. Washington, USA). By pretrial power analysis of the first three patients, we calculated that 15 matched pairs were necessary for obtaining statistical significance. The Friedman test, the Wilcoxon signed rank test and Mann-Whitney U tests were used as post-hoc tests.

A value of $P \leq 0.05$ was considered to be significant, $p \leq 0.01$ very significant, and $p \leq 0.001$ highly significant. These different levels of significance are marked by 1 to 3 stars (*) in Figures 1–4.

The study is approved by the local Ethical Committee of the board of Medical Profession of Rhineland-Palatinate (837.368.10/7377). All participants gave their written informed consent, and the data were analyzed anonymously with matching numbers. The study was conducted according to the principles of the declaration of Helsinki.

Results

Bone Turnover Markers

The results of the laboratory analyses of BAP, TGFβ1, β-CTX and TRAP5b are presented graphically in Figures 1–4.

The levels of the bone formation marker BAP showed a remarkable difference between the two groups that could be detected at the first time point. The control group showed a higher level of BAP (16.6 μg/l) than osteoporotic patients, who had a value of 11.8 μg/l. In the first week after surgery, a decrease of BAP to 7.8 μg/l was detected in the control group, whereas the level of the low bone mineral density group differed significantly at 13.6 μg/l. Until the fourth week after surgery, the BAP levels in both groups showed a constant increase, with a maximum value of 16.1 μg/l in the low BMD group, which surpassed the maximum value of the control group significantly (9.5 μg/l). Until the eighth postoperative week, a slight decrease was observed in the control group, while the levels of BAP in the low BMD group decreased slightly.

The results of measuring the levels of TGFβ1 revealed an increase in the first week, followed by a slight decrease up to eight weeks in both groups. The measurements of TGFβ1 levels in the patients with low BMD were at all time points higher than those in the patients with a normal BMD, but without significance.

The β-CTX levels were only slightly different between both groups at the first time point (the day after the fracture occurred), with values of 0.49 μg/l in those with low BMD and 0.44 μg/l in

Table 1. Table of matched pairs.

Patient No.	Sex	Age	Fracture localization	Fracture Type	Osteosyn-thesis	Osteopo-rosis
1	female	57	Distal radius fracture	A	plate	healthy
1	female	59	Distal radius fracture	A	plate	**diseased**
2	female	62	Distal radius fracture	A	plate	healthy
2	female	61	Distal radius fracture	A	plate	**diseased**
3	female	57	Distal radius fracture	A	plate	healthy
3	female	57	Distal radius fracture	A	plate	**diseased**
4	female	63	Distal radius fracture	A	plate	healthy
4	female	67	Distal radius fracture	A	plate	**diseased**
5	female	66	Distal radius fracture	A	plate	healthy
5	female	68	Distal radius fracture	A	plate	**diseased**
6	female	65	Distal radius fracture	A	plate	healthy
6	female	64	Distal radius fracture	A	plate	**diseased**
7	female	56	Distal radius fracture	B	plate	healthy
7	female	69	Distal radius fracture	B	plate	**diseased**
8	female	60	proximal humeral fractures	A	plate	healthy
8	female	59	proximal humeral fractures	A	plate	**diseased**
9	female	68	proximal humeral fractures	C	plate	healthy
9	female	71	proximal humeral fractures	C	plate	**diseased**
10	female	74	proximal humeral fractures	C	plate	healthy
10	female	78	proximal humeral fractures	C	plate	**diseased**
11	male	72	femoral neck fractures	A	screws	healthy
11	male	75	femoral neck fractures	A	screws	**diseased**
12	male	64	femoral neck fractures	A	DHS	healthy
12	male	68	femoral neck fractures	A	DHS	**diseased**
13	female	59	Intertrochanteric fracture	B	DHS	healthy
13	female	63	Intertrochanteric fracture	B	DHS	**diseased**
14	female	66	Intertrochanteric fracture	C	IFN	healthy
14	female	70	Intertrochanteric fracture	C	IFN	**diseased**
15	male	64	Intertrochanteric fracture	B	IFN	healthy
15	male	68	Intertrochanteric fracture	B	IFN	**diseased**

Matching criteria were age (+/−5 years), sex (male, female), fracture localization (proximal humerus, distal radius, proximal femur), fracture type (according to AO-classification; A-, B- or C-type fractures) and operation method (plate, intramedular nail).

the control group. Within the control group, β-CTX levels constantly increased up to the eighth week after surgery, reaching a maximum value of 0.62 μg/l. The values of β-CTX from the control group were always higher during the healing process than the values from the low BMD group. In the control group, CTX

Table 2. Table of demographic data of the included and matched patients.

	mean		standard deviation		p-values (t-test)
parameter	**normal BMD**	**low BMD**	**normal BMD**	**low BMD**	
age	63.40	66.0	5.27	6.11	0.226
BMI (kg/m^2)	26.01	27.11	5.27	4.75	0.556
weight (kg)	73.37	76.13	18.39	12.17	0.631
height (cm)	168.87	168.53	9.21	7.31	0.913
creatinin (mg/dl)	0.7613	0.78	0.145	0.093	0.678

There were no significant differences in base line demographics. Statistics were performed using the software SPSS 11.0.0 (IBM Germany, Munich, Germany), $P \leq 0.05$ was considered to be significant.

Table 3. Fracture consolidation was scored according to the Lane-Sandhu Score by 2 independent examiners.

Points	Callus and Fracture line
0	no callus tissue, fracture line clear
1	25% callus tissue, fracture line still clearly visible
2	50% callus tissue, fracture line blurred
3	75% callus tissue, fracture line barely visible
4	100% callus tissue, no remaining fracture line visible

The score provides 5 levels of consolidation. The results are shown in Figure 5.

levels decreased initially and stayed at a level of approximately 0.3 μg/l.

The level of TRAP5b in both groups showed an initial increase until the first week after the fracture and remained steady at this level up to the eighth week. At all time points, the values of the control group surpassed those of the low BMD group, and this increase was highly significant.

Fracture Consolidation

The consolidation was scored using the Lane-Sandhu Score (Table 3). There was a mean score of 2.6 after four weeks in the control group and 3.43 after eight weeks. In the groups of patients with a low level BMD, the score after four weeks was 2.07 and after eight weeks was 2.86. At both time points, there was a significantly reduced score in the low level BMD group (Figure 5). The normal BMD level group showed better callus production, which is a sign of a better fracture healing. None of the patients developed pseudarthrosis. Twice, an endoprosthesis had to be implanted after a failure of the primary osteosynthesis.

Discussion

Because osteoporosis represents one of the increasing health problems in the world, it is important to examine the mechanisms underlying the qualitatively and quantitatively reduced healing processes [17,18] of typical metaphyseal fractures in osteoporotic bone.

Bone is remodeled by formation and resorption processes that can be studied by biochemical analyses of the enzymatic activities, degradation products and neosynthesized constituents produced during bone changes [19].

When a fracture occurs, increased resorption and formation are needed to support bone repair and fracture healing [20]. Because bone turnover is increased during fracture healing, biochemical markers of bone metabolism are useful surrogate markers for monitoring fracture healing.

Previous studies showed increased levels of markers of bone resorption in patients with vertebral or hip fractures at an early stage of fracture healing [21,22], although biochemical markers of bone formation increased at a later stage [23]. Our study showed interesting variations in the levels of the markers of bone metabolism that have not been described in the literature before.

In bone that is of normal BMD, the course of resorption markers β-CTX and TRAP5b showed a slight increase in the first weeks of the fracture healing period and remained at a stable level during the remodeling process in the 4th and up to the 8th week [18,19,23]. However, there are significant differences in the levels of bone metabolism markers in bone that is of low BMD. At nearly all time points of the fracture healing process, resorption markers β-CTX and TRAP5b are clearly and significantly reduced compared to bone markers in patients with normal BMD. This could be a result of the disturbed osteoclastic activity in the osteoporotic situation and may be a first explanation of the delayed healing process: the initially necessary bone resorption processes do not occur physiologically (Figures 1, 2).

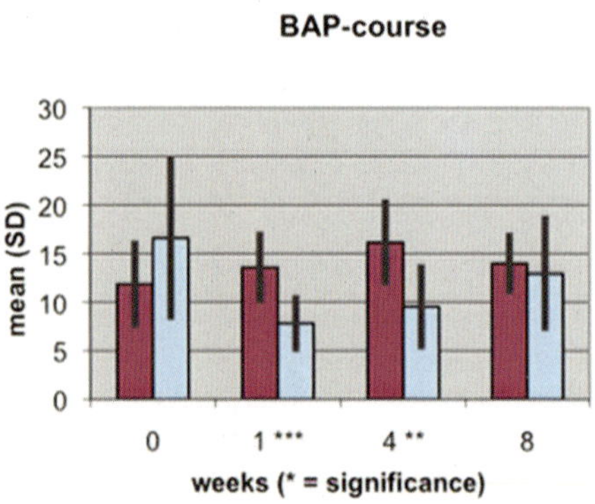

Figure 1. Course of BAP serum concentration during fracture healing of eight weeks in low BMD versus normal BMD patients. Statistics were performed using the software SPSS 11.0.0 (IBM Germany, Munich, Germany), P≤0.05 was considered to be significant, p≤0.01 as very significant, and p≤0.001 as highly significant. Different levels of significance are marked by one to three stars.

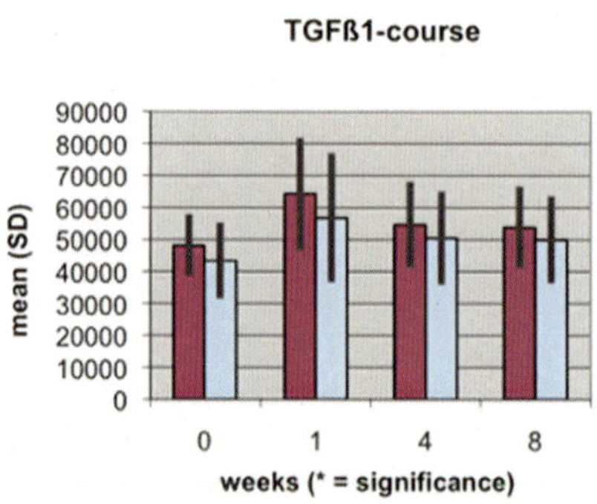

Figure 2. Course of TGFβ1 serum concentration during fracture healing of eight weeks in low BMD versus normal BMD patients. Statistics were performed using the software SPSS 11.0.0 (IBM Germany, Munich, Germany), P≤0.05 was considered to be significant, p≤0.01 as very significant, and p≤0.001 as highly significant. Different levels of significance are marked by one to three stars.

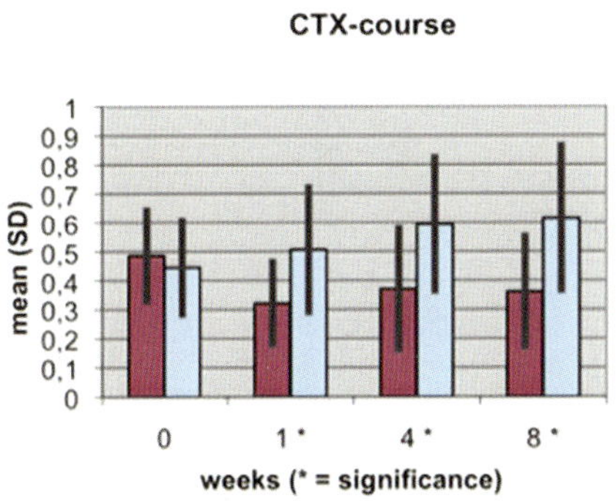

Figure 3. Course of CTX serum concentration during fracture healing of eight weeks in low BMD versus normal BMD patients. Statistics were performed using the software SPSS 11.0.0 (IBM Germany, Munich, Germany), P≤0.05 was considered to be significant, p≤0.01 as very significant, and p≤0.001 as highly significant. Different levels of significance are marked by one to three stars.

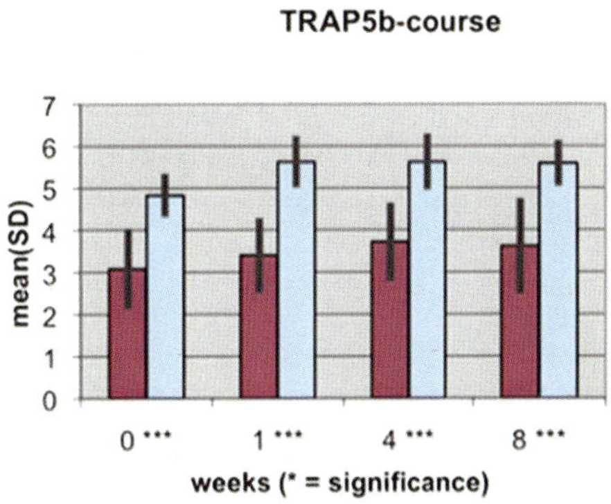

Figure 4. Course of TRAP5b serum concentration during fracture healing of eight weeks in low BMD versus normal BMD patients. Statistics were performed using the software SPSS 11.0.0 (IBM Germany, Munich, Germany), P≤0.05 was considered to be significant, p≤0.01 as very significant, and p≤0.001 as highly significant. Different levels of significance are marked by one to three stars.

β-CTX additionally has a high clinical relevance, since it shows very fast and dynamically the changes in bone transforming processes. This marker therewith could be implemented as a special monitoring option for control of therapies. TRAP 5 belongs to the most abundant enzymes in osteoclasts and therefore specific determination of TRAP 5 activity can be essential for clinical assessment of bone metabolism, especially since our results have shown a significant difference to the processes in normal BMD bone.

BAP represents one of the most sensitive markers for bone formation. In our study, the concentration of BAP during the healing process in patients with either low or normal bone density levels shows interesting results. The decrease in BAP in the first week of fracture healing in normal bone is a new finding that is not yet reported in the medical literature. One reason for the decrease in BAP may be that the initial focus of the healing organism is on resorption processes of the bony structure on the side of the fracture (Figure 4). Therefore, resorption markers β-CTX and TRAP5b increase during this first week (Figures 1, 2). BAP is located in the membranes of osteoblasts. In the first week after the fracture, the reactive phase, the amount of soft-tissue cells (endothelial cells, macrophages, granulocytes and fibroblasts) surpasses the number of osteoblasts, perhaps temporarily displacing them, which may explain our findings.

In the patients with low BMD, BAP shows a different concentration curve, with increasing levels up to the 4th week after the injury and then slight decreases until the 8th week of fracture healing. Apart from the first week, BAP levels in the group with low BMD always exceed those in the group with normal BMD, which is partly significant. This result could mean that in bone of normal BMD, there are less active osteoblasts necessary to achieve sufficient fracture healing. More BAP is needed in bone of low BMD and osteoblasts are more activated to balance the remodeling processes in osteoporotic bone (Figure 4).

The chosen second bone formation parameter was TGFβ1, which has been implicated as a regulator of enchondral ossification during skeleton formation, but also during fracture healing. TGFβ is known to be expressed during all stages of fracture repair, and endogenous TGFβ has strong effects on gene expression and differentiation of bone cells during bone repair [24,25]. Furthermore, in vivo administration of TGFβ induces rapid closure of callus formation in normal bone, and increased bone formation and strength during rat tibial fracture repair of non-osteoporotic [24,25]. Taken together, these findings illustrate that TGFβ can regulate bone formation cell function in vitro and in vivo, but the roles of endogenous TGFβ in the activities of these cell types and in bone remodeling in a situation of low BMD remained unclear so far.

When considering the evaluated levels of TGFβ1 in our study, the findings are more discrete than the BAP-results, but follow the same structure. At all time points, TGFβ1-activation in bone of patients with low BMD surpasses that of patients with normal BMD. There is a clear increase in the first week of fracture healing that slowly decreases up to the 8th week as the fracture stabilizes (Figure 4). This could be explained as a result of an increased activation of bone formation cells in the osteoporotic situation in order to balance the disturbed microarchitecture especially in the first time period.

Other than the significant differences in bone formation markers between the groups with low BMD and normal BMD, we also found differences in the fracture healing itself as measured by the Lane-Sandhu Scoring System. While the scoring system is inherently subjective, two independent examiners nevertheless rated the patients with low BMD significantly lower in fracture healing than those with normal BMD.

To achieve a more detailed image of these complex processes, further studies are necessary to examine more bone specific markers, as well as fibroblastic and angiogenetic factors. The aim is to establish decision criteria for treatment of fractures and for monitoring osteoporotic fracture healing. These studies are currently in process in our department.

Limitations

However the study design was planned carefully, the study has some limitations, which were not preventable.

Our study lacks a control group that matches the demographics of individuals without fractures. We had to accept this flaw in our study design because we rarely see patients without fractures in our trauma department.

Additionally, the number of patients included in our study does not reflect the proportion of patients who are treated with metaphyseal fractures in our department. Nearly 60% of the patients asked had no interest in taking part in the study or in

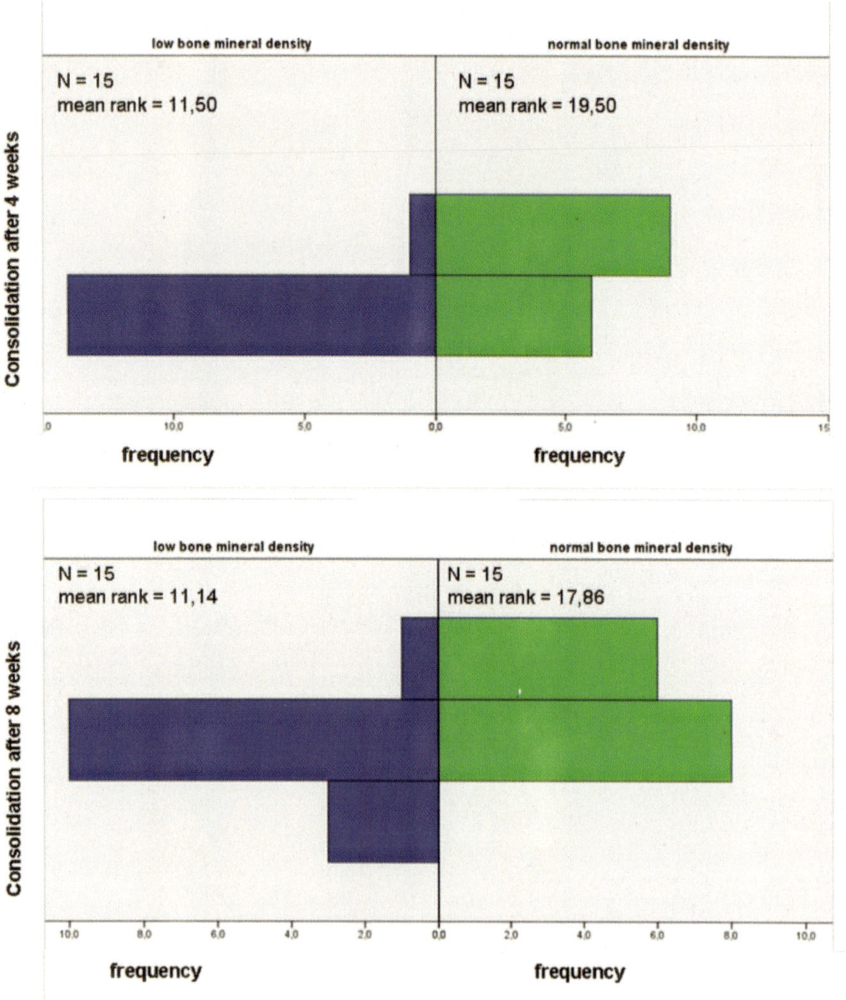

Figure 5. Consolidation of the fractures following the Lane-Shandu-scoring after 4 and 8 weeks, assessed by two independent examiners.

further diagnostics, such as DEXA measurements of bone density; by this, we had to accept the use of the matched pair analysis with the included low number of patients.

Conclusions

With this study, we give first insights to the molecular biology of fracture healing in osteoporotic bone that may explain the mechanisms of fracture healing. The conspicuously elevated osteoanabolic proteins and decreased osteocatabolic proteins during the healing period of patients with low BMD bone compared to patients with normal BMD could be a result caused by disturbed remodeling metabolism and leading to the qualitatively reduced healing process. Further studies are necessary to achieve a more detailed knowledge of fracture healing and the creation of decision criteria for fracture therapy and for monitoring fracture healing.

Supporting Information

Document S1 Exemplary profile of DEXA and laboratory measurements of one study patient.

Document S2 Positive vote of the Ethical Committee of the board of Medical Profession of Rhineland-Palatinate (837.368.10/7377).

Acknowledgments

We would like to thank Dr. Arash Moghaddam for his previous works which inspired us to let this study follow. Thanks are due to the whole team of the departments for their support in this study.

Author Contributions

Conceived and designed the experiments: CW LK. Performed the experiments: CW DS CT. Analyzed the data: CW LK BH TG PAG UK. Wrote the paper: CW LK.

References

1. Ivaska KK, Gerdhem P, Akesson K, Garnero P, Obrant KJ (2007) Effect of Fracture on Bone Turnover Markers: A Longitudinal Study Comparing Marker Levels Before and After Injury in 113 Elderly Women. JBMR 22: 1155–64.
2. Garnero P (2008) Biomarkers for osteoporosis management: utility in diagnosis, fracture risk prediction and therapy monitoring. Mol Diagn Ther 12: 157–70.
3. Garnero P, Delmas PD (2004) Contribution of bone mineral density and bone turnover markers to the estimation of risk of osteoporotic fracture in postmenopausal women. J Musculoskelet Neuronal Interact 4: 50–63.
4. Joerring S, Jensen LT, Andersen GR, Johansen JS (1992) Types I and III procollagen extension peptides in serum respond to fracture in humans. Arch Orthop Trauma Surg 111: 265–7.
5. Joerring S, Krogsgaard M, Wilbek H, Jensen LT (1994) Collagen turnover after tibial fractures. Arch Orthop Trauma Surg 113: 334–6.
6. Akesson K, Vergnaud P, Delmas PD, Obrant KJ (1995) Serum osteocalcin increases during fracture healing in elderly women with hip fracture. Bone 16: 427–30.
7. Kurdy NM, Bowles S, Marsh DR, Davies A, France M (1998) Serology of collagen types I and III in normal healing of tibial shaft fractures. J Orthop Trauma 12: 122–6.
8. Obrant KJ, Ivaska KK, Gerdhem P, Alatalo SL, Pettersson K (2005) Biochemical markers of bone turnover are influenced by recently sustained fracture. Bone 36: 786–92.
9. Ingle BM, Hay SM, Bottjer HM, Eastell R (1999) Changes in bone mass and bone turnover following distal forearm fracture. Osteoporos Int 10: 399–407.
10. Ingle BM, Hay SM, Bottjer HM, Eastell R (1999) Changes in bone mass and bone turnover following ankle fracture. Osteoporos Int 10: 408–15.
11. Veitch SW, Findlay SC, Hamer AJ, Blumsohn A, Eastell R (2006) Changes in bone mass and bone turnover following tibial shaft fracture. Osteoporos Int 17: 364–72.
12. Obrant KJ (1984) Trabecular bone changes in the greater trochanter after fracture of the femoral neck. Acta Orthop Scand 55: 78–82.
13. Nyman MT, Paavolainen P, Forsius S, Lamberg-Allardt C (1991) Clinical evaluation of fracture healing by serum osteocalcin and alkaline phosphatase. Ann Chir Gynaecol 80: 289–93.
14. Kurdy NM (2000) Serology of abnormal fracture healing: The role of PIIINP, PICP, and BsALP. J Orthop Trauma 14: 48–53.
15. Heiss C, Hoesel LM, Pausch M, Meissner SA, Horas U, et al. (2008) Biochemical bone resorption markers during the healing of osteoporotic fractures. Unfallchirurg 111: 695–702.
16. Kanis JA, Johnell O, Oden A, Dawson A, De Laet C, et al. (2001) Ten year probabilities of osteoporotic fractures according to BMD and diagnostic thresholds. Osteoporos Int 12: 989–95.
17. Lill CA, Gerlach UV, Eckhardt C, Goldhahn J, Schneider E (2002) Bone changes due to glucocorticoid application in an ovariectomized animal model for fracture treatment in osteoporosis. Osteoporos Int 13: 407–14.
18. Mallmin H, Ljunghall S, Larsson K (1993) Biochemical Markers of Bone Metabolism in Patients With Fracture of the Distal Forearm. Clin Orthop Rel Res 295: 259–63.
19. Hoesel LM, Wehr U, Rambeck A, Schnettler R, Heiss C (2005) Biochemical Bone Markers Are Useful to Monitor Fracture Repair. Clin Orthop Rel Res 440: 226–32.
20. Hoshino H, Takahashi M, Kushida K, Ohishi T, Inoue T (1998) Urinary excretion of type I collagen degradation products in healthy women and osteoporotic patients with vertebral and hip fractures. Calcif Tissue Int 62: 36–9.
21. Sato Y, Kaji M, Higuchi F (2001) Changes in bone and calcium metabolism following hip fracture in elderly patients. Osteoporos Int 12: 445–9.
22. Emami A, Larsson A, Petren-Mallmin M, Larsson S (1999) Serum bone markers after intramedullary fixed tibial fractures. Clin Orthop Relat Res 368: 220–9.
23. Ohishi T, Takahashi M, Kushida K (1998) Changes of biochemical markers during fracture healing. Arch Orthop Trauma Surg 118: 126–30.
24. Bostrom MPG, Asnis P (1998) Transforming growth factor in fracture repair. Clin. Orthop. Rel. Res 355: 124–131.
25. Rosier RN, O'Keefe RJ, Hicks DG (1998) The potential role of transforming growth factor in fracture healing. Clin. Orthop. Rel. Res 355: 294–300.

Effects of Negative Pressure Wound Therapy on Mesenchymal Stem Cells Proliferation and Osteogenic Differentiation in a Fibrin Matrix

Jin Zhu, Aixi Yu*, Baiwen Qi, Zonghuan Li, Xiang Hu

Department of Micro-Orthopedics, Zhongnan Hospital of Wuhan University, Wuhan, China

Abstract

Vacuum-assisted closure (VAC) negative pressure wound therapy (NPWT) has been proven to be an effective therapeutic method for the treatment of recalcitrant wounds. However, its role in bone healing remains to be unclear. Here, we investigated the effects of NPWT on rat periosteum-derived mesenchymal stem cells (P-MSCs) proliferation and osteoblastic differentiation in a 3D fibrin matrix. P-MSCs underwent primary culture for three passages before being used to construct cell clots. The fibrin clots were incubated with NPWT under continuous suction at −125 mmHg in a subatmospheric perfusion bioreactor. Clots exposed to atmospheric pressure served as the static control. Compared to the control group, cell proliferation significantly increased in NPWT group after incubation for 3 days. There was no statistical difference in apoptosis rate between two groups. The ALP activity and mineralization of P-MSCs all increased under continuous suction. The expressions of collagen type 1 and transcription factor Cbfa-1 were higher at the 1-, 3-, and 7-day timepoints and the expressions of osteocalcin and integrin β5 were higher at the 3-, and 7-day timepoints in the NPWT group. These results indicate that a short time treatment with NPWT, applied with continuous suction at −125 mmHg, can enhance cellular proliferation of P-MSCs and induce the differentiation toward an osteogenic phenotype. The mechanotransduction molecule integrin β5 was found to be highly expressed after NPWT treatment, which indicates that NPWT may play a positive role in fracture healing through enhance bone formation and decrease bone resorption.

Editor: Takuya Matsumoto, Department of Biomaterials, Japan

Funding: This study was supported by the National Natural Science Foundation of China (no. 81171713) and the Hubei Provience's Outstanding Medical Academic Leader Program. The funders had no role in study design, data collection and analysis, decision to publish, or preparation of the manuscript.

Competing Interests: The authors report no conflicts of interest. The authors alone are responsible for the content and writing of the paper.

* Email: yuaixi666@hotmail.com

Introduction

Negative pressure wound therapy (NPWT) has been proven to be effective at treating complex wounds [1–4]. This therapy can promote granulation tissue formation and improve wound healing through reducing tissue edema, removing factors that inhibit wound healing, increasing wound perfusion, and reducing incidence of infection [5–8]. However, controversy still remains regarding the benefits of NPWT on bone tissue, though there have been many clinic and basement reports about its application in treatment of open fracture or osseous defect combined with soft tissue injury, and these studies nearly all show that NPWT can effectively improve wound and bone healing or has no deleterious effect on fracture healing [9–12].

Bone regeneration is a complex process involving many cells and factors from different compartments of the bone. Mesenchymal stem cells (MSCs) from periosteum, endosteum and bone marrow play a pivotal role in bone healing. They may contribute to healing through osteogenic and chondrogenic differentiation, endochondral ossification, and/or through the release of paracine factors resulting in recruitment and activation of host osteoprogenitor cells [13]. Except for the above factors, mechanical strain is also one important factor in the regulation of bone modeling and remodeling [14]. Yamazaki et al [15] showed that a lack of mechanical stress can significantly reduce the capability of MSCs to differentiate into an osteoblast. Numerous in vitro researches have also demonstrated that mechanical stimuli and hydrostatic pressure can enhance cellular viability and improve osteogenic differentiation and maturation of MSCs [16–20]. Swain et al [21] reported NPWT activates within mature dura a natural healing cascade that results in osseous tissue formation using a rabbit cranial critical-size defects model, they reasoned that negative pressure-induced mechanical signals (tissue stretching) may promote the process that progenitor cells from the dura differentiate to osteoblasts and then synthesize bone matrix with subsequent mineralization. Therefore, we hypothesize that the application of NPWT in traumatic wound with fracture or segmental bone loss may result in the transduction of strain to the underlying periosteum, with concomitant cell stretching, stimulating osseous healing in an analogous manner.

Wilkes et al [22] firstly described an in vitro NPWT system. They developed a fibrin matrix to support cellular growth, withstand the suction forces generated during subatmospheric pressure application, and allow culture medium flow through the matrix. This new culture system mimics the wound microenvironment and permits the study of the cellular changes under NPWT in vitro. In this study, to show the correlation between NPWT and osteogenic differentiation of periosteum-derived mesenchymal stem cells (P-MSCs), we assembled a bioreactor which is similar to the above report, and then investigated the effects of NPWT on P-MSCs that were the initial stage in the process of osteogenic differentiation by induction with dexamethasone, ascorbic acid and β-glycerophosphate. As this experiment here is the first to explore the effects of NPWT on P-MSCs, we chose the subatmospheric value −125 mmHg, which is most effective for soft-tissue wounds [2,5,23]. We examined cellular viability, alkaline phosphatase (ALP) activity, mineralization and the expression levels of ostoblast-related genes and proteins under NPWT or static control. The aim of this work was to detect the possible role of NPWT in bone healing.

Materials and Methods

Ethics statement

All experiments were approved by the Institutional Animal Care and Use Committee of Wuhan University, and the animal procedures were performed in strict accordance with institutional and national guidelines. All efforts were made to minimize suffering.

Cell isolation and culture

Twelve 4-week-old male Sprague-Dawley rats were sacrificed for the present study. P-MSCs were isolated and characterised in accordance with published techniques [24]. Briefly, the rats were sacrificed by cervical dislocation and sterilized in 75% ethanol for 5 min before surgery. The periosteum was stripped off mechanically from femora and tibiae using forceps, then minced, digested for 2 h at 37°C with 0.2% type II collagenase (Sigma-Aldrich, St.Louis, MO, USA). The released cells were collected by centrifugation (1,000 rpm for 5 minutes) after filtration by 40-μm cell strainers, and maintained in expansion medium consisting of L-DMEM (Hyclone) and 10% FBS (Gibco) supplemented with 2 mM L-glutamine, 100 U/ml penicillin and 100 U/ml streptomycin in a humidified atmosphere containing 5% CO_2 at 37°C. For subculture, cells were detached with 0.25% trypsin (Amresco) and passaged at a ratio of 1:2 plates when cells grew to 70–80% confluence. P-MSCs were identified as CD44(+), CD90(+), and CD34(−); furthermore, these cells cultured in adipogenic or osteogenic media differentiated into adipocytes and osteoblasts, respectively (Figure S1). P-MSCs were used for experiments from the second to third passages.

Fibrin matrix and cell clots preparation

Fibrin clots were prepared as described [22]. Briefly, porcine plasma (Lampire Biological Laboratories Inc, Pipersville, PA) supplemented with fibrinogen (Sigma) to a final fibrinogen concentration of 9.8 mg/ml was prepared. To form the bottom layer, 600 μl porcine plasma was added to each insert (BD Falcon: 6-well format, 1 μm pore size) and then was clotted by 150 μl of thrombin solution (1800 U/ml). The top layer was formed by adding 600 μl porcine plasma with 20,000 P-MSCs on the top of first clot layer. Another 150 μl of thrombin was then added to encapsulate the cells. Double-layered clots were incubated at 37°C for 1 hour before adding cell culture medium.

NPWT treatment using a bioreactor

We assembled the bioreactor modifying from the previous report [22]. Briefly, the inserts were placed through one O-sealing ring and then into the well of a 6-well plate. A layer of foam (VSD Inc, Wuhan, China) was placed on the top of the clot. To create a seal, a drape was placed on the top of the wells. One needle accessed through a 3 M bumpon was inserted into the foam and connected to a vacuum pump (VSD Inc.) that generated continuously suction at −125 mmHg. Another needle with an adhesive-backed elastomeric disc was placed in the O-ring and reached the bottom of the plate. This needle was used to inject media through a peristaltic pump (Longer, Baoding, China) at 8 ml per 24 hours per well. As a comparator, control inserts were cultured in the same bioreactor without suction. For osteogenic differentiation assays, all cell clots were initially maintained with osteogenic medium (serum-containing DMEM supplemented with 50 mg/ml ascorbic acid, 10 mM β-glycerophosphate, and 0.1 mM dexamethasone [all from Sigma]) at 37°C and 5% CO_2 for 7 days, and then were cultured in the same medium with or without NPWT for another 7 days. As for other experiments, constructs were evaluated after 3 days of incubation using expansion medium. All experiments were repeated 3 times in each of the following assays.

Cell counting kit-8 assay

Following 72 hours of treatment with NPWT or static conditions, the cell clots were fed with fresh media containing a water soluble tetrazolium salt from the cell counting kit-8 (CCK-8, Dojindo, Japan). The experiment was carried out according to the manufacturer's protocol. The absorbance at 450 nm was measured on a microplate reader.

TUNEL Assay

Following 72 hours of treatment with NPWT or static conditions, the cell clots were fixed with 4% paraformaldehyde, and then were permeabilized in 0.5% Triton X-100, followed by freshly prepared TUNEL reaction mixture for 1 h in a dark room. The nuclei were stained by DAPI in mounting medium. Cells in clots were visualized and photographed using a confocal microscope (LSM710, ZEISS, Germany). Percent apoptosis was determined by counting the number of $TUNEL^+$ cells and dividing by the total number of cells in randomly selected areas.

ALP staining and activity assay

Following treatment with or without NPWT for 3 and 7 days, ALP staining was performed using leukocyte alkaline phosphatase (LAP) kits (Sigma) according to the manufacturers' instruction. ALP activity was determined by measuring the OD values for absorbance at 405 nm after incubation with p-nitrophenyl phosphate (Sigma) for 15 min. The calibration curve was derived from a standard dilution series of p-nitrophenol (pNP, Sigma) which was prepared with concentrations ranging from 0 to 0.2 μmol/ml. ALP activity was expressed as nanomoles of pNP/μg DNA×min.

Matrix Mineralization

Alizarin red staining was used to characterize mineralization of the cells. Following treatment with or without NPWT for 3 and 7 days, the clots were incubated with 2% Alizarin red S (Sigma) for 30 min. After that, they were washed with PBS and imaged using an Olympus Inverted Microscope. Following imaging, the stain was eluted off the cells with 10% cetylpyridinium chloride in 10 mM sodium phosphate solution for 15 min at room temperature. The absorbance was then measured at 590 nm using a spectrophotometer.

Immunofluorescence staining

Following treatment with or without NPWT for 3 and 7 days, the cell clots were collected and fixed in 4% paraformaldehyde and permeabilized with 0.5% Triton X-100 at room temperature. Then they were blocked with goat serum, and incubated with the specific rat primary antibodies against collagen type 1 (COL1) (1:100, BOSTER, Wuhan, China) overnight at 4°C. The clots were then incubated with a red fluorescently labeled goat anti-mouse secondary antibody for another 30 minutes at 37°C. The nuclei were stained with DAPI. After washing three times with PBS, the clots were viewed under a confocal laser-scanning microscope.

Real-time PCR analysis

Following treatment with or without NPWT for 3 and 7 days, total RNA was extracted using Trizol (Invitrogen). Reverse transcription was carried out using 1 μg total RNA in final volume of 20 μL with PrimeScript RT reagent kit (Takara Bio, Shiga, Japan) according to the manufacturer's recommendations. Real-time PCR was performed in an ABI 7900HT system using a real-time PCR kit (Takara Bio). The settings were as follows: denaturation at 95°C for 10 sec, and then 40 cycles (10 sec at 95°C, 30 sec at 60°C). A dissociation curve was constructed using the system software program v2.1 to confirm that there was no non-specific amplification. The housekeeping gene β-actin was used to be endogenous control for normalization. The primer sequences used in this study were listed in Table 1.

Western-blot analysis

Following treatment with or without NPWT for 3 and 7 days, the cells in fibrin clots were lysed using the protein extractiong reagent RIPA (Beyotime, Shanghai, China) containing 1 mM phenylmethylsulfonyl fluoride (Sigma) and a phosphatase-inhibitor cocktail (Sigma). Samples (50 ng protein) were separated by SDS polyacrylamide gel electrophoresis and electrotransferred onto Hybond-polyvinylidene fluoride (PVDF) membrane. The membranes were then incubated with rabbit anti-RUNX2 antibody (1:200) (Santa Cruz, Inc.), rabbit anti-osteocalcin (OC) antibody (1:400) (Abcam, Inc.), rabbit anti-integrin β5 (ITGB5) antibody (1:1000) (Santa Cruz, Inc.) or rabbit anti-β-actin antibody (1:1000) (BOSTER) in TBST overnight at 4°C. Horseradish peroxidase conjugated goat anti-rabbit IgG Ab (1:1000) (Santa Cruz, Inc.) were used as secondary antibody. The protein bands were detected by ECL chemiluminescence. The results were quantified by Image J software.

Statistical analysis

In all experiments, data were expressed as mean ± standard. Statistical comparisons were performed using Student's *t*-test which was carried out using SPSS, v.18.0. P-value<0.05 was considered statistically significant.

Results

Cell morphology

Visual inspection of the cells using Wright–Giemsa staining revealed morphological differences between the two groups. The cells in Figure 1A are representative of static P-MSCs, thin with elongated spindle shape. Compared with control group, the cells in NPWT group appeared larger and thicker with dendrite-like branching and spread more (Figure 1B).

Cell proliferation

The CCK-8 assay showed that the proliferation of P-MSCs in NPWT group was significantly upregulated compared to the control (Figure 2). We also performed TUNEL assay to observe if NPWT induced P-MSCs apoptosis. As shown in Figure 3A, treatment with continuous suction at −125 mmHg for 72 hours didn't dramatically increase the number of $TUNEL^+$ cells in P-MSCs. There was no significant difference in the percentage of apoptosis cells between the NPWT group and control group (Figure 3B).

Osteogenic differentiation of P-MSCs

ALP staining showed that a deeper black-blue color could be seen in NPWT group than that in control group (Figure 4A). Alizarin Red staining showed that there were nearly no mineralization dots in control group, but sporadic, brownish red and opaque calcified nodules could be observed in the NPWT group after treated for 3 days. At day 7, the mineralization nodules were much bigger and denser in NPWT group (Figure 4C). Quantification assay showed significant increases in ALP activity and calcification in the NPWT group compared to the control (Figure 4B, D).

Immunofluorescence staining showed that many cells in the clots incubated with NPWT for 3 days were shown to be stained positive for COL1, and the more so at day 7. However, very little stain was observed in the cells cultured without suction at day 3 and only a part of cells were positive at day 7 (Figure 5).

In NPWT group, OC mRNA expression profiles showed an early increase at day 3, after that a significant upregulation at day 7 was detected. The mRNA expression of ALP, COL1 and Cbfa1/Runx2 peaked at day 3, and then slight decline was detected at day 7. The mRNA levels of ALP exhibited no significant differences among the two groups at day 7 (Figure 6). Western-blot analysis was used to confirm the expression changes of Cbfa1/Runx2 and OC, and the results were consistent with real-time RT-PCR (Figure 7A, B).

Table 1. Primer sequences for real-time RT-PCR.

Genes	Forward primer (5′-3′)	Reverse primer (5′-3′)
Alpl	TGGACGGTGAACGGGAGAAC	GCCATGACGTGGGGGATGTA
Bglap	CAAGTCCCACACAGCAACTC	TCACCACCTTACTGCCCTCC
Cbfa1/Runx2	GCTTCTCCAACCCACGAATG	GAACTGATAGGACGCTGACGA
Col1a1	CAGGCTGGTGTGATGGGATT	CCAAGGCATTCTGCCTCT
Itgb5	CGAGCTTGGGATAAAGCAAG	TCAACAGGCATCTCAACAGC
Actb	CGTTGACATCCGTAAAGACCTC	TAGGAGCCAGGGCAGTAATCT

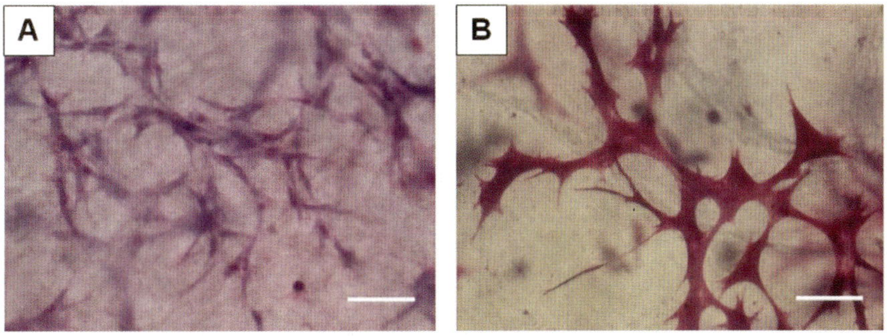

Figure 1. Effects of NPWT on morphological change. Control cells were thin with elongated spindle shape (A). The cells that were applied with NPWT were larger and thicker with many dendrite-like branches (B). Scale bar represents 100 μm.

ITGB5 mRNA and protein expression

Compared to the control group, the ITGB5 mRNA expression was significantly increased at day 3 and 7 (Figure 6E). Western-blot also showed that its protein expression was increasing slightly during 7 days treatment with NPWT (Figure 7C).

Discussion

It's well known that NPWT is a highly successful and widely used therapeutic method for wound healing. To date, many papers have been published on its action mechanism and application in various acute, chronic and complex wounds. However, little is known about its effect on bone healing. In this in vitro study, we provide new evidence that NPWT may play a positive role in the process of bone reconstruction and remodeling by strengthening the contribution of P-MSCs in fracture repair. This is supported by a) the enhanced proliferation of P-MSCs observed under NPWT treatment for 3 days; b) the significantly increased ALP activity and cell mineralization after treatment with NPWT for 3 and 7 days; c) the elevated expression of the osteoblastic-related markers at mRNA and protein levels after application of NPWT to P-MSCs.

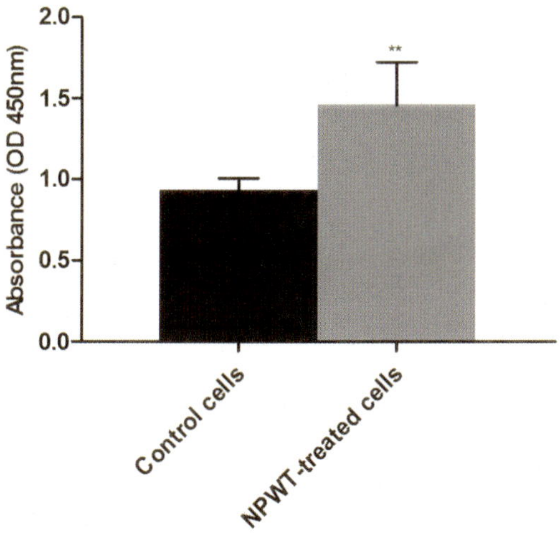

Figure 2. Cell proliferation assay. Following 72 hours of treatment with suction or static conditions, clots were exposed to water soluble tetrazolium salt-8-containing medium for 4 hours and optical density values at 450 nm were measured. Compared with control cells, NPWT-treated cells had a higher OD value (**$p<0.01$).

As far as we know, this may be the first study about the effects of NPWT (continuous suction at −125 mmHg) on P-MSCs using a perfusion bioreactor which was designed by K.C.I. research group [22]. Many researchers have reported that fibroblasts treated with NPWT exhibit greater cell survival, migration, proliferation and levels of growth factors using this bioreactor [25,26]. In our study, NPWT also increased the proliferation of P-MSCs at 72 h in continuous suction manner. There is no significant difference about cell apoptosis rate between two groups at this timepoint. However, this result may differ from previous reports [27,28]. They showed that the proliferation of bone marrow-derived MSCs (B-MSCs) was inhibited and apoptosis was induced under low-intensity and intermittent negative pressure incubation. Except for the different pressure value, suction manner and laboratory environment, we hypothesize that other two reasons may contribute to these differences.

First, the bioreactor used in our experiment may be better for investigating the application of NPWT in vitro. As the report from K.C.I., we assembled multiple units of NPWT system and applied them on P-MSCs clots. Though the action mechanisms of NPWT are not fully understood, many studies have pointed that cell response is related to the polyurethane foam, whereas the tissue strain induced by the NPWT system stimulate cell proliferation [29]. McNulty et al [25] compared the viability, chemotactic signaling and proliferation of fibroblasts with different dressing, their results indicated that the dressing material has a significant effect on cell response following NPWT, the in vitro application of NPWT with foam support cell growth, proliferation and without increasing apoptosis. The mechanical stress created by application of NPWT principally thought to be via mechanical stretch and fluid-shear stress [30]. The effect of mechanical strain or hydrostatic pressure on the proliferation of osteoblastic cells is still controversial. In some studies, appropriate mechanical stress can increase proliferation of B-MSCs [16], while in others, the proliferation rate was reduced [31]. In our study, the cells in clots treated with NPWT may be stimulated by mechanical stretch and fluid-shear stress together. Mechanical stimuli through the suction of negative pressure source and hydrostatic pressure created by fluid media controlled by the peristaltic pump may conjointly cause the proliferation of P-MSCs in fibrin matrix.

Second, as we know, cell growth is related to cell shape [32]. Application of NPWT to P-MSCs induced the changes in their morphology. This change was consistent with the previous report [26]. How the cell shape control cell-cycle is unclear. Huang and Ingber [33] showed that changes in cell shape were related to the configuration of internal cell structures, including microfilaments and microtubules. For cells to respond to soluble mitogenic factors, they must extend and generate isometric tension by adherence to a

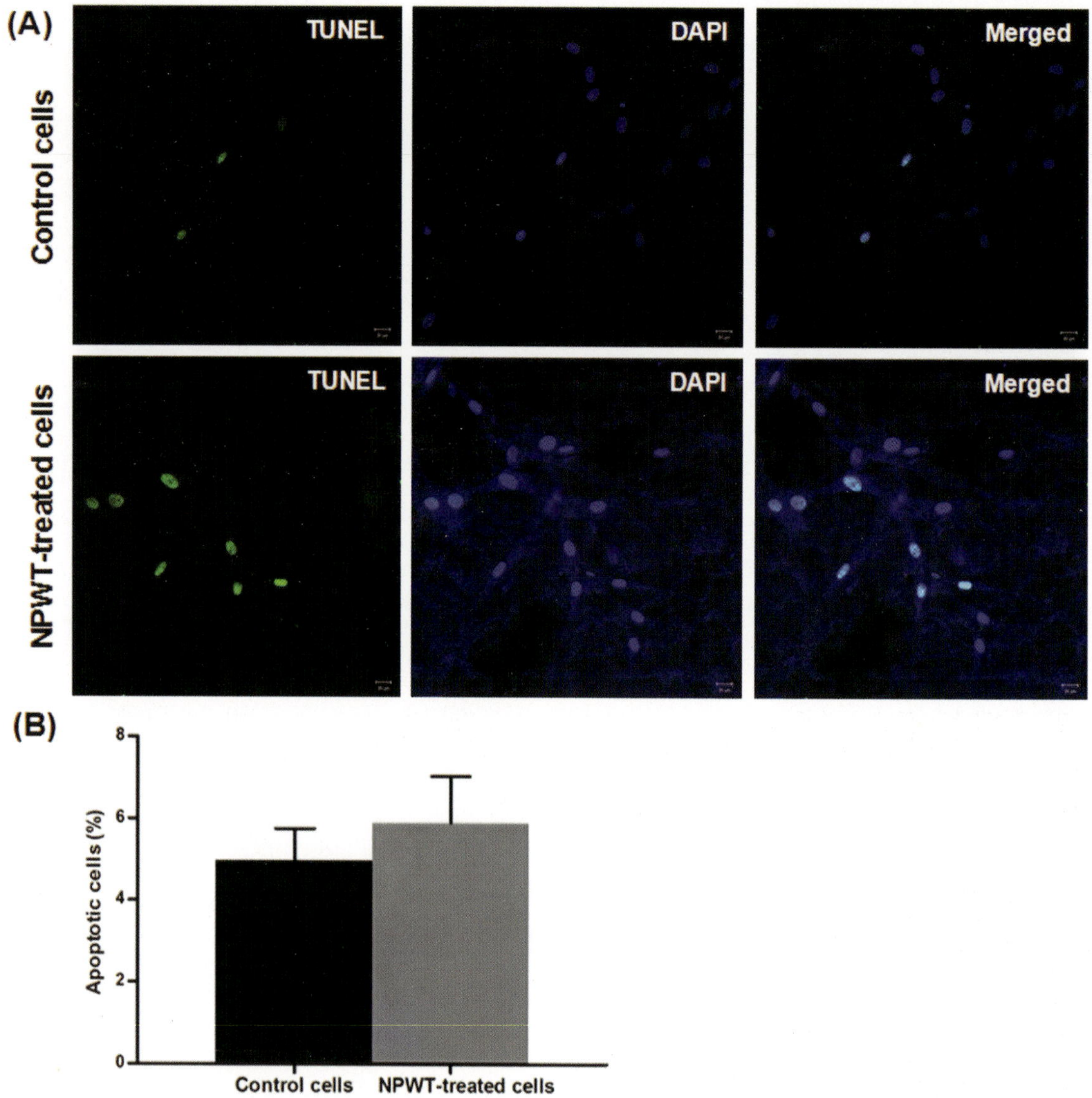

Figure 3. Cell apoptosis assay. Following 72 hours of treatment with suction or static conditions, apoptosis of MSCs was evaluated by TUNEL assay. The images of TUNEL^{+} cells was shown in (A, bars = 20 μm). Percentages of apoptotic cells in clots are shown in (B). Compared with control group, 72 hours of suction didn't result in a significant increase in cell apoptosis ($p>0.05$).

stiff substrate or extracellular application of mechanical force. The cellular adhesion to ECM, cell shape and mechanical tension in cytoskeleton are very important for the local control of cell-cycle progression. In this study, P-MSCs were cultured in a three-dimensional fibrin matrix. So, we hypothesize that micromechanical deformation of the fibrin matrix induced by foam and suction results in extracellular matrix (ECM) distortion, then may change single cell shape and make the cellular proliferation response.

To further explore the events involved during osteogenic differentiation of P-MSCs under treatment with NPWT in vitro, characterization of the expression of several osteogenic markers was performed. ALP and Alizarin Red S staining denoted early differentiation and production of mineralized matrix nodules. The results showed that increased ALP expression and significant enhancement of mineralization in P-MSCs treated with NPWT compared to control cells. Cbfa1/Runx2 is a key transcription factor in osteoblastogenesis. Our data showed that production of Cbfa1/Runx2 initially increased but then decreased in response to a long period of NPWT treatment. This result was consistent with the report from Huang and Rei [17], and opposite to the reports about osteogenic response of MSCs to continuous mechanical strain [16,34]. We hypothesize that both mechanical stretch and hydrostatic pressure contribute to the osteoblastic differentiation of P-MSCs, and the cells in fibrin matrix were more sensitive to fluid-shear stress, which may play a leading role in the mechanical stimuli created by NPWT. Detection of other osteogenic markers, such as COL1 and OC, also showed marked increase when P-MSCs were treated with NPWT.

Integrins are important mechanotransduction molecules that connect the major ECM components with the intracellular cytoskeleton and control ostoblasts differentiation and fate. Many studies reported the role of α5β1 and β1 subunits in osteoblasts differentiation and maturation. The integrin-ECM interactions could trigger many kinds of downstream signal pathways that converge to promote early osteoblast-specific gene expression in state with mechanical loading [35]. Huang et al [17] firstly

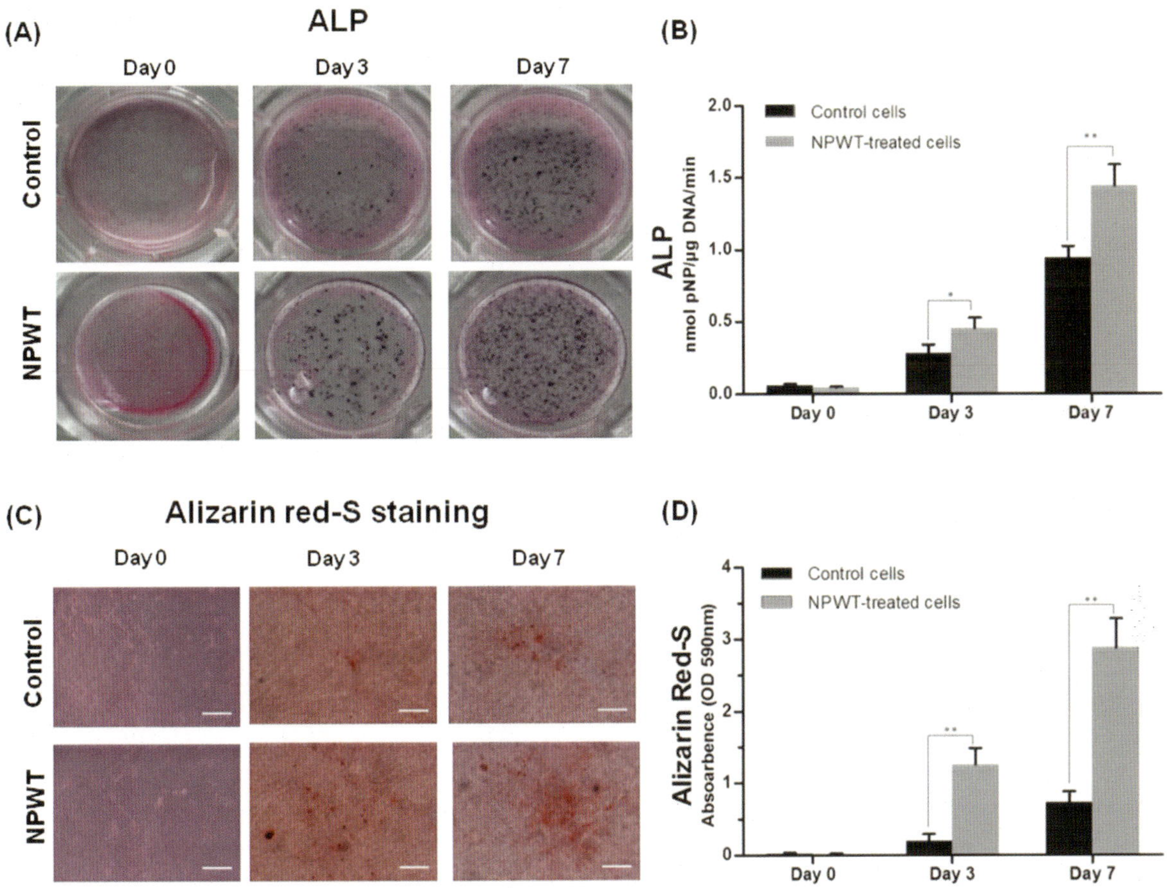

Figure 4. The expression of ALP and alizarin red-S staining. (A) Images of ALP staining of rat P-MSCs with or without NPWT treatment of different daily duration for 7 days. (B) ALP activity in P-MSCs treated with NPWT was notably higher than that in control group (*$p<0.05$, **$p<0.01$). (C) Result of alizarin red-S staining was in accordance with ALP staining (Bars = 50 µm). (D) Result of semi-quantitative analysis of alizarin red-S showed that absorbance index in NPWT group was significantly higher than that in control group (**$p<0.01$).

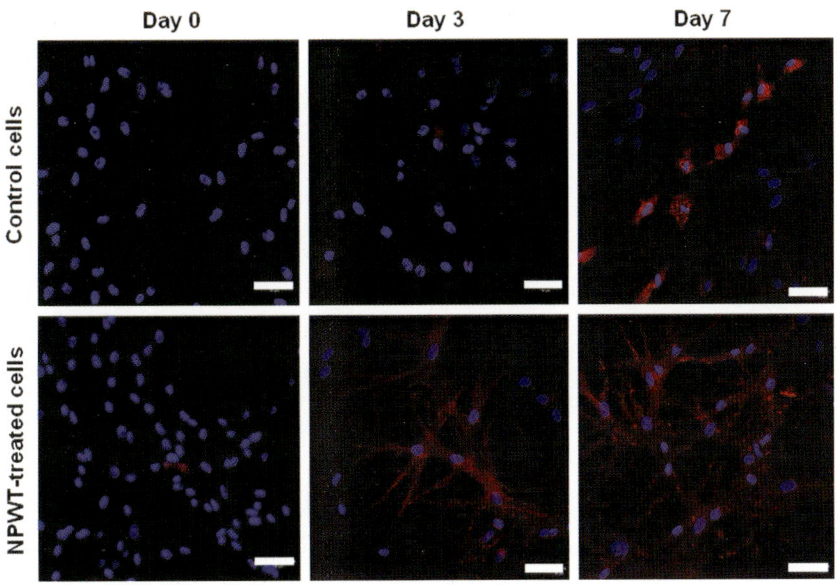

Figure 5. Immunofluorescence staining for COL1. Immediately before and 3, 7 days after incubation, cell clots were harvested and confocal microscopy was performed to detect fluorescent immunostaining for COL1. Results showed that the expression of COL1 was absent or weak in two groups before incubation, but stronger in NPWT group at day 3 and 7 after incubation. Bars = 50 µm.

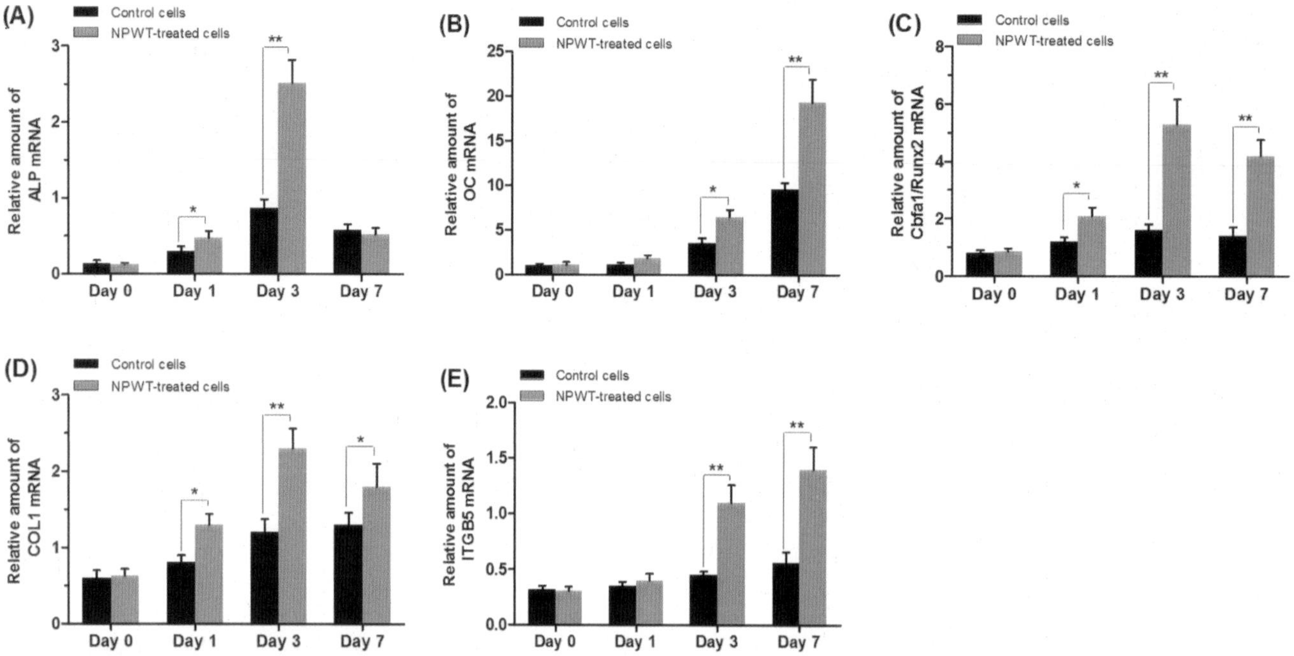

Figure 6. Real-time RT-PCR analysis. NPWT-treated and static control group cell clots were harvested before and 1, 3, and 7 days after incubation (n = 3 per timepoint for each group) and analyzed by real-time RT-PCR. The expressions of the specific osteogenic genes (A) ALP, (B) OC, and (D) COL1 were higher in NPWT group than those in control group (*$p<0.05$, **$p<0.01$). The NPWT group also expressed higher levels of the osteogenic transcription factor Cbfa1 (also known as Runx2) and the mechanosignaling molecule integrin β5 (ITGB5) (C) and (E) (*$p<0.05$, **$p<0.01$).

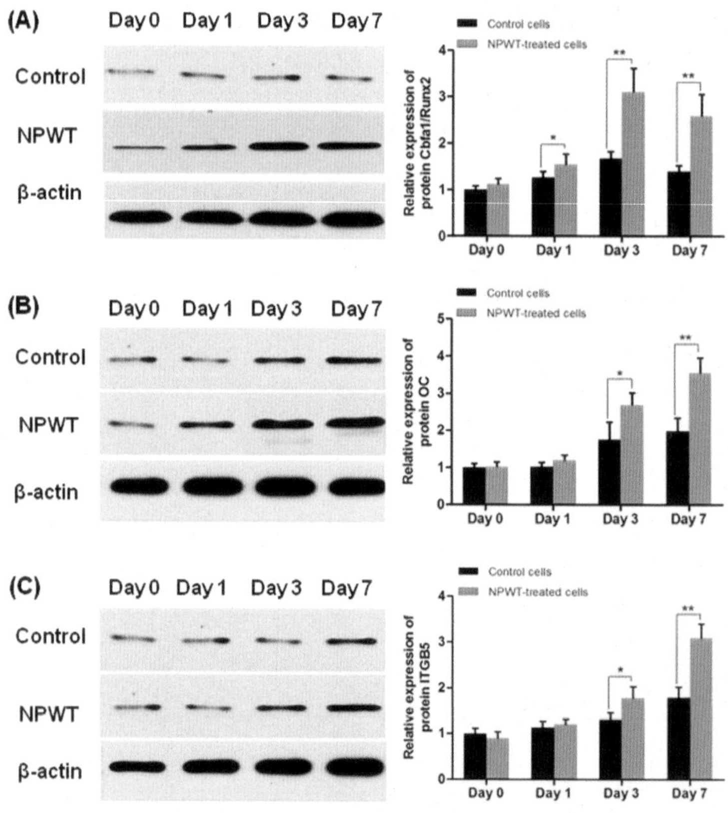

Figure 7. Western-blot assay. Protein expression levels of osteogenic factors in P-MSCs treated with NPWT at different time points were shown in (A) and (B). (A) Cbfa1/Runx2 was statistically overexpressed at day 1 after treatment with NPWT, with the increase being more significant after day 3. (B) Compared with control group, the expression of OC was markedly upregulated in NPWT group after day 3. ITGB5 protein level was shown in (C), it was not affected at day 1, but was strikingly upregulated after day 3 in NPWT group. (*$p<0.05$, **$p<0.01$).

reported that the β5 subunit of integrin was expressed in response to mechanical stimulation in MSCs. They suggested that integrin β5 may serve as a mechanotransducer in the osteogenic differentiation of MSCs promoted by hydrostatic pressure. In this study, we detected the expression of integrin β5 in two groups, and also found it expressed at a higher level after treatment with NPWT for 3 and 7 days. It has been proven that osteoclast maturation is accelerated in mice that lack integrin β5 subunit [36]. And, the expression level of integrin β5 in osteoclast from autosomal dominant osteopetrosis type II (ADO II) patients is higher than normal donors [37]. These results indicate that integrin β5 could inhibit osteoclast formation and may participate in NPWT driven oseogenesis through enhance osteoblastic differentiation and decrease osteoclast formation. This may be one possible mechanism for the promoted osteoblastic differentiation process of P-MSCs induced by NPWT in vitro.

We believe that the osteogenic induction of P-MSCs treated with NPWT is very complex. Many signals may participate in this process. The detailed mechanism studies are required to fully elucidate the mechanosignaling pathways at RNA and protein levels. It's also essential to try other pressure values and time of treatment to find optimal conditions for promoting osteogenesis. Further work will be conducted using an animal model of fracture to confirm the role of NPWT in bone healing in vivo.

Conclusion

In summary, we explored the influence of NPWT on P-MSCs proliferation and osteogenic differentiation in a 3D fibrin matrix. Our results show that a short time treatment with continuous suction at −125 mmHg could induce the differentiation of P-MSCs toward an osteogenic phenotype associated with enhancement of cellular proliferation. The mechanotransduction molecule integrin β5 was found to be highly expressed after NPWT treatment, which indicates that NPWT may promote fracture healing through enhancing bone formation and decreasing bone resorption. We hope this pilot study provided a scientific basis to prove the positive role of NPWT in bone healing and find the most beneficial waveforms of application in, treatment of complex wound with fracture or bone defect.

Supporting Information

Figure S1 Characterization of P-MSCs. A: Cell surface markers of P-MSCs (Passage 3) were analyzed by Fluorescence-activated cell sorting (FACS). P-MSCs expressed CD44 and CD90, but not CD34, CD45. **B**: Adipogenic differentiation was confirmed using Oil Red-O staining (×100). **C** and **D**: Osteogenic differentiation was revealed with ALP staining and alizarin red staining (×100).

Author Contributions

Conceived and designed the experiments: AXY JZ. Performed the experiments: JZ BWQ ZHL XH. Analyzed the data: JZ ZHL. Contributed to the writing of the manuscript: JZ AXY.

References

1. Bee TK, Croce MA, Magnotti LJ, Zarzaur BL, Maish GO 3rd, et al. (2008) Temporary abdominal closure techniques: a prospective randomized trial comparing polyglactin 910 mesh and vacuum-assisted closure. J Trauma 65: 337–42; discussion 342–4.
2. Morykwas MJ, Argenta LC, Shelton-Brown EI, McGuirt W (1997) Vacuum-assisted closure: a new method for wound control and treatment: animal studies and basic foundation. Ann Plast Surg 38: 553–62.
3. Armstrong DG, Lavery LA (2005) Negative pressure wound therapy after partial diabetic foot amputation: a multicentre, randomised controlled trial. Lancet 366: 1704–10.
4. Fleck T, Gustafsson R, Harding K, Ingemansson R, Lirtzman MD, et al. (2006) The management of deep sternal wound infections using vacuum assisted closure (V.A.C.) therapy. Int Wound J 3: 273–80.
5. Argenta LC, Morykwas MJ (1997) Vacuum-assisted closure: a new method for wound control and treatment: clinical experience. Ann Plast Surg 38: 563–76; discussion 577.
6. Weed T, Ratliff C, Drake DB (2004) Quantifying bacterial bioburden during negative pressure wound therapy: does the wound VAC enhance bacterial clearance? Ann Plast Surg 52: 276–9; discussion 279–80.
7. Orgill DP, Bayer LR (2011) Update on negative-pressure wound therapy. Plast Reconstr Surg 127 Suppl 1: 105S–115S.
8. Liu Y, Zhou Q, Wang Y, Liu Z, Dong M, et al. (2014) Negative pressure wound therapy decreases mortality in a murine model of burn-wound sepsis involving Pseudomonas aeruginosa infection. PLoS One 9: e90494.
9. Takeuchi N, Mae T, Hotokezaka S, Sasaki K, Matsushita A, et al. (2011) A Gustilo type IIIB open forearm fracture treated by negative pressure wound therapy and locking compression plates: a case report. Fukuoka Igaku Zasshi 102: 293–7.
10. Babiak I (2012) Open tibial fractures grade IIIC treated successfully with external fixation, negative-pressure wound therapy and recombinant human bone morphogenetic protein 7. Int Wound J.
11. Deng K, Yu AX, Xia CY, Li ZH, Wang WY (2013) Combination of negative pressure wound therapy with open bone grafting for bone and soft tissue defects. Mol Med Rep 8: 468–72.
12. Suzuki T, Minehara A, Matsuura T, Kawamura T, Soma K (2014) Negative-pressure wound therapy over surgically closed wounds in open fractures. J Orthop Surg (Hong Kong) 22: 30–4.
13. Wang X, Wang Y, Gou W, Lu Q, Peng J, et al. (2013) Role of mesenchymal stem cells in bone regeneration and fracture repair: a review. Int Orthop 37: 2491–8.
14. Duncan RL, Turner CH (1995) Mechanotransduction and the functional response of bone to mechanical strain. Calcif Tissue Int 57: 344–58.
15. Yamazaki S, Mizumoto T, Nasu A, Horii T, Otomo K, et al. (2011) Regulation of osteogenetic differentiation of mesenchymal stem cells by two axial rotational culture. J Artif Organs 14: 310–7.
16. Koike M, Shimokawa H, Kanno Z, Ohya K, Soma K (2005) Effects of mechanical strain on proliferation and differentiation of bone marrow stromal cell line ST2. J Bone Miner Metab 23: 219–25.
17. Huang C, Ogawa R (2012) Effect of hydrostatic pressure on bone regeneration using human mesenchymal stem cells. Tissue Eng Part A 18: 2106–13.
18. Wu Y, Zhang X, Zhang P, Fang B, Jiang L (2012) Intermittent traction stretch promotes the osteoblastic differentiation of bone mesenchymal stem cells by the ERK1/2-activated Cbfa1 pathway. Connect Tissue Res 53: 451–9.
19. Kang MN, Yoon HH, Seo YK, Park JK (2012) Effect of mechanical stimulation on the differentiation of cord stem cells. Connect Tissue Res 53: 149–59.
20. Song G, Ju Y, Shen X, Luo Q, Shi Y, et al. (2007) Mechanical stretch promotes proliferation of rat bone marrow mesenchymal stem cells. Colloids and Surfaces B: Biointerfaces 58: 271–277.
21. Swain LD, Cornet DA, Manwaring ME, Collins B, Singh VK, et al. (2013) Negative pressure therapy stimulates healing of critical-size calvarial defects in rabbits. Bonekey Rep 2: 299.
22. Wilkes RP, McNulty AK, Feeley TD, Schmidt MA, Kieswetter K (2007) Bioreactor for application of subatmospheric pressure to three-dimensional cell culture. Tissue Eng 13: 3003–10.
23. Morykwas MJ, Faler BJ, Pearce DJ, Argenta LC (2001) Effects of varying levels of subatmospheric pressure on the rate of granulation tissue formation in experimental wounds in swine. Ann Plast Surg 47: 547–51.
24. Rosales-Rocabado JM, Kaku M, Kitami M, Akiba Y, Uoshima K (2014) Osteoblastic differentiation and mineralization ability of periosteum-derived cells compared with bone marrow and calvaria-derived cells. J Oral Maxillofac Surg 72: 694 e1–9.
25. McNulty AK, Schmidt M, Feeley T, Kieswetter K (2007) Effects of negative pressure wound therapy on fibroblast viability, chemotactic signaling, and proliferation in a provisional wound (fibrin) matrix. Wound Repair Regen 15: 838–46.
26. Lu F, Ogawa R, Nguyen DT, Chen B, Guo D, et al. (2011) Microdeformation of three-dimensional cultured fibroblasts induces gene expression and morphological changes. Ann Plast Surg 66: 296–300.
27. Zhang YG, Yang Z, Zhang H, Wang C, Liu M, et al. (2010) Effect of negative pressure on human bone marrow mesenchymal stem cells in vitro. Connect Tissue Res 51: 14–21.
28. Yang Z, Yao JF, Xu P, Zhang JB, Zhang YM, et al. (2014) Functions and mechanisms of intermittent negative pressure for osteogenesis in human bone marrow mesenchymal stem cells. Mol Med Rep 9: 1331–6.

29. Scherer SS, Pietramaggiori G, Mathews JC, Prsa MJ, Huang S, et al. (2008) The mechanism of action of the vacuum-assisted closure device. Plast Reconstr Surg 122: 786–97.
30. Banwell PE, Musgrave M (2004) Topical negative pressure therapy: mechanisms and indications. Int Wound J 1: 95–106.
31. Puetzer J, Williams J, Gillies A, Bernacki S, Loboa EG (2013) The effects of cyclic hydrostatic pressure on chondrogenesis and viability of human adipose- and bone marrow-derived mesenchymal stem cells in three-dimensional agarose constructs. Tissue Eng Part A 19: 299–306.
32. Folkman J, Moscona A (1978) Role of cell shape in growth control. Nature 273: 345–9.
33. Huang S, Ingber DE (1999) The structural and mechanical complexity of cell-growth control. Nat Cell Biol 1: E131–8.
34. Zhang P, Wu Y, Jiang Z, Jiang L, Fang B (2012) Osteogenic response of mesenchymal stem cells to continuous mechanical strain is dependent on ERK1/2-Runx2 signaling. Int J Mol Med 29: 1083–9.
35. Thompson WR, Rubin CT, Rubin J (2012) Mechanical regulation of signaling pathways in bone. Gene 503: 179–93.
36. Lane NE, Yao W, Nakamura MC, Humphrey MB, Kimmel D, et al. (2005) Mice lacking the integrin beta5 subunit have accelerated osteoclast maturation and increased activity in the estrogen-deficient state. J Bone Miner Res 20: 58–66.
37. Coudert AE, Del Fattore A, Baulard C, Olaso R, Schiltz C, et al. (2014) Differentially expressed genes in autosomal dominant osteopetrosis type II osteoclasts reveal known and novel pathways for osteoclast biology. Lab Invest 94: 275–85.

17

Computed Tomographic Imaging of Subchondral Fatigue Cracks in the Distal End of the Third Metacarpal Bone in the Thoroughbred Racehorse Can Predict Crack Micromotion in an Ex-Vivo Model

Marie-Soleil Dubois[1], Samantha Morello[1], Kelsey Rayment[1], Mark D. Markel[1], Ray Vanderby Jr[2], Vicki L. Kalscheur[1], Zhengling Hao[1], Ronald P. McCabe[2], Patricia Marquis[1,3], Peter Muir[1]*

1 Comparative Orthopaedic Research Laboratory, School of Veterinary Medicine, University of Wisconsin-Madison, Madison, Wisconsin, United States of America, **2** Department of Orthopedics & Rehabilitation, School of Medicine & Public Health, University of Wisconsin-Madison, Madison, Wisconsin, United States of America, **3** Gulfstream Park, Hallandale Beach, Florida, United States of America

Abstract

Articular stress fracture arising from the distal end of the third metacarpal bone (MC3) is a common serious injury in Thoroughbred racehorses. Currently, there is no method for predicting fracture risk clinically. We describe an ex-vivo biomechanical model in which we measured subchondral crack micromotion under compressive loading that modeled high speed running. Using this model, we determined the relationship between subchondral crack dimensions measured using computed tomography (CT) and crack micromotion. Thoracic limbs from 40 Thoroughbred racehorses that had sustained a catastrophic injury were studied. Limbs were radiographed and examined using CT. Parasagittal subchondral fatigue crack dimensions were measured on CT images using image analysis software. MC3 bones with fatigue cracks were tested using five cycles of compressive loading at -7,500N (38 condyles, 18 horses). Crack motion was recorded using an extensometer. Mechanical testing was validated using bones with 3 mm and 5 mm deep parasagittal subchondral slots that modeled naturally occurring fatigue cracks. After testing, subchondral crack density was determined histologically. Creation of parasagittal subchondral slots induced significant micromotion during loading ($p<0.001$). In our biomechanical model, we found a significant positive correlation between extensometer micromotion and parasagittal crack area derived from reconstructed CT images ($S_R = 0.32$, $p<0.05$). Correlations with transverse and frontal plane crack lengths were not significant. Histologic fatigue damage was not significantly correlated with crack dimensions determined by CT or extensometer micromotion. Bones with parasagittal crack area measurements above 30 mm^2 may have a high risk of crack propagation and condylar fracture in vivo because of crack micromotion. In conclusion, our results suggest that CT could be used to quantify subchondral fatigue crack dimensions in racing Thoroughbred horses in-vivo to assess risk of condylar fracture. Horses with parasagittal crack arrays that exceed 30 mm^2 may have a high risk for development of condylar fracture.

Editor: Damian Christopher Genetos, University of California Davis, United States of America

Funding: This research [Project AOVET-12-05M] was supported by a grant from the AO Foundation. The funders had no role in study design, data collection and analysis, decision to publish, or preparation of the manuscript.

Competing Interests: Please note that although Patricia Marquis is affiliated with the Gulfstream Park company in Florida.

* Email: muirp@vetmed.wisc.edu

Introduction

Parasagittal fracture of the condyles of the third metacarpal/metatarsal bone (MC3/MT3), or condylar fracture, is common in Thoroughbred and Standardbred racehorses and is often identified as part of a syndrome of fetlock breakdown injury. Some of these injuries are catastrophic and require euthanasia of the horse [1,2]. In horses where surgical treatment is indicated, prognosis for return to athletic activity is not always favorable [2–4]. Risk of catastrophic injury may be as high as 2.17%, or 1 in every 46 race starts at some National Hunt racecourses in the United Kingdom [5]. Metacarpal fracture is the second most common cause of fatalities arising from a fracture in United States [6]. In the United Kingdom, condylar fractures are the most common type of fracture associated with racing and the most common reason for euthanasia of Thoroughbred racehorses with fracture [7].

Over the last 30 years, various etiologies for condylar fracture have been proposed. These theories fall into three main categories: first, accidental injury from mechanical overload [8]; second, pathological fracture associated with traumatic osteochondrosis [9–10]; and third, failure of functional adaptation and development of stress fracture [11–14]. Functional adaptation is a process by which bone remodels in response to mechanical loading. Bones are typically adapted to normal loads, but may be poorly designed to resist propagation of macroscopic fatigue cracks [15]. Although research data are primarily associative, it is now widely accepted that condylar fractures are site-specific articular stress fractures that essentially represent failure of functional adaptation to protect the subchondral bone plate of affected joints from cumulative fatigue injury [11–16]. Functional strains normally range from −1,500 to −3,000 microstrain in cursorial mammals [17]. However, in-vivo strains of more than −5,000 microstrain have been recorded in the MC3 mid-diaphysis of Thoroughbreds during galloping [18].

Functional adaptation is readily detectable by 4 months of race training [19]. Contact stresses on the palmar or plantar regions of the distal end of the MC3/MT3 bones from the proximal sesamoid bones are more than twice the stresses imposed on the dorsal region at the canter; this is a result of more load being shifted to the suspensory apparatus during increased fetlock joint extension [20]. As training increases, adaptation in the subchondral plate leads to sclerosis of the trabecular bone in the palmar/plantar aspect of the condyles, endochondral ossification of the joint surface, and advancement of the tidemark to the articular surface [11,14]. These changes are associated with site-specific microdamage accumulation in calcified cartilage and the underlying subchondral bone of the parasagittal condylar grooves [11,12,14]. Microcrack initiation occurs in the calcified cartilage layer [14] and stimulates a targeted remodeling response that results in the formation of resorption spaces containing activated osteoclasts in the damaged bone [14]. This reparative response is associated with an increase in bone porosity, and may make horses more vulnerable to stress fracture if athletic activity is ongoing [14]. Accumulation and coalescence of these microcracks leads to development of macroscopic crack arrays in the subchondral bone of the condylar grooves [11,12,14]. Crack propagation through porous bone compromises the overlying cortical shell at the distal end of the MC3/MT3 bone [15,21]. Once the cortical shell of the distal end of the MC3/MT3 bone is mechanically compromised, crack propagation proximally along trabecular planes can easily develop, thereby rendering the horse at high risk of developing condylar stress fracture [15,21].

Currently, there are differing opinions in the field regarding the etiology of fetlock breakdown injury in the racing Thoroughbred. The causative mechanism is likely complex and involves all of the joint structures, the third metacarpal or metatarsal, the proximal sesamoids, and the proximal phalanx. Very little is known about the mechanical stability of the fatigue cracks in the subchondral bone plate that precede development of a condylar stress fracture. It is likely that condylar stress fracture is preceded by cracks in the subchondral plate that become sufficiently severe to permit development of micromotion at the high joint loads associated with training or racing. Therefore, knowledge of the relationship between crack dimensions determined by cross-sectional imaging and crack micromotion at high load may facilitate early identification of horses that are at high risk of condylar stress fracture. Ultimately, this knowledge could help reduce the incidence of serious or catastrophic injuries at the racetrack.

Multiple imaging methods relevant to the distal limb are available to the equine clinician. Radiography is inferior to computed tomography (CT) and magnetic resonance imaging (MRI) for identification of pathologic features in subchondral bone and articular cartilage, such as fatigue cracks in the subchondral bone plate [22,23]. In addition to increased sensitivity for identifying pathologic changes in the articular surface of the fetlock joint, CT allows for multi-planar analysis of cross-sectional images of bone, facilitating a more accurate determination of size or extent of specific structures, such as subchondral fatigue cracks.

The objective of the present study was to develop an ex-vivo biomechanical model in which subchondral crack micromotion at high loads could be measured in distal MC3. We then used this model to determine the relationship between subchondral crack dimensions measured using CT and crack micromotion. We hypothesized that subchondral crack micromotion would be commonly detectable in the distal end of the MC3 bone in Thoroughbred racehorses at joint loads that model racing activity. Such a result would suggest that athletic Thoroughbred horses commonly train and race with incipient condylar stress fracture and are vulnerable to fracture propagation during athletic activity. A secondary objective was to study detection of fetlock joint abnormalities by CT imaging.

Materials and Methods

Thoroughbred racehorses

Thirty-six pairs of entire distal forelimbs and 4 individual limbs from 40 Thoroughbred racehorses that died or were euthanatized for reasons unrelated to the present study were given for use in this work (**Fig. 1**). Horses were euthanatized humanely by a veterinarian at the racetrack using an intravenous anesthetic overdose. Euthanasia was performed for clinical reasons because of serious injury during racing. Only thoracic limbs were used for this study. Condylar fractures most commonly affect the thoracic limbs [2,3,24,25]. Limbs were transected at the level of the carpus, sealed in plastic bags, and stored at -20C until needed. The age, gender, and racing history were collected from the Jockey Club Information Systems, Inc. Thoroughbred racehorse database (www.equineline.com) for horses with parasagittal subchondral cracks that were tested mechanically.

Digital radiography (DR)

DR radiographs of the metacarpophalangeal joint of each limb specimen were made using a single dorsopalmar radiographic view (70 kVp, 0.08 Ms, EDR3-MFA, Sound-Eklin, Carlsbad, CA) to determine whether fractures of the MC3 bone, proximal sesamoid bones or proximal phalanx were present. Limbs were excluded if a fracture of the MC3 bone was present.

Computed tomography (CT)

CT imaging was performed at high-resolution using 0.625 mm contiguous slices (64 slices GE Discovery CT750 HD, GE Healthcare Technologies, Waukesha, WI, USA). CT images were reconstructed in the sagittal, transverse, and frontal planes using a 64-bit Dicom viewer (OsiriX, Pixmeo SARL, Bernex, Switzerland). CT images were examined for evidence of pathological changes, including the presence of subchondral sclerosis, fractures, defects in the joint surface, and parasagittal fatigue cracks within the condylar grooves. The presence of palmar osteochondral disease (POD), initially referred to in the literature as traumatic osteochondrosis [26,27], was defined by the presence of subchondral bone lysis in the palmar condyle area [22]. The dimensions of subchondral cracks were measured radiographically on transverse and reconstructed frontal plane CT images (**Fig. 2**). In addition, crack area was measured in the parasagittal plane using image analysis (Image J, NIH) (**Fig. 2**). Using commercially available software (Mimics 13.1 Materialise, Ann Arbor, Michigan), the distal end of each MC3 bone with a parasagittal condylar groove lesion was segmented manually. A 3D volumetric model of the subchondral crack lesion was then created from the segmented images on a voxel-by-voxel basis to yield measurements of subchondral crack volume and the surface area of the subchondral crack volume.

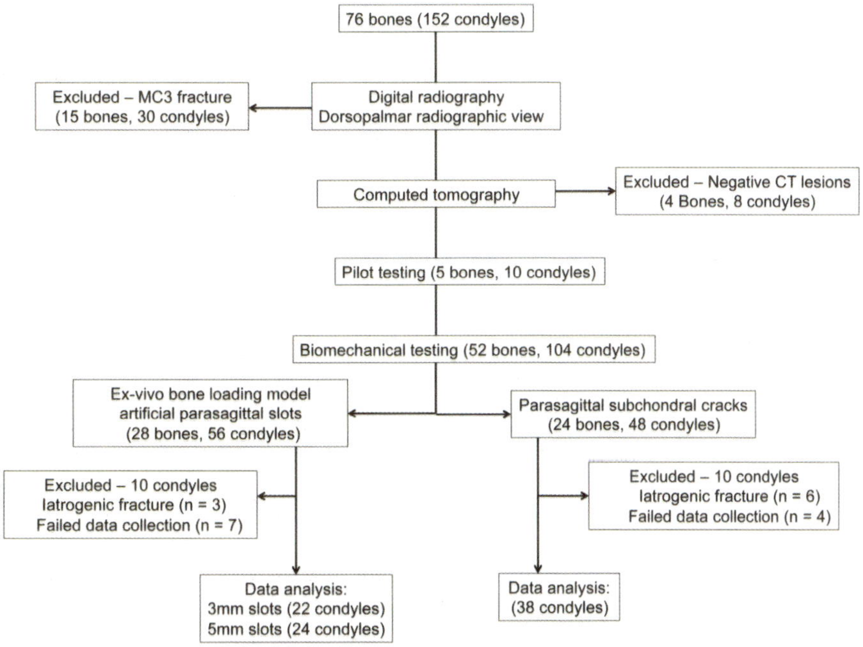

Figure 1. Flow diagram for limb inclusion and exclusion. Of the 152 condyles from 76 limbs horses initially screened, 38 condyles with naturally occurring subchondral fatigue cracks were ultimately studied in detail.

Visual examination and photography

After CT imaging, all soft tissue was removed from each MC3 bone. The shaft was cut with a band saw in the mid-diaphysis, 12 cm proximal to the dorsal articular margin of the distal end of the bone. The second and fourth metacarpal bones were removed. The articular surface at the distal end of the bone was photographed and the articular cartilage and remaining soft tissues were then digested using 0.15–0.2 M sodium hydroxide at 37°C. The solution was changed as needed every 1 to 3 days. Once the soft tissues were removed, bones were fixed in 70% ethanol and additional photographs of the distal articular surface were made. Severity of the parasagittal crack arrays was graded using a visual analogue scale as previously described [12]. The articular surface was also evaluated for any other pathology before and after digestion. The presence of POD was considered positive if there was discoloration of the cartilage or subchondral bone of the palmar condyle, ulceration/collapse of the cartilage, or presence of subchondral defect in the palmar region of the condyle [26,27]. Severity of POD was also graded using a visual analogue scale [12].

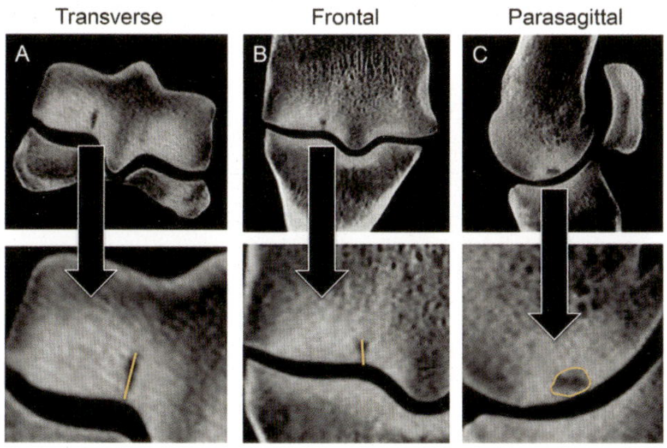

Figure 2. Subchondral fatigue crack dimensions were measured in transverse (**A**) and reconstructed frontal plane (**B**) computed tomography (CT) images. In addition, the area of the crack array was measured in the parasagittal plane (**C**).

Ex-vivo bone loading model

To study subchondral crack micromotion at high loads associated with athletic performance, we developed a non-destructive MC3 bone-loading model. An isolated single bone model was chosen for this work because of the high compressive load used for mechanical testing. Each bone was potted in an aluminum cylinder that was 10 cm long using epoxy (Evercoat 100156 Lite Weight Autobody Filler, Fiber Glass-Evercoat, Cincinnati, OH, USA). An 8 mm hole was drilled in the proximal end of the potted bone and the surrounding cylinder approximately 2 cm from the end of the cylinder, perpendicular to the long axis of the bone and the joint surface, and a stainless steel pin was inserted for additional stability.

Bone specimens without detectable CT lesions in the condylar grooves were used to validate the biomechanical model. Holes, 1.25 mm in diameter, were drilled at the distal palmar aspect of the sagittal ridge and 1 mm abaxial to the condylar groove in the same oblique frontal plate to span the region-of-interest. The potted bone specimen was then positioned in a custom jig (**Fig. 3**). The bones were oriented obliquely in the jig with the palmarodistal aspect facing up in order to mimic compressive loading by the proximal sesamoid bones from weight-bearing. Hypodermic needles (18 gauge) were placed in the drill holes and connected to an extensometer (MTS Systems Corp., Model 632-120-20, Eden Prairie, MN). Lateral and medial condyles of each bone were tested separately. As the bones were not tested destructively each specimen acted as it's own control. Each intact condyle was tested once, in order to obtain a baseline extensometer measurement

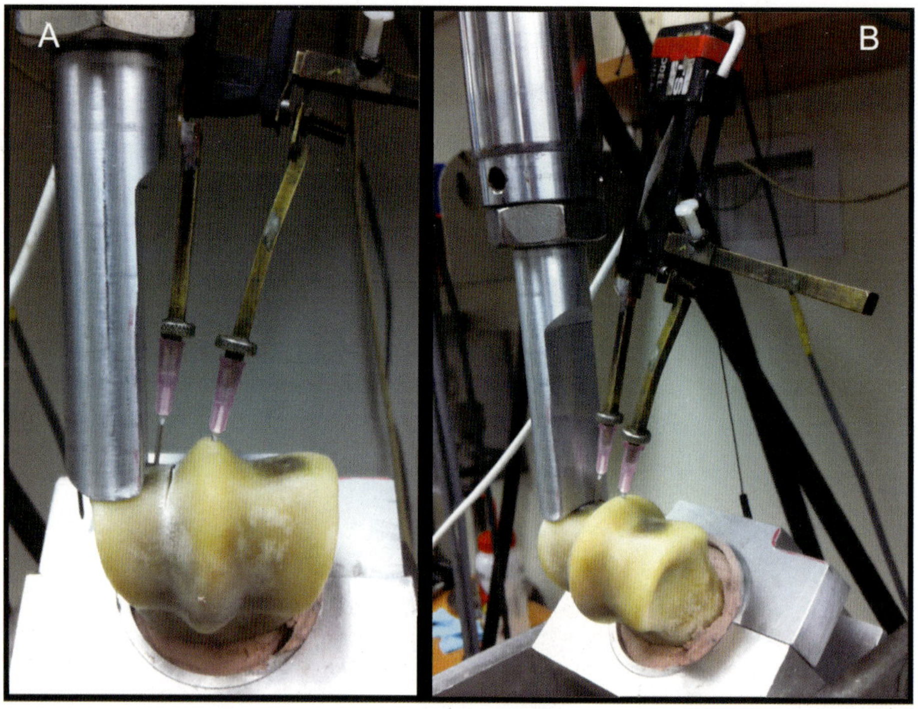

Figure 3. Photograph illustrating the custom-made jig that secures the distal end of the MC3 bone to the platen of a materials testing machine (MTS 858, Minneapolis, MN). (A) Drill holes 1.25 mm in diameter were made on the lateral and medial side of the artificial slot or crack array in the parasagittal condylar groove. (B) Hypodermic needles (18 g) were then placed in the drill holes and attached to an extensometer to measure motion across the slot or crack. The actuator consisted of a metal rod that was contoured to conform to the curved surface of the condyle.

before creation of an artificial subchondral slot to model an in-vivo fatigue crack.

Crack micromotion was measured using a materials testing system (modified MTS Bionics 858 hydraulic test machine; MTS Systems Corp, Eden Prairie, Minneapolis, MN) under load control. Before the mechanical test, each bone was pre-loaded at 100 N. Five cycles of compressive load of 7,500 N were then applied to the condyle abaxial to the extensometer at 0.1 Hz. This load was selected based on biomechanical modeling of fetlock joint loading [20]. Data were collected at 30 Hz for all channels (load, displacement and extensometer motion) and stored on a computer in a data file for future analysis. Mean micromotion for each test was determined by peak-to-peak measurements for the five load cycles. It has been previously estimated that the peak compressive load on the palmar surface of the distal end of the MC3 bone exerted by each proximal sesamoid bone on its respective condyle is at least 7,500 N for a 500 kg horse at the canter, giving rise to a peak stress of 23.9 MNm^{-2} [20].

After an initial baseline testing, an artificial slot was created in the palmar region of the condylar groove using a high-speed rotary tool with a circular diamond wheel, 0.6 mm thick (Dremel 545, Racine, WI) to model a naturally occurring parasagittal array of fatigue cracks. Lateral and medial condyles were randomly assigned to slots that were either 3 mm or 5 mm deep and approximately 18 mm long in a dorsopalmar direction. Mechanical testing was then repeated.

Mechanical testing of parasagittal subchondral fatigue cracks

Bone specimens that were found to have macroscopic parasagittal crack arrays in the condylar groove after cartilage digestion and corresponding lesions detectable on CT cross-sectional images were also tested biomechanically. In order to separate pre-existing fatigue cracking from artifactual damage induced by mechanical testing, a bulk-staining method was used [28]. The entire distal end of the MC3 bone was bulk-stained in 1% basic fuchsin for three days, changing the solution daily. The bones were then placed in 100% ethyl alcohol for 20 minutes before being incrementally rehydrated and then placed in 0.9% saline. The bones were mounted and tested as described above. Movement during loading of the condyle was detected by placement of the extensometer across the array of cracks in the condylar groove. Lateral and medial condyles were again tested separately, but testing was not repeated.

Bone morphometry

After mechanical testing, 1.1 mm thick oblique frontal sections of the distal end of each MC3 bone were prepared using a diamond saw. Sections were cut in a proximodorsal distopalmar plane to pass through the palmar crack array in the condylar groove [12]. Microradiographs (Faxitron, Wheeling, IL, USA) of each section were made for comparison with equivalent frontal plane CT images.

Bone sections were examined for condylar groove cracking [14]. Subchondral cracks that were stained with basic fuchsin were counted within the condylar groove region and normalized to the length of the regional bone boundary to give a crack boundary density (N.Cr/B.Bd, #/mm) by a single observer (KR) [14]. Sections were also examined for unstained artifactual subchondral cracks associated with mechanical testing and bone sectioning. In addition, stained subchondral cracks were examined for evidence of crack extension during mechanical testing.

Statistical analysis

The Shapiro-Wilk test was used to determine whether data approximated a normal distribution. To validate the ex-vivo bone-loading model, baseline extensometer motion was subtracted from extensometer motion recorded after slot creation. Because data did not approximate a normal distribution, the Wilcoxon Signed Rank test was used to determine whether data for each slot group differed from a theoretical median of zero (no extensometer displacement). Distribution of condyles between groups was examined using the Chi-squared test. The Wilcoxon Signed Rank test or the Student's t test for paired data, as appropriate, were used to analyze pathological change in the lateral and medial joint regions. The correlative relationships between measurements of fatigue crack dimensions on CT images and extensometer micromotion and subjective and objective measures of pathologic change in the joint surface were examined using the Spearman Rank test. Baseline micromotion for bones with naturally occurring fatigue cracks was determined from extensometer measurements of all condyles without fatigue cracks evident on CT examination (n = 14 condyles). A mean baseline extensometer reading was subtracted from the mean micromotion value for each bone before analysis. The Spearman Rank test was also used to determine whether a correlative relationship existed between athletic history (horse age, number of race starts, number of career wins, and racing surface [turf or dirt]) and fatigue crack dimensions measured by CT. A similar analysis was performed for crack micromotion measured by mechanical testing, and subjective and objective measurement of pathologic change.

The relationship between fatigue crack micromotion from mechanical testing and crack dimensions was also examined using logistic regression. Extensometer micromotion was coded as 1 – motion is >15% above baseline, or 0 – ≤15% above baseline for condyles without CT evidence of subchondral fatigue cracks from the pool of bones with naturally occurring fatigue crack arrays. 15% above baseline was arbitrarily chosen to create a conservative assessment of crack micromotion within the statistical model. Horse identity and the presence or absence of a proximal sesamoid bone fracture were included as variables in the logistic regression model. For crack measurement methods with significant results in the logistic regression model, postestimation was used to determine probability of a positive outcome for each CT measurement. Results were considered significant at $p<0.05$. Fatigue cracks with a probability estimate >0.8 for micromotion 15% above baseline were considered clinically relevant.

Results

Digital radiography

DR radiographs were made of 76 forelimbs (**Fig. 1**). Fifteen limbs (20%) revealed a fracture of MC3. Eleven limbs (14%) had a condylar fracture (9 lateral and 2 medial). A comminuted diaphyseal fracture was seen in 4 limbs (5%). These limbs were excluded from further analysis (**Fig. 1**). Lesions other than a fracture were identified in distal MC3 bone in 2 of 76 limbs. In one limb, a small radiolucency in the lateral condylar groove was seen, which, subsequently, was associated with a fatigue crack in the subchondral plate identified using CT. Severe POD of both condyles characterized by a subchondral bone defect and associated radiolucency adjacent to the joint surface was seen in another limb. These changes were also visible on CT. Biaxial proximal sesamoid fracture was seen in 12 of 76 limbs (16%) and uniaxial proximal sesamoid fracture was seen in 6 of 76 limbs (8%). Condylar fracture was seen concurrently in three limbs with proximal sesamoid fracture.

Metacarpophalangeal joint osteoarthritis was seen in three limbs, and evidence of rupture of the intersesamoidian ligament (abnormal distance between both proximal sesamoid bones) was seen in one limb. Lateral condylar fracture was also seen concurrently with a comminuted fracture of the proximal phalanx in one limb.

Computed tomography

Sixty-one bones were examined via CT imaging (see Fig. 1 for exclusions). Palmar subchondral bone sclerosis was identified in all condyles studied. Parasagittal crack arrays in the palmar subchondral plate of the distal end of the MC3 bone were identified in 42 of 122 condyles (34%), or 27 of 61 limbs (44%) (Table 1). Of those, 24 were located in a lateral condyle, and 18 in a medial. Fifteen limbs had cracks in both the medial and lateral grooves. The appearance of these subchondral lesions within the condylar grooves varied tremendously in shape and density, ranging from a faint lucency to a distinctive crack in the subchondral plate (Figs. 4, 5). POD was found in 46 of 122 condyles (38%), or 28 of 61 limbs (46%) (Fig. 6). In addition, several other fetlock joint abnormalities were identified, including fractures of the proximal sesamoid bone (15 limbs), osteoarthritis (10 limbs), dorsoproximal proximal phalanx fracture (7 limbs), irregularities on the dorsoproximal aspect of the proximal phalanx (5 limbs), irregularities of the distal mid-sagittal ridge (3 limbs), enthesophytosis of the proximal sesamoid bone (2 limbs), and frontal proximal phalanx fracture (1 limb). Fractures of 26 proximal sesamoid bones were seen. Of the 26 fractures, 12 were comminuted, 7 were mid-body, 5 were basilar, and 2 were apical. Four limbs were not studied further because of the absence of CT lesions (Fig. 1).

Visual examination and photography

The distal end of the MC3 bone was examined in 57 limbs, after exclusion for MC3 fracture (15 limbs) and absence of CT lesions (4 limbs) (**Fig. 1**). On gross examination of the joints before digestion of articular cartilage, multiple different pathologies were identified (**Table 1**).

Wear lines. Wear lines were identified on the cartilage of the distal end of 24 MC3 bones (42%).

Parasagittal subchondral crack arrays. Results are summarized in **Table 2**. Focal or linear cartilage defects were present in the condylar grooves of 58 of 114 condyles (51%). Of these 58 condyles, parasagittal subchondral crack arrays were identified in 33 (57%) after articular cartilage digestion (**Figs. 4, 5**). No cracks in the subchondral plate were seen in the other 25 condyles. After cartilage digestion, subchondral bone crack arrays were identified in 51 of 114 condyles (45%), of which 33 were also identified before cartilage digestion. Of those 51 condyles with visible cracks after removal of the articular cartilage, 28 were evident with CT imaging (55%). Subchondral cracking identified in 11 condyles using CT imaging had no visible lesions in the joint surface of the condylar grooves. Median (range) severity scores for lateral and medial parasagittal linear cartilage defects were 8 (0,48) and 10 (0,42) respectively; severity of disease was not significantly different between lateral and medial condyles. Median (range) severity scores for lateral and medial parasagittal fatigue crack arrays in the subchondral plate were 21.5 (0,92) and 1 (0,90) respectively. Severity of subchondral fatigue damage was increased in the lateral condyle, compared with the medial condyle ($p<0.05$). Severity of subchondral fatigue damage assessed by subjective scoring was not significantly correlated with crack dimensions measured on reconstructed CT images or extensometer micromotion during mechanical testing.

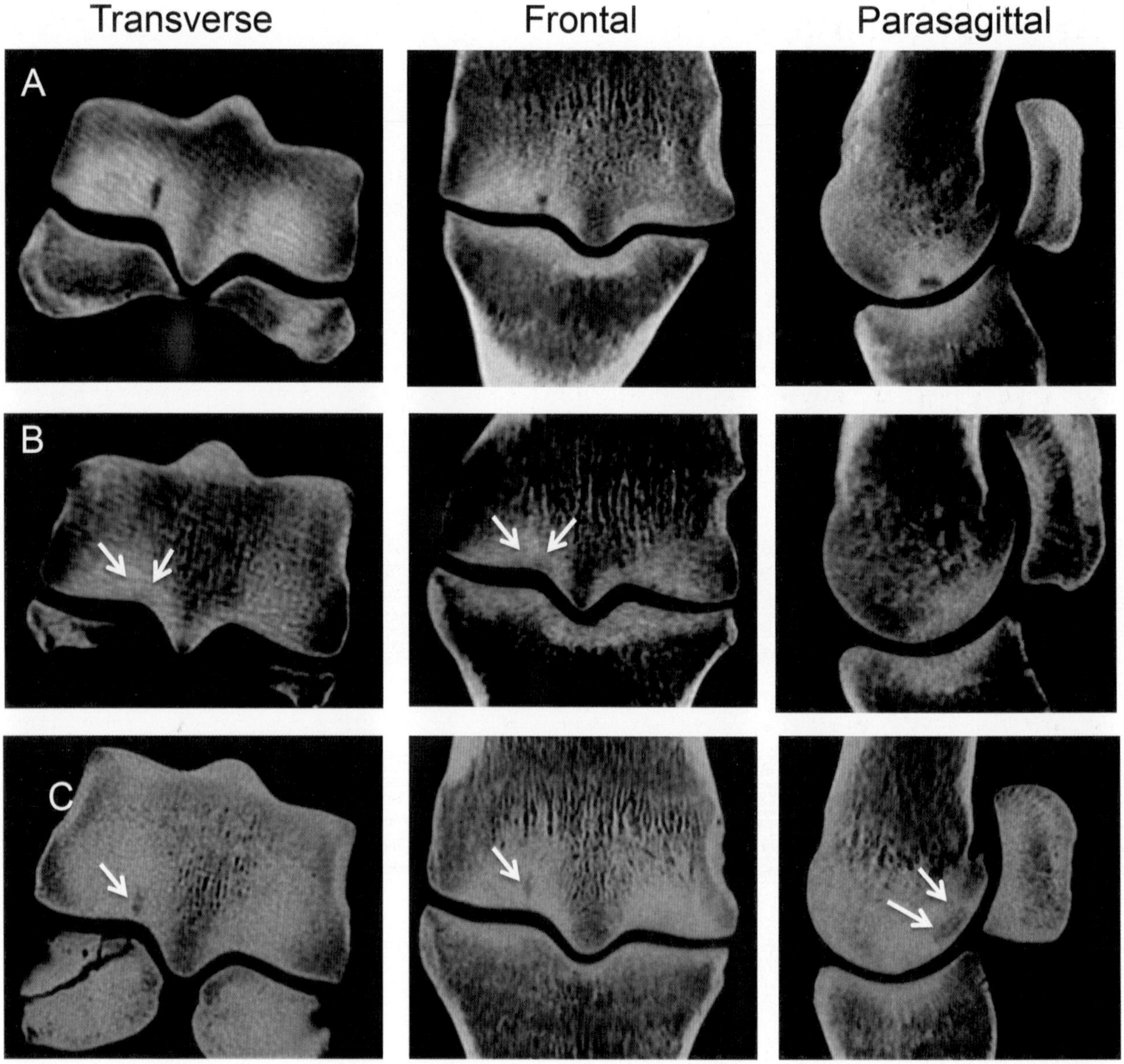

Figure 4. Representative computed tomography images of the distal end of the third metacarpal bone illustrating variation in appearance of parasagittal subchondral crack arrays in the condylar grooves of racing Thoroughbreds. (**A**) A large subchondral crack is evident within the lateral condylar groove. The crack is evident in all three planes. (**B**) In this horse, a small radiolucency is evident in the subchondral plate in the condylar groove (arrows) associated with the presence of a smaller array of fatigue cracks in the transverse and frontal plane images (arrows). (**C**) In this horse, a small well-defined crack is present in the subchondral bone of the medial condylar groove (arrow), which was associated with a large parasagittal crack area that exceeded 30 mm^2. Fracture of the adjacent proximal sesamoid is also evident.

Palmar osteochondral disease. POD was identified in 67 of 114 condyles (59%) after cartilage digestion. Abnormality in the cartilage overlying the subchondral bone lesion was evident in 50 (75%) of these condyles (**Fig. 6, 7**). Of the 67 condyles in which POD was identified after removal of the articular cartilage, 39 were evident with CT imaging (58%). Median (range) severity scores for lateral and medial parasagittal fatigue crack arrays in the subchondral plate were 5 (0,54) and 8 (0,48) respectively. Severity of POD was increased in the medial condyle, compared with the lateral condyle ($p<0.05$).

Ex-Vivo Bone Loading Model

In the 3 mm slot group, there were 22 condyles (14 medial and 8 lateral) analyzed from 19 MC3 bones. In the 5 mm slot group, there were 24 condyles (11 medial and 13 lateral) analyzed from 20 MC3 bones. Three condyles did not yield interpretable data and were excluded due to fracture of the bone during biomechanical testing. Six other condyles were excluded because of failure of extensometer data collection (**Fig. 1**).

There was no significant difference in the distribution of medial to lateral condyles in both groups. In both the 3 mm and 5 mm groups, significant micromotion was detected with compressive

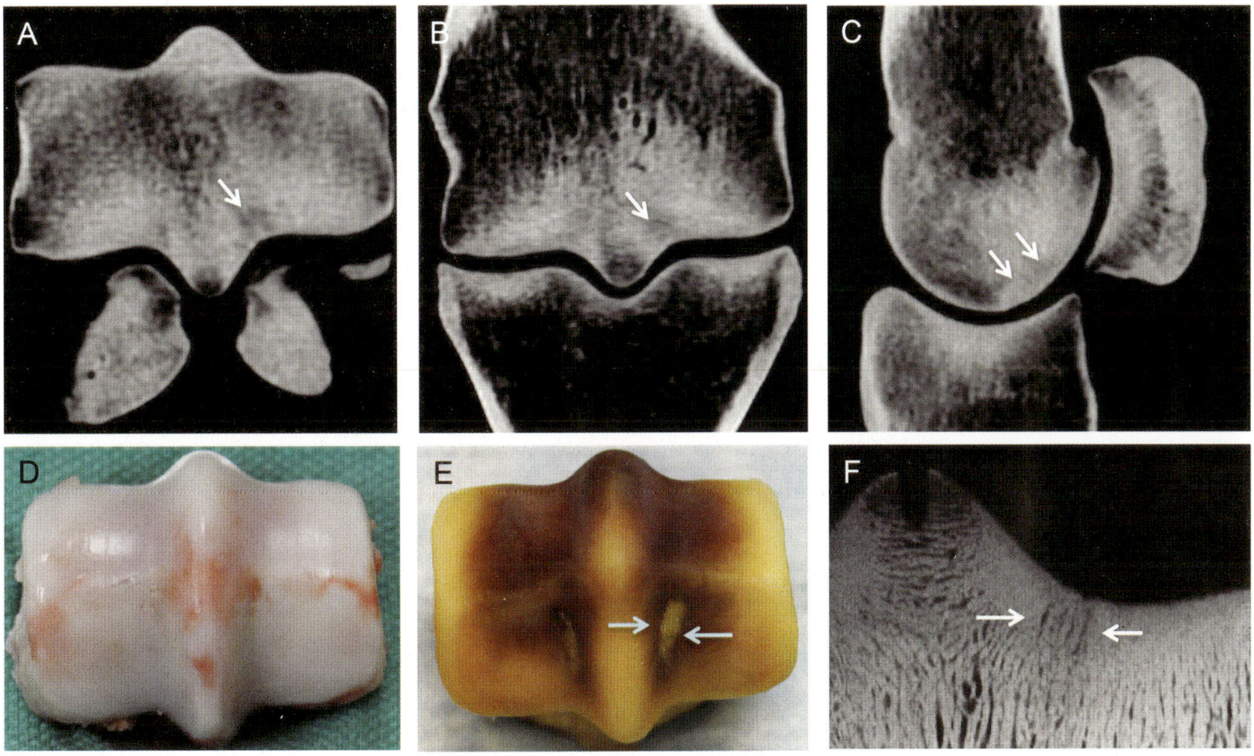

Figure 5. Representative images of the distal end of the third metacarpal bone illustrating the appearance of a large parasagittal subchondral crack array in the lateral condylar groove of the joint surface (arrows) evident on transverse (**A**), frontal (**B**), and parasagittal reconstructed computed tomography images (**C**). A large array of subchondral cracks is present in the subchondral bone of lateral condylar groove (arrows) with relatively little change in the overlying cartilage (**D, E**). An array of fatigue cracks that extend into the proximal part of the subchondral plate is also evident (arrows) on a microradiograph of an oblique frontal bone section (**F**).

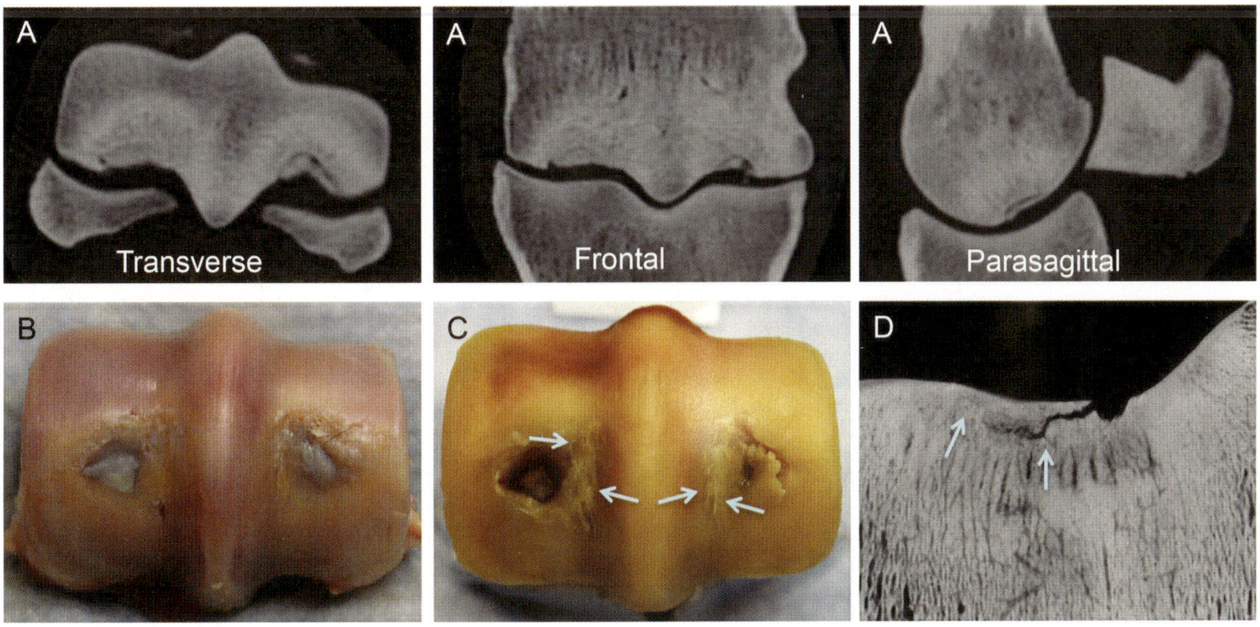

Figure 6. Representative images of the distal end of the third metacarpal bone illustrating articular saucer stress fracture formation in a racing Thoroughbred horse with severe palmar osteochondral disease. (**A**) In reconstructed computed tomography images, a circular articular saucer fracture is present in both condyles. A halo of reduced bone density adjacent to the saucer fracture is caused by the reparative remodeling response in the subchondral plate. Extensive adaptive subchondral sclerosis is also evident. (**B**) Hyaline cartilage overlying the stress fracture has been replaced by fibrocartilage. (**C**) Extensive fatigue damage to the underlying subchondral plate is also evident, including parasagittal cracks in the condylar grooves (arrows). (**D**) Propagation of the fracture line at the interface of the vascular remodeling response to the fatigue injury in the subchondral plate is evident (arrows) on a microradiograph of an oblique frontal bone section.

Table 1. Distribution of fetlock joint abnormalities in Thoroughbred racehorses identified by radiographic imaging and direct observation.

	Digital radiography	Computed tomography	Observation of articular cartilage	Observation of the subchondral plate
	Wear lines			
Horses (n = 38)	n/a	n/a	20 (53%)	n/a
Bones (n = 57)	n/a	n/a	24 (42%)	n/a
Condyles (n = 114)	n/a	n/a	46 (40%)	n/a
	Parasagittal subchondral crack array			
Horses (n = 38)	1 (3%)	21 (55%)	23 (61%)	25 (66%)
Bones (n = 57)	1 (2%)	27 (47%)	31 (54%)	31 (54%)
Condyles (n = 114)	1 (1%)	42 (37%)	58 (51%)	51 (45%)
	Palmar osteochondral disease			
Horses (n = 38)	1 (3%)	19 (50%)	23 (61%)	29 (76%)
Bones (n = 57)	1 (2%)	27 (47%)	32 (56%)	41 (72%)
Condyles (n = 114)	2 (2%)	42 (37%)	53 (46%)	67 (59%)
	Proximal sesamoid fracture			
Horses (n = 38)	15 (39%)	15 (39%)	n/a	n/a
Bones (n = 57)	15 (26%)	15 (26%)	n/a	n/a
Condyles (n = 114)	27 (24%)	27 (24%)	n/a	n/a

Note: One hundred fourteen condyles from 57 MC3 bones from 38 horses were dissected and digested to evaluate the articular surface (see also Fig. 1). Subchondral plate observations were made after cartilage digestion.

loading, ($p<0.001$), with median values of 0.008 mm and 0.038 mm, respectively. Micromotion was significantly increased in the 5 mm slot group when compared with the 3 mm slot group ($p<0.001$) (**Fig. 8**).

Relationship between crack micromotion and crack dimensions derived from computed tomographic imaging

MC3 bones from 24 limbs were used for mechanical testing. Of the 48 condyles, 6 did not yield interpretable data and were excluded because the bone sustained a fracture during mechanical testing. Iatrogenic fractures did not propagate from the condylar groove, and affected either the potted region of the bone shaft (n = 2) or the region of the condyle in direct contact with the actuator (n = 4). Four other condyles were excluded because of failure of extensometer data collection. Mechanical data were acquired for the remaining 38 condyles (**Fig. 1**). These condyles were derived from 21 bones from 18 Thoroughbred horses.

Micromotion 15% above baseline was detected in 18 of 38 condyles (47%) (**Fig. 9**). Median micromotion corrected for the baseline value was 0.007 mm, with a maximum value of 0.103 mm. There was a significant positive correlation between extensometer micromotion and parasagittal crack area measured from reconstructed CT images ($S_R = 0.32$, $p<0.05$). Correlations with transverse and frontal plane crack lengths were not significant. Similarly, correlations with volumetric and surface measurements on 3D reconstructed images were not significant. All CT measurements were significantly correlated with each other ($S_R>0.74$, $p<0.001$). When extensometer motion data were transformed into a binary format, we found a significant relationship between crack dimensions on CT and the presence of fatigue crack micromotion ($p<0.05$ for frontal plane crack length, parasagittal crack area, crack volume, and crack surface area, when data were corrected for motion 15% above baseline (**Table 3**); significance was greatest for parasagittal crack area. For parasagittal crack area, a similar result was obtained with a simple baseline correction ($p = 0.06$). Comparisons of other CT measurements with baseline-corrected crack micromotion were not significant. The presence of a proximal sesamoid fracture was not significantly correlated with subchondral crack micromotion and was not a significant factor in the logistic regression model.

Table 2. Identification of parasagittal subchondral crack arrays in the distal end of the third metacarpal bone of Thoroughbred racehorses by computed tomography and direct observation.

	Computed tomography	Observation of articular cartilage	Observation of the subchondral plate
Computed tomography	42 (37%)		
Observation of articular cartilage	30 (26%)	58 (51%)	
Observation of the subchondral plate	28 (25%)	33 (29%)	51 (45%)

Note: One hundred fourteen condyles from 57 MC3 bones from 38 different horses were dissected and digested to evaluate the articular surface (see also Fig. 1). Data represent number of condyles. Percentages represent proportion of total (114 condyles).

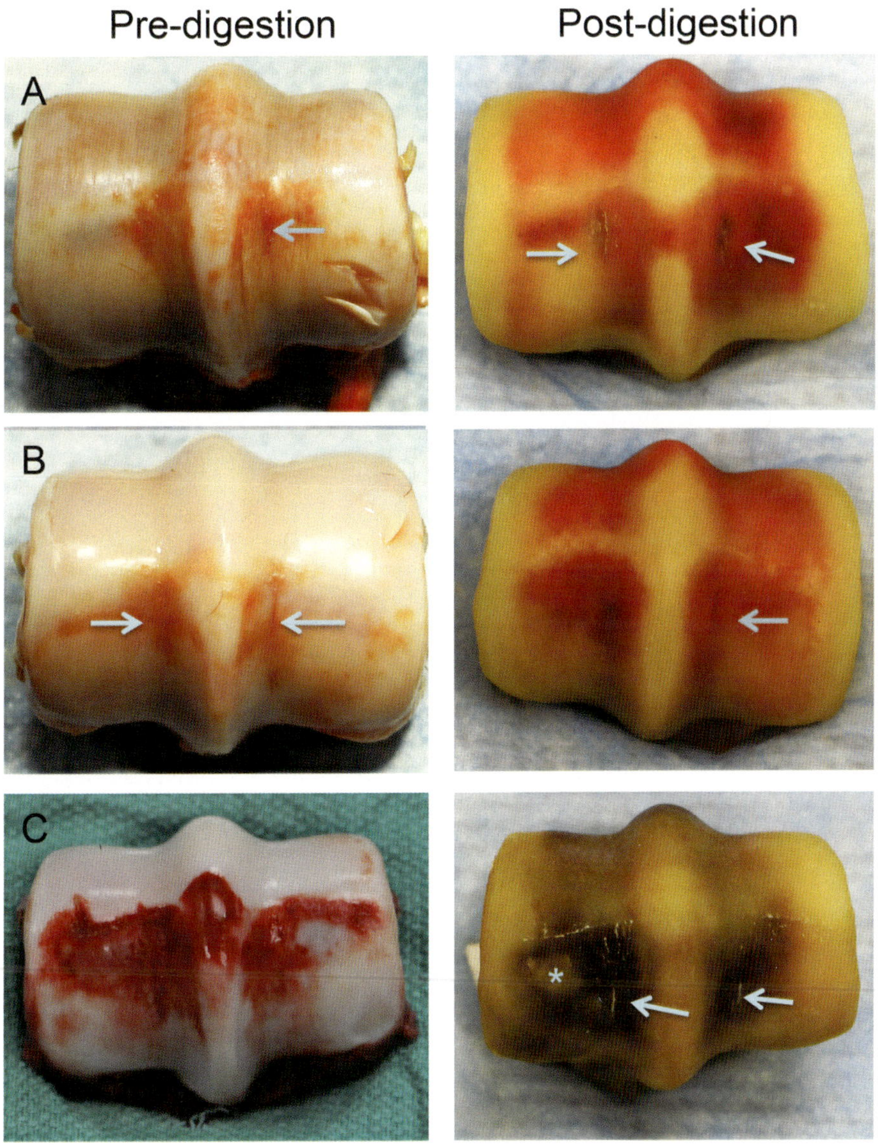

Figure 7. Representative images of the distal end of the third metacarpal bone before and after cartilage digestion illustrating fetlock abnormalities commonly associated with the presence of subchondral fatigue crack arrays. Extensive wear lines in hyaline cartilage (**A**), subchondral bruising (**A–C**) and flattening of the palmar region of the condyles (**C**) were commonly found. In some horses parasagittal defects in the hyaline articular cartilage of the condylar grooves were of mild severity and associated with varying degrees of fatigue cracking of the underlying subchondral plate (arrows) (**A–C**). Palmar osteochondral disease was commonly associated with condylar groove fatigue cracks (* in **C**). Images obtained from the same horses as Figure 4.

In the logistic regression model, 3 of 38 condyles (7.9%) in the limbs of three different horses had parasagittal fatigue cracks in the condylar groove with a parasagittal crack area measurement that exceeded 30 mm^2. Specimens with parasagittal crack area measurements above this value had a probability of >0.8 that crack micromotion in our biomechanical model would exceed baseline +15% and be deemed clinically significant (**Figs. 4,5,7**).

Subchondral fatigue crack histomorphometry

Mean ± standard deviation N.Cr/B.Bd was 0.62±0.34 and 0.55±0.32 respectively for the lateral and medial condyles; severity of histologic fatigue damage was not significantly different between lateral and medial condyles. Severity of histologic fatigue damage was not significantly correlated with crack dimensions measured on reconstructed CT images or extensometer micromotion during mechanical testing. Examination of the oblique frontal bone sections after mechanical loading did not reveal any evidence of crack extension from mechanical testing. One or two unstained cracks were identified in the articular surface of the condylar groove in 6 of 38 condyles after mechanical testing.

Relationship between athletic history and severity of subchondral fatigue damage

Mechanical data were obtained for 38 condyles from 22 limbs of 18 horses. Of these 18 Thoroughbreds, a racing history was available for 15 animals. The study group was comprised of 7 females and 8 males consisting of 5 stallions and 3 geldings. The median age was 4 years old (range of 2 to 8). Median number of career starts was 12 (range of 0 to 46). Seven horses were racing on

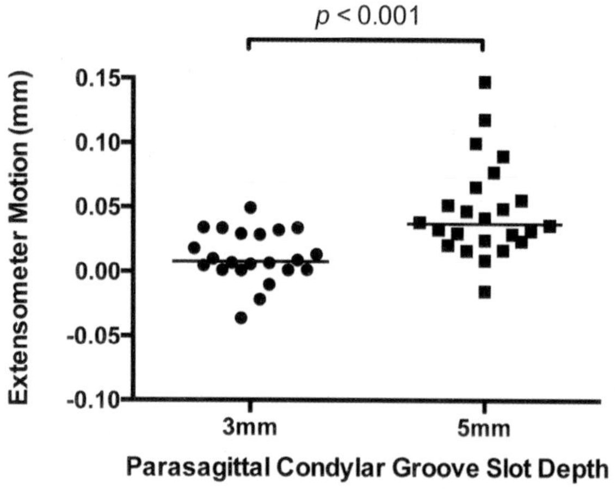

Figure 8. In our ex-vivo biomechanical model, extensometer micromotion associated with creation of shallow parasagittal slots in the palmar region of the condylar groove was used to model naturally occurring arrays of fatigue cracks. In both the 3 mm and 5 mm groups, baseline-corrected extensometer motion was significantly different from zero (no motion) ($p<0.001$). Increased slot depth was associated with increased micromotion. In our model, the condyle was loaded at −7,500 N in compression. In the scatterplot, the horizontal bar represents the median value for each group.

dirt and 4 on turf. One horse never raced. Athletic history was not available for the other three horses. There were no significant correlations between athletic history and the magnitude of parasagittal fatigue crack dimensions from CT imaging of the distal end of the MC3 bone. Similarly, there were no significant correlations between athletic history and detection of crack micromotion. Subjective scoring and histomorphometric assessment of parasagittal subchondral fatigue damage, but not severity of POD, was significantly correlated with horse age and athletic activity (**Table 4**). Significant correlations between severity of subchondral fatigue damage and racing surface were not detected.

Discussion

Collectively, past observations suggest that condylar stress fractures arise from site-specific accumulation of fatigue damage in the subchondral plate of the distal end of the MC3/MT3 bone [12–16]. However, the mechanism by which fatigue damage ultimately precipitates structural failure of the MC3/MT3 bone during athletic activity is poorly understood and little investigated. Results from our ex-vivo model suggest that it is likely that some degree of fatigue crack micromotion is present in a large proportion of Thoroughbred racehorses during training and racing. Although subchondral crack micromotion may not be the only determinant of a stress fracture, microcrack propagation, as opposed to initiation, is likely an important component of stress fracture development [29]. Microstructural features of the subchondral plate, such as resorption spaces, may also have an important role in crack propagation [14,29]. Our results suggest that CT imaging could be used to quantify subchondral fatigue crack dimensions in racing Thoroughbred horses and assess risk of condylar fracture in clinical longitudinal studies. Horses with parasagittal crack arrays that exceed 30 mm^2 may have a high risk for development of condylar fracture; based on our results it is likely that fatigue crack arrays exceeding these dimensions are exposed to micromotion during high speed running and are, therefore, vulnerable to catastrophic crack propagation [14,15].

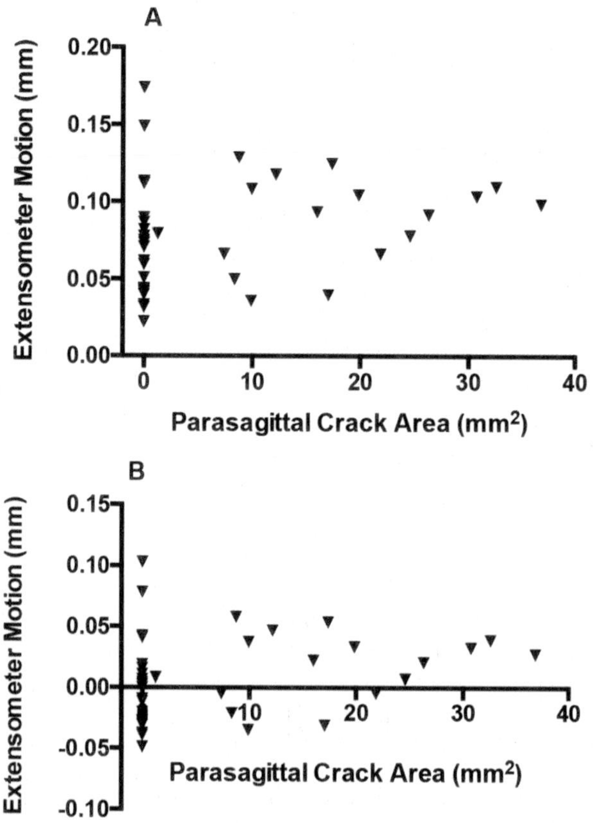

Figure 9. In our ex-vivo biomechanical model, extensometer micromotion associated with naturally occurring parasagittal fatigue cracks in the palmar region of the condylar groove was also determined. (**A**) There was a significant correlation between extensometer motion and parasagittal crack area measured from reconstructed computed tomographic images ($S_R=0.32$, $p<0.05$). (**B**) Extensometer motion corrected for baseline. Micromotion 15% above baseline was detected in 18 of 38 condyles (47%).

During initial screening with DR, we found that condylar fracture was present in 14% of limbs of the Thoroughbred horses in this study. This observation is similar to other epidemiological studies that suggest that condylar stress fracture is commonly associated with catastrophic injuring in racing Thoroughbreds [5–7]. Fractures of the proximal sesamoid bones were also commonly detected using DR and CT imaging in the Thoroughbred horses of the present study. The majority of these were comminuted. Similar observations have been made in clinical studies in Thoroughbred racehorses with catastrophic injuries [6,7].

The lesions we identified on examination of the articular surface before and after cartilage digestion were similar to earlier studies [11,12,23,30] and support the concept that pathological changes to the fetlock joint are common in racing Thoroughbreds, including young horses at the beginning of their racing career.

Previous work from our laboratory suggests that cross-sectional imaging, particularly with CT, is superior to digital radiography for lesion identification in the fetlock joint of racing Thoroughbreds [22,23]. This observation was reaffirmed in the present study. However, CT imaging was only able to identify 55% of condyles with visible subchondral cracking after cartilage digestion. This might be explained by the fact that some visible crack arrays are small and only affect the subchondral bone plate superficially, thus preventing identification on CT examination. Histologic examination of the distal joint surface of the MC3 bone

Table 3. Relationship between computed tomography measurement of parasagittal fatigue crack dimensions and detection of crack micromotion during mechanical loading.

	Statistical Model	Odds ratio	95% Confidence Interval	Likelihood Ratio Chi-square	Significance
Crack length in the transverse plane	Crack length + horse			5.57	0.06
	Crack length				0.41
Crack length in the frontal plane	Crack length + horse			7.79	0.02
	Crack length				0.1
Parasagittal crack area	Crack area + horse			9.53	0.01
	Crack area	1.08	1.00–1.16		0.05
Crack volume	Crack volume + horse			6.90	0.03
	Crack volume				0.17
Crack surface	Crack surface + horse			7.43	0.02
	Crack surface				0.13

Note: A logistic regression model was used to determine whether there was a significant relationship between fatigue crack dimensions determined by measurement from computed tomography images and crack micromotion under clinically relevant joint loads in an ex-vivo model (micromotion corrected to 15% above baseline) (n = 38 condyles from 21 bones from 18 horses). Within the multivariate models of CT measurement parameter and horse identity, parasagittal crack area was the only CT measurement that yielded a significant result.

from racing Thoroughbreds suggests that fatigue injury is initiated in the calcified cartilage of the joint surface [14]. However, in the present study, we found that subchondral cracking identified in 11 condyles on CT imaging had no visible lesions in the joint surface of the condylar grooves after cartilage digestion. This may suggest site-specific remodeling in the subchondral plate proximal to the articular surface is also an early event in the disease mechanism. Alternatively, crack initiation may occur deeper within the subchondral plate in some horses. It should be noted that our evaluation of these condyles occurred at a specific point in time, and cannot consider how adaptive remodeling may lead to changes in pathological features within the subchondral plate over time. Therefore, it is possible that some of these lesions represent the early phase of the damage process before development of a more extensive crack array in the subchondral plate, or alternatively the beginning of a healing process.

The appearance of parasagittal subchondral crack arrays in the condylar grooves of the MC3 joint surface was quite variable using CT imaging. Subchondral cracks surrounded by radiolucency may have a greater area or volume than cracks with more clearly defined margins. This is likely important, as stressed volume is thought to be an important factor in the pathogenesis of stress fracture [31]. Our regression analyses suggested that measurement of parasagittal crack area, as opposed to transverse or frontal plane measurements of crack length, yielded the best predictor of crack micromotion. Detection of radiolucency in the parasagittal condylar groove on CT may suggest that the array of interconnected fatigue cracks occupies a larger volume in the subchondral plate. This concept could be examined by more detailed histomorphometric examination of fatigue-damaged bone with this CT abnormality. In the present study, we did not identify a significant correlation between crack array dimensions on CT and

Table 4. Relationship between athletic history and severity of pathologic change observed in the joint surface of the distal end of the third metacarpal of racing Thoroughbreds.

Parameter	S_R	Significance
Horse age		
Condylar groove cartilage defect severity score	−0.25	NS
Condylar groove subchondral bone damage severity score	0.61	$p<0.001$
N.Cr/B.Bd, #/mm	0.57	$p<0.001$
Number of race starts		
Condylar groove cartilage defect severity score	−0.38	$p<0.05$
Condylar groove subchondral bone damage severity score	0.50	$p<0.005$
N.Cr/B.Bd, #/mm	0.37	$p<0.05$
Number of career wins		
Condylar groove cartilage defect severity score	−0.30	NS ($p=0.09$)
Condylar groove subchondral bone damage severity score	0.35	$p=0.05$
N.Cr/B.Bd, #/mm	0.37	$p<0.05$

Note: Correlations with severity scoring of palmar osteochondral disease were not significant for any athletic history parameter (n = 32 condyles).

objective measurement of histologic fatigue damage or subjective grading of joint pathology. Even though CT imaging was performed at high resolution, precise determination of crack margins was not always straightforward. Improvements in image resolution may help to identify horses with more subtle fatigue damage in the subchondral plate of the distal end of the MC3/MT3 bone.

CT imaging was also able to identify POD in a large proportion of the condyles studied. However, not all POD lesions seen on examination of the subchondral plate after cartilage digestion were evident with CT imaging. The main reason for this discrepancy is that those POD lesions not identified on CT imaging were mostly a discoloration of the palmar condyle area, and not a bony defect. Ten of 24 limbs in the naturally occurring crack group were affected by POD, potentially complicating measurement of subchondral crack motion during mechanical testing. In specimens with this lesion, care was taken to place the extensometer needle axial to the POD lesion. By doing so, any POD-associated micromotion should not be included in the motion measured by the extensometer. Although subchondral bone cracks and POD are different clinical entities, they have a similar etiology and both represent fatigue injury to the joint surface [16]. They are a consequence of repetitive stresses from strenuous exercise [12–14,16,26,27], which predisposes them to occurring simultaneously in the same condyle. It is unclear why some horses develop POD instead of parasagittal subchondral fatigue cracks, or vice versa.

To validate our ex-vivo model, we measured micromotion before and after creation of parasagittal slots of two different depths in the palmar region of the condylar groove. Data from this initial experiment supported the validity of our biomechanical model and yielded micromotion values that approximated the values obtained from bones with naturally occurring fatigue crack arrays. Loading conditions for the model were based on earlier studies [20]. Although removal of the articular cartilage may have influenced load distribution during testing, cartilage removal was necessary to observe parasagittal subchondral crack arrays, if present.

We found evidence of fatigue crack micromotion in 47% of condyles, suggesting that a large proportion of racing Thoroughbreds may experience some degree of crack micromotion in vivo. This is an important observation, since it is unlikely that articular fatigue damage will heal well clinically in the face of ongoing instability from habitual training and racing. Horses with parasagittal crack areas that exceed 30 mm^2 are likely to experience substantial crack micromotion under high joint loads, based on our regression analysis. This result was identified in 7.9% of horses, suggesting that a large number of Thoroughbreds racing in the United States are vulnerable to condylar stress fracture during racing.

In this experiment, extensometer motion was detected in condyles without detectable subchondral crack arrays. This is likely a consequence of the large compressive load that was applied to the joint surface during testing to model weight-bearing during high-speed running. Rotational motion and creep of some of the bones inside the potting cylinder was noticed during the mechanical testing and there was a tendency for some degree of extensometer drift during the five loading cycles of each test. To account for this limitation, mechanical data were baseline-corrected before statistical analysis. Further, we chose to only consider crack micromotion as relevant when it increased ≥15% above baseline. As there is no established model to determine what amount of motion is truly relevant, this value was chosen arbitrarily as a conservative approach to data interpretation. Development of an improved method for measurement of crack motion during mechanical testing may be help improve precision of mechanical testing in future work.

Histomorphometric quantification and severity scoring of subchondral cracking were significantly correlated with horse age and number of race starts, suggesting that accumulation of MC3 subchondral fatigue injury is related to habitual athletic activity. Cumulative cyclic loading of the fetlock is influenced by accumulation of racing starts as well as high-speed timed workout. Another important component of fetlock loading history is the frequency of these events, which can significantly influence risk of a catastrophic musculoskeletal injury [32]. Severity of the defect in the condylar groove cartilage was significantly and inversely related to number of race starts suggesting that cartilage damage is an early feature of joint injury from habitual athleticism. We did not identify any significant correlation between the cumulative racing history and the magnitude of parasagittal fatigue crack dimensions from CT imaging of the distal end of the MC3 bone, or detection of crack micromotion. However, data were only collected from a limited number of horses, so this finding should be interpreted with caution in the absence of relevant data describing the training activity, as the amount and intensity of workout sessions is likely important to accumulation of subchondral fatigue damage over time. More work is needed to comprehensively understand the relationship between athletic history and subchondral fatigue injury. Clinically, condylar fractures are more common in younger horses that may not have an extensive racing history [1,3,25].

A limitation of this project in accurately modeling an *in vivo* scenario was our use of frozen limbs collected from catastrophically injured racing Thoroughbreds. Limbs were thawed for DR and CT imaging and then refrozen until further dissection, digestion, and basic fuchsin staining. It is possible that post-mortem change and freeze-thaw effects could have influenced our results. Such effects are likely relatively small in a high load biomechanical model. Furthermore, all specimens tested were treated in a similar manner. Removal of the articular cartilage was necessary to appreciate the subchondral crack array in the condylar grooves. Another limitation is that we studied an isolated single bone model with our mechanical testing. Therefore, our study does not address the role of the first phalanx in loading of the distal MC3 bone. It is likely that the articulation between the proximal phalanx and the metacarpus and the loading pattern resulting from this is of importance in the pathogenesis of condylar fracture. Although currently unknown, this interaction, as well as the forces placed on the condyles by the adjacent soft tissues structures (collateral ligaments) probably plays a role in the formation and propagation of these fractures. Our goal was to isolate one portion of the bone that is of known importance in condylar fractures to estimate crack micromotion during direct loading via the articulation between the condyle and the sesamoid. While of great importance, addressing the roles of other anatomical structures is outside the scope of this study, but relevant to future work. The presence of a proximal sesamoid fracture was not significantly related to detection of crack micromotion in our model. Although actuator placement modeled the position of the proximal sesamoid during mechanical testing, in-vivo loading of the distal MC3 bone by the proximal sesamoid may be different. This may explain the iatrogenic fracture that occurred in some bones during testing. Finally, athletic history was obtained from a relatively limited number of horses. Additional epidemiological work is needed to comprehensively understand the relationship between habitual athleticism and fetlock injuries, such as accumulation of MC3 subchondral fatigue damage.

The current design of equine CT scanners requires general anesthesia, which limits the use of CT as a diagnostic modality for equine athletes in race training. However, CT scanning of the foot in the standing horse using a gantry in a horizontal orientation has been performed [33]. Results of the present study suggest that this approach to equine CT imaging needs to be expanded to include the fetlock. With cross-sectional imaging of the fetlock, particularly if available as a standing modality, longitudinal screening of a population of Thoroughbred racehorses in training or racing could improve our ability to recognize and monitor the progression of specific pathologic features in vivo. This would be extremely informative to understanding and treatment of distal MC3/MT3 injury or disease. While reduction in joint loading may contribute to bone healing, it is unknown whether healing of condylar groove subchondral cracks occurs if habitual athletic activity is withdrawn.

In conclusion, condylar stress fractures are common in Thoroughbred racehorses. Parasagittal arrays of fatigue cracks in the subchondral plate of the condylar grooves of the distal end of the MC3 bone are readily detectable by CT. Our results suggest that measurement of crack area on reconstructed parasagittal CT images is a predictive marker for crack micromotion at joint loads associated with high-speed running. Consequently, this parameter may prove to be a useful predictive marker for condylar fracture risk in longitudinal in-vivo studies of Thoroughbred racehorses. Improved determination of fracture risk promises reduction in serious injuries during racing and better clinical management of horses with incipient condylar fracture. Furthermore, such knowledge promises improved understanding of the epidemiological relationship between habitual athletic activity and fetlock breakdown injury.

Acknowledgements

The authors gratefully acknowledge the help of all the Comparative Orthopaedic Research Laboratory students who contributed to this project. Molly VanBommel provided assistance with bone sectioning.

Author Contributions

Conceived and designed the experiments: P. Muir MDM RV RPM. Performed the experiments: MSD SM KR VK ZH RPM P. Muir. Analyzed the data: MSD P. Muir. Wrote the paper: MSD SM P. Muir. Contributed limb specimens for analysis: P. Marquis.

References

1. Richardson DW (1984) Medial condylar fractures of the third metatarsal bone in horses. J Am Vet Med Assoc 185: 761–765.
2. Bassage LH, Richardson DW (1998) Longitudinal fractures of the condyles of the third metacarpal and metatarsal bones in racehorses: 224 cases (1986–1995). J Am Vet Med Assoc 212: 1757–1764.
3. Ellis DR (1994) Some observations on condylar fractures of the third metacarpus and third metatarsus in young Thoroughbreds. Equine Vet J 26: 178–183.
4. Zekas LJ, Bramlage LR, Embertson RM, Hance SR (1999) Results of treatment of 145 fractures of the third metacarpal/metatarsal condyles in 135 horses (1986–1994). Equine Vet J 31: 309–313.
5. McKee SL (1995) An update on racing fatalities in the UK. Equine Vet Educ 7: 202–204.
6. Stover SM, Murray A (2008) The California Postmortem Program: Leading the Way. Vet Clin North Am Equine Pract 24: 21–36.
7. Clegg PD (2011) Musculoskeletal disease and injury, now and the future. Part 1: Fractures and fatalities. Equine Vet J 43: 643–649.
8. Rooney JR (1974) Distal condylar fractures of the cannon bone in the horse. Mod Vet Pract 55: 113–114.
9. Kaneko M, Oikawa M, Yoshihara T (1993) Pathological analysis of bone fractures in racehorses. J Vet Med Sci 55: 181–183.
10. Krook L, Maylin G (1988) Fractures in Thoroughbred racehorses. Cornell Vet 78: 7–133.
11. Riggs CM, Whitehouse GH, Boyde A (1999) Pathology of the distal condyles of the third metacarpal and third metatarsal bone of the horse. Equine Vet J 31: 140–148.
12. Radtke CL, Danova NA, Scollay MC, Santschi EM, Markel MD, et al. (2003) Macroscopic changes in the distal ends of the condyles of the third metacarpal and third metatarsal bone in Thoroughbred racehorses with condylar fracture. Am J Vet Res 64: 1110–1116.
13. Stepnik MW, Radtke CL, Scollay MC, Oshel PE, Albrecht RM, et al. (2004) Scanning electron microscopic examination of third metacarpal/third metatarsal bone failure surfaces in Thoroughbred racehorses with condylar fracture. Vet Surg 33: 2–10.
14. Muir P, McCarthy J, Radtke CL, Markel MD, Santschi EM, et al. (2006) Role of endochondral ossification of articular cartilage and functional adaptation of the subchondral plate in the development of fatigue microcracking of joints. Bone 38: 342–349.
15. Currey JD (2003) How well are bones designed to resist fracture? J Bone Miner Res 18: 591–598,
16. Muir P, Peterson AL, Sample SJ, Scollay MC, Markel MD, et al. (2008) Exercise-induced metacarpophalangeal joint adaptation in the Thoroughbred racehorse. J Anat 213: 706–717.
17. Rubin CT, Lanyon LE (1982) Limb mechanics as a function of speed and gait: A study of function strains in the radius and tibia of the horse and dog. J Exp Biol 101: 187–211.
18. Nunamaker DM, Butterweck DM, Provost MT (1990) Fatigue fractures in Thoroughbred racehorses: Relationships with age, peak bone strain, and training. J Orthop Res 8: 604–611.
19. Reilly GC, Currey JD, Goodship AE (1997) Exercise of young Thoroughbred horses increases impact strength of the third metacarpal bone. J Orthop Res 15: 862–868.
20. Riggs CM, Whitehouse GH, Boyde A (1999) Structural variation of the distal condyles of the third metacarpal bone and third metatarsal bone in the horse. Equine Vet J 31: 130–139.
21. Boyde A, Haroon Y, Jones SJ, Riggs CM (1999) Three dimensional structure of the distal condyles of the third metacarpal bone of the horse. Equine Vet J 31: 122–129.
22. Morgan JW, Santschi EM, Zekas LJ, Scollay-Ward MC, Markel MD, et al. (2006) Comparison of radiography and computed tomography to evaluate metacarpo/metatarsophalangeal joint pathology of paired limbs of Thoroughbred racehorses with severe condylar fracture. Vet Surg 35: 611–617.
23. O'Brien T, Baker TA, Brounts SH, Sample SJ, Markel MD, et al. (2011) Detection of articular pathology of the distal aspect of the third metacarpal bone in Thoroughbred racehorses: Comparison of radiography, computed tomography, and magnetic resonance imaging. Vet Surg 40: 942–951.
24. Zekas LJ, Bramlage LR, Embertson RM, Hance SR (1999) Characterization of the type and location of fractures of the third metacarpal/metatarsal condyles in 135 horses in central Kentucky (1986–1994). Equine Vet J 31: 304–308.
25. Jacklin BD, Wright IM (2012) Frequency distributions of 174 fractures of the distal condyles of the third metacarpal and metatarsal bones in 167 Thoroughbred racehorses (1999–2009). Equine Vet J 44: 707–713.
26. Hornof WJ, O'Brien TR, Pool RR (1981) Osteochondritis dissecans of the distal metacarpus in the adult racing Thoroughbred horse. Vet Radiol 22:98–106.
27. Pool RR (1996) Pathologic manifestations of joint disease in the athletic horse. In: McIlwraith CW, Trotter GW, editors. Joint Disease in the Horse. Philadelphia: W.B Saunders. pp 87–104.
28. Burr DB, Hooser M (1995) Alterations to the en bloc basic fuchsin staining protocol for the demonstration of microdamage produced in vivo. Bone 17: 431–433.
29. Taylor D, O'Reilly P, Vallet L, Lee TC (2003) The fatigue strength of compact bone in torsion. J Biomech 36:1103–1109.
30. Barr ED, Pinchbeck GL, Clegg PD, Boyde A, Riggs CM (2009) *Post mortem* evaluation of palmar osteochondral disease (traumatic osteochondrosis) of the metacarpo/metatarsophalangeal joint in Thoroughbred racehorses. Equine Vet J 41:366–371.
31. Taylor D (1998) Fatigue of bone and bones: An analysis based on stress volume. J Orthop Res 16:163–169.
32. Estberg L, Gardner IA, Stover SM, Johnson BJ (1998) A case-crossover study of intensive racing and training schedules and risk of catastrophic musculoskeletal injury and lay-up in California Thoroughbred racehorses. Prev Vet Med 33:159–170.
33. Desbrosse FG, Vandeweerd JMEF, Perrin RAR, Clegg PD, Launois MT, et al (2008) A technique for computed tomography (CT) of the foot in the standing horse. Equine Vet Educ 20:93–98.

The Mechanical Benefit of Medial Support Screws in Locking Plating of Proximal Humerus Fractures

Wen Zhang[1], **Langqing Zeng[2]**, **Yanjie Liu[1]**, **Yao Pan[1]**, **Wei Zhang[1]**, **Changqing Zhang[1]**, **Bingfang Zeng[1]**, **Yunfeng Chen[1]***

1 Department of Orthopaedic Surgery, Shanghai Jiao Tong University Affiliated Sixth People's Hospital, Shanghai Jiao Tong University, Shanghai, China, 2 Department of Orthopaedics, Zhuhai People's Hospital, Jinan University Affiliated Zhuhai Hospital, Guangdong, China

Abstract

Background: The purpose of this study was to evaluate the biomechanical advantages of medial support screws (MSSs) in the locking proximal humeral plate for treating proximal humerus fractures.

Methods: Thirty synthetic left humeri were randomly divided into 3 subgroups to establish two-part surgical neck fracture models of proximal humerus. All fractures were fixed with a locking proximal humerus plate. Group A was fixed with medial cortical support and no MSSs; Group B was fixed with 3 MSSs but without medial cortical support; Group C was fixed with neither medial cortical support nor MSSs. Axial compression, torsional stiffness, shear stiffness, and failure tests were performed.

Results: Constructs with medial support from cortical bone showed statistically higher axial and shear stiffness than other subgroups examined ($P<0.0001$). When the proximal humerus was not supported by medial cortical bone, locking plating with medial support screws exhibited higher axial and torsional stiffness than locking plating without medial support screws ($P\leq0.0207$). Specimens with medial cortical bone failed primarily by fracture of the humeral shaft or humeral head. Specimens without medial cortical bone support failed primarily by significant plate bending at the fracture site followed by humeral head collapse or humeral head fracture.

Conclusions: Anatomic reduction with medial cortical support was the stiffest construct after a simulated two-part fracture. Significant biomechanical benefits of MSSs in locking plating of proximal humerus fractures were identified. The reconstruction of the medial column support for proximal humerus fractures helps to enhance mechanical stability of the humeral head and prevent implant failure.

Editor: Mikko Lammi, University of Eastern Finland, Finland

Funding: There were no funding sources for this study.

Competing Interests: The authors have declared that no competing interests exist.

* Email: chenyunfeng1969@163.com

These authors contributed equally to this work.

Introduction

Proximal humerus fractures account for approximately 5% of all fractures [1–3]. Surgical intervention is generally accepted for unstable fractures, including displaced fractures and fractures associated with osteoporosis. Recent research noted a high failure rate(8.6%–22.0%) after open reduction and internal fixation (ORIF) of proximal humerus fractures [4–7]. Fixation without the reconstruction of medial support is considered one of the risk factors of implant failure [5]. Gardner et al. demonstrated the direct association between medial support and subsequent loss of reduction [8]. Zhang et al. found that insertion of a medial support screw (MSS) into the medio-inferior region increased the stability of fixation of complex fractures and reduced the risk of implant failure[9]. When medial comminution and malreduction are present at the proximal humerus, the insertion of a MSS precisely to the medio-inferior region of the humeral head is one method to reconstruct the medial column support.

Investigation into the value of MSSs in the treatment of proximal humerus fractures has been limited to clinical outcome studies. No biomechanical studies have been reported. The purpose of this study was to evaluate the biomechanical advantages of MSSs in the locking plate for the treatment of proximal humerus fractures and to use this information to guide clinical practice.

Methods

A total of 30 adult synthetic left humeri (HI-C type, Orthobone, Hangzhou, China) and 30 sets of proximal humerus locking plates and screws (Double medical, Xiamen, China) (Fig. 1) were prepared. All the mechanical tests were performed on an Axial-Torsional Biomechanical Testing System (301.6 Shore Western Manufacturing, California,USA) with the following load cell characteristics: a maximum force rating of 3,200 pounds (14.2 kN) and a stroke of four inches (100 mm). The torsional

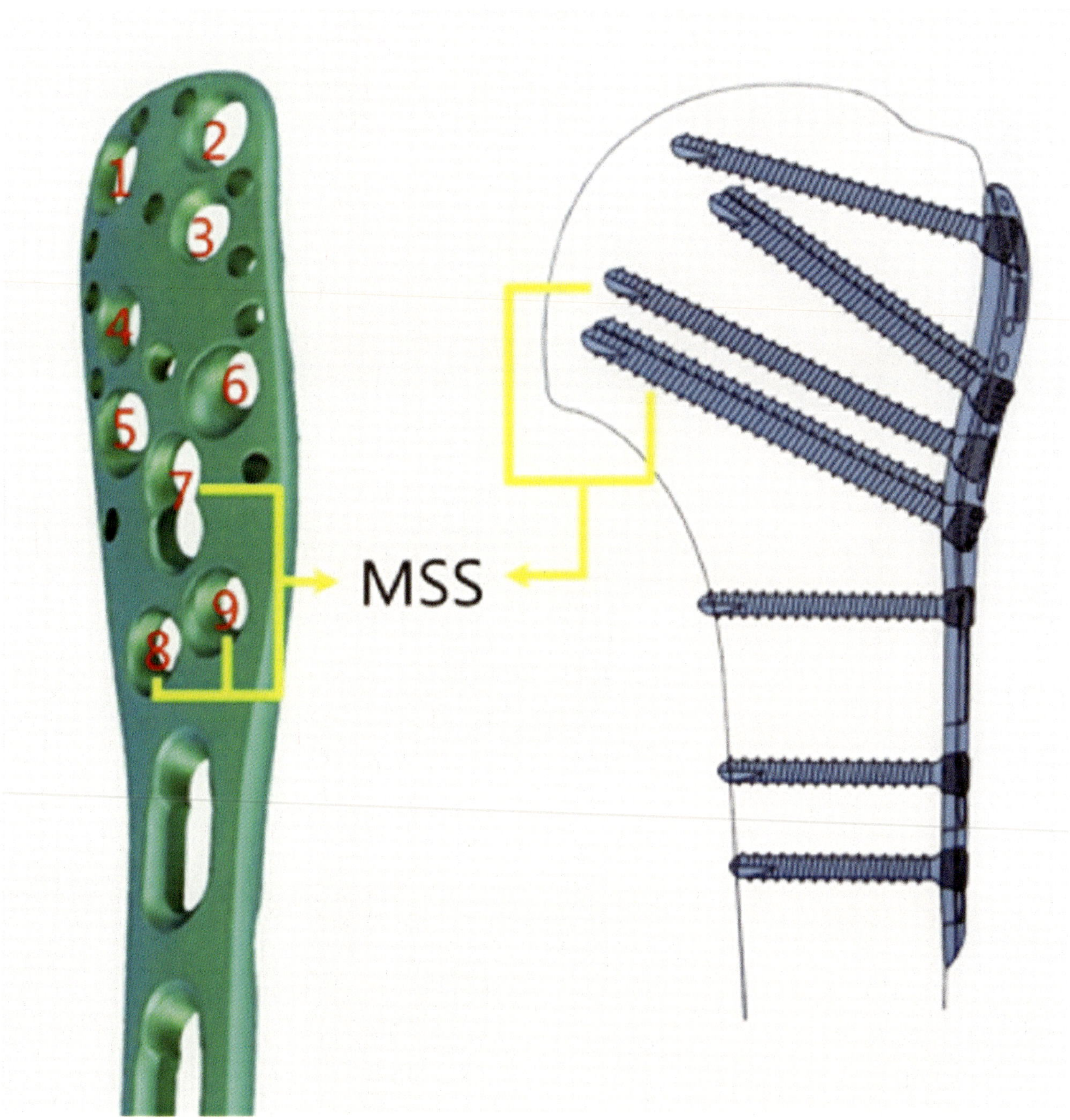

Figure 1. The proximal screw distribution and the medial support screws (MSS) for the locking proximal humerus plate.

rating on this unit is 1,000 inch-pounds (120 Nm) with a rotary motion capability of ±140°.

The 30 synthetic humeri were randomly divided into three groups (*ie*, Groups A, B, and C with 10 specimens/group). A two-part surgical neck fracture was created in each proximal humerus, and all fractures were fixed with a locking proximal humerus plate.

Fracture groups

Group A (Fig. 2a and Fig. 2d). Ten proximal humerus fractures were fixed with medial cortical support; however, MSSs were not used. A horizontal line (line A) was made 1 cm distal to the humeral head, and transverse osteotomies were created along this line using an industrial bandsaw to simulate a two-part surgical neck fracture of the proximal humerus. Fractures were anatomically reduced and fixed with a locking proximal humerus plate. Six locking screws were inserted into the proximal holes of the plate from No. 1 to No. 6. (Fig 1).

Group B (Fig. 2b and Fig. 2e). Ten proximal humerus fractures were fixed with 3 MSSs; however, no medial cortical support was provided. A horizontal line (line A) was made 1 cm distal to the humeral head. The intersection of line A and the lateral cortex of the proximal humeral metaphysis was identified, and a line (line B) was drawn from this point to the most medio-inferior point of the humeral head. Wedge osteotomies were created along lines A and

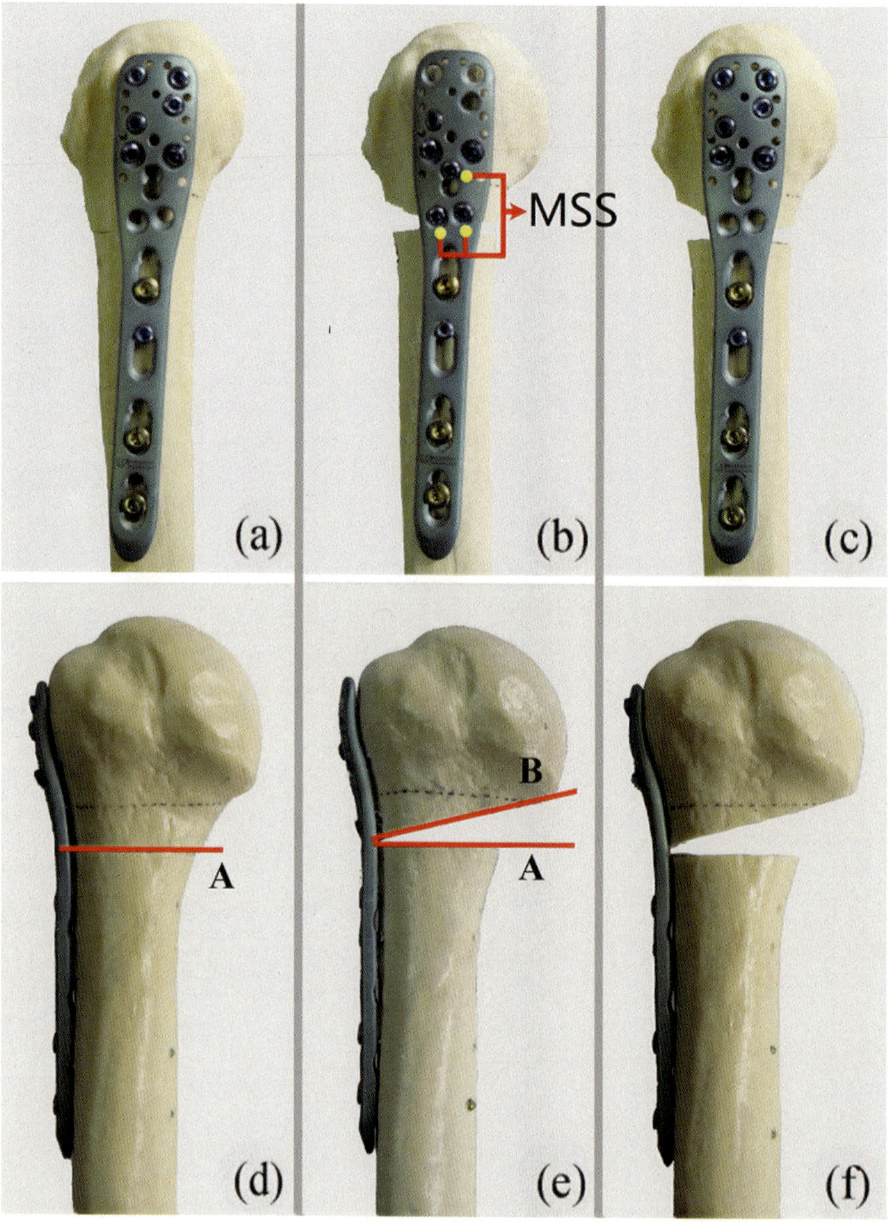

Figure 2. Division of the proximal humerus fracture models. In group A, proximal humerus fractures were fixed without MSSs (Fig.2a); transverse osteotomies were created along a horizontal line (line A) (Fig. 2d). In group B, proximal humerus fractures were fixed with 3MSSs(Fig.2b); wedge osteotomies were created along a horizontal line(line A) and an oblique line (line B) to simulate medial comminution of the proximal humerus(Fig. 2e). In group C, proximal humerus fractures were fixed without medial cortical support or MSSs(Fig.2c); wedge osteotomies were created identical to group B (Fig. 2f).

B to simulate medial comminution of the proximal humerus. Three locking screws were inserted through holes No. 7–9(Fig 1) into the medio-inferior region of the humeral head at the proximal part of the plate. Another three screws were randomly inserted into the other six holes (No. 1–6) of the proximal part of the plate.

Group C (Fig. 2c and Fig. 2f). Ten proximal humerus fractures were fixed without medial cortical support or MSSs. The fracture model was constructed identical to Group B. However, six locking screws were inserted into holes No. 1 to 6 of the proximal part of the plate.

The proximal screws in all three groups were inserted 5 to 8 mm below the subchondral bone to simulate clinical practice [10]. Humeral shafts were fixed with one cortical screw and three locking screws. Plate-bone gap was not present in all experimental models. The distal part of the humeri were removed 15 cm distal to line A. Specimens were 20 cm long, and the distal portion of each specimen was fixed by a square steel chamber filled with a commercially-available anchoring cement to a depth of 12 cm.

Biomechanical testing

Axial stiffness. Each humerus was oriented vertically in the coronal and sagittal planes. Using a plate attached to the mechanical tester, axial compression was applied with a vertical load at the apex of the humeral head using displacement control (max deflection = 0.5 mm; load rate = 5 mm/min [11]; preload = 50 N). The maximum load was recorded, and the slope of the load-deflection curve was used to compute the axial baseline stiffness. Each test was repeated three times, and the average maximum load and average stiffness were calculated (Fig. 3a). Every specimen was kept within the linear elastic region to prevent any permanent damage (average linearity coefficient R^2>0.99). No visual evidence of damage was noted.

Torsional stiffness. Each humerus was positioned inside the cup of a cylindrical stainless steel block and secured using three 4.0 mm screws that were inserted into the humeral head. A torque was applied using displacement control (maximum angulation = 5°; rate = 12°/min; pre-torque = 0 Nm) to simulate rotation of the humeral head. The maximum torque was recorded, and the slope of the torque-angulation graph was used to determine torsional stiffness. The application of torque was repeated three times, and an average maximum torque and average torsional stiffness were calculated (Fig. 3b). All specimens were kept within the linear elastic region to avoid permanent specimen damage (average linearity coefficient R^2>0.99). No visual evidence of damage was noted.

Shear stiffness. Each humerus was mounted distally in a vice with the shaft axis in 20° of abduction(Fig.3c) as recommended by Koval et al. in order to simulate the shear loading across a proximal fracture site experienced when rising out of a chair or crutch weight bearing [11].The same test procedure as that with axial stiffness testing was performed, except that maximum displacement was 1.0 mm. Load levels were chosen to prevent permanent damage to the specimens. All specimens remained within the linear elastic region to avoid permanent damage (average linearity coefficient R^2>0.99). No visual damage was noted.

Strength testing. Load-to-failure in shear for each of the three groups was determined using displacement control (load rate = 5 mm/min; preload = 50 N) to apply a vertical force to generate shear compression on each specimen oriented 20° in abduction (Fig.3c). The force was applied until catastrophic failure of the implant occurred. The highest peak load was determined to indicate significant structural collapse [11]. Catastrophic fracture patterns of the bone and implant were examined and recorded.

Statistical analysis

For the statistical analysis, the SAS 11.0 (SAS Institute Inc, North Carolina, USA) was used. Statistical analyses were performed by an independent statistician blinded to surgical outcomes. The Student's t-test was employed with the one-way analysis of variance (ANOVA) test used for continuous variables. The Turkey *post hoc* test was used to differentiate groups for statistical differences. The level of statistical significance was set to $P<0.05$. The chi-square test or the Fisher's exact test was employed for binary variables with the level of statistical significance set to $P<0.05$.

Results

There was no evidence of plate or screw loosening or breakage. No fractures occurred during axial, torsional and shear stiffness tests. The results of four different load tests for the three groups are shown in Table 1.

Axial stiffness

The maximum load (max displacement = 0.5 mm) and the axial stiffness showed statistical differences between the groups (Group A> Group B> Group C; $P\leq0.0207$) (Fig. 4a, Fig 4b).

The maximum loads were 240.88 N±19.13 in Group A, 169.04 N±19.26 in Group B, and 128.58 N±17.53 in Group C. The axial stiffness was 424.4 N/mm ±101.2 for Group A, 230.7 N/mm ±40.54 for Group B, and 147.0 N/mm ±29.2 for Group C.

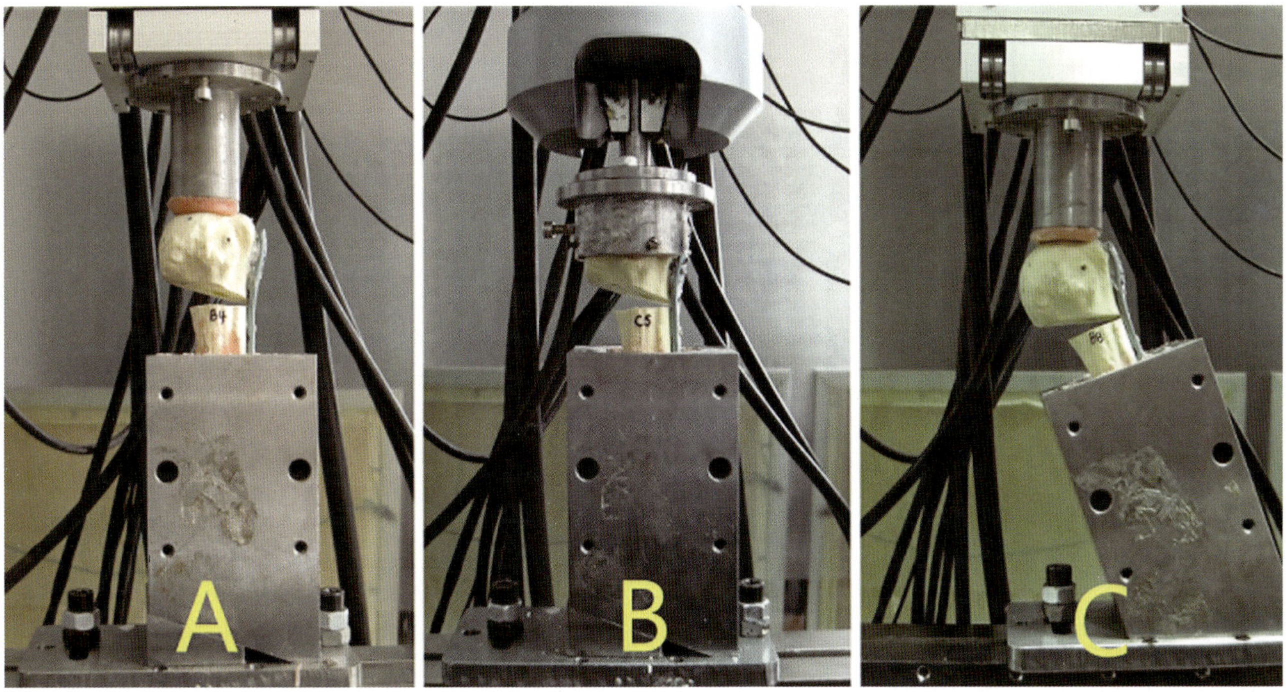

Figure 3. Mechanical test modes used to assess the (A) axial stiffness; (B) torsional stiffness; and (C) shear stiffness and load-to-failure of the plated humeral constructs.

Table 1. The results under four different load tests for the three groups ($\bar{x}\pm sd$, n = 10).

Group	Torsional stiffness test (max angulation = 5°)		Axial stiffness test (max displacement = 0.5 mm)		Shear stiffness test (max displacement = 1 mm)		Shear failure test
	Maxtorque (NM)	Torsional stiffness (NM/deg)	Max load (N)	Axial stiffness (N/mm)	Max load (N)	Shear stiffness (N/mm)	Shear failure load (N)
Group A	8.92±0.25	1.80±0.07	240.9±19.1	424.4±101.2	444.7±20.9	470.0±54.4	2949.8±355.1
Group B	9.09±0.31	1.86±0.07	169.0±19.3^{a}	230.7±40.54^{a}	228.8±29.0^{a}	183.9±29.6^{a}	2448.1±402.4^{a}
Group C	7.57±0.53^{a,b}	1.53±0.10^{a,b}	128.6±17.5^{a,b}	147.0±29.2^{a,b}	188.7±26.2^{a,b}	140.2±32.1^{a}	2222.6±336.4^{a}
F value	47.06	45.14	92.94	47.67	290.53	198.05	10.36
P value	<.0001	<.0001	<.0001	<.0001	<.0001	<.0001	0.0005
Comparison	A vs B: 0.6086	A vs B: 0.2738	A vs B: <0.001	A vs B: <0.001	A vs B: <0.001	A vs B: <0.001	A vs B: 0.0131
of three	A vs C: <0.001	A vs C: <0.001	A vs C: <0.001	A vs C: <0.001	A vs C: <0.001	A vs C: <0.001	A vs C: 0.0004
group	B vs C: <0.001	B vs C: <0.001	B vs C: <0.001	B vs C: 0.0207	B vs C: 0.0044	B vs C: 0.0561	B vs C: 0.3655

[a]compared with group A, P<0.05;
[b]compared with group B, *P*<0.05.

Torsional stiffness

The maximum load of Group C (7.57 Nm ±0.53) was statistically different from both Group A (8.92 Nm ±0.25) and Group B (9.09 Nm ±0.31) (Group A> Group C, Group B> Group C; $P<0.0001$). The torsional stiffness of Group C (1.53 Nm/deg ±0.10) was statistically different from both Group A (1.80 Nm/deg ±0.07) and Group B (1.86 Nm/deg ±0.07) (Group A> Group C, Group B> Group C; $P<0.0001$); however, the comparisons of Groups A and B for maximum load ($P = 0.6086$) and torsional stiffness ($P = 0.2738$) were not significantly different (Fig 4c, Fig 4d).

Shear stiffness

The maximum load between subgroups showed statistical differences (Group A> Group B> Group C; $P\leq0.0044$)(Fig 4e). The values were 444.7 N ±20.9 for Group A, 228.8 N±29.0 for Group B, and 188.7 N±26.2 for Group C.

The shear stiffness of Group A(470.0 N/mm ±54.4) was statistically different from both Group B(183.9 N/mm ±29.6) and Group C(140.2 N/mm ±32.1)(Group A>Group B, Group A>Group C; P<0.001); however, the comparisons of Group B and Group C for shear stiffness were not significantly different(P = 0.056). (Fig 4f).

Shear failure

The load-to-failure of Group A (2949.76 N±355.08) was statistically different from both Group B (2448.13 N±402.39) and Group C (2222.55 N±336.41) (Group A> Group B, Group A > Group C; $P\leq0.0131$); however, no statistical differences were noted between Group B and Group C ($P = 0.3655$). (Fig. 4g).

Shear failure mode

In group A, seven specimens failed by humeral shaft fracture (Fig. 5A), and three specimens failed by humeral head fracture. No plate bending occurred in Group A. In group B, five specimens failed by plate bending with humeral head collapse, and five specimens failed by humeral head fracture (Fig. 5B). In group C, six specimens failed by significant plate bending with humeral head collapse (Fig. 5C), and four specimens failed by humeral head fracture.

Discussion

Biomechanical tests are currently being used in studies of fracture fixation [11–14]. In the current study, biomechanical tests showed that medial support from cortical bone in the proximal humerus provided the best stability when locking plates were used to treat proximal humerus fractures. When the proximal humerus was not supported by medial cortical bone, locking plating with MSSs exhibited higher biomechanical performance than locking plating without MSSs. There were differences among the three groups in the mode of failure. When the proximal humerus was supported by medial cortical bone, specimens showed no evidence of plate bending and failed primarily by fracture of the humeral shaft or humeral head. When the proximal humerus was not supported by medial cortical bone, specimens failed primarily by significant plate bending at the fracture site during axial loading. The humeral head was then crushed by the medial cortical bone of the humeral shaft, which caused a humeral head fracture.

A recent biomechanical study by Lescheid et al. also demonstrated that locking plating with medial cortical support was more resistant to axial compression and shear force compared with locking plating without medial cortical support [12]. However, there was no significant difference between specimens with medial

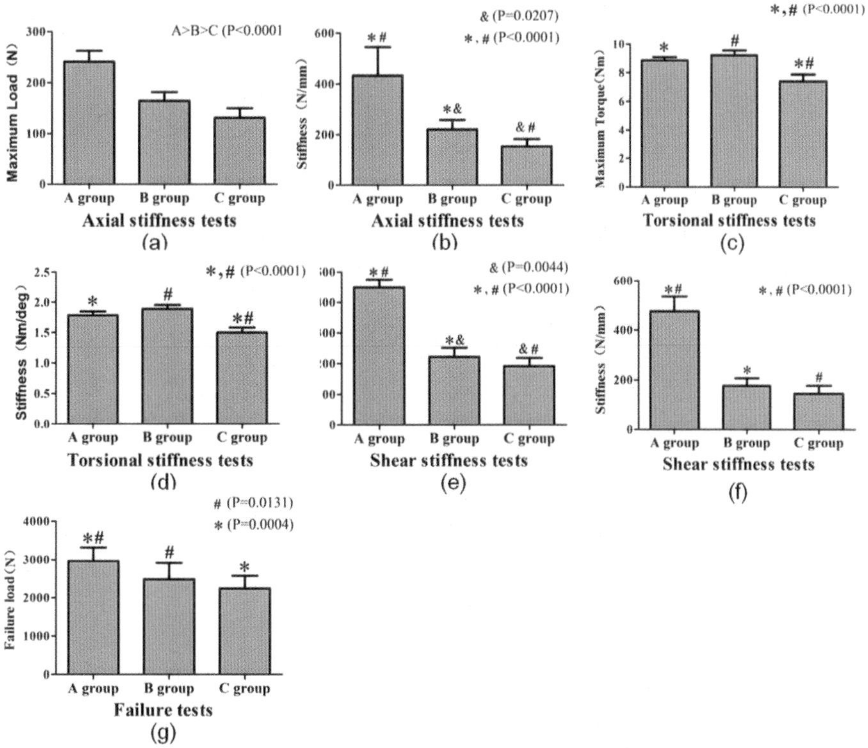

Figure 4. Comparison of stiffness tests among three groups under four load steps (a,b) axial stiffness test, (c, d) torsional stiffness test, (e, f) shear stiffness test, (g) failure test. Fig 4 a, Fig4 b Axial stiffness data for all subgroups. The maximum load and the axial stiffness showed statistical differences between the groups (Group A> Group B> Group C; $P \leq 0.0207$) Fig 4 c Torsional stiffness data for all subgroups. The maximum load of Group C was statistically different from both Group A and Group B, (Group A> Group C, Group B> Group C; *,#, $P < 0.0001$). The comparisons of Groups A and B for maximum load were not significantly different ($P = 0.6086$). Fig 4 d Torsional stiffness data for all subgroups. The torsional stiffness of Group C was statistically different from both Group A and Group B (Group A> Group C, Group B> Group C; *,#, $P < 0.0001$). The comparisons of Groups A and B for torsional stiffness were not significantly different ($P = 0.2738$). Fig 4 e Shear stiffness data for all subgroups. The maximum load showed statistical differences between the groups (Group A> Group B> Group C; $P \leq 0.0044$). Fig4 f Shear stiffness data for all subgroups. The shear stiffness of Group A was statistically different from both Group B and Group C (Group A> Group B, Group A> Group C; *,#, $P < 0.0001$). The comparisons of Groups B and C for shear stiffness were not significantly different ($P = 0.0561$). Fig 4 g The load-to-failure of Group A was statistically different from both Group B and Group C (Group A> Group B, Group A> Group C; *,#, $P \leq 0.0131$); however, no statistical differences were noted between Group B and Group C ($P = 0.3655$).

cortical contact and other subgroups, which was different to our results. This difference may be resulted from the small number of specimens included in their research, only 6–7 specimens were included in each subgroup. In addition, the supporting role of MSS was not studied in their research. The effect of the MSS was limited to the clinical literature with no evidence of biomechanical research. Our study was conducted to verify the biomechanical benefits of the MSSs in proximal humerus locking plates and to use this information to guide clinical practice.

Based on our results, strong medial support should be reconstructed in every case. When treating two-part proximal humerus fractures, anatomical reduction of the medial cortical bone should be obtained. When the medial cortical bone is comminuted or cannot be anatomiacally reduced, 2 or 3 MSSs can be inserted in order to help the reconstruction of the medial support. If medial support is not reconstructed, the resistance to axial compression and torsional force decreases, and early failure of the fracture fixation can occur.

Compared with traditional fixation methods, the fixed-angle devices can provide a greater ability to resist angular and rotational forces, especially in osteoporotic patients [15,16]. Friess et al. also found that locking plates showed higher performance on both the functional range of motion and American Shoulder and Elbow Surgeons (ASES) scores after a mean 45-month follow-up [16]. However, locking plating still has early failures, especially in patients with comminuted and osteoportic fractures or fixation without reconstruction of medial support [5,6]. Common complications include varus deformity (16%), humeral head necrosis (10%), and screw cut out (8%) [17]. Fixation without reconstruction of medial support is one of the risk factors for implant failure [5]. Reconstruction of the medial support increases the stability of fixation by providing effective support to the humeral head [8], sharing the varus deforming force, and decreasing the cutting force between the screws and the bone. Therefore, it is advisable to reconstruct the medial support of proximal humerus during the operation.

Anatomical reduction of the medial cortical bone of the proximal humerus is one of the methods to reconstruct the medial column support of the proximal humerus [8]. The current study confirmed that the medial cortical bone support of the proximal humerus has the best biomechanical stability. When the medial cortical bone of the proximal humerus is anatomically reduced, the cortical bone contacts, and the supporting forces are created to increase axial, torsional, and shear stiffness. Therefore, for a simple fracture of the proximal humerus, attempts should be made to achieve anatomical reduction of the medial cortical bone to gain

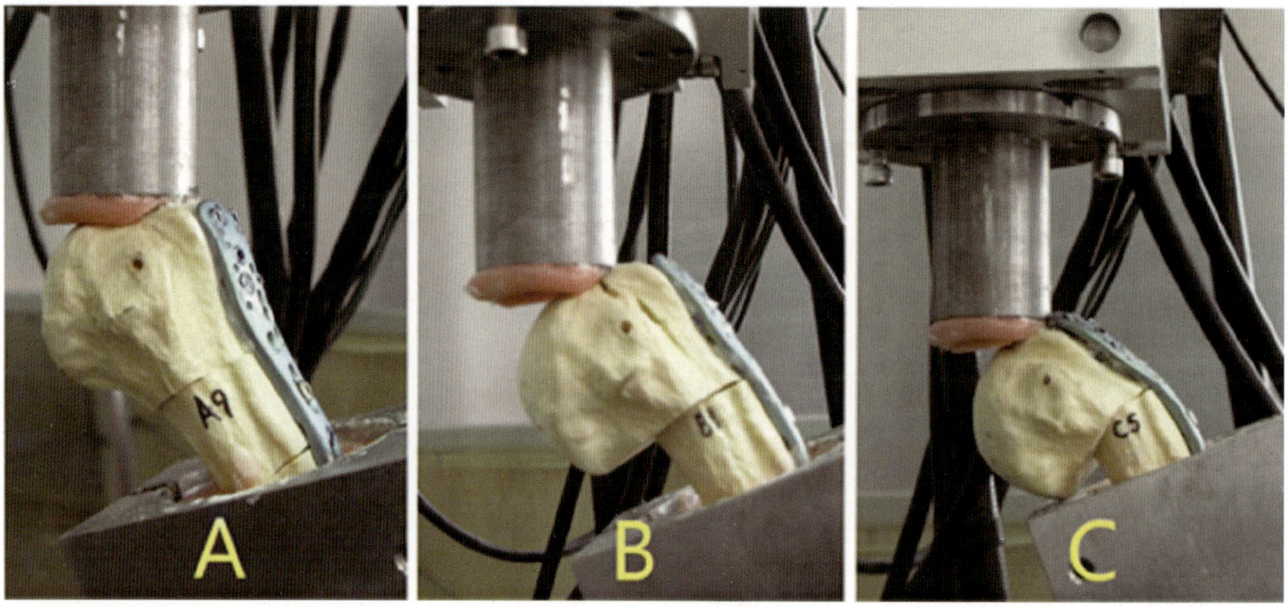

Figure 5. Shear Failure Mode: humeral shaft fracture (A), humeral head fracture (B) and specimens failed by significant plate bending (C).

medial column support and help avoid implant failure. When the medial metaphysis of the proximal humerus is comminuted, fractured with a bony defect, or the fracture is malreduced, one or two additional locking screws can be inserted obliquely into the medio-inferior region of the humeral head to reconstruct medial column support of the proximal humerus [10]. A cadaveric biomechanical study by Liew et al. found that the grasping force of a screw placed under the subchondral bone of the medial and inferior region was comparably stronger than that of a screw placed either in the middle of the humeral head or in the lateral and superior region[18]. Another histomorphometric study by Hepp et al. showed the highest bone strength to be in the medial and dorsal aspects of the proximal humeral head[19]. As a result, the optimal fixation of a screw is in the posterior-medial-inferior aspect of the humeral head to prevent screw cut out and implant loosening. Furthermore, MSSs in hole No. 7~9 were comparably closer to the fracture line than that of a screw placed in hole No. 1~6, and MSSs were relatively upwards inserted. These screws would support the proximal fragment directly from the medio-inferior part of the humeral head and might be conducive to the resistance to varus deforming force. Zhang et al. and Hardeman et al. found MSSs increase the stability of proximal humerus fractures [9,20]. However, their studies were limited to clinical outcomes with no evidence of biomechanical study. Through biomechanical tests, our study proved when the medial cortical bone of the proximal humerus is fractured with comminution, MSSs could help to increase the stability of fixation and should be strongly considered.

Several methods exist for the reconstruction of medial column support in comminuted proximal humerus fractures with bony defects. Egol et al. performed fracture site augmentation with calcium phosphate cement to increase stability after ORIF of the proximal humerus fractures [21]. Micic et al. achieved anatomical reduction with autogenous bone graft into the area of medial comminution [22], while Hettrich et al. augmented the fixation with a fibular allograft inserted medially[23]. However, there is still no gold standard treatment for reconstruction of medial column support in comminuted proximal humerus fractures. And to some extent, the bone graft methods mentioned above need more stripping of soft tissue at the medial side of the proximal humerus, which is important for the blood supply of the humeral head. In our opinion, inserting two to three MSSs will help the reconstruction of the medial support if the supporting screws can be inserted precisely into the medio-inferior region of the humeral head. To achieve this, we need to adjust the locking plate to the appropriate height and confirm the position of the tips of the MSSs by intraoperative fluoroscopy. This procedure does not require stripping a wide range of soft tissue or excessive manipulation of the fracture fragments. For comminuted and osteoporotic fractures, tension band suture is routinely used as supplemental fixation to improve the stability of the humeral head[24,25].

There are a number of limitations in this study. First, the effect of the surrounding soft tissues on the mechanical stability of the construct was not evaluated. Second, synthetic bone may more closely simulate normal, rather than osteoporotic, bone. The biomechanical characteristics were likely different from the complicated proximal humerus fractures seen in osteoporotic patients, especially the failure mode. More specimens might have failed by humeral head fracture or humeral head collapse if osteoporotic specimen were used. However, under the same objective conditions, the same experimental procedure was used to assess the mechanical stiffness and strength of each proximal humerus fracture fixation for three subgroups (medial cortical support, MSSs, and no medial column support). Third,the effect of cyclic loading was not investigated, which may be more predictive of the long-term performance of the construct than static load. Fourth, in order to make the study closer to clinical practice, we did not specify which three holes to be used for screw insertion in No. 1~6 in group B. Clinically, the number of holes selected depends on the specific condition in the operation such as fracture configuration. While screw position of the aforementioned three holes might have impacted on our results, we are unable to quantify its contribution. Future studies using finite element method will be undertaken to further investigate this.

Conclusions

Proximal humerus fracture fixation with medial cortical contact demonstrated the best biomechanical characteristics. Every effort should be made to achieve anatomical reduction of the medial cortical bone of the proximal humerus. Constructs with three MSSs showed statistically higher axial, torsional, and shear stiffness than constructs without medial support. Therefore, it is recommended that if the medial comminution is present with bony defect or the medial cortical bone is malreduced, three MSSs should be inserted to reconstruct medial column support of the proximal humerus to prevent postoperative implant failure.

Acknowledgments

We warmly acknowledge the supporting from Dr. Luyuan Sun in Shanghai Jiao Tong University Affiliated Sixth People's Hospital, Shanghai Jiao Tong University.

Author Contributions

Conceived and designed the experiments: Wen Zhang LQZ CQZ BFZ YFC. Performed the experiments: Wen Zhang LQZ. Analyzed the data: Wei Zhang. Contributed reagents/materials/analysis tools: YJL YP YFC. Wrote the paper: Wen Zhang LQZ.

References

1. Court-Brown CM, Caesar B (2006) Epidemiology of adult fractures: A review. Injury 37: 691–697.
2. Agudelo J, Schürmann M, Stahel P, Helwig P, Morgan SJ, et al. (2007) Analysis of efficacy and failure in proximal humerus fractures treated with locking plates. J Orthop Trauma 21: 676–681.
3. Volgas DA, Stannard JP, Alonso JE (2004) Nonunions of the humerus. Clin Orthop Relat Res 419: 46–50.
4. Helmy N, Hintermann B (2006) New trends in the treatment of proximal humerus fractures. Clin Orthop Relat Res442: 100–108.
5. Krappinger D, Bizzotto N, Riedmann S, Kammerlander C, Hengg C, et al. (2011) Predicting failure after surgical fixation of proximal humerus fractures. Injury 42: 1283–1288.
6. Solberg BD, Moon CN, Franco DP, Paiement GD (2009) Locked plating of 3- and 4-part proximal humerus fractures in older patients: the effect of initial fracture pattern on outcome. J Orthop Trauma 23: 113–119.
7. Bogner R, Hübner C, Matis N, Auffarth A, Lederer S, et al. (2008) Minimally-invasive treatment of three- and four-part fractures of the proximal humerus in elderly patients. J Bone Joint Surg (Br) 90: 1602–1607.
8. Gardner MJ, Weil Y, Barker JU, Kelly BT, Helfet DL, et al. (2007) The importance of medial support in locked plating of proximal humerus fractures. J Orthop Trauma 21: 185–191.
9. Zhang L, Zheng J, Wang W, Lin G, Huang Y, et al. (2011) The clinical benefit of medial support screws in locking plating of proximal humerus fractures: a prospective randomized study. Int Orthop 35: 1655–1661.
10. Schulte LM, Matteini LE, Neviaser RJ (2011) Proximal periarticular locking plates in proximal humeral fractures: functional outcomes. J Shoulder Elbow Surg 20: 1234–1240.
11. Koval KJ, Blair B, Takei R, Kummer FJ, Zuckerman JD (1996) Surgical neck fractures of the proximal humerus: a laboratory evaluation of ten fixation techniques. J Trauma 40: 778–783.
12. Lescheid J, Zdero R, Shah S, Kuzyk PR, Schemitsch EH (2010) The biomechanics of locked plating for repairing proximal humerus fractures with or without medial cortical support. J Trauma 69: 1235–1242.
13. Weeks CA, Begum F, Beaupre LA, Carey JP, Adeeb S, et al. (2013) Locking plate fixation of proximal humeral fractures with impaction of the fracture site to restore medial column support: a biomechanical study. J Shoulder Elbow Surg 22(11):1552–1557.
14. Osterhoff G, Baumgartner D, Favre P, Wanner GA, Gerber H, et al. (2011) Medial support by fibula bone graft in angular stable plate fixation of proximal humeral fractures: an in vitro study with synthetic bone. J Shoulder Elbow Surg 20: 740–746.
15. Brunner F, Sommer C, Bahrs C, Heuwinkel R, Hafner C, et al. (2009) Open reduction and internal fixation of proximal humerus fractures using a proximal humeral locked plate: a prospective multicenter analysis. J Orthop Trauma 23: 163–172.
16. Friess DM, Attia A (2008) Locking plate fixation for proximal humerus fractures: a comparison with other fixation techniques. Orthopedics 31.
17. Sproul RC, Iyengar JJ, Devcic Z, Feeley BT (2011) A systematic review of locking plate fixation of proximal humerus fractures. Injury 42: 408–413.
18. Liew AS, Hohnson JA, Patterson SD, King GJ, Chess DG (2000) Effect of screw placement on fixation in the humeral head. J Shoulder Elbow Srug 9: 423–426.
19. Hepp P, Lill H, Bail H, Korner H, Niederhagen M, et al. (2003) Where should implants be anchored in the humeral head? Clin Orthop Relat Res 415: 139–147.
20. Hardeman F, Bollars P, Donnelly M, Bellemans J, Nijs S (2012) Predictive factors for functional outcome and failure in angular stable osteosynthesis of the proximal humerus. Injury 43: 153–158.
21. Egol KA, Sugi MT, Ong CC, Montero N, Davidovitch R, et al. (2012) Fracture site augmentation with calcium phosphate cement reduces screw penetration after open reduction-internal fixation of proximal humeral fractures. J Shoulder Elbow Surg 21: 741–748.
22. Micic ID, Kim KC, Shin DJ, Shin SJ, Kim PT, et al. (2009) Analysis of early failure of the locking compression plate in osteoporotic proximal humerus fractures. J Orthop Sci 14: 596–601.
23. Hettrich CM, Neviaser A, Beamer BS, Paul O, Helfet DL, et al. (2012) Locked plating of the proximal humerus using an endosteal implant. J Orthop Trauma 26: 212–215.
24. Badman B, Frankle M, Keating C, Henderson L, Brooks J, et al. (2011) Results of proximal humeral locked plating with supplemental suture fixation of rotator cuff. J Shoulder Elbow Surg 20: 616–624.
25. Voigt C, Hurschler C, Rechi L, Vosshenrich R, Lill H. (2009) Additive fiber-cerclages in proximal humeral fractures stabilized by locking plates: no effect on fracture stabilization and rotator cuff function in human shoulder specimens. 80: 465–471.

Low-Dose X-Ray Irradiation Promotes Osteoblast Proliferation, Differentiation and Fracture Healing

Ming Chen[1]⁹, Qun Huang[2]⁹, Wei Xu[2], Chang She[2], Zong-Gang Xie[2], Yong-Tao Mao[2], Qi-Rong Dong[2]*, Ming Ling[1]*

1 Department of Orthopedics, Shaanxi Provincial Peoples Hospital, Xi'an, Shaanxi, China, **2** Department of Orthopedics, Second Affiliated Hospital of Soochow University, Suzhou, Jiangsu, China

Abstract

Great controversy exists regarding the biologic responses of osteoblasts to X-ray irradiation, and the mechanisms are poorly understood. In this study, the biological effects of low-dose radiation on stimulating osteoblast proliferation, differentiation and fracture healing were identified using in vitro cell culture and in vivo animal studies. First, low-dose (0.5 Gy) X-ray irradiation induced the cell viability and proliferation of MC3T3-E1 cells. However, high-dose (5 Gy) X-ray irradiation inhibited the viability and proliferation of osteoblasts. In addition, dynamic variations in osteoblast differentiation markers, including type I collagen, alkaline phosphatase, Runx2, Osterix and osteocalcin, were observed after both low-dose and high-dose irradiation by Western blot analysis. Second, fracture healing was evaluated via histology and gene expression after single-dose X-ray irradiation, and low-dose X-ray irradiation accelerates fracture healing of closed femoral fractures in rats. In low-dose X-ray irradiated fractures, an increase in proliferating cell nuclear antigen (PCNA)-positive cells, cartilage formation and fracture calluses was observed. In addition, we observed more rapid completion of endochondral and intramembranous ossification, which was accompanied by altered expression of genes involved in bone remodeling and fracture callus mineralization. Although the expression level of several osteoblast differentiation genes was increased in the fracture calluses of high-dose irradiated rats, the callus formation and fracture union were delayed compared with the control and low-dose irradiated fractures. These results reveal beneficial effects of low-dose irradiation, including the stimulation of osteoblast proliferation, differentiation and fracture healing, and highlight its potential translational application in novel therapies against bone-related diseases.

Editor: Jan Peter Tuckermann, University of Ulm, Germany

Funding: This work was supported by the National Natural Science Foundation of China (81171730) and the Plans for Graduate Research and Innovation in Colleges and Universities of Jiangsu Province (CXZZ12_0841). The funders had no role in study design, data collection and analysis, decision to publish, or preparation of the manuscript.

Competing Interests: The authors have declared that no competing interests exist.

* Email: dongqirong@hotmail.com (QRD); lingming029@163.com (ML)

⁹ These authors contributed equally to this work.

Introduction

Bone development and homeostasis are maintained through the balance between bone-forming osteoblasts and bone-resorbing osteoclasts. Osteoblasts are the chief bone-making cells that are responsible for the production of bone extracellular matrix during bone remodeling or healing [1]. During the process of bone formation, osteoblasts must proliferate, differentiate and induce mineralization of the bone extracellular matrix. A variety of genes in osteoblasts, including fluctuations in type I collagen (Col1), alkaline phosphatase (ALP), osteopontin (OPN), osteonectin (ON), osteocalcin (OCN) and others, undergo characteristic sequential changes in phenotypic gene expression during this series of events [2].

It is well known that high-dose irradiation delivers deleterious effects to bone tissue, including osteoradionecrosis, sclerosis, loss of bone mass and bone fracture, in a dose- and time-dependent manner [3–6]. Damage to osteoblasts and osteocytes is thought to be a primary contributor to the reduced bone mineral density that is observed following irradiation. Previous studies have suggested that irradiation can impair bone formation by impeding osteoblast proliferation and differentiation, inducing cell-cycle arrest, reducing collagen production and increasing the sensitivity to apoptotic agents [7,8]. However, the effects of low-dose irradiation, especially at levels less than 1Gy, on bone responses and healing have rarely been described in the literature. Orthopedic patients are more often subjected to radiation exposure, such as radiography, computed tomography or fluoroscopy during surgery, where the exposure to ionizing radiation is typically at low-dose levels (<1 Gy) [9,10]. In addition, several studies have revealed the detrimental effects of low-dose irradiation (<1 Gy) through various molecular mechanisms, including increases in reactive oxygen species formation, DNA double-strand breaks and chromosomal breakage [11–13]. Conversely, other studies have reported contrasting results concerning low-dose irradiation. For example, Li *et al.* reported that 75 mGy X-ray irradiation induced maximal stimulation of bone marrow hematopoietic progenitor cell proliferation and a significant increase in the mobilization of these cells to the peripheral blood post-irradiation [14]. In addition, Liang *et al.* reported that the proliferative capacity of bone marrow-derived mesenchymal stem cells (BM-MSCs) exposed to low-dose X-rays was significantly enhanced compared with the non-irradiated control group [15]. Nevertheless, the biological response of osteoblast lineage cells to low-dose X-ray irradiation remains controversial. Recently, the study performed by Pramojanee *et al.* showed that 1.5 mGy X-ray irradiation decreased oxidative stress in osteoblasts and did not alter cell viability, cellular proliferation or cellular apoptosis [11]. A previous study demonstrated that 2 Gy X-ray ionizing radiation induced time-dependent cell cycle arrest and had no significant effects on osteoblast proliferation and differentiation in an osteoblastic cell line [16,17]. However, Park *et al.* [18] reported that 2 Gy X-ray irradiation not only increased differentiation and mineralization of the cells but also upregulated the expression of ALP, Col1, OPN and OCN in the early stage of differentiation.

It is generally considered that sequential proliferation and differentiation of osteoblasts is indispensable for bone remodeling and healing. Our preliminary studies surprisingly demonstrated that 1 Gy X-ray irradiation promoted callus formation and mineralization in a rat model [19], and this type of radiation was also shown to have different effects on the proliferation and differentiation of osteoblasts in vitro (0.5–1 Gy) [20]. However, the underlying mechanism has not been evaluated in osteoblasts exposed to low-dose irradiation. In this study, we investigated the mechanism by which low-dose X-ray irradiation (0.5 Gy) influences the proliferation and differentiation of osteoblasts and promotes fracture healing. Osteogenic gene expression patterns were evaluated to explore the possible mechanisms involved in irradiation-stimulated osteoblast differentiation *in vivo* and *in vitro*. Our findings provide a greater understanding of the biological responses of osteoblasts exposed to low-dose X-ray irradiation and highlight the potential positive effects of this treatment.

Methods

Cell culture and irradiation

MC3T3-E1 subclone 14 cells were purchased from the Chinese Academy of Sciences Cell Bank. The same procedures, such as seeding time, cell numbers and replacing osteogenic medium, were performed during our study. Cells were cultured in α-MEM (HyClone, USA) containing 10% fetal bovine serum (Gibco, USA), 100 U/ml penicillin and 100 µg/ml streptomycin. In the osteoblast differentiation experiments, the culture media was replaced with osteogenic medium supplemented with 50 µg/ml ascorbic acid (Sigma-Aldrich, USA) and 10 mM β-glycerophosphate (Sigma-Aldrich, USA) after the cells had achieved 70–80% confluence. The cells were exposed to a single 0.5 Gy (low-dose) or 5 Gy (high-dose) dose of X-ray irradiation at a rate of 200 cGy/min using a medical linear accelerator with a 6 MV radiation source (Siemens Primus, Concord, CA, USA). All irradiations were performed at room temperature, and the control samples were treated similarly but were not irradiated. The time at irradiation was termed day 0. The cells were maintained in a 5% CO_2 atmosphere at 37°C, and the medium was exchanged every 3 days.

Fracture model establishment and irradiation

All animal studies were performed in strict accordance with the recommendations in the Guide for the Care and Use of Laboratory Animals of the National Institutes of Health. The protocol was approved by the Committee on the Ethics of Animal Experiments of the Second Affiliated Hospital of Soochow University. All surgeries were performed under chloral hydrate anesthesia, and all efforts were made to minimize suffering.

Male Sprague-Dawley rats (body weight 220±20 g) were obtained from the Animal Unit Center of Soochow University. A total of 96 rats were used in our *in vivo* studies. The animals were acclimated for 7 days prior to the experiments and were administered food and water ad libitum. Closed femur fractures were created as described previously [19]. Briefly, the rats were anesthetized with 3.6% chloral hydrate (360 mg/kg, intraperitoneal injection). A lateral parapatellar knee incision was made to expose the distal femoral condyles. A 1.2-mm diameter K-wire was inserted into the length of the medullary canal of the femur from the trochlear groove until the wire exited through the greater trochanter and the skin. The distal end was positioned deeply into the articular surface of the knee, and a mid-diaphyseal fracture was created via three-point bending with a custom-made guillotine-like fracture apparatus. Clear oblique fracture lines or comminuted fractures were excluded based on radiography performed after the surgery. Then, the established fracture animal models were randomized into the irradiation and control groups. The animals in the irradiation group were administered a single dose (0.5 or 5 Gy) of X-ray irradiation locally to the operated thigh using a linear accelerator with a 6 MV radiation source. Control rats were treated in the same manner as the irradiation groups; however, these rates were not exposed to X-ray irradiation.

CCK-8 assay for cell viability

MC3T3-E1 cells after irradiation were seeded in 96-well plates at a density of 3000 cells/well and cultured in an incubator for 1- to 7-day periods. The Cell Counting Kit-8 (CCK-8; Dojindo, Japan) was employed to quantitatively evaluate cell viability. Briefly, α-MEM (100 µl) with 10 µl CCK-8 was added to each pre-cultured well, and the plates were then incubated for 2 h at 37°C. The absorbance was determined at a wavelength of 450 nm using a TECAN Infinite M200 microplate reader (Tecan Group Ltd., Switzerland).

Bromodeoxyuridine (BrdU) incorporation for cell proliferation

The cells were plated and treated as described above for 2, 4 or 6 days. A BrdU ELISA kit (Roche, Germany) was used to determine cell proliferation according to the manufacturer's instructions. First, BrdU was added to the medium, and the plates were incubated for 2 h at 37°C. Then, the cells were fixed, and the DNA was denatured for 30 min at room temperature after removal of the culture medium. The anti-BrdU antibody was then added to bind to the BrdU that had been incorporated into the newly synthesized cellular DNA. Finally, the immune complexes were detected by the subsequent substrate reaction, and the absorbance of each well was measured using a TECAN Infinite M200 microplate reader at 370 nm (492 nm reference wavelength).

Flow cytometric analysis

The cell cycle progression of MC3T3-E1 cells was analyzed by flow cytometry. After irradiation, the cells were incubated for 3 days. The harvested cells were washed twice with PBS, fixed with ice-cold 70% ethanol and stored at 4°C overnight. The fixed cells were then washed with PBS again and incubated in 100 µl RNase A/PBS (200 µg/ml) at 37°C for 30 min. Intracellular DNA was labeled with 300 µl propidium iodide (PI, 10 µg/ml) at 4°C for 15 min, and the stained cells were analyzed on a flow cytometer for relative DNA content based on increased red fluorescence. The data were presented as percentages of the total population.

Table 1. List of Oligonucleotide Primer Sequences for Real-Time PCR.

Gene	Primer Sequences
β-actin	Forward: 5′- GAGAGGGAA ATCGTGCGTGAC-3′
	Reverser: 5′- CATCTGCTGGAAGGTGGACA-3′
Col1α1	Forward: 5′-AAGGCCCACGGGGACCTGTT-3′
	Reverser: 5′-GGGCCAGGCACGGAA ACTCC-3′
Col2α1	Forward: 5′-CTACGGCGACGGCAACCTGG-3′
	Reverser: 5′-TGCCCTCGGCCCTCATCTCC-3′
OCN	Forward: 5′-GCGCATCTATGGCACCACCGT-3′
	Reverser: 5′-TTTGGA GCAGCTGTGCCGTCC-3′
ALP	Forward: 5′-GCCCAGGCA ACCTCGAGCAG-3′
	Reverser: 5′-TCCGACCCACGGAGGGTTCC-3′
Runx2	Forward: 5′-TCCAGGAGGACAGCAAGGAGGC-3′
	Reverser: 5′-TCGGTTGGTCTCGGTGGCTGG-3′
Osterix	Forward: 5′- AGAAGATCCCTCCCAGCGCCC-3′
	Reverser: 5′- GGGTTGGCTGTCCCGTCTCC-3′
OPG	Forward: 5′-ATCGGCCACGCGAACCTCAC-3′
	Reverser: 5′-GCTGCTCGCTGGGTTTGCAG-3′
RANKL	Forward: 5′-GGGCCA ACCGAGACTACGGC-3′
	Reverser: 5′-GGATGCAGCGGACCCTCGTG-3′

Greater than 1×10^4 cells were analyzed per sample, and 3 independent experiments were conducted.

Alizarin Red staining

The degree of mineralization in MC3T3-E1 cells was determined in 24-well plates by Alizarin Red staining. Irradiated osteoblasts were fixed for 1 h in ice cold 70% ethanol 21 days after irradiation. The cells were then washed thoroughly with deionized H_2O, and mineralization was detected with 40 mM Alizarin red (pH 4.2) for 15 min. Following staining, cells were washed thoroughly with deionized H_2O to remove non-specific Alizarin red staining. After air-drying, the cell culture plates were evaluated by light microscopy.

Western blot analysis

The cells were homogenized in RIPA lysis buffer (Beyotime, China) using a sonic dismembrator containing protease and phosphatase inhibitors (Roche, Switzerland). Freshly isolated cell homogenates were centrifuged for 10 min at 12,000×g and 4°C. The supernatant was collected, and the protein concentration was determined using a bicinchoninic acid (BCA) protein assay kit (Beyotime, China). All samples were then diluted to an equal concentration in PBS and boiled for 5 min. Equal amounts of protein (30 μg) were subjected to 8–15% SDS-PAGE and then transferred onto polyvinylidene fluoride (PVDF) membranes. After blocking with 5% w/v non-fat dry milk for 1 h at room temperature, the membranes were incubated overnight with primary antibodies against β-actin (ab133626, Abcam, USA; dilution 1:3000), Col1α (ab34710, Abcam, USA; dilution 1:5000), ALP (ab95462, Abcam, USA; dilution 1:2000), OCN (AB10911, Millipore, USA; dilution 1:1000), Runx2 (sc-10758, Santa Cruz, USA; dilution 1:500) and Osterix (ab22552, Abcam, USA; dilution 1:2000) at 4°C with gentle shaking. After washing thrice in PBST, the blots were incubated with a 1:2000 dilution of goat anti-rabbit IgG horseradish peroxidase (HRP)-conjugated secondary antibody (ab97200, Abcam, USA) for 2 h at room temperature. The blots were washed thrice and visualized using a chemiluminescence kit (BioInd, Israel). Images were then captured with a chemiluminescence imaging system (Syegene, UK). Given that protein levels differ in relative abundance, exposure times or image intensities were varied to produce linear stain-to-background ratios.

Real-time quantitative PCR analysis

Rats were euthanized at 7, 14, 21 and 28 days after irradiation (4 rats per group). The fracture callus and 1–2 mm of the normal bone margin were carefully excised from the soft tissue using a scalpel. The samples were frozen in liquid N_2, pulverized using a nitrogen-cooled mortar and pestle apparatus and purified for total RNA using the Trizol system (Invitrogen, USA) according to the manufacturer's instructions. First-strand cDNA was obtained from the total RNA (1 μg) using RevertAid M-MuLV reverse transcriptase and oligo (dT) primer (Fermentas, Lithuania). Real-time PCR was performed in a total volume of 20 μl, which consisted of 1 μl of cDNA (500 ng), 1 μl of gene-specific 10 μM PCR primer-pair stock and 10 μl of SsoFast EvaGreen Mix (Bio-Rad, USA), using the Bio-Rad CFX96 system according to the manufacturer's protocol. The primer sequences for β-actin, Col1a1, Col2α1, OCN, ALP, Runx2 and Osterix are presented in Table 1. The PCR conditions consisted of an initial step at 95°C for 30 s to activate the DNA polymerase followed by 40 cycles of 5 s at 95°C and 5 s at 60°C, which were subsequently followed by the melting curve test. The relative amount of mRNA expression normalized to β-actin was expressed as a fold change, which was calculated using the comparative Ct ($2^{-\Delta\Delta C_t}$) method using the control group as a reference with $2^{-\Delta\Delta C_t} = 1$. Each sample was assayed in triplicate, and each experiment was independently repeated thrice.

Histology and analysis

The fractured femurs were harvested on days 7, 14, 21 and 28 post-irradiation (4 rats per group). Excess muscle and soft tissue were excised and fractured femurs were assessed by radiography. Four specimens from each group were fixed in 10% neutral buffered formalin. The specimens were decalcified for 4–5 weeks in 10% EDTA (pH 7.2), embedded in paraffin and sectioned at a thickness of 3 μm. The sections were cut through the long axis of each femur in the sagittal plane and stained with Masson's trichrome stain and TRAP stain (three levels per animal). Osteoclast counts were obtained from the number of TRAP-positive cells. The total callus area, total cartilage area and total woven bone area were quantified using Image Pro Plus 6.0 software as described previously [21].

Immunohistochemistry was also performed on these sections using a previously described method [22]. The sections were mounted on poly-L-lysine-coated glass slides and then air-dried overnight at room temperature. The sections were then deparaffinized with xylene and hydrated with serial concentrations of 100, 95, 80 and 70% alcohol. Endogenous peroxidase activity was blocked with 0.5% hydrogen peroxide in methanol for 60 min. Following a Tris-buffered saline (TBS)/0.1% bovine serum albumin (BSA) wash, hyaluronidase treatment (hyaluronidase 1 mg/ml in sodium acetate buffer, pH 5.5, 0.85% NaCl) was performed for 30 min at 37°C. After washing with TBS/0.1% BSA, the sections were incubated with blocking solutions (fresh 10 ml of TBS/0.5% BSA containing 130 μl of normal horse serum) at room temperature for 15 min. The sections were then incubated with the proliferating cell nuclear antigen (PCNA) monoclonal antibody (PC10; sc-56, Santa Cruz, USA) and OCN polyclonal antibody (AB10911, Millipore, USA) at a 1:100 dilution. A subsequent reaction was performed using a Vectastain avidin/biotin-peroxidase complex (ABC) kit. The sections were reacted with diaminobenzidine (DAB) solution and were then counterstained with methyl green. We identified the cell type in the histological analyses based on tissue types, callus areas and cellular morphology [23]. Briefly, in the early stages after fracture, the calluses were mainly composed of soft tissue, including cell debris and mesenchymal cells, which exhibited a high proliferation activity. Chondrocytes were detected in the cartilage island. The premature cells were located in the margin of the cartilage adjacent to the soft tissue and were small and round in shape. The hypertrophic or mature chondrocytes were located in the center of the cartilage tissue or adjoined to the woven bone and displayed vacuole morphology. The vessel located in the soft tissue presented a cavity structure, which was encircled by flat endothelial cells.

Statistical analysis

Statistical analyses were performed using SPSS version 17.0 (IBM SPSS, USA). All data are expressed as the means ± SD. One-way or two-way analysis of variance (ANOVA) and post-hoc multiple comparisons were used for statistical analyses. A difference was considered significant if the *p*-value was <0.05.

Results

Low-dose X-ray irradiation increases the cell viability and proliferation of osteoblastic MC3T3-E1 cells

We performed cell viability CCK-8 assays at days 1 through 7 following irradiation. As shown in Fig. 1, no statistically significant differences in CCK-8 activity in MC3T3-E1 cells were noted between the individually irradiated groups and the non-irradiated controls at day 1 post-irradiation. However, cells irradiated with a single, low dose (0.5 Gy) exhibited an increased in cell viability at days 2 to 6 ($p<0.05$), whereas high-dose (5 Gy) X-ray irradiation significantly reduced cell viability at days 2 to 7 ($p<0.05$). In addition, 0.5 Gy of irradiation exhibited no significant effect by day 7, and this result might be attributed to the notion that MC3T3-E1 cell growth had plateaued in both the control and the low-dose irradiation cultures. To determine whether this variation in cell viability was due to cell proliferation, BrdU incorporation was measured after irradiation. The results indicated that low-dose (0.5 Gy) X-ray irradiation promoted cell proliferation on days 2, 4 and 6 post-irradiation compared with the 0 Gy control ($p<0.05$), whereas high-dose (5 Gy) irradiation inhibited MC3T3-E1 cell proliferation (Fig. 2A). Cell cycle analysis by flow cytometry revealed that single, low-dose (0.5 Gy) X-ray irradiation induced a decrease in the proportion of cells at the sub-G1 phase, which indicates active apoptosis (6.75%±0.21%, $p<0.05$ *vs.* control), whereas increasing levels of cell death by apoptosis were observed in the high-dose irradiation group (14.26%±0.41%, $p<0.05$ *vs.* control). Moreover, our results indicated that low-dose irradiation caused a 5.85% increase in the S+G2/M phases of the cell cycle in osteoblasts compared with control ($p<0.05$), whereas high-dose irradiation had no effect (Fig. 2B). These results indicated that low-dose X-ray irradiation potentially promotes osteoblast survival and renewal.

Low-dose X-ray irradiation promotes osteoblasts differentiation and mineralization in *vitro*

After X-ray irradiation, MC3T3-E1 cells were further cultured in osteogenic medium, and the expression levels of proteins associated with osteoblast differentiation were examined by Western blot at 4, 7, 10 and 14 days after irradiation. The statistical analysis histograms are presented in Fig. 3A–F. Osteoblast differentiation markers, such as OCN, Runx2 and Osterix, were inhibited temporarily at 4 days post-irradiation in both the low- and high-dose groups, with the levels of Runx2 and Osterix demonstrating the most prominent decreases in the low-dose group (Fig. 3A, D–F). The levels of Col1α were decreased at 4 and 14 days but were elevated at 10 days post-irradiation in the low-dose group, whereas a continual decrease in Col1α levels was observed in the high-dose group from days 4 to 14 after irradiation (Fig. 3A, B). Irradiation-stimulated increases in alkaline ALP levels occurred at 7 and 10 days after 0.5 Gy and 5 Gy X-ray irradiation (Fig. 3A, C). In addition, both the 0.5 Gy and 5 Gy radiation doses led to significant increases in OCN levels at 10 days, with the increases in the 0.5 Gy group continuing through 14 days post-irradiation (Fig. 3A, F). Decreased Runx2 levels were detected in the high-dose group at 7 days and in the low-dose group at 10 days; however, both low- and high-dose irradiation stimulated increases in Runx2 protein levels at 14 days after irradiation (Fig. 3A, D). In addition, the expression of Osterix in the low-dose group was significantly increased at 7, 10 and 14 days compared with the non-irradiated control group (Fig. 3A, E). These findings indicate that X-ray irradiation induced dynamic variations in the differentiation of pre-osteoblastic cells. Although we observed temporary reductions in osteogenic markers of early osteoblast differentiation after single-dose X-ray irradiation, dramatic increases in the related differentiation markers occurred at the medium differentiation. In addition, Alizarin Red staining demonstrated that low-dose irradiation promoted mineralization in MC3T3-E1 cells. For cells irradiated with high-dose irradiation, the mineralized bone nodules decreased in number (Fig. 2C). Together, low-dose X-ray irradiation promoted osteoblasts differentiation and mineralization in *vitro*.

Low-dose X-ray irradiation accelerates endochondral and intramembranous ossification in fracture healing

A rat femur fracture model was employed to study fracture healing after irradiation. Fracture calluses from irradiated and non-irradiated rats, which were age- and sex-matched, were examined by radiography assessment and Masson's trichrome staining at days 7, 14, 21 and 28 following irradiation (Fig. 4). The radiographs indicate that 0.5 Gy X-ray irradiation accelerated callus mineralization and fractures repair, whereas 5 Gy X-ray irradiation delayed fracture healing (Fig. 4B). Histology sections of the calluses confirmed accelerated fracture healing and remodeling in low-dose (0.5 Gy) irradiated rats compared with the non-irradiated control group. However, the fractures in high-dose (5 Gy) animals demonstrated delayed healing. On day 7 following irradiation, low-dose irradiated rats presented increased callus areas and cartilage formation compared with non-irradiated rats. In contrast, decreased callus areas and less bone and cartilage formation were detected in high-dose irradiation rats (Fig. 4A, C–D). By day 14, the calluses in the high-dose group were also composed of less cartilage and woven bone area compared with the control group (Fig. 4A, D, E). On days 21 to 28, fractures in the low-dose irradiated and control rats were healed, and cartilage tissue was essentially absent in the calluses. However, healing was incomplete in the fractures of high-dose irradiated rats where a central area of cartilage tissue persisted (Fig. 4A, D). In addition to the accelerated osteogenesis, the fractures in the low-dose group underwent more rapid remodeling. In particular, low-dose irradiated rats exhibited abundant woven bone formation that peaked at 14 days; this event occurred earlier than the bone formation observed in the non-irradiated group, in which peak bone area was measured at 21 days. Subsequently, the bone areas

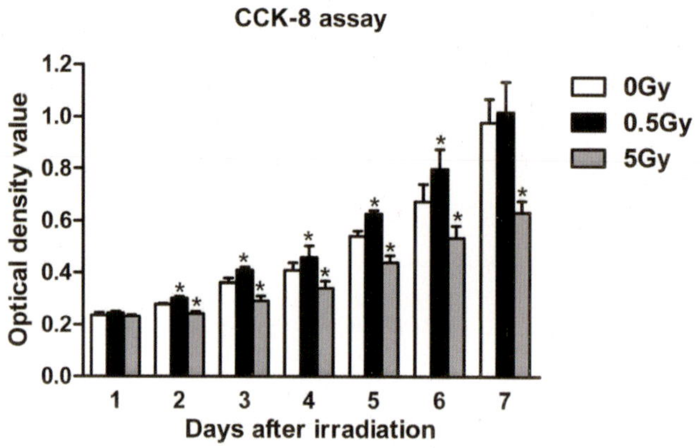

Figure 1. MC3T3-E1 cell viability as determined by the CCK-8 assay. Compared with the control cells (0 Gy), single low-dose (0.5 Gy) irradiation significantly increased cell viability from days 2 to 6, whereas high-dose (5 Gy) irradiation significantly reduced cell viability from days 2 to 7. *$p<0.05$ *vs.* the control group.

of both groups progressively decreased (Fig. 4A, E). Beginning on day 21, low-dose-irradiated rats demonstrated decreased callus area, and most of the initial woven bone within the calluses had been remodeled with lamellar bone, which persisted through 28 days post-irradiation (Fig. 4A, C). By 28 days, the fractures in the low-dose irradiated rats had essentially undergone complete remodeling, and the femurs exhibited a similar morphology to non-fractured bone. In the control group, extensive remodeling was not observed until 28 days post-irradiation. Moreover, abnormal mineralization and remodeling were involved in fracture healing after high-dose irradiation. Fracture calluses in high-dose irradiated rats remained enlarged and contained areas of woven bone where greater amounts of mature collagen (red stained) were deposited at 28 days (Fig. 4A).

Immunohistochemistry revealed increased numbers of proliferating cells during fracture repair in low-dose (0.5 Gy) irradiated rats. This increase in proliferating cells included periosteal cells, osteoblasts and mesenchymal cells or chondrocytes, which are known to contribute to intramembranous ossification, chondrogenesis and endochondral ossification during fracture repair. On day 7, near the fracture site, the periosteal cells stained by PCNA antibodies in the fibrous layer were increased in the low-dose group compared with the non-irradiated group. In contrast, the high-dose irradiated group displayed significantly decreased numbers of PCNA-positive periosteal cells (Fig. 5A, B). In soft calluses, greater chondrogenesis was observed in the 0.5 Gy group on day 7; small, round, premature chondrocytes and mesenchymal cells were detected near the cartilage tissue. The proliferating

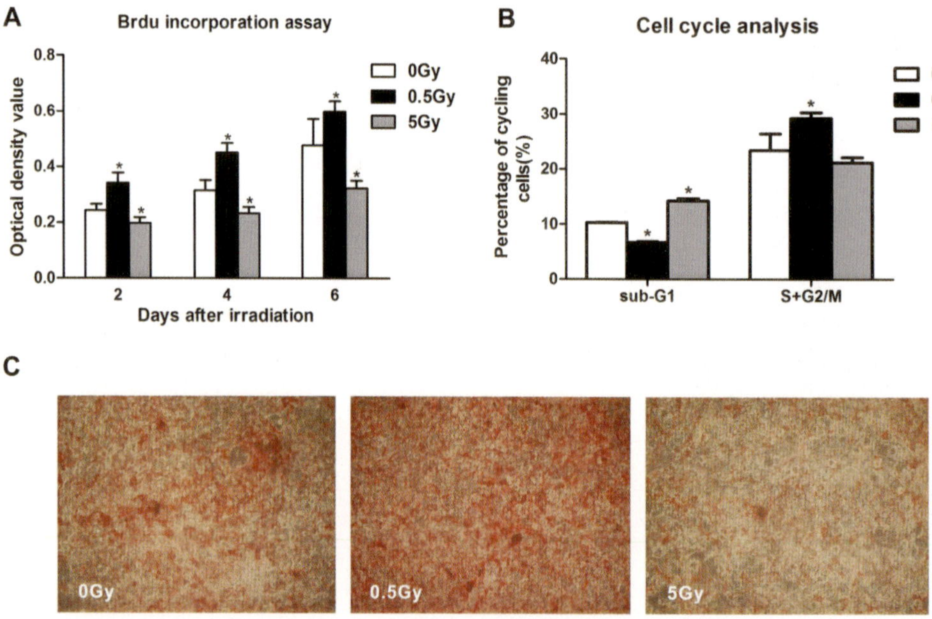

Figure 2. MC3T3-E1 cell proliferation and mineralization after irradiation. Low-dose (0.5 Gy) irradiation significantly promoted cell proliferation from days 2 to 6 compared with control cells (0 Gy), whereas high-dose (5 Gy) irradiation inhibited cell proliferation (A). Low-dose (0.5 Gy) irradiation resulted in an approximate 6.75% decrease in the percentage of cells in the sub-G1 phase, whereas high-dose (5 Gy) irradiation elicited an approximate 14.26% increase in the percentage of cells in the sub-G1 phase (B). Low-dose (0.5 Gy) irradiation accelerated osteoblasts mineralization 21 days after irradiation, and high-dose (5 Gy) irradiation decreased alizarin red staining (C). *$p<0.05$ *vs.* the control group.

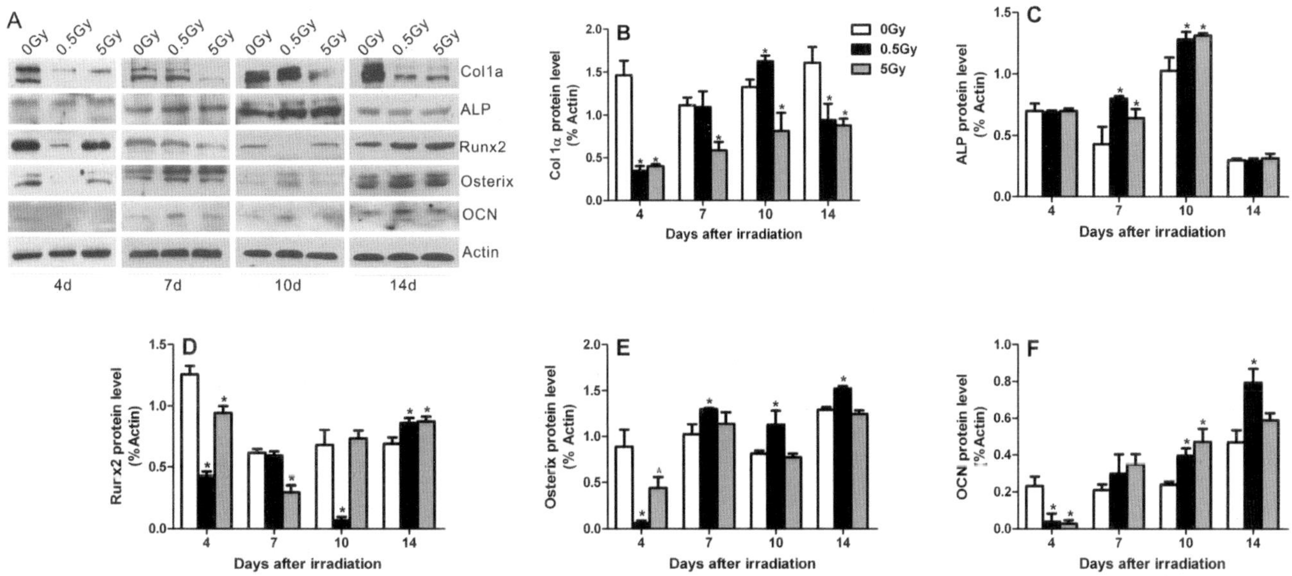

Figure 3. The effects of irradiation on the expression of osteoblast differentiation markers *in vitro*. The expression of Col1α, ALP, Runx2, Osterix and OCN proteins was assessed by Western blot on post-irradiation days 4, 7, 10 and 14 (A). The Col1α (B), ALP (C), Runx2 (D), Osterix (E) and OCN (F) protein levels were normalized to β-actin expression. *$p<0.05$ *vs.* the control group.

premature chondrocytes stained by PCNA antibodies were significantly increased in the low-dose group compared with the non-irradiated group. In contrast, deceased PCNA-positive cells, of which mesenchymal cells were predominant, were observed in the high-dose group (Fig. 5C, D). On day 14, a greater reduction in PCNA-positive cells was detected in each group compared with the early phase. The proliferating chondrocytes in the non-irradiated control were more numerous compared with the irradiated groups (Fig. 5C, D). In addition, vascularization was observed in the fibrous calluses, and fewer PCNA-positive mesenchymal cells were noted in the low-dose and control groups. Furthermore, the majority cells in the soft callus area differed in appearance from the hypertrophic chondrocytes observed in the high-dose group, and fibrous tissue was observed in a criss-cross pattern in the cartilage calluses on day 14 (Fig. 5C). In addition, immunohistochemistry demonstrated that low-dose irradiation also increased the expression of OCN protein among proliferating cells on day 14 after irradiation (Fig. 6A, B). PCNA is a protein involved in the major DNA replication repair machinery of cells. When not engaged in DNA replication, PCNA (most often under the control of p53) commits cells to cell cycle arrest and repair of DNA damage. Alternatively, when repair is not possible, absent or low levels of functional PCNA may drive cells to apoptosis [24]. On the one hand, the suppression of PCNA signaling promotes cellular apoptosis [25]. In contrast, PCNA activation suppresses osteoblast apoptosis during *in vitro* culture [26]. These facts reveal that PCNA is also related to cellular apoptosis. Our results indicate that low-dose irradiation increased PCNA protein expression in the calluses. To some degree, this that low-dose irradiation protects cells against apoptosis during fracture repair.

Osteoblast differentiation was accelerated in the fractures of low-dose irradiated rats

The expression of genes involved in osteoblast differentiation was also examined in the callus tissue of fractures from irradiated and non-irradiated rats (Fig. 7). Col2a1 expression was elevated earlier in fractures from low-dose irradiated rats compared with non-irradiated control rats. This observation was consistent with the increase in cartilage observed in low-dose irradiated rats by histomorphometry at day 7, signifying the acceleration of the endochondral phase of fracture repair (Fig. 7B). Moreover, Col2a1 expression was absent in low-dose irradiated and non-irradiated rats by day 21, whereas Col2a1 expression persisted until day 28 in high-dose irradiated rats. Additionally, the expression of the osteoblast-specific transcription factors Runx2 and Osterix was elevated in fracture calluses from low-dose irradiated rats, whereas Runx2 and Osterix expression in the fracture calluses appeared to be not effected by high-dose irradiation (Fig. 7D, E). Furthermore, the expression of the osteoblast differentiation markers ALP and OCN was elevated earlier in fractures from irradiated rats (both low- and high-dose), which is consistent with accelerated osteoblast differentiation (Fig. 7C, F). In the fractures from low-dose irradiated rats, Col1a1 expression appeared earlier, and peak levels were observed by days 14–21 compared with the maximal expression observed at day 28 in non-irradiated control rats (Fig. 7A). ALP expression in fractures from irradiated rats was significantly increased compared with non-irradiated rats on day 14 (Fig. 7C). Furthermore, OCN expression levels were also elevated earlier in fractures from irradiated rats compared with non-irradiated rats, and this increase persisted to 28 days post-irradiation (Fig. 7F). These findings suggest that osteoblasts undergo more rapid differentiation in low-dose irradiated rats; in contrast, high-dose irradiation results in unnatural osteoblast differentiation that is characterized by delayed collagen expression and collagen maturation. Furthermore, this type of rapid osteoblast differentiation in low-dose irradiated rats is consistent with the more rapid completion of endochondral and intramembranous ossification.

Low-dose irradiation accelerates callus remodeling via enhanced osteoclast-induced signals

The fracture calluses were stained for TRAP expression, which is an osteoclast marker. In day 14, 0.5 Gy X-ray irradiation increased the number of osteoclasts in the fracture calluses by

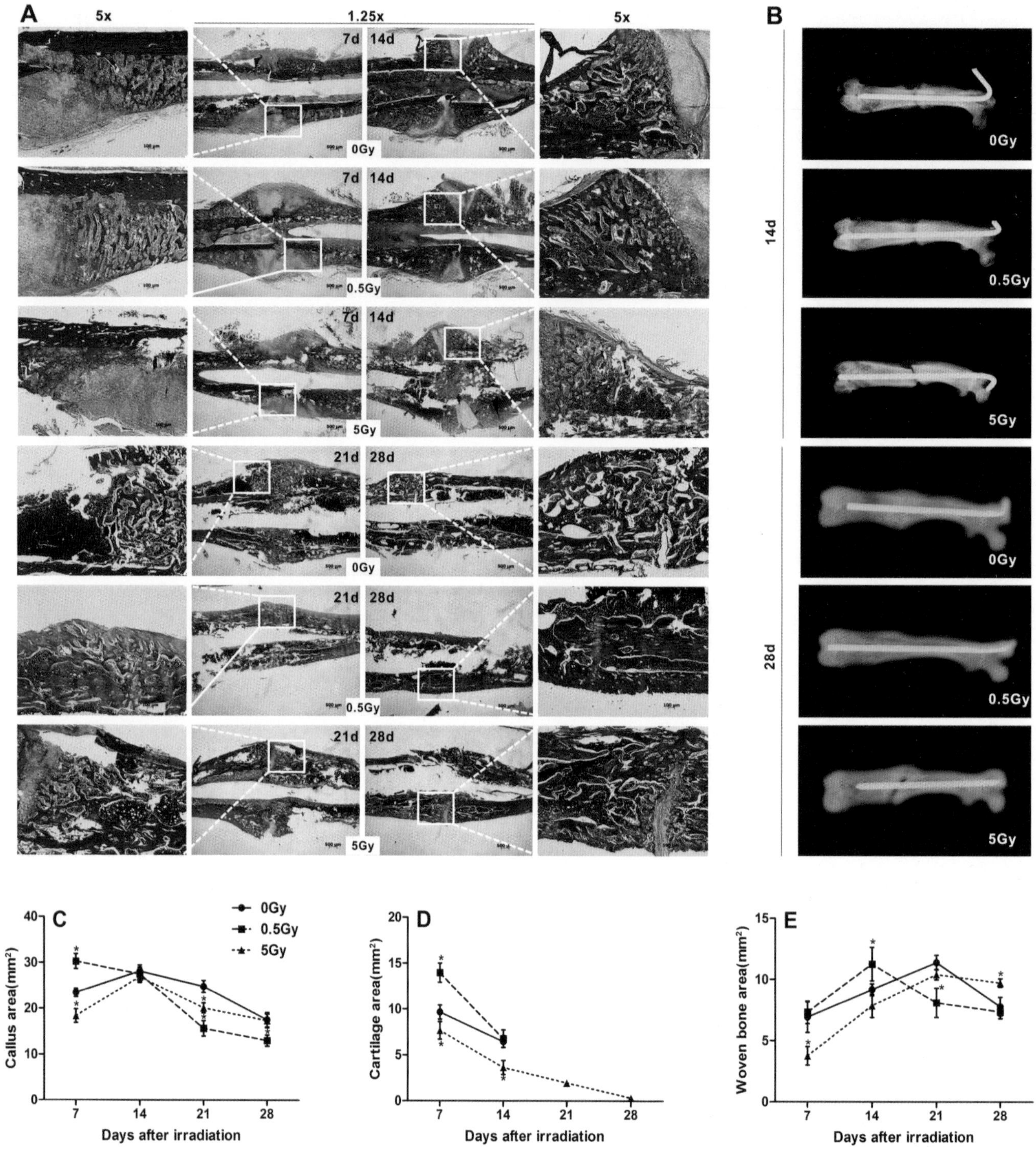

Figure 4. The effects of irradiation on fracture healing. Fractured femurs were harvested and immediately assessed by radiography. Representative histologies of fractured femurs stained with Masson's trichrome staining is depicted at 7, 14, 21 and 28 days after X-ray irradiation; accelerated remodeling on day 21 in fractures irradiated with low-dose X-ray irradiation was evident comparing the contracted calluses to the broad calluses that remained in the control fractures, whereas non-union on day 28 was observed in fractures that received high-dose X-ray irradiation (A). Radiographs demonstrated the accelerated callus mineralization and fracture repair (B). Histomorphometric measurements (total callus area, cartilage area, woven bone area) were performed, and the results are presented as a diagram (C, D, E). n = 4 rats/group, **p*<0.05 *vs.* the control group.

61.9% ($p<0.01$) compared with non-irradiated fractures. This observation was consistent with accelerated bone remodeling. By day 21, fractures in the non-irradiated rats contained a certain number of osteoclasts. Surprisingly, few osteoclasts were observed in 21 day-old fractures from 0.5 Gy X-ray irradiated rats. However, high-dose (5 Gy) X-ray irradiation decreased osteoclast numbers at each time-point (Fig. 8A, B). Real-time PCR was performed to measure the expression of the osteoclast-inducing

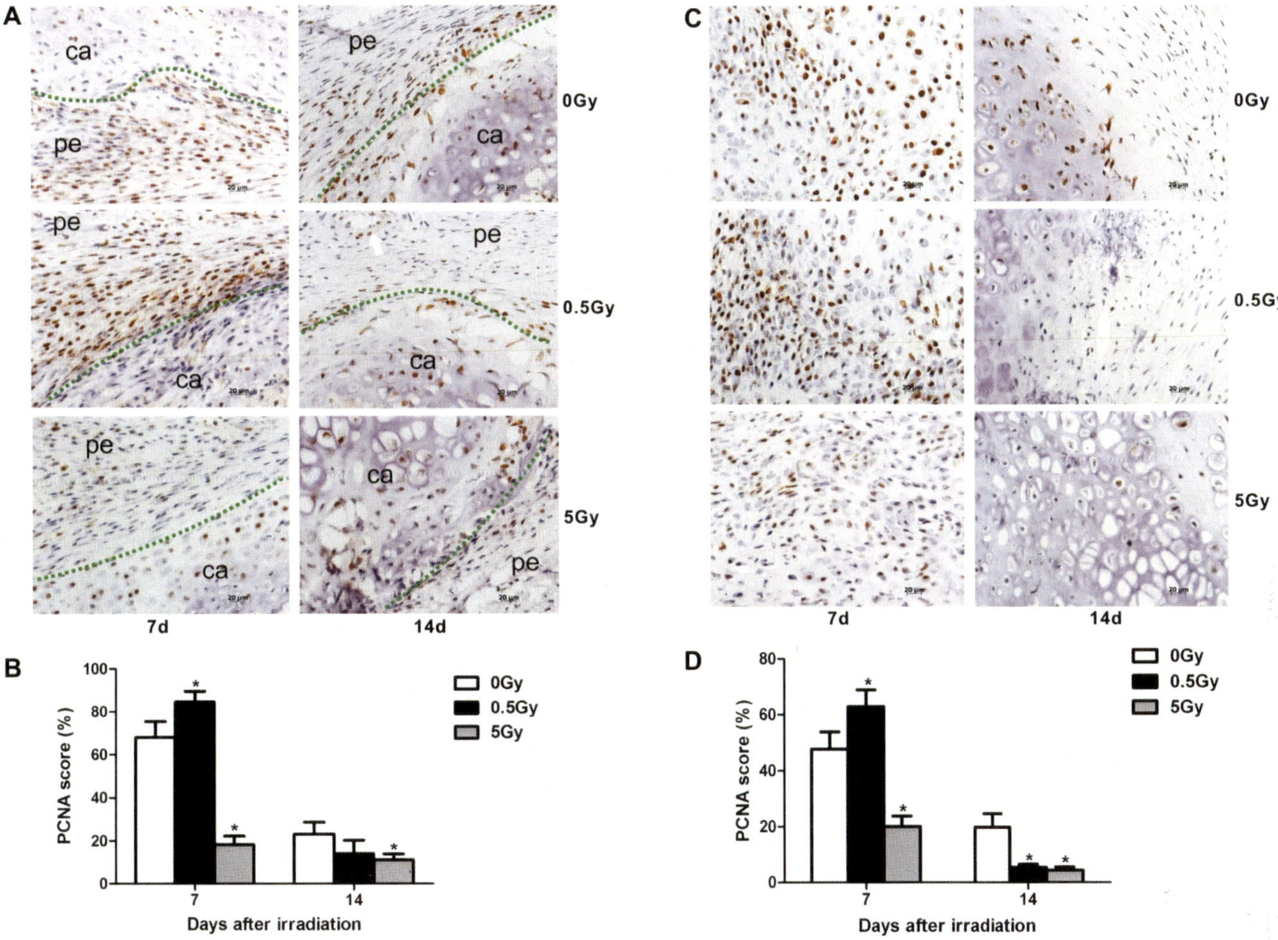

Figure 5. Cell proliferation during intramembranous osteogenesis and chondrogenesis. PCNA immunostaining was performed at 7 and 14 days after X-ray irradiation. Low-dose X-ray irradiation promoted the proliferation of periosteum cells and chondrocytes at day 7 after irradiation in fracture sites, whereas high-dose X-ray irradiation inhibited the proliferation of these cells at both days 7 and 14 post-irradiation (A, C). Quantification of cell proliferation in each group (B, D). The green dot represents the demarcation between the soft tissue and cartilage, and the white arrow denotes a vessel. pe: periosteum, ca: cartilage, n = 4 rats/group,*$p<0.05$ *vs.* the control group.

gene RANKL and its receptor antagonist OPG. The fracture calluses from 0.5 Gy irradiated rats exhibited an increased overall expression of both RANKL and OPG, and both genes were elevated earlier in fractures in 0.5 Gy irradiated rats compared with non-irradiated rats (Fig. 8C, D). The maximum expression levels of RANKL occurred at 14 days in the fracture tissue from the 0.5 Gy X-ray group and at 21 days in the control. RANKL expression exhibited a sharp peak in facture tissues from the 0.5 Gy X-ray group, whereas the control group exhibited a lower order of magnitude of expression that was more sustained. The RANKL/OPG radio in 0.5 Gy group was significantly increased compared with non-irradiated group at 14 days. However, the ratio of RANKL/OPG was reduced during fracture repair in the 5 Gy irradiated rats (Fig. 8E). These data were consistent with the differences observed in osteoclast numbers in the fracture calluses. Thus, our results suggest that 0.5 Gy irradiation accelerates callus remodeling by enhanced osteoclast-induced signals.

Discussion

In this study, we observed increased proliferation and differentiation among osteoblasts in cell culture and fracture healing models stimulated by low-dose irradiation. Given that osteoblasts exhibit a developmental sequence of events, including distinct proliferative, differentiating and mineralizing stages, we selected different time points for the proliferation and differentiation analyses in our study. After single-dose 0.5 Gy X-ray irradiation, osteoblastic cell activity was enhanced, consistent with increased osteoblast proliferation. Similarly, increased numbers of PCNA-positive cells were detected in calluses early during the fracture-healing process. In addition, low-dose (0.5 Gy) X-ray irradiation promoted osteoblastic cell survival and reduced apoptotic cell death based on the sub-G1 cell cycle analysis of cultured cells. Furthermore, low-dose irradiation induced accelerated osteoblast differentiation and fracture healing by triggering the expression of osteoblast-specific differentiation markers and inhibiting apoptosis. These results demonstrated the stimulatory effect of low-dose irradiation on osteogenesis, which was mediated through increased osteoblast proliferation and differentiation.

Despite accumulating evidence highlighting the biological effects of irradiation on bone, a series of controversies remain in this field. For example, although previous researchers have demonstrated the detrimental effects of irradiation on bone [7,27–29], other reports demonstated positive effects of irradiation on osteoblastic differentiation and bone-specific gene expression [16,18,20,30]. Furthermore, a few studies have reported stimula-

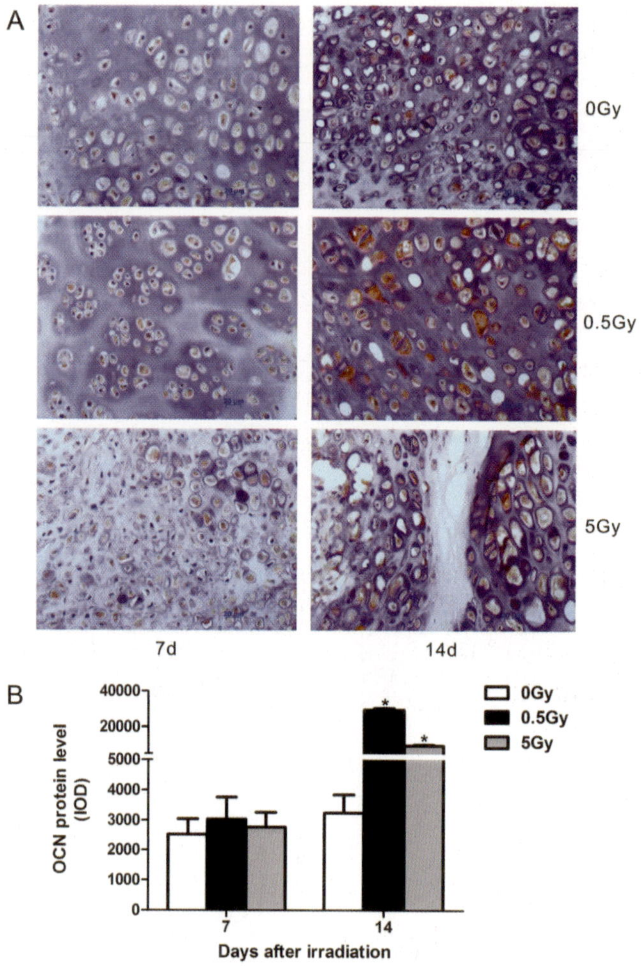

Figure 6. Irradiation increased OCN-positive cells in calluses on day 14 after irradiation. Representative immunohistochemistry of the calluses stained with OCN antibody at 7 and 14 days after X-ray irradiation (A). Quantification of OCN protein expression in each group (B). n = 4 rats/group,**p*<0.05 *vs.* the control group.

tory effects of low-dose X-ray irradiation (<0.2 Gy) on the proliferation of BM-MSCs, which are osteoblast progenitors and may undergo osteoblastic differentiation in osteogenic medium [16]. These contradictory conclusions may be due to differences in cell lines, irradiation doses and time points used in the gene expression analyses. Our study primarily focused on the effects of low-dose X-ray irradiation on osteoblast proliferation and differentiation both *in vivo* and *in vitro*. Given that the radiosensitivity of cells differs according to cell type and differentiation stage, the relatively low dose of 0.5 Gy was used in our experiments. After 0.5 Gy irradiation, Osteoblast proliferation increased for increased BrdU incorporation and PCNA-positive cells were detected *in vivo* and *in vitro*. The consistent inhibitory effect of high-dose (5 Gy) irradiation on osteoblast proliferation was also reported in this study. A variety of types of DNA damage, including single-strand breaks, double-strand breaks and base damage, occur in response to radiation, and the DNA repair process is activated to address such damage. However, high-dose radiation can induce extensive DNA damage that is difficult to repair and might interfere with cell cycle progression, at which point cells undergo programmed cell death [16,17,31]. Adaptive protection against DNA damage and bystander effects might also occur in response to low-dose radiation, generally in terms of the protective mechanisms associated with hormesis [11,15,32,33]. Our results indicate that low-dose irradiation elicited DNA synthesis in osteoblastic cells with an increase in proliferation activity and apoptosis suppression. Although the effect of 0.5 Gy irradiation on osteoblast viability and proliferation was mild, the differences between the control and 0.5 Gy groups were statistically significant. At a minimum, this result indicates that osteoblasts can complete DNA repair at the early stage in response to 0.5 Gy irradiation and that osteoblast proliferation is not inhibited. As demonstrated in our previous study, ≤1.0 Gy irradiation had no significant effect on cell proliferation, viability and apoptosis [20]. This contradiction was attributed to the modulation of the irradiation procedure. In the previous experiment, osteoblasts were irradiated the day after seeding. However, in the present study, we performed an irradiation schedule whereby the irradiated osteoblasts in the logarithmic phase of growth were immediately seeded onto a plate. It is known that different cell types and stages of differentiation exhibit varying susceptibility and responses to radiation exposure.

The osteoblast differentiation process is tightly controlled by bone-specific regulatory factors. Col1 is the main structural component of bone matrix. ALP is important in stabilizing the matrix. OCN is another non-collagenous protein that is almost exclusively expressed in bone and is upregulated during matrix mineralization [34,35]. In the case of bone, the dynamic and well-

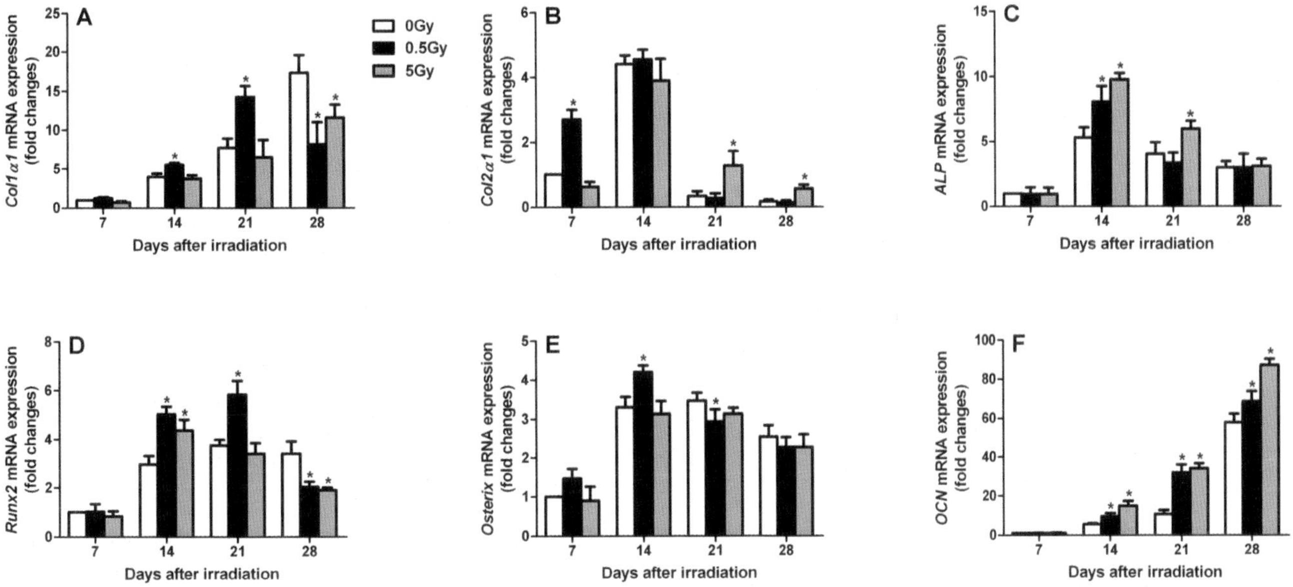

Figure 7. Irradiation-stimulated changes in mRNA expression patterns of osteoblast differentiation-related genes in fracture callus tissues. Real-time PCR was performed at various time points after X-ray irradiation. The following primer sets were used: Col1a1 (A), Col2a1 (B), ALP (C), Runx2 (D), Osterix (E) and OCN (F). n = 4 rats/group,**p*<0.05 *vs.* the control group.

regulated expression patterns of these marker genes depend on the differentiation stage of the osteoblasts [18,35]. For example, Col1 is expressed from the beginning of osteoblast differentiation, whereas only mature osteoblasts in the matrix calcification stage secrete OCN. From our experiments, X-ray irradiation induced significant differentiation effects on osteoblasts. For example, after relatively low-dose irradiation, Col1, ALP and OCN expression was increased in the mature stage of osteoblast differentiation. Similarly, high-dose irradiation also enhanced the expression of osteoblastic differentiation markers with the exception of Col1, which was clearly decreased at all time points. Interestingly, a temporary decline in the expression of several differentiation markers at 4 days after both low-dose and high-dose irradiation *in vitro* was noted, and the following reasons might contribute to this dynamic tendency. First, this decline in expression might represent a cellular survival strategy when radiation damage is present [17]. The major trigger of the cellular response to irradiation is the destruction of genome integrity, and cells can mount a coordinated response to genotoxic stresses, including irradiation, by activating a network of interacting signaling pathways collectively known as the DNA damage response [32]. In response to irradiation, osteoblasts immediately initiate DNA repair mechanisms. Lau et al. [17] reported that discrete γ-H2AX foci that reflect DNA damage were detected as early as 30 min after irradiation in osteoblasts, and approximately all double-strand breaks were effectively rejoined after a repair period of 24 h. As a survival strategy, osteoblasts either retain their proliferative capability and repair DNA damage or are programmed to die (or become senescent or prematurely terminally differentiated) if DNA is heavily damaged [17,32,33]. Therefore, cells primarily focus on DNA repair during the early stages after irradiation, whereas the differentiation potential is inhibited. Second, the progressive development of the osteoblastic phenotype, which requires precise coordination between cellular proliferation and differentiation, might play a critical role in the early stages after irradiation [17]. Cell fate is decided according to the balance between self-renewal and differentiation, where cell self-renewal blocks differentiation and supports cell division [36]. Our results revealed that low-dose irradiation stimulated pre-osteoblast proliferation, which may be related to the decreased expression of differentiation markers in the early stage after irradiation. Consistently, following low-dose irradiation, the expression of the transcription factors Runx2 and Osterix, which are key regulators in osteoblast differentiation, was significantly high-dose irradiation. In other words, the increased proliferation observed following low-dose irradiation may constrain the differentiation potentiality in the early stages after irradiation. Although high-dose irradiation increased terminal differentiation among osteoblasts, it inhibited cell proliferation and reduced production of the extracellular matrix. Thus, the cells' bone forming capacity was weakened in response to high-dose irradiation. However, low-dose irradiation enhanced osteoblast proliferation in the early stages, increased the expression of osteogenic markers and promoted the terminal differentiation process. This result demonstrates that low-dose X-ray increases the osteogenic potential of osteoblast.

Fracture healing is a complex process during which mesenchymal stem cells are recruited to the site of injury and subsequently undergo proliferation and differentiation into bone-forming cells [37]. The present study reveals that low-dose irradiation acts as a positive factor in the fracture-healing process given that it promoted cell proliferation, differentiation and fracture healing in animal models. Accelerated intramembranous bone formation and endochondral bone formation were observed in low-dose irradiated fractures. Low-dose irradiation also accelerated callus remodeling by enhanced osteoclast-induced signals. Furthermore, low-dose irradiation enhanced the expression of osteoblast differentiation genes in the fracture calluses. Our *in vivo* experimental results were consistent with the results of osteoblast culture *in vitro*. For example, the number of proliferating cells increased in calluses from fractures irradiated with low-dose X-ray radiation, and gene expression studies from fracture callus tissues demonstrated an enhanced rate of chondrocyte and osteoblast differentiation after low-dose irradiation. Maximal expression of Col2a1 occurred early after low-dose irradiation, demonstrating

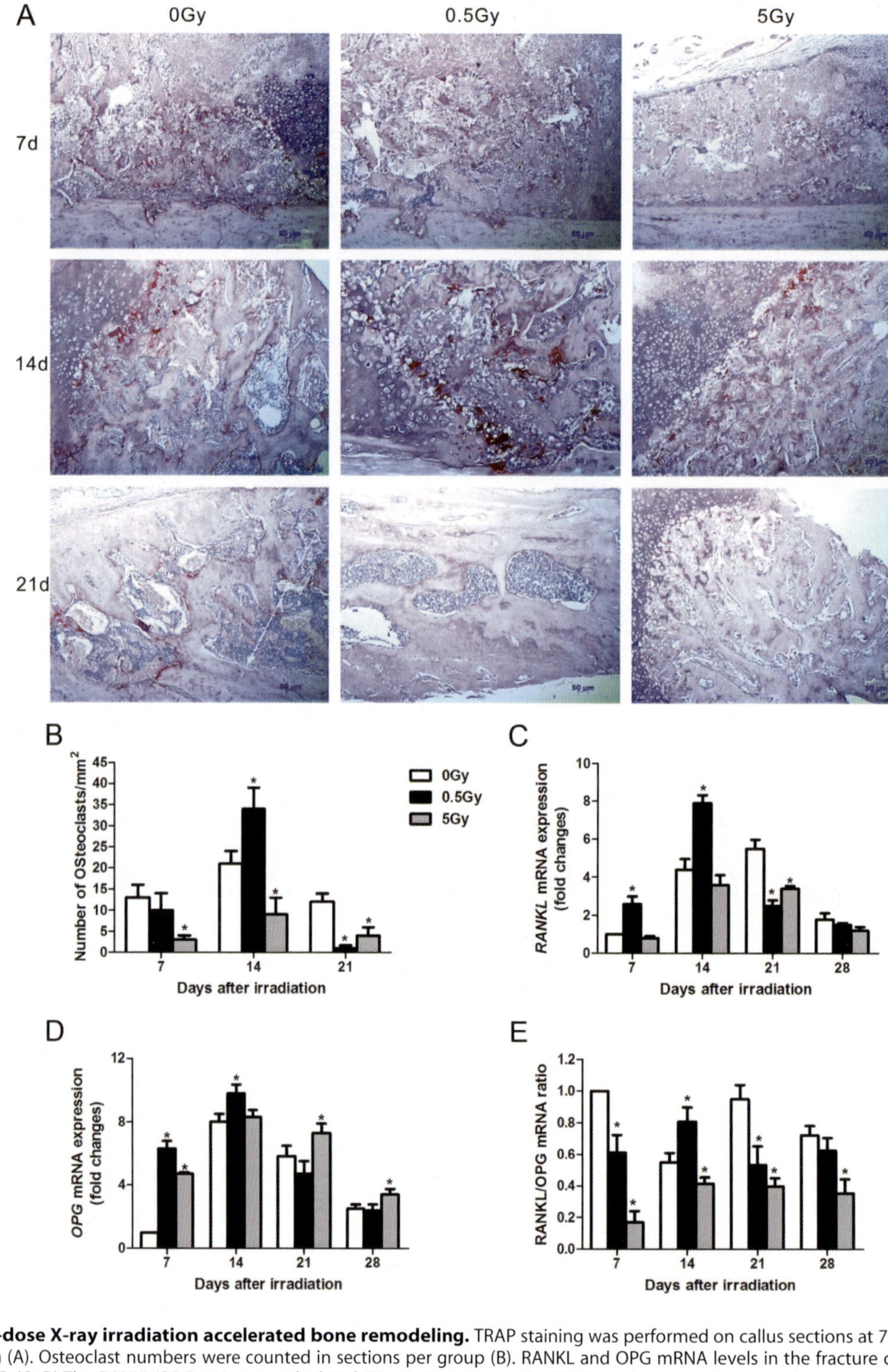

Figure 8. Low-dose X-ray irradiation accelerated bone remodeling. TRAP staining was performed on callus sections at 7, 14 and 21 days after X-ray irradiation (A). Osteoclast numbers were counted in sections per group (B). RANKL and OPG mRNA levels in the fracture callus were examined by real-time PCR (C, D).The RANKL/OPG ratio was calculated (E). n = 4 rats/group,*$p<0.05$ *vs.* the control group.

the acceleration of complete endochondral ossification. These mature, calcified cartilage tissues may act as a template for bone formation and remodeling. Consistent with the acceleration of the cartilage phase of fracture repair, the expression of osteogenic genes, such as ALP, OCN, Col1a1, Runx2 and Osterix, peaked early or were increased in the low-dose irradiated callus tissues. These results document that low-dose X-ray irradiation enhances the bone formation potential of osteoblast in *vitro* and *vivo*. In addition to enhanced bone formation, our findings also suggest that callus remodeling was accelerated upon low-dose irradiation. We performed TRAP staining to determine whether low-dose X-ray irradiation-induced callus remolding was associated with the potential for accelerated osteoclast formation. Our study reveals that the calluses from the rats irradiated by low-dose X-ray irradiation had more osteoclastogenesis. The RANKL/OPG ratio was consistently increased in the fractures after low-dose X-ray radiation. Finally, fracture union was rapid, and the rate of remodeling was enhanced in low-dose irradiated fractures. Our findings are consistent with previous descriptions indicating that low-dose X-ray irradiation promotes the mineralization of fracture callus tissue in rats [19]. However, callus formation and fracture union were delayed in high-dose X-ray-irradiated fractures, and greater collagenous fiber senescence occurred in high-dose irradiated fracture callus tissue. The following reasons contributed to this observation. On one hand, the discoordination between reduced proliferation and abnormal expression of osteogenic genes might result from decreased bone formation. On the other hand, the reduced number of osteoclasts affected callus remodeling, leading to bone matrix aging or sclerosis.

One limitation of this study was that over-active cell proliferation and tumorigenicity should be addressed for all low-dose irradiation interventions. In fact, because current hospital medical imaging procedures may increase patient exposure to low-dose radiation, the risk of cancer development represents a serious concern. Additionally, human epidemiological data warn that irradiation might trigger abnormal cell proliferation and thus promote tumor growth [10]. Nevertheless, our data show that low-dose X-ray irradiation may induce middle and late osteoblast differentiation simultaneously. Another limitation was that we exclusively focused on the effects of radiation on the fracture healing process using a rat fracture model *in vivo* in the present study. However, we failed to detect changes in the distinct regions or non-fractured sites. Irradiation affects bone tissues by both cellular and physicochemical processes, including bone metabolism and fracture healing. The altered compositions of bone tissues lead to differential response to irradiation [38]. Different local environments and components were noted in the fracture or non-fractured sites. In other words, irradiation had different effects on distinct regions of bone. Given the lack of investigations focused on non-fractured bones, the generalization of our conclusion should be interpreted with caution. In addition, low-dose irradiation appeared to accelerate age-related changes in skeletal micro-architecture [39]. In this study, limited passages of osteoblasts and adult animals were employed for *in vitro* and *in vivo* studies. However, it remains unclear whether the stimulatory effects of low-dose irradiation on osteoblasts and fracture healing represent an age-related phenomenon.

Conclusion

In summary, our experiments revealed that X-ray irradiation at low- or high-doses exhibited opposing effects on osteogenesis. Low-dose (0.5 Gy) X-ray irradiation presented certain beneficial effects on osteoblast proliferation, differentiation and fracture repair. Although high-dose (5 Gy) X-ray irradiation increased terminal differentiation among osteoblasts, it weakened the bone formation capacity of osteoblasts by inhibiting cell proliferation and reducing extracellular matrix production. These findings provide a better understanding of low-dose irradiation-induced biological responses during bone formation and might lead to the development of improved strategies with translational applications for bone-related diseases in humans.

Author Contributions

Performed the experiments: MC QH. Wrote the paper: MC QH QRD ML. Designed and led the study: QRD. Conducted irradiation: MC WX CS. Conducted statistical analysis: WX ML CS. Contributed reagents and fracture model establishment: ZGX YTM.

References

1. Matsumura S, Hiranuma H, Deguchi A, Maeda T, Jikko A, et al. (1998) Changes in phenotypic expression of osteoblasts after X irradiation. Radiat Res 149: 463–471.
2. Long F (2012) Building strong bones: molecular regulation of the osteoblast lineage. Nat Rev Mol Cell Biol 13: 27–38.
3. Phulpin B, Dolivet G, Marie PY, Poussier S, Gallet P, et al. (2010) Re-assessment of chronic radio-induced tissue damage in a rat hindlimb model. Exp Ther Med 1: 553–560.
4. Takahashi S, Sugimoto M, Kotoura Y, Sasai K, Oka M, et al. (1994) Long-term changes in the haversian systems following high-dose irradiation. An ultrastructural and quantitative histomorphological study. J Bone Joint Surg Am 76: 722–738.
5. Peyre HM, Coffigny H, Reillaudou M, Beaumatin J, Morin M, et al. (2000) Transformation by radiation of rat foetal glial cells. Int J Radiat Biol 76: 87–94.
6. Jia D, Gaddy D, Suva LJ, Corry PM (2011) Rapid loss of bone mass and strength in mice after abdominal irradiation. Radiat Res 176: 624–635.
7. Szymczyk KH, Shapiro IM, Adams CS (2004) Ionizing radiation sensitizes bone cells to apoptosis. Bone 34: 148–156.
8. Sakurai T, Sawada Y, Yoshimoto M, Kawai M, Miyakoshi J (2007) Radiation-induced reduction of osteoblast differentiation in C2C12 cells. J Radiat Res 48: 515–521.
9. Theocharopoulos N, Perisinakis K, Damilakis J, Papadokostakis G, Hadjipavlou A, et al. (2003) Occupational exposure from common fluoroscopic projections used in orthopaedic surgery. J Bone Joint Surg Am 85-A: 1698–1703.
10. Fazel R, Krumholz HM, Wang Y, Ross JS, Chen J, et al. (2009) Exposure to low-dose ionizing radiation from medical imaging procedures. N Engl J Med 361: 849–857.
11. Pramojanee SN, Pratchayasakul W, Chattipakorn N, Chattipakorn SC (2012) Low-dose dental irradiation decreases oxidative stress in osteoblastic MC3T3-E1 cells without any changes in cell viability, cellular proliferation and cellular apoptosis. Arch Oral Biol 57: 252–256.
12. Sangsuwan T, Haghdoost S (2008) The nucleotide pool, a target for low-dose gamma-ray-induced oxidative stress. Radiat Res 170: 776–783.
13. Asaithamby A, Chen DJ (2009) Cellular responses to DNA double-strand breaks after low-dose gamma-irradiation. Nucleic Acids Res 37: 3912–3923.
14. Li W, Wang G, Cui J, Xue L, Cai L (2004) Low-dose radiation (LDR) induces hematopoietic hormesis: LDR-induced mobilization of hematopoietic progenitor cells into peripheral blood circulation. Exp Hematol 32: 1088–1096.
15. Liang X, So YH, Cui J, Ma K, Xu X, et al. (2011) The low-dose ionizing radiation stimulates cell proliferation via activation of the MAPK/ERK pathway in rat cultured mesenchymal stem cells. J Radiat Res 52: 380–386.
16. He J, Qiu W, Zhang Z, Wang Z, Zhang X, et al. (2011) Effects of irradiation on growth and differentiation-related gene expression in osteoblasts. J Craniofac Surg 22: 1635–1640.
17. Lau P, Baumstark-Khan C, Hellweg CE, Reitz G (2010) X-irradiation-induced cell cycle delay and DNA double-strand breaks in the murine osteoblastic cell line OCT-1. Radiat Environ Biophys 49: 271–280.
18. Park SS, Kim KA, Lee SY, Lim SS, Jeon YM, et al. (2012) X-ray radiation at low doses stimulates differentiation and mineralization of mouse calvarial osteoblasts. BMB Rep 45: 571–576.
19. Zhou XZ, Zhang G, Dong QR, Chan CW, Liu CF, et al. (2009) Low-dose X-irradiation promotes mineralization of fracture callus in a rat model. Arch Orthop Trauma Surg 129: 125–132.
20. Xu W, Xu L, Chen M, Mao YT, Xie ZG, et al. (2012) The effects of low dose X-irradiation on osteoblastic MC3T3-E1 cells in vitro. BMC Musculoskelet Disord 13: 94.
21. Naik AA, Xie C, Zuscik MJ, Kingsley P, Schwarz EM, et al. (2009) Reduced COX-2 expression in aged mice is associated with impaired fracture healing. J Bone Miner Res 24: 251–264.
22. Iwaki A, Jingushi S, Oda Y, Izumi T, Shida JI, et al. (1997) Localization and quantification of proliferating cells during rat fracture repair: detection of proliferating cell nuclear antigen by immunohistochemistry. J Bone Miner Res 12: 96–102.
23. Srivastava UK, Srivastava SR, Guru PY (1989) Rat luteal cells in tissue culture: a technique for obtaining primary cell culture without enzymatic dissociation. Indian J Exp Biol 27: 602–606.
24. Paunesku T, Mittal S, Protic M, Oryhon J, Korolev SV, et al. (2001) Proliferating cell nuclear antigen (PCNA): ringmaster of the genome. International journal of radiation biology 77: 1007–1021.
25. Yu YL, Chou RH, Liang JH, Chang WJ, Su KJ, et al. (2013) Targeting the EGFR/PCNA signaling suppresses tumor growth of triple-negative breast cancer cells with cell-penetrating PCNA peptides. PloS One 8: e61362.
26. Schnoke M, Midura SB, Midura RJ (2009) Parathyroid hormone suppresses osteoblast apoptosis by augmenting DNA repair. Bone 45: 590–602.
27. Tsai CJ, Hofstede TM, Sturgis EM, Garden AS, Lindberg ME, et al. (2013) Osteoradionecrosis and radiation dose to the mandible in patients with oropharyngeal cancer. Int J Radiat Oncol Biol Phys 85: 415–420.

28. Lee IJ, Koom WS, Lee CG, Kim YB, Yoo SW, et al. (2009) Risk factors and dose-effect relationship for mandibular osteoradionecrosis in oral and oropharyngeal cancer patients. Int J Radiat Oncol Biol Phys 75: 1084–1091.
29. Williams HJ, Davies AM (2006) The effect of X-rays on bone: a pictorial review. Eur Radiol 16: 619–633.
30. Chae HJ, Chae SW, Kang JS, Bang BG, Han JI, et al. (1999) Effect of ionizing radiation on the differentiation of ROS 17/2.8 osteoblasts through free radicals. J Radiat Res 40: 323–335.
31. Smialek MA, Moore SA, Mason NJ, Shuker DE (2009) Quantification of radiation-induced single-strand breaks in plasmid DNA using a TUNEL/ELISA-based assay. Radiat Res 172: 529–536.
32. Sugrue T, Brown JA, Lowndes NF, Ceredig R (2013) Multiple facets of the DNA damage response contribute to the radioresistance of mouse mesenchymal stromal cell lines. Stem Cells 31: 137–145.
33. Feinendegen LE (2005) Evidence for beneficial low level radiation effects and radiation hormesis. Br J Radiol 78: 3–7.
34. Caetano-Lopes J, Canhao H, Fonseca JE (2007) Osteoblasts and bone formation. Acta Reumatol Port 32: 103–110.
35. Choi JY, Lee BH, Song KB, Park RW, Kim IS, et al. (1996) Expression patterns of bone-related proteins during osteoblastic differentiation in MC3T3-E1 cells. J Cell Biochem 61: 609–618.
36. Singh AM, Reynolds D, Cliff T, Ohtsuka S, Mattheyses AL, et al. (2012) Signaling network crosstalk in human pluripotent cells: a Smad2/3-regulated switch that controls the balance between self-renewal and differentiation. Cell Stem Cell 10: 312–326.
37. Zhang M, Ho HC, Sheu TJ, Breyer MD, Flick LM, et al. (2011) EP1(−/−) mice have enhanced osteoblast differentiation and accelerated fracture repair. J Bone Miner Res 26: 792–802.
38. Green DE, Adler BJ, Chan ME, Lennon JJ, Acerbo AS, et al. (2013) Altered composition of bone as triggered by irradiation facilitates the rapid erosion of the matrix by both cellular and physicochemical processes. PloS One 8: e64952.
39. Alwood JS, Kumar A, Tran LH, Wang A, Limoli CL, et al. (2012) Low-dose, ionizing radiation and age-related changes in skeletal microarchitecture. J Aging Res 2012: 481983.

The Effect of Naturally Occurring Chronic Kidney Disease on the Micro-Structural and Mechanical Properties of Bone

Anna Shipov[1*¶], Gilad Segev[1¶], Hagar Meltzer[1], Moran Milrad[1], Ori Brenner[2], Ayelet Atkins[1], Ron Shahar[1]

1 Koret School of Veterinary Medicine, Hebrew University of Jerusalem, Rehovot, Israel, **2** Department of Veterinary Resources, Weizmann Institute, Rehovot, Israel

Abstract

Chronic kidney disease (CKD) is a growing public health concern worldwide, and is associated with marked increase of bone fragility. Previous studies assessing the effect of CKD on bone quality were based on biopsies from human patients or on laboratory animal models. Such studies provide information of limited relevance due to the small size of the samples (biopsies) or the non-physiologic CKD syndrome studied (rodent models with artificially induced CKD). Furthermore, the type, architecture, structure and biology of the bone of rodents are remarkably different from human bones; therefore similar clinicopathologic circumstances may affect their bones differently. We describe the effects of naturally occurring CKD with features resembling human CKD on the skeleton of cats, whose bone biology, structure and composition are remarkably similar to those of humans. We show that CKD causes significant increase of resorption cavity density compared with healthy controls, as well as significantly lower cortical mineral density, cortical cross-sectional area and cortical cross-sectional thickness. Young's modulus, yield stress, and ultimate stress of the cortical bone material were all significantly decreased in the skeleton of CKD cats. Cancellous bone was also affected, having significantly lower trabecular thickness and bone volume over total volume in CKD cats compared with controls. This study shows that naturally occurring CKD has deleterious effects on bone quality and strength. Since many similarities exist between human and feline CKD patients, including the clinicopathologic features of the syndrome and bone microarchitecture and biology, these results contribute to better understanding of bone abnormalities associated with CKD.

Editor: Luc Malaval, Université Jean Monnet, France

Funding: This work was supported by the Israel Science Foundation (Grant No 151/08) to RS. The funders had no role in study design, data collection and analysis, decision to publish, or preparation of the manuscript.

Competing Interests: The authors have declared that no competing interests exist.

* Email: anna.shipov@mail.huji.ac.il

¶ These authors contributed equally to this work.

Introduction

Chronic kidney disease (CKD) is a growing public health concern worldwide, with increasing incidence in all age groups. The prevalence of moderate to severe CKD in the general population is reported to be as high as 8.5% [1,2]. The disease is irreversible and progressive in nature, and as it progresses, metabolic derangements worsen. This is particularly true in the ageing population, where CKD has become a major cause of morbidity and mortality.

CKD-associated bone diseases include several different types of bone pathologies, such as adynamic bone disease and osteomalacia which are characterized by low bone turnover, osteitis fibrosa cystica which is characterized by high bone turnover (due to secondary hyperparathyroidism) and mixed uremic osteodystrophy which is characterized by either high or low turnover and abnormal mineralization [3].

One of the inevitable metabolic consequences of CKD is secondary renal hyperparathyroidism (SRH) [4]. The pathophysiology of SRH is complex and involves phosphorus retention leading to hyperphosphatemia, ionized hypocalcemia, decreased circulating 1,25-dihydroxyvitamin D (calcitriol) concentration and increased concentrations of parathyroid hormone (PTH) and fibroblast growth factor 23 [FGF23, [5]]. FGF23, which has been shown to have a pivotal role in mineral homeostasis, is produced mainly by osteocytes and osteoblasts [6]. Serum levels of FGF23 increase already in the early stages of CKD, when patients are still normo-phosphatemic and have normal PTH levels [7–9]. When PTH levels increase, they promote bone resorption, and persistently high PTH concentrations, as documented in CKD patients, eventually lead to, osteopenia, and increased risk of pathological fractures [10].

It is widely recognized that bone fragility increases markedly in patients with CKD, and that fracture risk increases with progression of the disease [11–13]. The risk of pathological fractures has been reported to increase by 9% with each 200-pg/mL increase in PTH concentration, and by 72% with PTH concentrations above 900 pg/mL (reference range, 150–300 pg/mL), [10], Furthermore, the United States Renal Data System

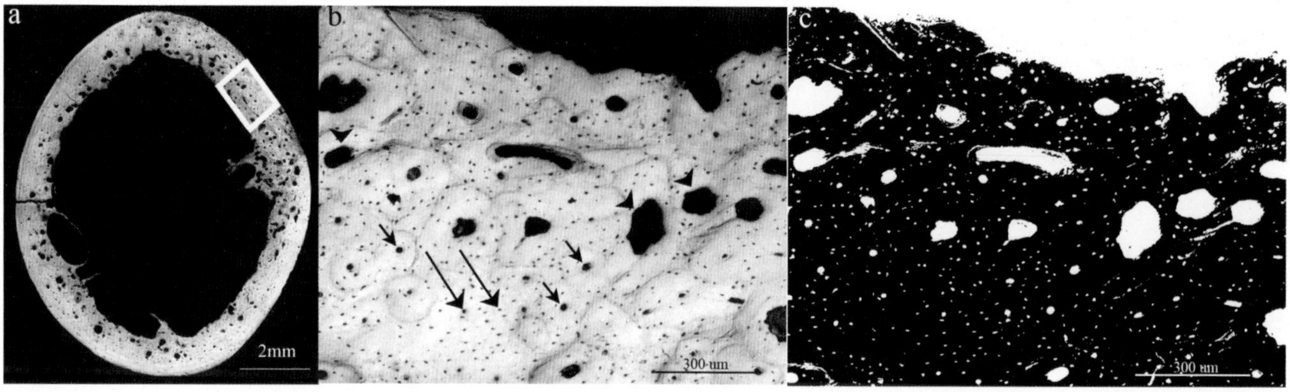

Figure 1. Bone cavity analysis. (a) Light microscopy image of a typical transverse cross section of the bone created by stitching together of many individual images. Classification of voids was performed on based on their size. (b) An individual image from the cross sectional image (marked by a white rectangle in image a). (c) Each image was first binarized, separating it into 'bone' (white) and 'void' (black) (right image). Cavities within the range of 9–50 μm^2 were considered to be lacunae (long arrows), cavities within the range of 151–2000 μm^2 were considered to be Haversian canal (short arrows) and cavities larger than 2000 μm^2 were considered resorptive lesions (arrowheads).

identified a 4-fold greater risk of hip fractures in human dialysis patients as compared to the general population [11].

The precise structural and compositional changes in the skeleton that occur in CKD patients, are not entirely clear. Data regarding the nature of these changes is crucial to the understanding of the skeletal consequences of CKD, since they determine the quality of bone material and the quantitative deterioration of material's mechanical properties. Most previous studies were based on data collected from human patients or from rodent models. For obvious reasons, studies conducted on human patients are subjected to severe inherent limitations, primarily the need to rely on non-invasive or minimally invasive (biopsy) methods. Biopsies, while a valuable diagnostic tool, by their nature provide data relevant to a very small region in a bone, and therefore can provide only limited information. Noninvasive methods used in human patient studies, such as determination of bone mass (or apparent mineral density) by dual x-ray absorptiometry (DEXA) provide imprecise information because of technical limitations, as described eloquently by Parfitt [14]. The main limitations of DEXA include its reliance on a 2-D proxy of mineral density (g/cm^2) measurement rather than true 3-D density, and the inability to obtain separate data for cortical and trabecular bone. Peripheral quantitative computed tomography (pQCT) provides true 3-D information and is therefore a valuable tool, however its resolution is in the mm range.

On the other hand, use of model animals (almost exclusively mice and rats), while allowing the use of a wide array of testing methods, is hindered by the fact that in most studies, CKD is induced by non-physiologic means, mostly partial nephrectomy [15]. This obviously does not mimic with precision the disease in human patients, and may affect the skeleton in ways which are subtly (or even substantially) different from those caused by the natural course of the disease in humans. Moreover, the structure and architecture of rat and mouse cortical bone differs greatly from that of human cortical bone, as shown recently by Shipov *et al* and Bach-Gansmo *et al* [16,17]. Therefore, the ability to directly extend the observed effects of artificially-induced CKD in the rat skeleton to the effects of naturally-occurring CKD in the human skeleton is limited.

The course, pathology and pathophysiology, diagnosis and treatment of feline CKD mirror those of the human disease very closely, and the disease is very prevalent in the feline population [18]. Another major advantage of studying the effects of CKD in cats is that the bones of mature cats are structurally and compositionally very similar to those of humans, both consisting mostly of remodeled secondary osteons [19].

Here we present a detailed study of the skeletal changes, both structural and mechanical, in cats with naturally occurring CKD. In this study we compare the femora and vertebra of cats diagnosed with CKD and those of age-matched cats with normally functioning kidneys.

Materials and Methods

2.1 Animals and data collection

The study was prospective, based on the patient population of the Veterinary Teaching Hospital of the Hebrew University of Jerusalem, and was approved by the institutional animal care and use committee. Cats considered for the study either died or were euthanized at their owners' request after medical management had failed. Euthanasia was performed using 200 mg/kg pentobarbital (CTS chemical industries LTD, Israel) administered intravenously. Cats were enrolled only after their owners had signed an informed consent form and donated the body to science. The study group consisted of 13 cats diagnosed with Stage III or IV CKD, based on the classification scheme of the International Renal Interest Society guidelines [20], for at least 6 months prior to death or euthanasia. These criteria included documentation of persistent azotemia (3 occasions, at least 2 weeks interval, serum creatinine concentration >2.8 mg/dL), urine specific gravity <1.020 and ultrasonographic changes consistent with CKD. CKD was additionally confirmed in all cats by histopathological examination showing moderate to severe interstitial nephritis accompanied by moderate to severe fibrosis.

The control group included 13 healthy cats without any clinicopathologic signs of CKD (e.g., normal creatinine, concentrated urine) that died or were euthanized in the Veterinary Medical Teaching Hospital due to reasons unrelated to diseases of the urinary system. Cats with concurrent metabolic diseases that could potentially affect the skeleton were excluded, as were cats that were treated for more than 2 weeks during the 6 months prior to their death with medications that could alter bone metabolism (e.g., vitamin D derivatives, corticosteroids).

Table 1. Morphometric characteristics of cortical bone of the distal femur in CKD and healthy controls by light microscopy.

Light microscopy morphometry	CKD (mean ±SD)	Controls (mean ±SD)	*P* value
Oseteocytic lacunae			
Size [μm²]	33.9±3.1	33.1±3.9	0.60
Density [mm⁻²]	510±55	524±106	0.70
Haversian canals			
Size [μm²]	481±115	411±48	0.10
Density [mm⁻²]	22.3±4.3	23.3±4.6	0.58
Resorption cavities			
Size [μm²]	10,342±11,888	12,406±25,258	0.78
Density [mm⁻²]	2.2±2.4	0.4±0.1	**0.04**

2.2 Sample collection and preparation

Blood and serum samples from all cats were collected *antemortem* for complete blood count and biochemical analysis. Sera were stored at −80°C for determination of PTH and vitamin D levels.

Tissue sample collection was performed within 12 hours of death. The right femora and lumbar vertebrae were carefully removed and cleaned of all soft tissue, wrapped in saline-soaked gauze, placed in a sealed plastic bag and stored at −20°C until testing. Kidney samples were harvested and stored in 10% formalin for histologic evaluation.

2.3 Light microscopy

Thin transverse slices (400 microns thick) of the mid-diaphyseal region of all right femora were cut by a water-cooled slow-speed diamond saw (Buehler Isomet low Speed saw, USA). The slices were then polished by increasingly fine grit (Buehlet Minimet Polisher, USA), from 320 grit to 1 μm diamond paste. Transverse cross-sections of all cortical samples were viewed by reflective light microscopy (Olympus BX-51) and their detailed architecture characterized by analysis of images captured by a dedicated high-resolution camera (Olympus DP 71, 12 MegaPixels).

Quantitative analysis of the transverse cross-sectional images, particularly quantification of voids and their classification, was performed with a public domain image processing software (ImageJ, NIH, v. 1.44p). Several microstructural parameters were measured, such as the number, size and density of the osteocytic lacunae, Haversian canals and resorption cavities within each cross section [21]. Specifically, each cross-sectional image was first binarized by selection of an appropriate threshold, separating it into 'bone' (white) and 'void' (black) entities [22], (Fig. 1 a, b). Next, the ImagJ 'analyze particles' command was applied to each cross-section to identify all individual voids within it. This command analyzes each void by its size and reports the results in a tabular form (see Figure 1) [23]. Based on sizes of osteocytic lacuna and Haversian canals reported in the literature [24–27] voids with an area in the range of 9–150 μm² were considered to be osteocytic lacunae, voids with an area in the range of 151–2000 μm² were considered to be Haversian canals, while voids larger than 2000 μm² were considered resorption cavities which are in the process of remodeling [21]. Voids smaller than 9 μm² were considered to be artifacts. Images were also visually examined by two of the authors (AS and HM) and the results of thresholding and void categorization were manually corrected if indicated. Overall porosity was calculated as the ratio of total void area (i.e. resorption cavities, lacunae and blood vessels) to total bone area.

2.4 Mechanical testing

Mechanical properties of cortical bone were evaluated using four-point bending tests performed on bone beams prepared from the cranial aspect of the mid-diaphyseal cortical region of the right femora. Beam sizes were 20 mm×1.5 mm×1 mm (long dimension along the bone axis).

Mechanical testing was performed with the samples immersed in saline, using a custom-built micromechanical-testing device as previously described [28]. All samples were thawed immediately before testing for one hour at room temperature. The beams were placed within a saline-containing testing chamber that had a stationary anvil attached to its wall [28]. This anvil consisted of two supports which were 15 mm apart. A movable double-pronged loading anvil was attached to a load-cell (model 31, Honeywell Sensotec, Colombus, OH, USA), which was in turn attached to a high-precision linear motor (PI GmbH, Karlsruhe, Germany). The loading anvil had a span of 5 mm between its two prongs, which were centered between the two supports of the stationary anvil.

The upper prongs were brought into contact with the tested beams at a predetermined preload (2N), the chamber was filled with physiologic saline solution at room temperature until the

Table 2. Morphometry of cortical bone of the mid-diaphyseal femur in CKD and healthy controls.

Microtomography	CKD (mean ±SD)	Controls (mean ±SD)	*P* value
Cortical cross sectional area (mm²)	28.5±3.6	32.2±5.5	**0.04**
Cross-sectional thickness (mm)	1.1±0.2	1.2±0.2	**0.03**
Mean polar area of inertia (μm⁴)	432±95	520 ±154	0.08

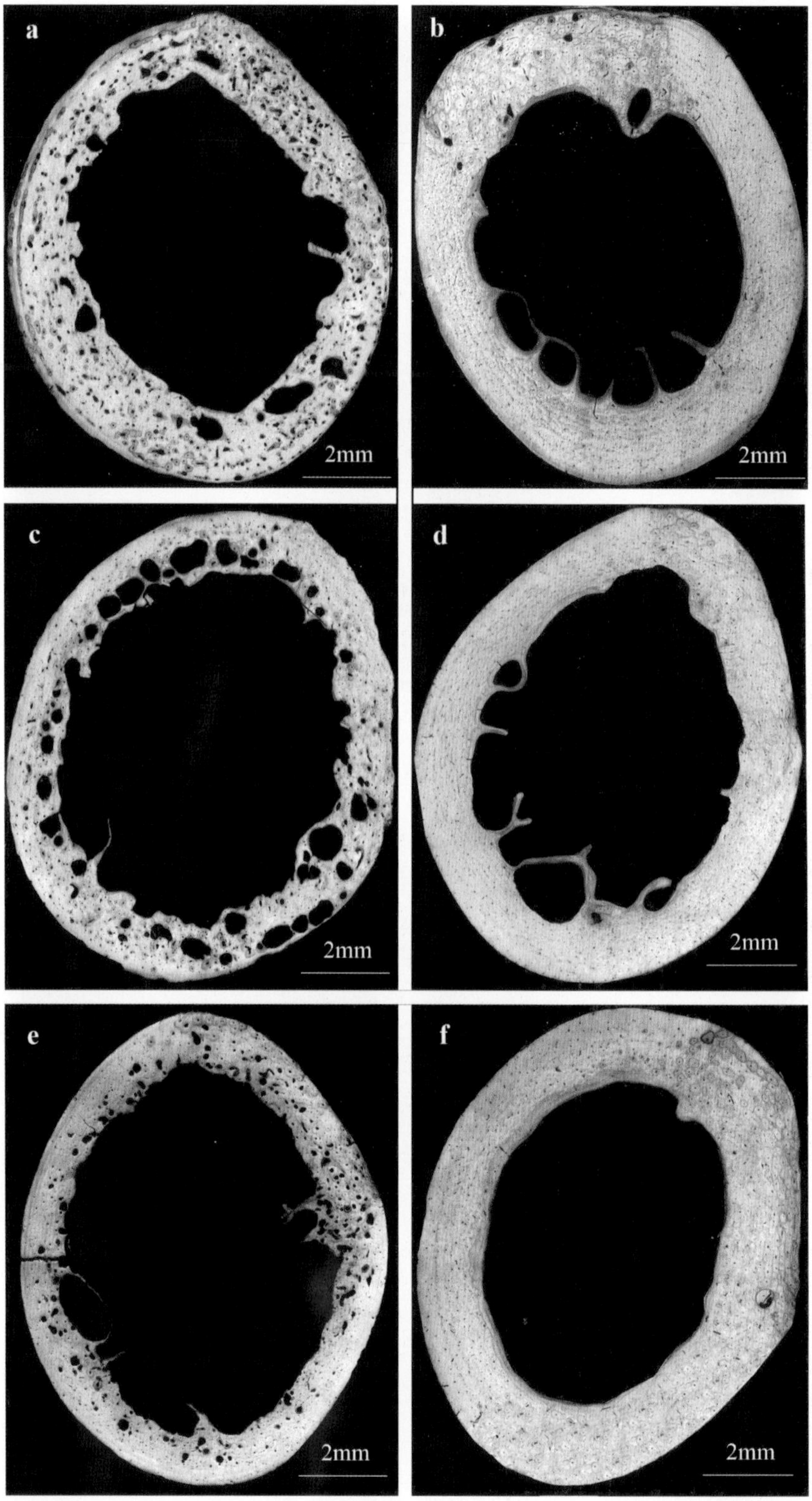

Figure 2. Light microscopy images of three transverse cross-sections of the femoral mid-diaphysis of (a, c, e) cats with CKD and (b, d, f) healthy cats. Note dramatic increase in unfilled resorption cavities in CKD cats compared to the healthy cats.

samples were fully immersed, and bending tests were conducted under displacement control at a rate of 500 μm/180 seconds up to failure. Force-displacement data were collected by custom-written software (LabView, National Instruments, Texas, USA) at 50 Hz. Load and displacement values were converted to stress and strain, respectively, based on beam theory [29]. The stress-strain curves were used to estimate Young's modulus of the beam material, as well as yield and failure stresses and strains. It should be noted that

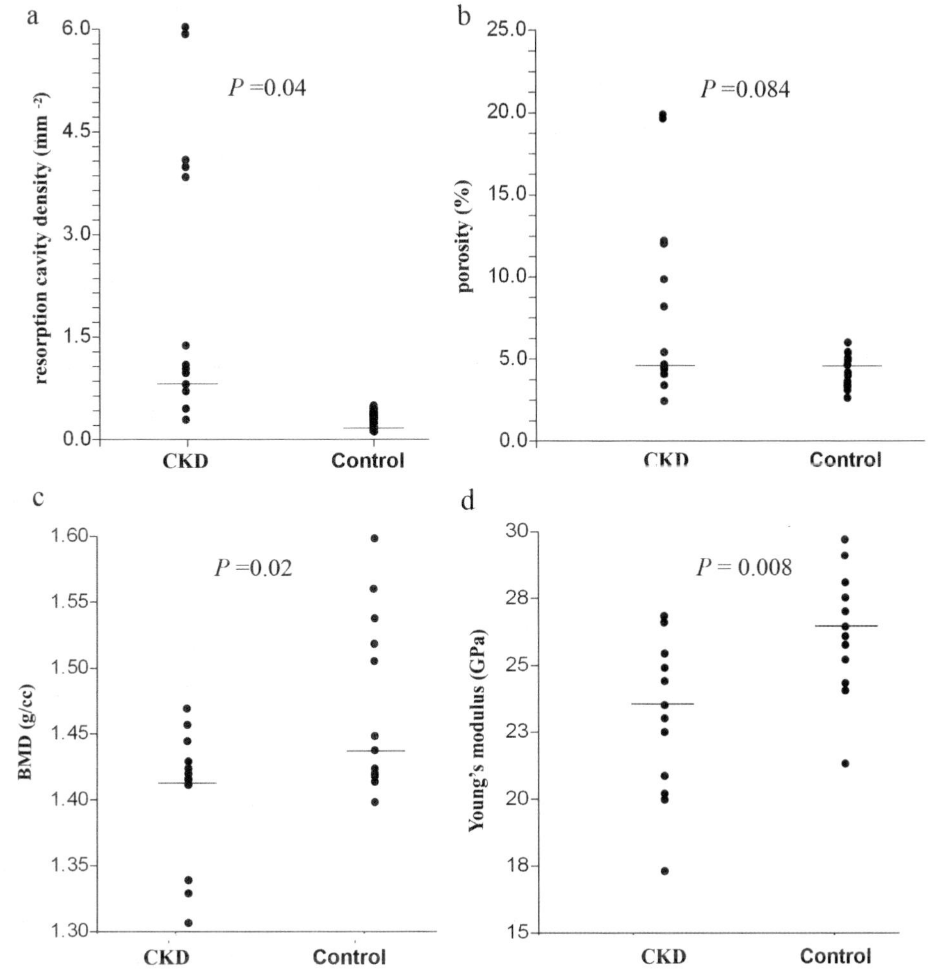

Figure 3. Dot plots depicting the data of CKD and control cats; the horizontal line represents the median. (a) resorption cavity density (b) porosity, (c) BMD and (d) Young's modulus.

care was taken to minimize shear deformation at the supports by maintaining a ratio of distance between supports/beam depth of 15:1 [30,31]. Yield point was determined for each beam as the point at which a line parallel with the linear portion of the stress-strain curve and offset by 0.03% strain intersected with this curve [32].

2.5 Microstructural characterization by Micro-CT

All cortical beams, the right femur and the 6th and 7th lumbar vertebrae were scanned by microCT (Skyscan 1174 compact micro-CT scanner, Belgium), with the beams scanned prior to mechanical testing. Analyses were performed on the entire beam, the mid-diaphyseal femoral cortex (cortical bone analysis), and in the distal femoral metaphyses and vertebral bodies (cancellous bone analysis).

The X-ray source was set at 50 kVp and 800 μA. A total of 450 projections were acquired over an angular range of 180°. The samples were scanned with an isotropic voxel size of 11.1 μm for the cortical bone beams and 19.6 μm for the femoral cortex and cancellous bone of both the femora and vertebrae. Integration time for all scans was 4500 ms, and a 0.25 mm aluminum filter was used. Scans were reconstructed and analyzed using commercial software (NRecon Skyscan software, version 1.6.1.2 and CT analyser Skyscan software, version 1.9.3.2, respectively). Cortical bone mineral density (BMD) of the beams was determined based on calibration with 2 phantoms of known mineral density (0.25 g/cm^3 and 0.75 g/cm^3) supplied by SkyScan, which were scanned under exactly the same condition as were the bone specimens.

2.6 Statistical analysis

The distribution of continuous parameters (normal vs. non-normal) was assessed using the Shapiro-Wilk's test. Normally and non-normally distributed continuous parameters were compared between the study and the control group using Student's t-test and Mann-Whitney U test, respectively. Gender proportion between the study group and the control groups was compared using the Fischer Exact test. Correlations between continuous parameters (e.g., biomechanical parameters and PTH concentration) were performed using the Pearson or the Spearman Rank correlation test, according to data distribution. For all tests $P<0.05$ was considered statistically significant. All calculations were performed using a statistical software (SPSS 17.0 for Windows, SPSS Inc; Chicago, IL, USA).

Results

3.1 Animals

The study population included 26 cats, of which 13 were diagnosed with CKD and 13 were healthy controls. There were eight males and five females in the study group and six males and seven females in the control group, with no gender proportion differences between the study groups. Mean body weight was significantly lower in cats with CKD compared with healthy controls (2.8±0.6 kg vs. 3.7±0.9 kg, respectively; $P = 0.01$). There was no statistically significant difference in mean age between the study and control groups (10.5±5.6 years compared to 9.7±3.9 years, respectively; $P = 0.7$).

3.2 Clinical pathology

Median serum creatinine concentration within the CKD group was 8.2 mg/dL (range 3.5–16.0 mg/dL) compared with a median of 0.9 mg/dL (range 0.6–1.2 mg/dL) [reference interval (RI), 0.5–1.6 mg/dL] of the control group. Three cats in the study group (23%) were classified as Stage III CKD, and the rest (77%) were classified as Stage IV CKD. Median phosphorous concentration in the study group was 8.8 mg/dL (range 5.3–21.7 mg/dL; RI, 3.0–6.2 mg/dL). Median concentration of ionized calcium in the study group was 0.80 mmol/L (range 0.65–1.01 mmol/L; RI, 0.9–1.4 mmol/L). PTH concentration, available for five cats of the study group, had a median concentration of 15.70 pmol/L (range, 0.9–32.9 pmol/L; RI, 0.4–2.5 pmol/L). Vitamin D concentration was below normal in five out of the seven cats in which it was measured (median 63 nmol/L, range 35–143 nmol/L; RI 65–170 nmol/L).

3.3 Cortical bone architecture

The results of the architectural analysis are presented in Table 1 (microscopy) and Table 2 (microCT). CKD-affected cats had significantly higher density of resorption cavities compared to healthy controls (Table 1, Figures 2, 3a). Other structural parameters were not significantly different between the groups. Porosity tended to be higher in the CKD group, however the difference between groups did not reach statistical significance ($P = 0.084$, Figure 3b).

Micro-CT analysis of cortical bone of the femoral diaphysis showed significantly lower cortical cross-sectional area and cross-sectional thickness in CKD cats (Table 2). Mean polar area moment of inertia tended to be lower in the CKD group, but the differences did not reach statistical significance ($P = 0.083$) (Table 2).

3.4 Cortical mineral density

Cortical mineral density of CKD cats was lower by 4.8% compared to controls, ($P = 0.02$, as shown in Figure 3c).

3.5 Mechanical properties of cortical bone

Table 3 and Figure 3 present a comparison of several mechanical properties of cortical bone material between the CKD and control groups. Bones from the CKD group were shown to have inferior mechanical properties compared to the control group, in particular lower stiffness (Young's modulus), lower yield stress, and lower ultimate stress (Table 3, Figure 3).

Correlation could not be demonstrated between PTH levels and any of the mechanical properties of the cortical bone.

3.6 Architecture of trabecular bone

Analysis of cancellous bone in the 6th and 7th lumbar vertebrae and in the distal femur revealed significantly lower trabecular thickness and bone volume over total volume (BV/TV) in bones belonging to the CKD group, compared with control cats (Figure 4).

Discussion

This study demonstrates that advanced CKD in cats results in deterioration of bone quality, in particular a dramatic increase of resorption cavities and decreased bone mineral density. These results provide insight into skeletal changes occurring in human CKD due to the similarity between cats and humans in terms of the pathophysiology of the syndrome and the type of bone architecture.

To the best of our knowledge, this is the first study to measure the detailed mechanical and structural effects of CKD on the skeleton of an animal model with *naturally occurring* CKD. Feline and human CKD have very similar clinicopathologic features and progression, therefore cats are superior models compared to rodents in which pharmaceutical and surgical interventions are usually employed to induce kidney disease [33–36]. Furthermore, the cat skeleton shows great similarities to human bone, in particular because it remodels continuously throughout life and therefore consists mostly of secondary osteons. Rodent bones on the other hand are remarkably different from those of human bones in terms of type, architecture, structure and biology. Most dramatically, rodent cortical bone does not remodel [16,17]. Therefore similar clinicopathologic circumstances, such as those occurring due to CKD, may affect rodent bones differently from human (or cat) bones.

We found that naturally occurring CKD results in several alterations to the architecture and morphology of the bones of the skeleton. Cortical thickness was found to be decreased by approximately 17% in CKD cats compared with controls. This change compromises the mechanical performance of long bones, by reducing their flexural stiffness and is likely to lead to increased fracture risk. Previous studies conducted in human patients with CKD showed similar tendencies, however with much smaller changes. For instance, a recent study documented 4.2% increase

Table 3. Mechanical properties of the cortical bone of CKD and control groups.

Parameter	CKD (mean ±SD)	Controls (mean ±SD)	*P* value
Young's modulus (GPa)	**23.5±2.9**	**27.1±2.8**	**0.01**
Yield stress (MPa)	**151±18**	**166±14**	**0.04**
Yield strain (millistrain)	5.6±0.8	5.6±0.4	.95
Ultimate stress (MPa)	**185±16**	**205±15**	**0.01**
Ultimate strain (millistrain)	8.6±1.0	8.1±0.4	0.37

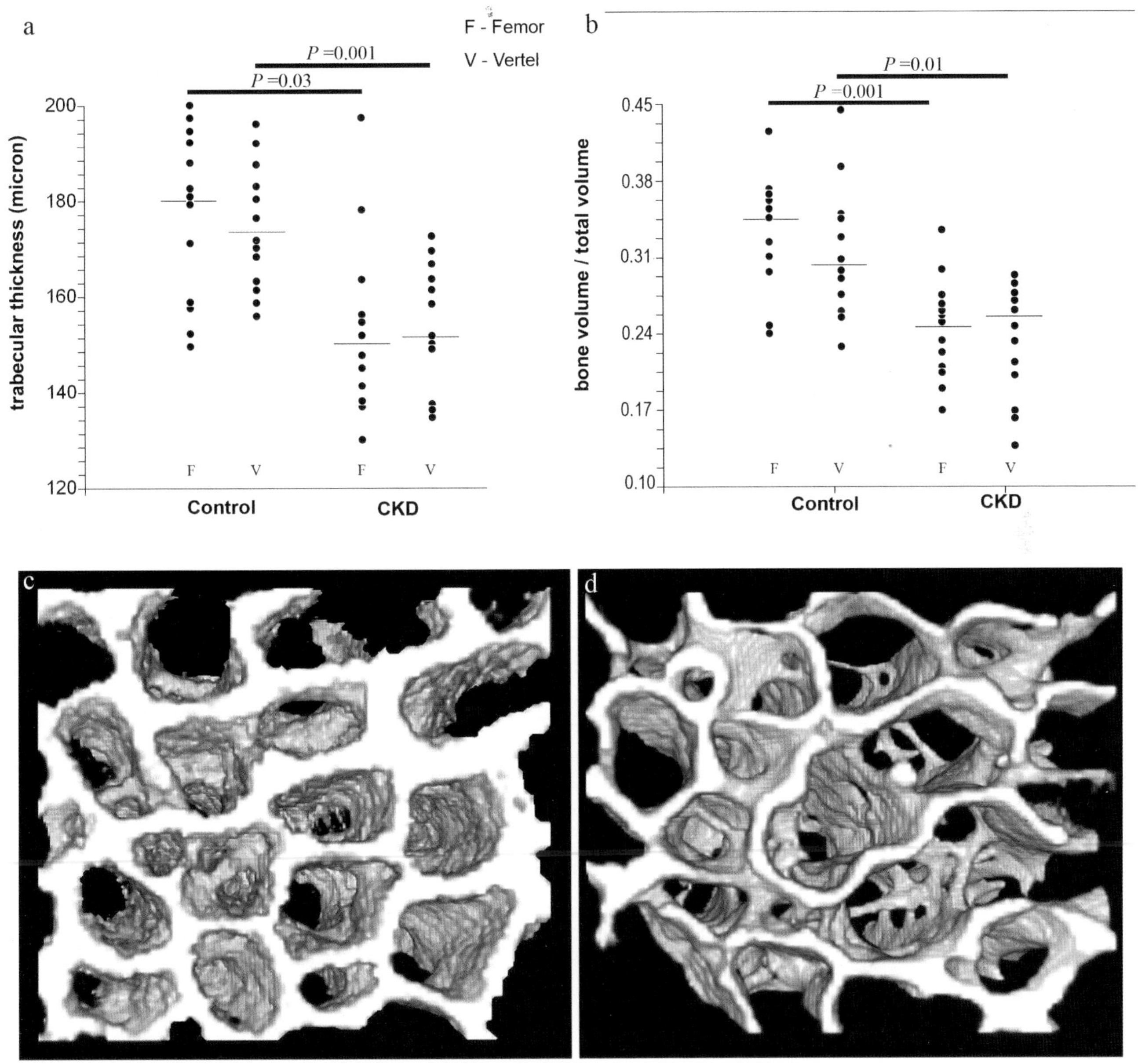

Figure 4. Trabecular bone analysis: Trabecular thickness (a) and bone volume/total volume (BV/TV, b) in the cancellous bone of CKD and control cats for both the femora (F) and the vertebrae (V). Data are presented as dot plots. The horizontal line represents the median. Data from the femur and vertebra are similar within the study groups; however, there is a significant difference for both parameters between the study and the control groups. Micro-CT scans of cancellous bone of a control (c) and CKD (d) cat.

in porosity, 2.9% decrease in cortical area and 2.8% decrease in cortical thickness, indicating progressive loss of cortical bone [37]. These results, like those of other human studies, were based on DEXA and high resolution peripheral quantitative CT. These methods have been shown to be limited in precision in terms of bone volume quantification due to inability to separate cortical from cancellous bone (DEXA), and low-resolution volumetric measurements, compared to microCT and whole bone sampling [38].

Overall cortical porosity in cats with advanced CKD tended to be somewhat higher compared with controls (Figure 3b), but this difference did not reach statistical significance, most likely due to small group size and biological variation. However, the density (number per unit area) of resorption cavities in CKD patients is greatly increased (5-fold, 2.22/mm^2 vs. 0.41/mm^2, $P = 0.04$). Such a difference is expected to affect mechanical behavior of long bones radically, and is likely to play an important role in the increased fragility of CKD patients. Previous studies in a rat model demonstrated that persistently elevated PTH concentrations result in high bone turnover, exhibited as elevated numbers and size of osteoclasts, increased osteoblastic activity and enhanced bone resorption [33]. Consequently, these studies found extensive endocortical, intracortical and periosteal resorption, resulting in a dramatic increase in cortical porosity (9.75% compared to 0%). It should be noted however that these results were observed in rat bone, which normally does not remodel, as oppose to cat (and human) bone.

Bone mineral density is another major determinant of bone quality, and the current clinical standard for prediction of fracture risk in osteoporotic patients [39]. Therefore, determining the influence of CKD on BMD was a major objective of this study. The cortical mineral density of cats with CKD was significantly lower compared to controls. It should be noted that despite appearing small, this decrease (4.8%) is clinically significant, as even a small decrease in BMD substantially decreases the stiffness of the bone and increases fracture risk [40], since the relationship between them is exponential [41]. A decrease in BMD was also reported in various studies in humans CKD patients, with a wide range of values [1.3% to 17.5%; [37,42,43]]. However, these studies were based on areal BMD (g/cm^2, using DEXA), histomorphometry or pQCT, while the current study measured volumetric BMD at high resolution and precision using microCT [38,44].

Reliable measurement of material properties requires precise and accurate mechanical testing. Such testing is difficult to achieve in rodents due to the small size of their bones, which are often tested by bending tests of whole bones, using the 3-point bending technique. Results are dependent upon the geometry of the bones and mechanical properties of the material, often leading to underestimation of Young's modulus [45,46]. The size of cat bones allowed us to prepare cortical bone beams, enabling accurate and reliable assessment of the material properties using four-point bending testing. Furthermore, four-point bending tests of beams allowed us also to measure other material properties, like yield and strength, and to document significant decrease in yield stress and failure stress in the cortical bone of the CKD cats compared to controls.

This study demonstrates that the cortical bone material of CKD cats is less stiff and more prone to micro-damage which occurs at lower loads, and will result in increased bone fragility. In particular, Young's modulus of the cortical bone, which reflects the stiffness of the material, was shown here to be significantly lower in the CKD group (23.5 GPa vs 27.1 GPa, respectively, $P = 0.008$). The lower Young's modulus in CKD cats compared with controls is most likely due to a combination of higher porosity and lower BMD.

Cancellous bone is also significantly affected by CKD, as reflected by decreased trabecular thickness and lower bone volume (BV/TV). Furthermore, the effect on cancellous bone was multi-site, shown to occur both in the vertebral bodies as well as in the long bones. Both changes (trabecular thickness and BV/TV) negatively affect bone quality and were shown to be associated with increased risk for fracture [47].

Since this study was based on cats with naturally occurring kidney disease, some variability existed among them in terms of the severity and the chronicity of the disease. Furthermore, the number of cats included in this study was relatively small, though comparable to numbers typically seen in published rodent model studies. It should also be noted that cats with advanced CKD often exhibit decreased appetite and thus might fail to consume enough food to meet their caloric requirements. Such nutritional deficiencies, as in human patients, might contribute to their decreased bone quality. Additionally, all of the cats in this study had a single etiology (interstitial nephritis, which is the etiology in more than 70% of cases with CKD in cats [18]), whereas human patients with CKD have multiple etiologies (e.g., diabetic nephropathy, transplant patients, etc.). Nevertheless, slowly progressive natural disease represents the human syndrome and its consequences, including renal osteopathy, much better than artificially-induced rodent models.

In conclusion, the current study demonstrates the deleterious effects of CKD on remodeled (secondary osteonal) bone quality and strength, including increased bone resorption, decreased BMD, and inferior mechanical and structural properties. Due to these changes, the bones of CKD patients become more fragile. Since many similarities have been demonstrated between human and feline CKD patients, in terms of the clinic-pathologic features of the syndrome, as well as bone-associated effects, cats are an extremely suitable and relevant animal model for studying the development of bone abnormalities in humans suffering from CKD.

Author Contributions

Conceived and designed the experiments: AS GS HM MM RS. Performed the experiments: AS GS HM MM AA OB RS. Analyzed the data: AS GS HM MM AA RS. Contributed reagents/materials/analysis tools: RS OB. Wrote the paper: AS HM GS MM OB AA RS.

References

1. Lora CM, Daviglus ML, Kusek JW, Porter A, Ricardo AC, et al. (2009) Chronic kidney disease in United States Hispanics: a growing public health problem. Ethn Dis 19: 466–472.
2. McClellan WM, Plantinga LC (2013) A public health perspective on CKD and obesity. Nephrol Dial Transplant 28 Suppl 4: iv37–iv42.
3. Spasovski GB, Bervoets AR, Behets GJ, Ivanovski N, Sikole A, et al. (2003) Spectrum of renal bone disease in end-stage renal failure patients not yet on dialysis. Nephrol Dial Transplant 18: 1159–1166.
4. Levin A, Bakris GL, Molitch M, Smulders M, Tian J, et al. (2007) Prevalence of abnormal serum vitamin D, PTH, calcium, and phosphorus in patients with chronic kidney disease: results of the study to evaluate early kidney disease. Kidney Int 71: 31–38.
5. Cozzolino M, Ciceri P, Volpi EM, Olivi L, Messa PG (2009) Pathophysiology of calcium and phosphate metabolism impairment in chronic kidney disease. Blood Purif 27: 338–344.
6. Nabeshima Y (2008) The discovery of alpha-Klotho and FGF23 unveiled new insight into calcium and phosphate homeostasis. Cell Mol Life Sci 65: 3218–3230.
7. Saito H, Kusano K, Kinosaki M, Ito H, Hirata M, et al. (2003) Human fibroblast growth factor-23 mutants suppress Na+ -dependent phosphate co-transport activity and 1 alpha,25-dihydroxyvitamin D-3 production. J Biol Chem 278: 2206–2211.
8. Shimada T, Hasegawa H, Yamazaki Y, Muto T, Hino R, et al. (2004) FGF-23 is a potent regulator of vitamin D metabolism and phosphate homeostasis. J Bone Miner Res 19: 429–435.
9. Ketteler M, Biggar PH, Liangos O (2013) FGF23 antagonism: the thin line between adaptation and maladaptation in chronic kidney disease. Nephrol Dial Transplant 28: 821–825.
10. Danese MD, Kim J, Doan QV, Dylan M, Griffiths R, et al. (2006) PTH and the risks for hip, vertebral, and pelvic fractures among patients on dialysis. Am J Kidney Dis 47: 149–156.
11. Alem AM, Sherrard DJ, Gillen DL, Weiss NS, Beresford SA, et al. (2000) Increased risk of hip fracture among patients with end-stage renal disease. Kidney Int 58: 396–399.
12. Coco M, Rush H (2000) Increased incidence of hip fractures in dialysis patients with low serum parathyroid hormone. Am J Kidney Dis 36: 1115–1121.
13. Stehman-Breen CO, Sherrard DJ, Alem AM, Gillen DL, Heckbert SR, et al. (2000) Risk factors for hip fracture among patients with end-stage renal disease. Kidney Int 58: 2200–2205.
14. Parfitt AM (1998) A structural approach to renal bone disease. J Bone Miner Res 13: 1213–1220.
15. Iwasaki Y, Kazama JJ, Yamato H, Shimoda H, Fukagawa M (2013) Accumulated uremic toxins attenuate bone mechanical properties in rats with chronic kidney disease. Bone 57: 477–483.
16. Bach-Gansmo FL, Irvine SC, Bruel A, Thomsen JS, Birkedal H (2013) Calcified Cartilage Islands in Rat Cortical Bone. Calcif Tissue Int 92: 330–338.
17. Shipov A, Zaslansky P, Riesemeier H, Segev G, Atkins A, et al. (2013) Unremodeled endochondral bone is a major architectural component of the cortical bone of the rat (Rattus norvegicus). J Struct Biol 183: 132–140.
18. Polzin DJ (2010) Chronic kidney disease. In: Ettinger SJ, Feldman EC, editors.Textbook of Veterinary Internal Medicine. 7th ed. St. Louis: Saunders. pp. 1990–2020.

19. Hillier ML, Bell LS (2007) Differentiating human bone from animal bone: A review of histological methods. J Forensic Sci 52: 249–263.
20. Segev G, Palm C, LeRoy B, Cowgill LD, Westropp JL (2013) Evaluation of neutrophil gelatinase-associated lipocalin as a marker of kidney injury in dogs. J Vet Intern Med 27: 1362–1367.
21. Zebaze RM, Ghasem-Zadeh A, Bohte A, Iuliano-Burns S, Mirams M, et al. (2010) Intracortical remodelling and porosity in the distal radius and post-mortem femurs of women: a cross-sectional study. Lancet 375: 1729–1736.
22. Bousson V, Meunier A, Bergot C, Vicaut E, Rocha MA, et al. (2001) Distribution of intracortical porosity in human midfemoral cortex by age and gender. J Bone Miner Res 16: 1308–1317.
23. Montanari S, Brusatte SL, De Wolf W, Norell MA (2011) Variation of osteocyte lacunae size within the tetrapod skeleton: implications for palaeogenomics. Biol Lett 7: 751–754.
24. Urbanova P, Novotny V (2005) Distinguishing between human and non-human bones: Histometric method for forensic anthropology. Anthropologie 43: 77–85.
25. Currey JD, Shahar R (2013) Cavities in the compact bone in tetrapods and fish and their effect on mechanical properties. J Struct Biol 183: 107–122.
26. Kuchler U, Pfingstner G, Busenlechner D, Dobsak T, Reich K, et al. (2013) Osteocyte lacunar density and area in newly formed bone of the augmented sinus. Clin Oral Implants Res 24: 285–289.
27. Tazawa K, Hoshi K, Kawamoto S, Tanaka M, Ejiri S, et al. (2004) Osteocytic osteolysis observed in rats to which parathyroid hormone was continuously administered. J Bone Miner Metab 22: 524–529.
28. Cohen L, Dean M, Shipov A, Atkins A, Monsonego-Ornan E, et al. (2012) Comparison of structural, architectural and mechanical aspects of cellular and acellular bone in two teleost fish. J Exp Biol 215: 1983–1993.
29. Sharir A, Barak MM, Shahar R (2008) Whole bone mechanics and mechanical testing. Vet J 177: 8–17.
30. Spatz HC, O'Leary EJ, Vincent JF (1996) Young's moduli and shear moduli in cortical bone. Proc Biol Sci 263: 287–294.
31. Draper ER, Goodship AE (2003) A novel technique for four-point bending of small bone samples with semi-automatic analysis. J Biomech 36: 1497–1502.
32. Turner CH, Burr DB (1993) Basic biomechanical measurements of bone: a tutorial. Bone 14: 595–608.
33. Miller MA, Chin J, Miller SC, Fox J (1998) Disparate effects of mild, moderate, and severe secondary hyperparathyroidism on cancellous and cortical bone in rats with chronic renal insufficiency. Bone 23: 257–266.
34. Cao HH, Nazarian A, Ackerman JL, Snyder BD, Rosenberg AE, et al. (2010) Quantitative P-31 NMR spectroscopy and H-1 MRI measurements of bone mineral and matrix density differentiate metabolic bone diseases in rat models. Bone 46: 1582–1590.
35. Iwasaki Y, Kazama JJ, Yamato H, Fukagawa M (2011) Changes in chemical composition of cortical bone associated with bone fragility in rat model with chronic kidney disease. Bone 48: 1260–1267.
36. Jokihaara J, Jarvinen TLN, Jolma P, Koobi P, Kalliovalkama J, et al. (2006) Renal insufficiency-induced bone loss is associated with an increase in bone size and preservation of strength in rat proximal femur. Bone 39: 353–360.
37. Nickolas TL, Stein EM, Dworakowski E, Nishiyama KK, Komandah-Kosseh M, et al. (2013) Rapid cortical bone loss in patients with chronic kidney disease. J Bone Miner Res 28: 1811–1820.
38. Barou O, Valentin D, Vico L, Tirode C, Barbier A, et al. (2002) High-resolution three-dimensional micro-computed tomography detects bone loss and changes in trabecular architecture early: comparison with DEXA and bone histomorphometry in a rat model of disuse osteoporosis. Invest Radiol 37: 40–46.
39. Nickolas TL, Leonard MB, Shane E (2008) Chronic kidney disease and bone fracture: a growing concern. Kidney Int 74: 721–731.
40. Yenchek RH, Ix JH, Shlipak MG, Bauer DC, Rianon NJ, et al. (2012) Bone mineral density and fracture risk in older individuals with CKD. Clin J Am Soc Nephrol 7: 1130–1136.
41. Wasnich RD, Ross PD, Davis JW, Vogel JM (1989) A Comparison of Single and Multi-Site Bmc Measurements for Assessment of Spine Fracture Probability. J Nucl Med 30: 1166–1171.
42. Balon BP, Hojs R, Zavratnik A, Kos M (2002) Bone mineral density in patients beginning hemodialysis treatment. Am J Nephrol 22: 14–17.
43. Rix M, Andreassen H, Eskildsen P, Langdahl B, Olgaard K (1999) Bone mineral density and biochemical markers of bone turnover in patients with predialysis chronic renal failure. Kidney Int 56: 1084–1093.
44. Leonard MB (2009) A Structural Approach to Skeletal Fragility in Chronic Kidney Disease. Semin Nephrol 29: 133–143.
45. van Lenthe GH, Voide R, Boyd SK, Muller R (2008) Tissue modulus calculated from beam theory is biased by bone size and geometry: implications for the use of three-point bending tests to determine bone tissue modulus. Bone 43: 717–723.
46. Torcasio A, Van Oosterwyck H, van Lenthe GH (2008) The systematic errors in tissue modulus of murine bones when estimated from three-point bending. J Biomech 41: S14.
47. Nickolas TL, Stein E, Cohen A, Thomas V, Staron RB, et al. (2010) Bone mass and microarchitecture in CKD patients with fracture. J Am Soc Nephrol 21: 1371–1380.

Biomechanical Comparison of Osteoporotic Distal Radius Fractures Fixed by Distal Locking Screws with Different Length

Xiong Liu[1,2], Wei-dong Wu[1,3], Ya-feng Fang[1], Mei-chao Zhang[1]*, Wen-hua Huang[1]

1 Department of Anatomy, Southern Medical University, Guangdong Provincial Key Laboratory of Medical Biomechanics, Guangzhou, Guangdong, P.R. China, **2** Department of Orthopaedics, Shilongboai Hospital (The Eight People's Hospital of Dongguan), Dongguan, Guangdong, P.R. China, **3** Department of Orthopaedics, Wuzhou Red Cross Hospital, Wuzhou, Guangxi, P.R. China

Abstract

Objectives: To evaluate the postoperative stability of osteoporotic distal radius fractures fixed with distal locking screws with different length.

Methods: A comminuted extra-articular dorsally unstable distal radius fracture, treated with volar locking plate system, was created. The 18 specimens were randomized into 3 groups based on distal locked screws with different length: Group A had unicortical screws with 50% length to the dorsal cortex. Group B had unicortical screws with 75% length to the dorsal cortex. Group C had bicortical screws. Axial compression and bending loads were imposed on the models before and after cycling testing as well as load to clinical and catastrophic failure.

Results: Minimum change in stiffness was observed before and after fatigue for all groups. The final stiffness to bending forces was statistically similar in all groups, but stiffness to axial compression was statistically significant different: Group A approached significance with respect to groups B and C ($P = 0.017$, 0.009), whereas stiffness in group B and C was statistically similar ($P = 0.93$). Load to clinical failure was significantly less for group A (456.54±78.59 N) compared with groups B (580.24±73.85 N) and C (591.07±38.40 N). Load to catastrophic failure was statistically similar between groups, but mean values for Group A were 18% less than means for Group C.

Conclusions: The volar locking plate system fixed with unicortical locking screws with at least 75% length not only produced early stability for osteoporotic distal radius fractures, but also avoided extensor tendon complications due to dorsal screw protrusion.

Editor: Carlos M. Isales, Georgia Regents University, United States of America

Funding: This research was supported by 863 Project of National Ministry of Science and Technology (http://www.most.gov.cn/) grant 2012AA02A603, National Natural Science Foundation of China (http://www.nsfc.gov.cn/Portal0/default152.htm) grant 31200708. The funders had no role in study design, data collection and analysis, decision to publish, or preparation of the manuscript.

Competing Interests: The authors have declared that no competing interests exist.

* Email: zmc@fimmu.com

Introduction

Distal radius fracture is a common type of skeletal injuries in clinical orthopedics, accounting for approximately 10% of all fractures. The incidence increases with the development of our aging society with increasing in osteoporosis. It consists of a compressive fracture of the dorsal cortex with comminution and tensile fracture of the volar cortex. Dorsal comminution is the most common fracture pattern observed with distal radius fractures [1,2,3,4,5,6,7,8]. The majority of cases have traditionally been treated by means of external fixation with plaster cast or splints after manual reduction, which often cannot maintain the biomechanical stability due to the unstable displaced distal radius fractures results in comminution. Thus treatment of open reduction and internal fixation is necessary for fractures with dorsal comminution [9,10,11].

Because of the lesser extensor tendon complications and increased stiffness of constructs, the fixations with volar locking plates, instead of dorsal plating have become more common. But the increased use of volar locking plates for distal radius fixation leads to several problems such as flexor tendon synovitis, extensor tenosynocitis, extensor pollicis longus rupture and so on, though only a few authors have reported these complications [12,13,14,15,16,17,18,19,20]. These dorsal extensor tendons may be injured by improper surgical technique such as inappropriate plate placement and drill penetration of the dorsal cortex to the overlying tendon during operation, or by dorsally prominent screw tips. The first improper technique can be minimized with extensive care, while the second one is tough because it's difficult for us to see the prominent screw tips dorsally with remarkable clarity with standard fluoroscopy resulting from the anatomic landmark of Lister's tubercle. So we wonder whether unicortial fixation with appropriate length can be used for distal radius fractures instead of bicortical fixation. If it can provide the equal fixation strength during early period of postoperation, it makes sense to avoid extensor tendon complications because of dorsal screw prominence. Accordingly, the purpose of this study was to clarify whether unicortical distal locked configurations could maintain postoperative biomechanical stability as for extra-articular osteoporotic distal radius fractures compared with bicortical locked fixation. Our null hypothesis was that there is no significant difference between unicortical screw fixation with appropriate lengths and distal bicortical screw fixation.

Materials and Methods

Ethics Statement

Ethical approval was obtained from the Human Research Ethics Committee, Southern Medical University, Guangzhou, China. The subjects gave informed consent. And all consent was written in nature regarding body donation for research.

Specimen preparation

18 embalmed cadaveric foreams without osseous defects and any history of upper extremity diseases including injury, arthritis, or tumor were obtained from the Department of Anatomy, Southern Medical University. Bone mineral density data were not available because the bones have been soaked with formalin for many years and may have a tendency to develop similar bone mineral density as well as low bone quality at last with the gradual loss of mineral substance. The specimens were randomized into 3 groups of 6 specimens according to the distal locked screws with different lengths in the distal fragment: Group A had unicortical locking screws with 50% length to the dorsal cortex. Group B had 75% length unicortical locking screws. Group C had bicortical locking screws (Fig. 1). The specimens were dissected of soft tissues maintaining the interosseous membrane and radioulnar ligaments intact. They were stored frozen (−20°C) in double plastic wrapping (Fig. 2A) and completely thawed for 2 hours at room temperature prior to experiment.

The plate is made up of medical titanium alloy (Ti6Al4V). All oblique angulated T-volar locking plates were placed according to the manufacturer's recommendation with position of the plate as distally as possible without risking penetration of the articular surface and bent manually to conform to the anatomy of the volar distal radius. Plates were temporarily partially affixed to the intact radius and holes were predrilled to assure restoration of alignment postosteotomy. Plates were removed, and a standard 1-cm-wide segment of bone, centered 2 cm proximal to the tip of radial styloid, was performed parallelly with a saw having both dorsal and volar cortex comminution to simulate comminuted extra-articular unstable distal radius fracture [21]. Volar locking plate was fixed with 3.5-mm threaded bicortical and unicortical locking screws with care to ensure that the locking screws were properly engaged into their threaded holes. The most distal diaphyseal hole of every plate in all groups was not filled as a result of the osteotomy cut as seen in actual clinical scenarios. The proximal radial and ulnar diaphyses were potted in acrylic thermoplastic resin in a vertical and neutral position.

Biomechanical testing

The cadaveric ulna and radius were kept moist with normal saline throughout the experimental procedure. Each specimen was placed in a materials testing machine (ElectroForce 3510, BOSE, USA) and was tested under 3 different conditions of axial compression, dorsal and volar bending. We created a custom-built device attached to the joint surface with acrylic resin powder and liquid to simulate axial load transmission in vivo (Fig. 2D). Cantilever model was applied during bending tests, and mean stiffness of the 3 groups were calculated under different loading conditions.

Each fixation construct was first tested under dorsal and volar bending loads of 50 N at a rate of 5 N/s, and then a static axial compression load was applied at 15 N/s to a maximum of 150 N (Fig. 2). The maximum load applied represents the upper end of estimated physiological forces with wrist motion. Each specimen was subsequently cycled 5000 times in axial compression (sinusoidal waveform, 10–150 N compression at 1 Hz), which was used to simulate physiologic loading over the initial 6-week healing time. For the stability of the whole fatigue process, the load we applied was conducted from a screw shaft attached to the testing machine (Fig. 2E). After cyclic loading, post-testing in the three prior loading conditions was repeated. Finally, destructive testing in axial compression was performed at a rate of 0.5 mm/s to determine load to clinical failure, which was defined as 2 mm of displacement at the osteotomy gap and subsequent catastrophic failure, defined as loosening of the screw-plate interfaces, fractures of distal radius near the location of the implant or deformation and breakage of the implant.

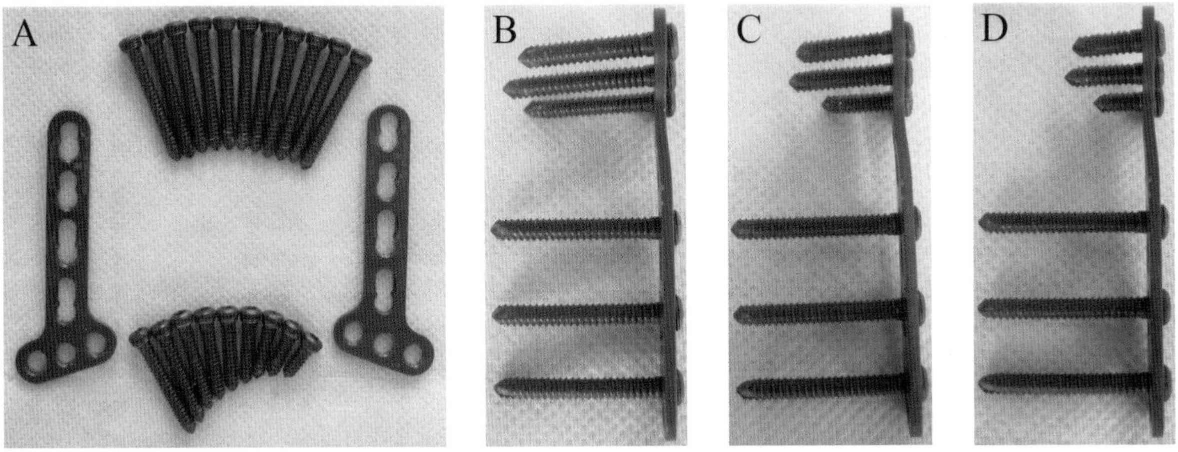

Figure 1. Different fixations in the distal fragment according to groups: (A) screws and plates used in the experiment, (B) fixation with bicortical screws, (C) fixation with 75% unicortical screws, (D) fixation with 50% unicortical screws.

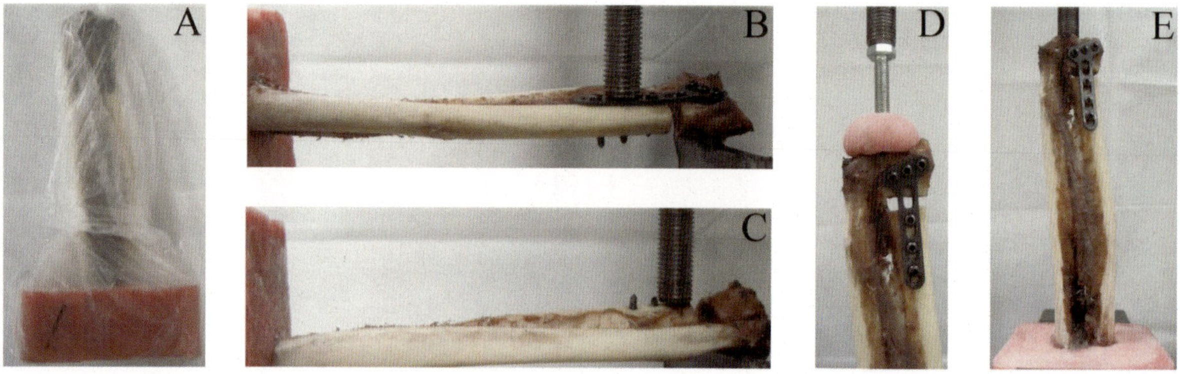

Figure 2. The specimens tested under different loading conditions in a materials testing machine: (A) A specimen was in double plastic wrapping, (B) volar bending, (C) dorsal bending, (D) axial compression, (E) A specimen under axial fatigue test.

Stiffness values of axial and bending loading were calculated as the slope of the straight-line region of the curve. The loads to clinical and catastrophic failure phenomena were observed and stiffness values were obtained according to characteristic load-displacement curves. Load to catastrophic failure was defined as a turning point in the continuous curve, usually denoted by a sudden drop in the force.

Statistical analysis

Means and standard deviations were calculated for descriptive purposes. One-way analysis of variance was performed and post hoc multiple comparisons with LSD and Dunnett T3 methods were used to distinguish statistical differences under each loading condition according to condition of homogeneity of variance. Independent-Samples T Test was conducted when two samples were from two independent populations. The 3 groups were compared for precycling and postcycling axial, volar and dorsal bending stiffness, clinical and catastrophic failure stiffness, load to 2-mm displacement and load to catastrophic failure. Statistically significant differences between the 3 groups were considered statistically significant with p value less than 0.05, and statistical analysis was performed with SPSS Statistics v20 software (IBM, Armonk, New York). Post-hoc analysis was carried out to help to explain the results if the study did not find any significant effects.

Results

There was no statistically significant difference in stiffness among the 3 groups under axial compression before and after cyclic testing (Fig. 3). Final mean stiffness under dorsal bending in group A was 100.66±67.91 N/mm, and under volar bending 101.62±50.58 N/mm. In group B the mean stiffness under dorsal bending was 128.41±83.75 N/mm, and under volar bending 106.74±86.79 N/mm; and in group C it was under dorsal bending 132.74±75.54 N/mm, and under volar bending 138.10±69.93 N/mm. Mean stiffness to dorsal and volar bending forces were statistically similar between different fixation constructions (Table 1) and each group (Fig. 4).

Final mean stiffness in axial loading for group A, group B, and group C was 423.01±14.64 N/mm, 497.42±42.51 N/mm, and 510.69±43.25 N/mm, respectively and there was statistically significant difference in all three groups ($P = 0.002$) as we can see from figure 5. The stiffness of group A decreased obviously and differences are statistically significant with group B and group C ($P = 0.017$, $P = 0.009$). However, mean axial stiffness in group B and group C was statistically similar ($P = 0.93$).

As for the axial loads to clinical failure, the mean values for group A, group B, and group C was 456.54±78.59 N, 580.24±73.85 N, and 591.07±38.40 N. There were statistically significant differences among all groups ($P = 0.013$) except between pair group B and C ($P = 0.80$) as we can see from figure 6, and a gradual decrease in axial load to clinical failure was observed when shortening screws to 50% of the distance to the dorsal cortex, with mean values for Group A are 27% and 29% less than those for Group B and C, respectively. As for the axial loads to catastrophic failure, the mean values for group A, group B, and group C were 969.33±205.01 N, 1074±141 N, 1142.67±145.91 N, and the differences were not statistically significant among all groups (Fig. 6). However, mean values for Group A were 18% less than means for Groups C. Phenomena of clinical and catastrophic failure were observed and recorded during the tests. In all specimens, clinical failure with 2-mm displacement occurred without fixation destruction. Catastrophic failure occurred via fractures of different locations of the bone close to the volar plate, uncoupling of the locking screw from the screw hole and slight deformation of the plate (Fig. 7).

Discussion

The dorsally angulated distal radius fracture is a common fracture that typically results from a fall with the forearm in pronation and the wrist in extension. The treatment goal should be anatomic reduction, stable fixation, and early mobilization of the wrist and forearm to avoid the potential disability caused by a malunion and/or prolonged immobilization. Obtaining and maintaining an anatomic reduction until the fracture is healed has resulted in a good clinical outcome. For this reason open reduction and internal fixation has become an increasingly common treatment for these injuries. Good outcomes have been reported with dorsal plates that can buttress the comminution of the dorsal cortex and maintain reduction of the dorsal displacement of the distal fragment [22,23,24]. It can be technically demanding, however, to place certain plates on the dorsal surface of the distal radius because of the irregularity of the distal dorsal radius. In addition there is limited soft tissue between the skin and bone surface, which can result in symptomatic hardware prominence. Besides, there also can be extensor tendon irritation or rupture from direct contact with a prominent dorsal plate or screws [25,26,27]. Thus in an attempt to avoid tendon irritation, it is suggested that dorsal plates should be low profile.

Volar locking plates have been designed to reduce extensor tendon complications observed with dorsal plates while still

Table 1. Results of Stiffness Under Different Conditions after Cyclic Testing.

Groups Compared	p Values for Axial Load	p Values for Volar Bending Load	p Values for Dorsal Bending Load
A versus B	.017	.902	.537
A versus C	.009	.385	.476
B versus C	.930	.454	.923

P<0.05 was considered to significant.

delivering stable fixation because volar plates with locking distal components can avoid the impaction of the cancellous bone in the distal fragment resulting in poor screw purchase and offer superior rigidity and axial loading strength, especially in the elderly [28,29]. A volar plate has less potential than a dorsal plate to cause tendon complications in part because of the ability to cover the plate with the pronator quadratus (PQ) muscle, thereby avoiding direct contact of the plate with the flexor tendons. Though pronator quadratus muscle is incised along distal radius border during surgery, the repaired PQ has little effect on the stability of whole fixation system and functional recovery [30,31,32,33]. However, with the increased use of volar locking plates, the tendon complications such as extensor tenosynovitis, extensor pollicis longus rupture have become more common owing to that fact that dorsally prominent screws and flexor tendon synovitis occurs occasionally when the volar plate is placed distal to the "watershed line" and prevents protection of flexor tendons by the pronator quadratus muscle. So we investigate whether it is necessary to use distal bicortical fixation and place the extensor tendons at potential risk, or whether unicortical distal fixation is sufficient

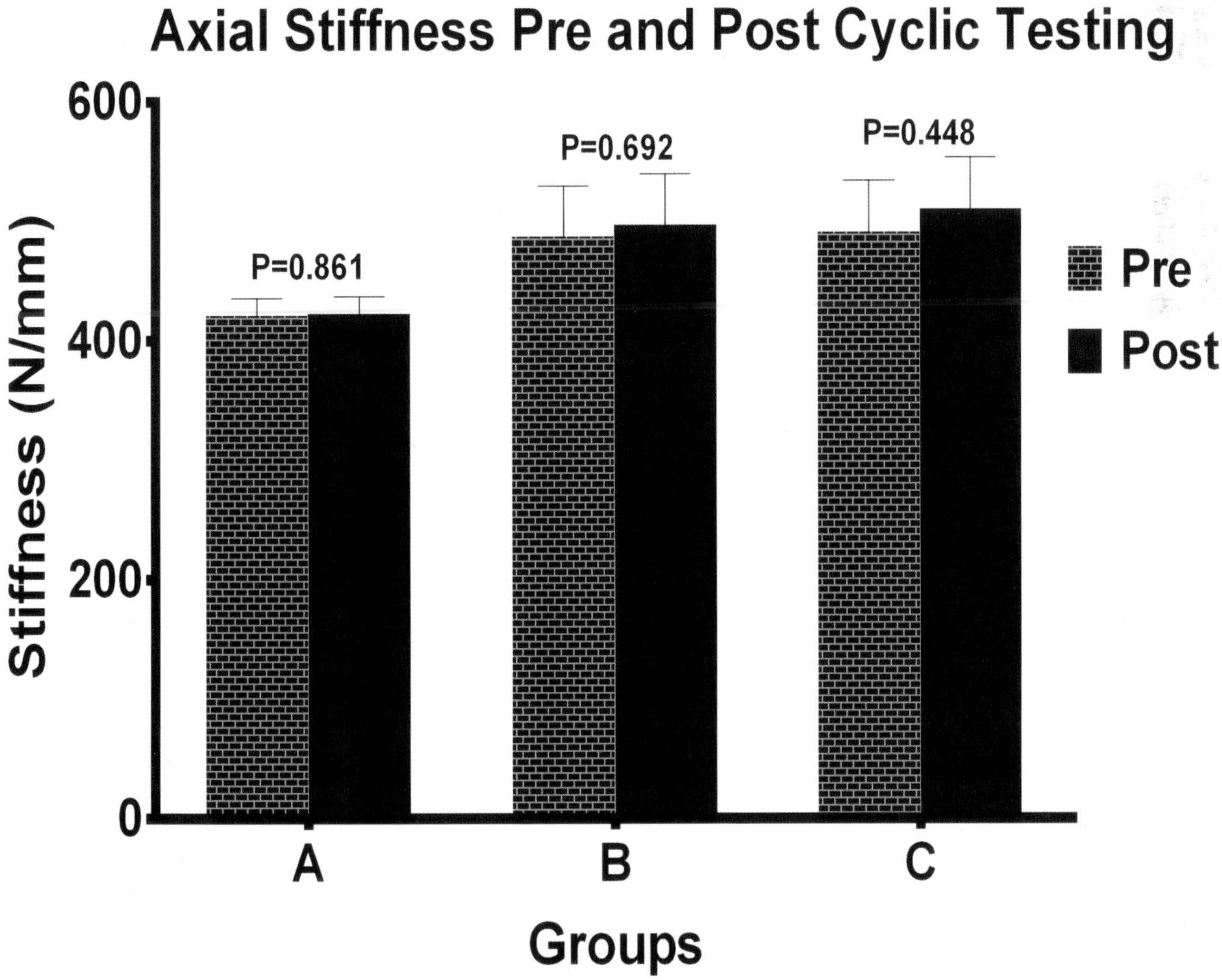

Figure 3. Axial stiffness before and after cyclic testing by different fixation groups. Mean stiffness of each group under axial loading condition were not significantly different (P>0.05). Numbers over bar indicated p values which were conducted through Independent-Samples T Test.

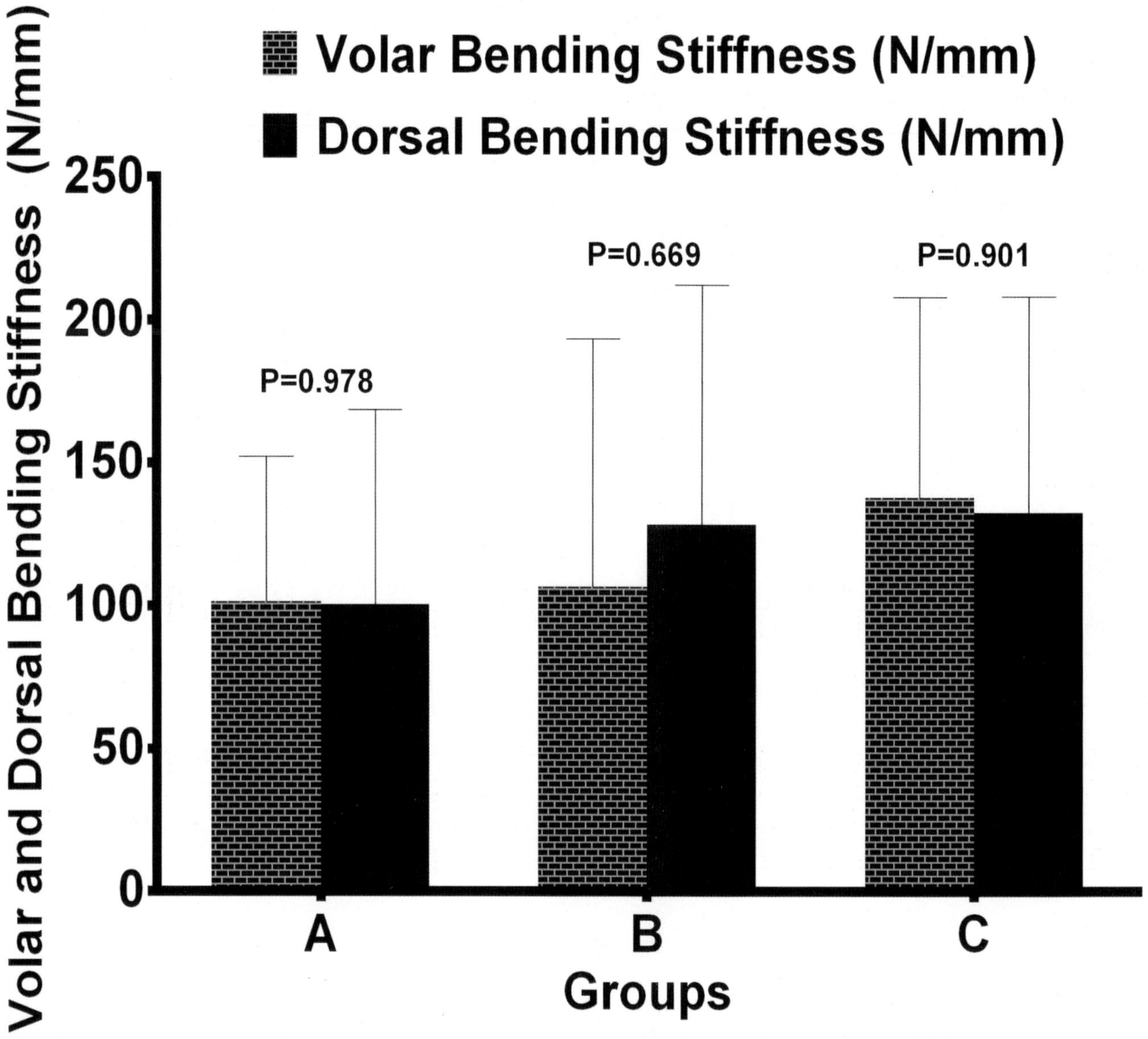

Figure 4. Mean stiffness results under volar and dorsal bending between groups. Stiffness values of each group under volar and dorsal bending load were not significantly different ($P>0.05$). P values were determined by way of independent sample test.

to provide early stability. The purpose of the present study was to compare the biomechanical properties of distal locking screws with different length in an extra-articular osteoporotic distal radius fracture model.

In this study, we removed a section of metadiaphyseal bone to simulate a comminuted distal radius fracture. Because the model was designed to study the effect of different locking screw lengths in the distal fragment in one volar plate system, we deliberately limited the fracture variables to a simple model to examine specific stability in fixation with different locking screw lengths. Contrary to earlier published studies with synthetic radial bone [24,34,35,36], we used true radial and ulnar bone with interosseous membrane and distal radioulnar ligaments undisturbed. Although a sawbone model can ensure consistency between specimens and obviate the need for computed tomography to assess for bone quality or substantial structural differences between specimens, these constructs cannot represent their in vivo states more closely.

The loads used in this study were designed comparable to the loads applied to the distal radius during early postoperative hand and wrist mobilization. Loads transmitted to the distal radius are about 50 N for each 10 N of grip forces with varies hand positions and radius lengths [37]. Although the forces of compression on the distal radius in vivo have not yet been clearly defined, several studies have suggested that compressive forces created by light active motion of the wrist do not exceed 100 N. Combined forces of motion of the wrist and the digits do not exceed more than 250 N [38,39,40,41]. So in the present study, the specimens were performed under load control to a force of 150 N for axial compression and a force of 50 N for volar and dorsal bending. Axial and bending stiffness before and after cyclic loading, load to failure of specimens with different lengths of fixation, has been measured in cadaveric models. Because the loads close to the

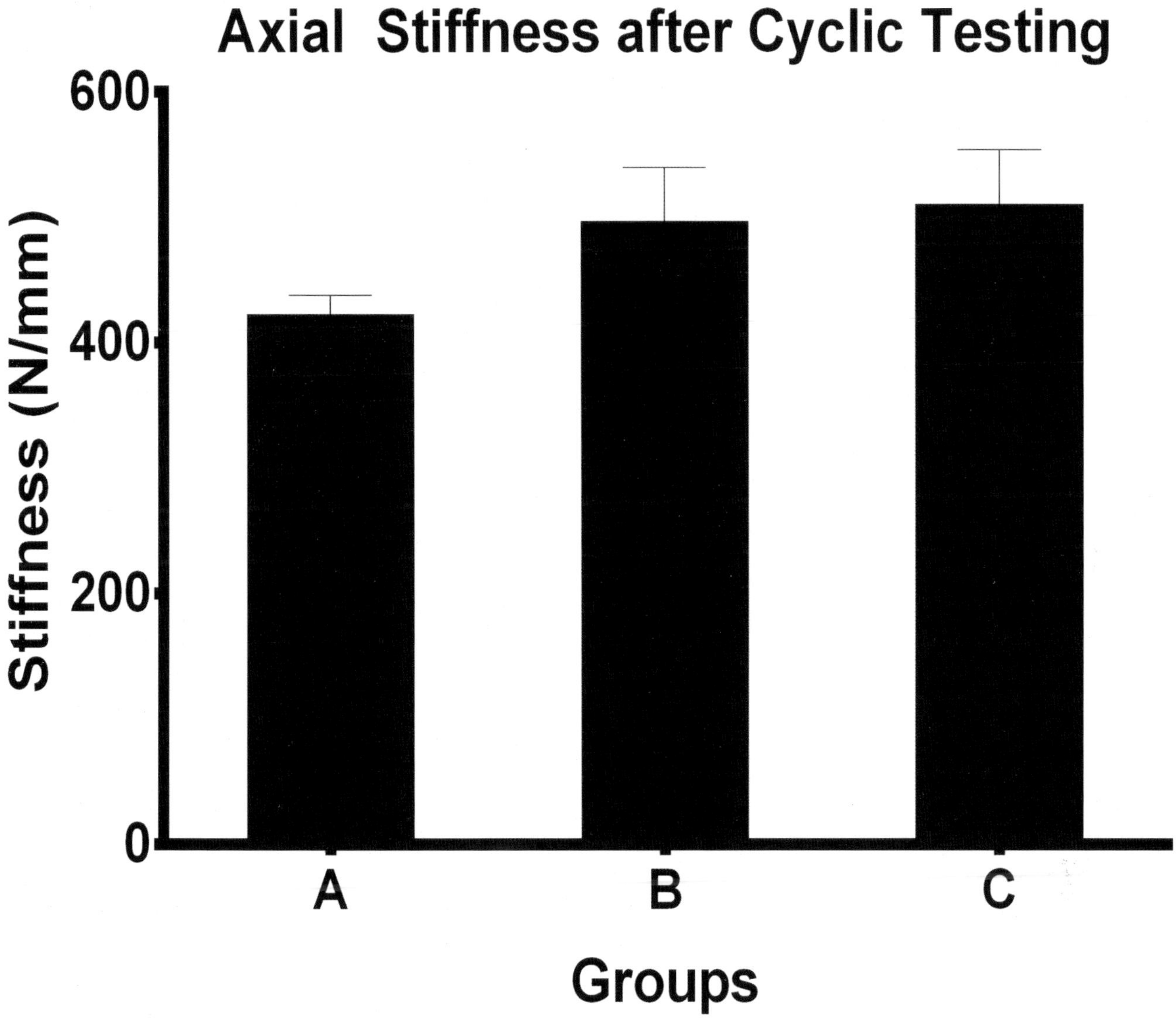

Figure 5. Comparison of postcycling axial stiffness among different groups. The stiffness were significantly different in all groups (P = 0.002) and P values were determined using One-way analysis of variance. While mean axial stiffness in group B and group C was statistically similar (*P* = 0.93).

fracture area are always changing and repeating when active mobilizations of the fingers are performed during the acute healing period, cyclic loading rather than single loading was included in the experiment, since it better simulates physiological loading. Matched pairs and equal numbers of right and left extremities were tested to minimize anatomic and bone quality differences as a confounding factor.

In order to determine the effect of fixation with different locking screw lengths, we compared the mechanical performance of 50%, 75% length and bicortical screws fixations. In the osteoporotic distal radius fracture model, it was demonstrated that 75% length unicortical distal locked fixation produces a construct that was as stiff as fixation with bicortical screws. After cyclic testing that simulated fatigue scenario during the initial healing period, both types of fixation had similar mean stiffness and load to clinical and catastrophic failure were not significantly different, while a gradual decrease in axial load to clinical failure was observed when shortening screws to 50% of the distance to the dorsal cortex. The load to clinical failure forces obtained in our study ranged from 323.83 to 673.74 N among all groups, so it was proved that all construct fixations would bear light active motion during early period of postoperation. We believe that the mechanical equivalence (clinically and statistically) of unicortical and bicortical distal fixation should be viewed as evidence in favor of placing unicortical fixation in clinical practice. Unicortical distal fixation of distal radius fractures is potentially advantageous to bicortical fixation for some reasons. First, bicortical fixation places the extensor tendons at risk for irritation, synovitis, and rupture as a result of dorsally protruding screws. Second, extensor tendons can be injured with drill penetration during operation treating dorsally comminuted fracture and this inciting injury may progress to tendinitis or tendon rupture.

Based on previous data analyses, we considered 6 specimens each experimental group to be sufficient to detect the difference in final axial stiffness between the constructs with 80% power. Although we planned and conducted this study with power

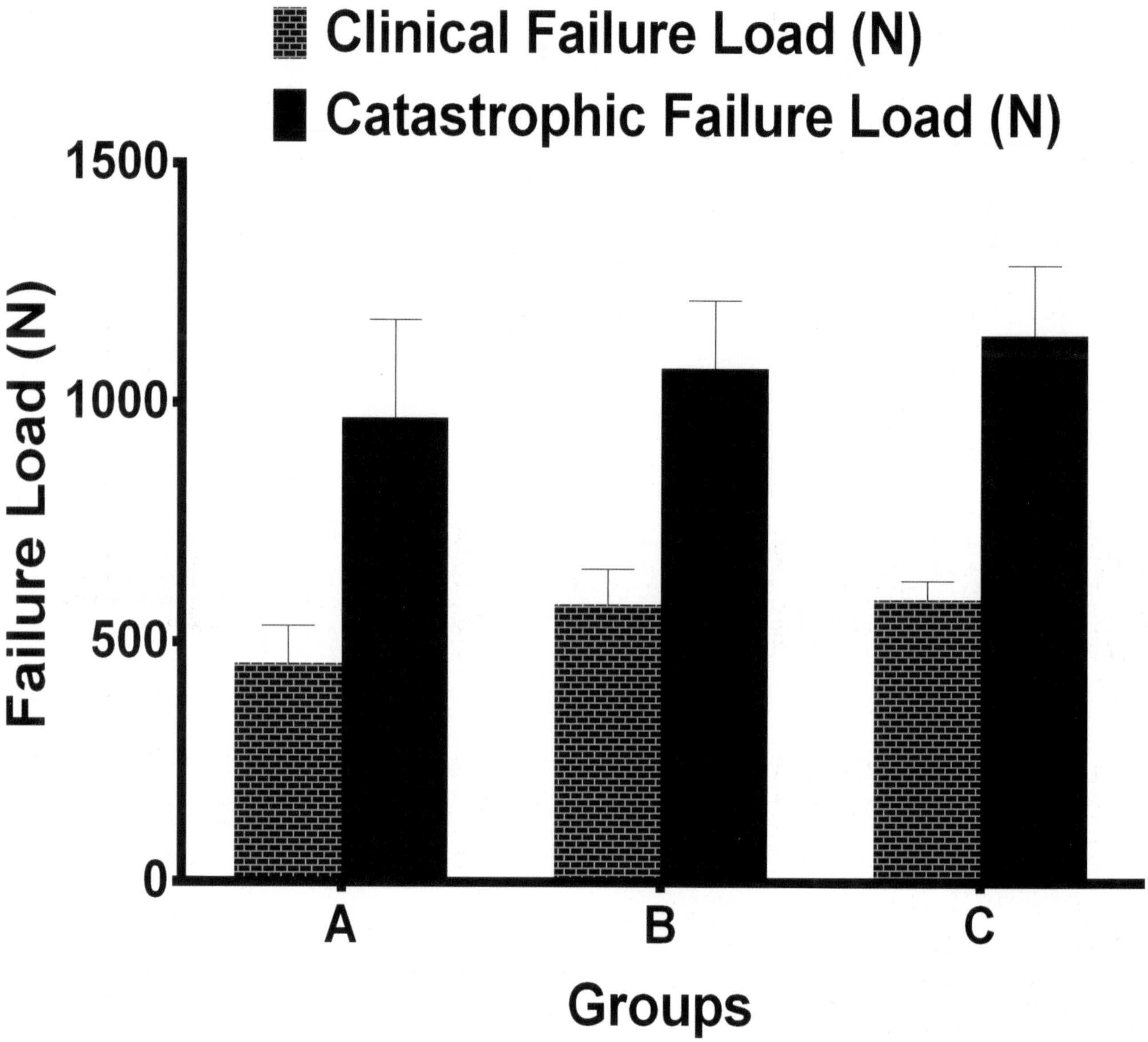

Figure 6. Comparison of mean load to clinical and catastrophic failure after cyclic conditioning by different fixation groups. As for load to clinical failure, there were statistically significant differences among all groups (P = 0.013), while the differences were not statistically significant for load to catastrophic failure (P = 0.483).

analyses consistent with prior investigations, several analyses were underpowered. Post-hoc analysis demonstrated appropriate power values when analyzing final axial stiffness and axial loading force to 2-mm displacement; however, we would have needed at least 19 specimens per group to detect whether the groups have difference as with final bending stiffness and axial loading to catastrophic failure. Even though, there is of less importance to detect the statistical significance of bending force condition because axial compression is just the main force transmitted to radius, as for axial loading to catastrophic failure, the result may be unreliable because of the poor bone quality of each group.

It is difficult to assess the penetration of bicortical screw tip dorsally during fracture fixation with standard lateral view. Because the dorsal surface of the distal radius has complex three-dimensional shape such as Lister tubercle which prevents recognize penetrating screws tips on a two-dimensional image. Several methods of radiological examination have been proposed such as oblique lateral view in pronation and supination and dorsally tangential view of distal radius [42,43,44]. However, both approaches have limitations to a certain degrees. On the other hand, distal comminuted fragments make it difficult or impossible to select appropriate screw lengths using a depth gauge. So distal bicortical fixation adopted in clinical practice in the metaphyseal and epiphyseal areas of the distal radius is at risk of screw prominence resulting in extensor tendon irritation.

In our study, almost all the constructs failed during catastrophic testing by collapse of the location of distal radius diaphysis or uncoupling of the locking screw from the screw hole. These kinds of failure have been observed after mechanical testing of cadavers with fractures of the distal radius in other published studies [45,46]. The outcome was directly related to the biological properties of the bone with osteoporosis, which can be dramatically improved via increases in sclerotin. A similar bone with more bone substance will resist collapsing failure.

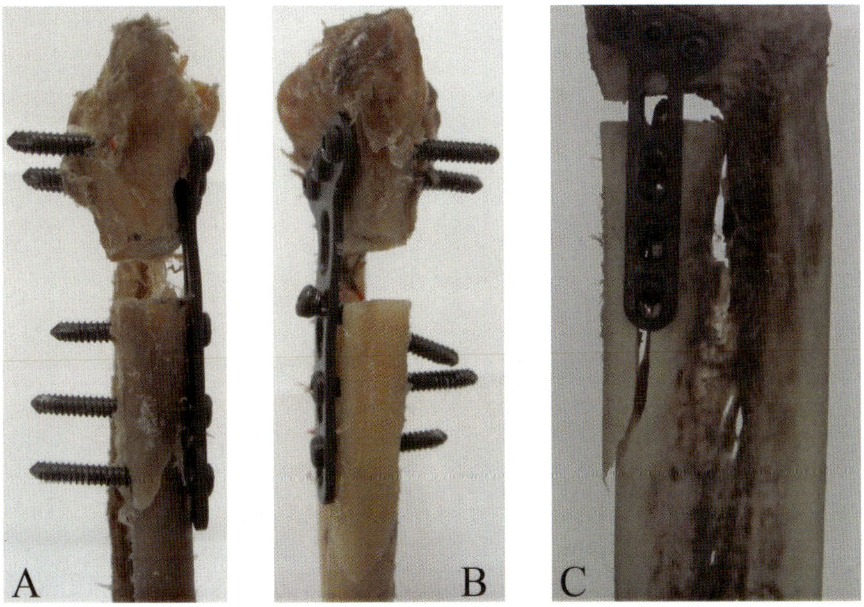

Figure 7. Catastrophic failure modes seen in specimens after failure testing: (A) A specimen failed by collapse of the location of distal radius diaphysis and slight deformation of mid-plate, (B) A specimen failed by collapse of the location of distal radius diaphysis and uncoupling of the proximal locking screw from the screw hole, (C) A specimen failed by collapse of the location of distal radius diaphysis.

This study has some limitations that are inherent with using a cadaver model for simulating the in vivo scenario. These shortcomings involve the usual concerns associated with a cadaveric study such as the limited number of specimens (open to type II error), the variability in specimen age, and bone mineral density (BMD). Secondly, the muscles and tendons were stripped from the specimens in the study and any dynamic stability that would normally be provided by the musculotendinous tissues was not present. Thirdly, although dorsal and volar bending was tested as well as axial compression, the in vivo loading will be more complex and a torsion component may be included. These rotational forces through the radius are commonly experienced during pronation–supination of the forearm, which are important components in most postoperative rehabilitation protocols. Finally, the fracture model in our research was limited to an extra-articular fracture in which no coronal and sagittal plane fracture, and cannot entirely represent various types of comminuted fractures of osteoporotic distal radius found in practice.

Conclusions

In summary, our study demonstrated that distal unicortical fixation with appropriate length screws provides adequate stiffness and strength for the internal fixation of extra-articular distal radius fractures during the acute healing period (6 weeks). So there is a thimbleful of effect on construct strength by decreasing screw length. We recommend at least 75% length unicortical screw fixation to minimize the risk of over-projection resulting in extensor tendon complications and suggested active range of motion should be instituted during the early period of post-operation to avoid wrist joint stiffness or disuse atrophy.

Acknowledgments

The authors thank Ze-yu Li and Jun Ouyang from the Department of Anatomy, Southern Medical University for assistance with specimen preparation; Mei-chao Zhang and Wei-dong Wu from the Department of Anatomy, Southern Medical University for their constructive suggestions in making this project possible; Ya-feng Fang for assistant with biomechanical experiments.

Author Contributions

Conceived and designed the experiments: MZ XL. Performed the experiments: XL WW YF. Analyzed the data: MZ XL. Contributed reagents/materials/analysis tools: MZ WH. Wrote the paper: XL. Obtained permission for use of materials testing machine: MZ WH.

References

1. Douthit JD (2005) Volar plating of dorsally comminuted fractures of the distal radius: a 6-year study. Am J Orthop (Belle Mead NJ) 34: 140–147.
2. Trease C, McIff T, Toby EB (2005) Locking versus nonlocking T-plates for dorsal and volar fixation of dorsally comminuted distal radius fractures: a biomechanical study. J Hand Surg Am 30: 756–763.
3. Blythe M, Stoffel K, Jarrett P, Kuster M (2006) Volar versus dorsal locking plates with and without radial styloid locking plates for the fixation of dorsally comminuted distal radius fractures: A biomechanical study in cadavers. J Hand Surg Am 31: 1587–1593.
4. Burkhart KJ, Nowak TE, Gradl G, Klitscher D, Mehling I, et al. (2010) Intramedullary nailing vs. palmar locked plating for unstable dorsally comminuted distal radius fractures: a biomechanical study. Clin Biomech (Bristol, Avon) 25: 771–775.
5. Konstantinidis L, Helwig P, Seifert J, Hirschmuller A, Liodakis E, et al. (2011) Internal fixation of dorsally comminuted fractures of the distal part of the radius: a biomechanical analysis of volar plate and intramedullary nail fracture stability. Arch Orthop Trauma Surg 131: 1529–1537.
6. Gondusky JS, Carney J, Erpenbach J, Robertson C, Mahar A, et al. (2011) Biomechanical comparison of locking versus nonlocking volar and dorsal T-plates for fixation of dorsally comminuted distal radius fractures. J Orthop Trauma 25: 44–50.
7. Jakubietz MG, Gruenert JG, Jakubietz RG (2011) The use of beta-tricalcium phosphate bone graft substitute in dorsally plated, comminuted distal radius fractures. J Orthop Surg Res 6: 24.
8. Chou YC, Chen AC, Chen CY, Hsu YH, Wu CC (2011) Dorsal and volar 2.4-mm titanium locking plate fixation for AO type C3 dorsally comminuted distal radius fractures. J Hand Surg Am 36: 974–981.
9. Chirpaz-Cerbat JM, Ruatti S, Houillon C, Ionescu S (2011) Dorsally displaced distal radius fractures treated by fixed-angle volar plating: Grip and

pronosupination strength recovery. A prospective study. Orthopaedics & Traumatology: Surgery & Research 97: 465–470.
10. Wilcke MK, Abbaszadegan H, Adolphson PY (2011) Wrist function recovers more rapidly after volar locked plating than after external fixation but the outcomes are similar after 1 year. Acta Orthop 82: 76–81.
11. Mignemi ME, Byram IR, Wolfe CC, Fan K, Koehler EA, et al. (2013) Radiographic Outcomes of Volar Locked Plating for Distal Radius Fractures. The Journal of Hand Surgery 38: 40–48.
12. Nunley JA, Rowan PR (1999) Delayed rupture of the flexor pollicis longus tendon after inappropriate placement of the pi plate on the volar surface of the distal radius. J Hand Surg Am 24: 1279–1280.
13. Koo SC, Ho ST (2006) Delayed rupture of flexor pollicis longus tendon after volar plating of the distal radius. Hand Surg 11: 67–70.
14. Rozental TD, Blazar PE (2006) Functional outcome and complications after volar plating for dorsally displaced, unstable fractures of the distal radius. J Hand Surg Am 31: 359–365.
15. Duncan SF, Weiland AJ (2007) Delayed rupture of the flexor pollicis longus tendon after routine volar placement of a T-plate on the distal radius. Am J Orthop (Belle Mead NJ) 36: 669–670.
16. Haug LC, Deml C, Blauth M, Arora R (2011) Dorsal screw penetration following implant removal after volar locked plating of distal radius fracture. Arch Orthop Trauma Surg 131: 1279–1282.
17. Cho CH, Lee KJ, Song KS, Bae KC (2012) Delayed rupture of flexor pollicis longus after volar plating for a distal radius fracture. Clin Orthop Surg 4: 325–328.
18. Kosiyatrakul A, Luenam S, Prachaporn S (2012) Flexor pollicis longus injury after corrective osteotomy of distal radius malunion with volar fixed-angle plating: case report and review literature of the flexor tendon injuries after volar plating. J Med Assoc Thai 95 Suppl 10: S213–S218.
19. Ward JP, Kim LT, Rettig ME (2012) Extensor indicis proprius and extensor digitorum communis rupture after volar locked plating of the distal radius–a case report. Bull NYU Hosp Jt Dis 70: 273–275.
20. Cho CH, Lee KJ, Song KS, Bae KC (2012) Delayed rupture of flexor pollicis longus after volar plating for a distal radius fracture. Clin Orthop Surg 4: 325–328.
21. Mehling I, Muller LP, Delinsky K, Mehler D, Burkhart KJ, et al. (2010) Number and locations of screw fixation for volar fixed-angle plating of distal radius fractures: biomechanical study. J Hand Surg Am 35: 885–891.
22. Lin CL, Lin YH, Chen AC (2006) Buttressing angle of the double-plating fixation of a distal radius fracture: a finite element study. Med Biol Eng Comput 44: 665–673.
23. Cheng HY, Lin CL, Lin YH, Chen AC (2007) Biomechanical evaluation of the modified double-plating fixation for the distal radius fracture. Clin Biomech (Bristol, Avon) 22: 510–517.
24. Chen AC, Lin YH, Kuo HN, Yu TC, Sun MT, et al. (2013) Design optimisation and experimental evaluation of dorsal double plating fixation for distal radius fracture. Injury 44: 527–534.
25. Trease C, McIff T, Toby EB (2005) Locking versus nonlocking T-plates for dorsal and volar fixation of dorsally comminuted distal radius fractures: a biomechanical study. J Hand Surg Am 30: 756–763.
26. Ruch DS, Papadonikolakis A (2006) Volar versus dorsal plating in the management of intra-articular distal radius fractures. J Hand Surg Am 31: 9–16.
27. Gondusky JS, Carney J, Erpenbach J, Robertson C, Mahar A, et al. (2011) Biomechanical comparison of locking versus nonlocking volar and dorsal T-plates for fixation of dorsally comminuted distal radius fractures. J Orthop Trauma 25: 44–50.
28. Ring D, Jupiter JB (2005) Treatment of osteoporotic distal radius fractures. Osteoporos Int 16 Suppl 2: S80–S84.
29. Mudgal CS, Jupiter JB (2008) Plate fixation of osteoporotic fractures of the distal radius. J Orthop Trauma 22: S106–S115.
30. Heidari N, Clement H, Kosuge D, Grechenig W, Tesch NP, et al. (2012) Is sparing the pronator quadratus muscle possible in volar plating of the distal radius? J Hand Surg Eur Vol 37: 402–406.
31. Swigart CR, Badon MA, Bruegel VL, Dodds SD (2012) Assessment of pronator quadratus repair integrity following volar plate fixation for distal radius fractures: a prospective clinical cohort study. J Hand Surg Am 37: 1868–1873.
32. Ahsan ZS, Yao J (2012) The importance of pronator quadratus repair in the treatment of distal radius fractures with volar plating. Hand (N Y) 7: 276–280.
33. Armangil M, Bezirgan U, Basarir K, Bilen G, Demirtas M, et al. (2013) The pronator quadratus muscle after plating of distal radius fractures: is the muscle still working? Eur J Orthop Surg Traumatol.
34. Drobetz H, Schueller M, Tschegg EK, Heal C, Redl H, et al. (2011) Influence of screw diameter and number on reduction loss after plating of distal radius fractures. ANZ J Surg 81: 46–51.
35. Konstantinidis L, Helwig P, Seifert J, Hirschmuller A, Liodakis E, et al. (2011) Internal fixation of dorsally comminuted fractures of the distal part of the radius: a biomechanical analysis of volar plate and intramedullary nail fracture stability. Arch Orthop Trauma Surg 131: 1529–1537.
36. Martineau PA, Waitayawinyu T, Malone KJ, Hanel DP, Trumble TE (2008) Volar plating of AO C3 distal radius fractures: biomechanical evaluation of locking screw and locking smooth peg configurations. J Hand Surg Am 33: 827–834.
37. Putnam MD, Meyer NJ, Nelson EW, Gesensway D, Lewis JL (2000) Distal radial metaphyseal forces in an extrinsic grip model: implications for postfracture rehabilitation. J Hand Surg Am 25: 469–475.
38. Chao EY, Opgrande JD, Axmear FE (1976) Three-dimensional force analysis of finger joints in selected isometric hand functions. J Biomech 9: 387–396.
39. Cooney WR, Chao EY (1977) Biomechanical analysis of static forces in the thumb during hand function. J Bone Joint Surg Am 59: 27–36.
40. Horii E, Garcia-Elias M, Bishop AT, Cooney WP, Linscheid RL, et al. (1990) Effect on force transmission across the carpus in procedures used to treat Kienbock's disease. J Hand Surg Am 15: 393–400.
41. Peine R, Rikli DA, Hoffmann R, Duda G, Regazzoni P (2000) Comparison of three different plating techniques for the dorsum of the distal radius: a biomechanical study. J Hand Surg Am 25: 29–33.
42. Maschke SD, Evans PJ, Schub D, Drake R, Lawton JN (2007) Radiographic evaluation of dorsal screw penetration after volar fixed-angle plating of the distal radius: a cadaveric study. Hand (N Y) 2: 144–150.
43. Joseph SJ, Harvey JN (2011) The dorsal horizon view: detecting screw protrusion at the distal radius. J Hand Surg Am 36: 1691–1693.
44. Ozer K, Toker S (2011) Dorsal tangential view of the wrist to detect screw penetration to the dorsal cortex of the distal radius after volar fixed-angle plating. Hand (N Y) 6: 190–193.
45. Koh S, Morris RP, Patterson RM, Kearney JP, Buford WJ, et al. (2006) Volar fixation for dorsally angulated extra-articular fractures of the distal radius: a biomechanical study. J Hand Surg Am 31: 771–779.
46. Gondusky JS, Carney J, Erpenbach J, Robertson C, Mahar A, et al. (2011) Biomechanical comparison of locking versus nonlocking volar and dorsal T-plates for fixation of dorsally comminuted distal radius fractures. J Orthop Trauma 25: 44–50.

Bone Health History in Breast Cancer Patients on Aromatase Inhibitors

Marilyn L. Kwan[1]*, Joan C. Lo[1], Li Tang[2], Cecile A. Laurent[1], Janise M. Roh[1], Malini Chandra[1], Theresa E. Hahn[2], Chi-Chen Hong[2], Lara Sucheston-Campbell[2], Dawn L. Hershman[3], Charles P. Quesenberry Jr.[1], Christine B. Ambrosone[2], Lawrence H. Kushi[1], Song Yao[2]

1 Division of Research, Kaiser Permanente Northern California, Oakland, California, United States of America, **2** Department of Cancer Prevention and Control, Roswell Park Cancer Institute, Buffalo, New York, United States of America, **3** Department of Medicine and the Herbert Irving Comprehensive Cancer Center, Columbia University, New York, New York, United States of America

Abstract

A cross-sectional study was performed to assess bone health history among aromatase inhibitor (AI) users before breast cancer (BC) diagnosis, which may impact fracture risk after AI therapy and choice of initial hormonal therapy. A total of 2,157 invasive BC patients initially treated with an AI were identified from a prospective cohort study at Kaiser Permanente Northern California (KPNC). Data on demographic and lifestyle factors were obtained from in-person interviews, and bone health history and clinical data from KPNC clinical databases. The prevalence of osteoporosis and fractures in postmenopausal AI users was assessed, compared with 325 postmenopausal TAM users. The associations of bone health history with demographic and lifestyle factors in AI users were also examined. Among all initial AI users, 11.2% had a prior history of osteoporosis, 16.3% had a prior history of any fracture, and 4.6% had a prior history of major fracture. Postmenopausal women who were taking TAM as their initial hormonal therapy had significantly higher prevalence of prior osteoporosis than postmenopausal AI users (21.5% vs. 11.8%, $p<0.0001$). Among initial AI users, the associations of history of osteoporosis and fracture in BC patients with demographic and lifestyle factors were, in general, consistent with those known in healthy older women. This study is one of the first to characterize AI users and risk factors for bone morbidity before BC diagnosis. In the future, this study will examine lifestyle, molecular, and genetic risk factors for AI-induced fractures.

Editor: Debashis Ghosh, SUNY Upstate Medical University, United States of America

Funding: Funded by the U.S. National Institutes of Health, National Cancer Institute (R01 CA166701 to M.L.K. and S.Y. and R01 CA105274 to L.H.K.). The funders had no role in study design, data collection and analysis, decision to publish, or preparation of the manuscript.

Competing Interests: The authors have declared that no competing interests exist.

* Email: Marilyn.L.Kwan@kp.org

Introduction

Aromatase inhibitors (AI) have been replacing tamoxifen (TAM) as adjuvant hormonal therapy for postmenopausal women diagnosed with early stage, hormone receptor (HR)-positive breast cancer. The current third-generation AIs inhibit 96–99% *in vivo* aromatase enzyme activity [1], thereby decreasing endogenous estrogen levels far below levels from natural menopause [2]. This highly efficient estrogen depletion by AIs benefits breast cancer patients by extending recurrence-free survival superior to TAM [3,4,5]. However, AIs put patients at high risk of fractures due to the central role of estrogen in maintaining normal bone metabolism [6]. In contrast, TAM is generally believed to be bone-conserving [2]. Several expert groups have developed guidelines for evaluating fracture risk in breast cancer patients who are planning to start AI therapy [7,8,9,10], so that the benefits and harms of AIs can be carefully assessed to make an educated decision on choice of hormonal therapy.

The aforementioned guidelines vary slightly but usually include bone mineral density (BMD) testing and clinical assessment of risk factors for fracture [7,8,9,10]. Although BMD remains a strong predictor for fracture risk, several studies have shown that a large proportion of patients who experienced fragility fractures had T-scores in the non-osteoporotic range [11,12], which highlights the importance of evaluation of BMD-independent risk factors, such as *a priori* bone health history, age, physical activity, smoking, and alcohol intake [13,14]. However, to our knowledge, only a few small studies have examined bone health history among AI users prior to breast cancer diagnosis [15,16], and no studies have investigated lifestyle factors and prior risk of fracture in this patient population. In a real-world clinical setting, it is unknown how bone health history would affect hormonal therapy choice among postmenopausal women with HR-positive breast cancer. These data will be important to inform treatment and prevention strategies for AI users as a high-risk population for bone morbidity. Furthermore, it is of clinical significance to also examine whether

Table 1. Baseline characteristics of study cohort by initial use of aromatase inhibitor (AI) or tamoxifen (TAM).

	Overall	Postmenopausal Only		
	AI (Initial Use)	**AI (Initial Use)**	**TAM (Initial Use)**	**p value[1]**
	n = 2157	**n = 2033**	**n = 325**	
	n (%)	**n (%)**	**n (%)**	
Age at Breast Cancer (BC) Diagnosis (years)				**<0.0001**
<50	80 (3.7)	28 (1.4)	47 (14.5)	
50–59	640 (29.7)	581 (28.6)	101 (31.1)	
60–69	891 (41.3)	883 (43.4)	99 (30.5)	
≥70	546 (25.3)	541 (26.6)	78 (24.0)	
Mean (SD)	64.4 (9.1)	65.2 (8.5)	62.0 (11.2)	
Menopausal Status				–
Premenopausal	118 (5.5)	0 (0)	0 (0)	
Postmenopausal	2033 (94.5)	2033 (100)	325 (100)	
AJCC Stage at BC Diagnosis				**0.0003**
I	1165 (54.0)	1120 (55.1)	218 (67.1)	
II	751 (34.8)	693 (34.1)	85 (26.2)	
III	206 (9.6)	187 (9.2)	20 (6.2)	
IV	35 (1.6)	33 (1.6)	2 (0.6)	
Race/Ethnicity				0.62
White	1541 (71.4)	1467 (72.2)	222 (68.3)	
African American	124 (5.8)	115 (5.7)	22 (6.8)	
Asian	221 (10.3)	202 (9.9)	31 (9.5)	
Hispanic	225 (10.4)	205 (10.1)	43 (13.2)	
Other	46 (2.1)	44 (2.2)	7 (2.2)	
BMI (kg/m^2)				**<0.0001**
<25	642 (30.0)	595 (29.5)	127 (39.4)	
25–29.9	680 (31.8)	645 (31.9)	108 (33.5)	
≥30	816 (38.2)	780 (38.6)	87 (27.0)	
Mean (SD)	29.0 (6.5)	29.0 (6.5)	27.6 (6.4)	
Mod-Vig Physical Activity (MET-hours/week)				
Mean (SD)	27.6 (28.6)	27.6 (28.9)	33.0 (34.0)	**0.03**
Median (IQR)	19.5 (7.3–39.1)	19.4 (7.1–39.1)	24.4 (9.3–45.4)	
Smoking History				0.28
Never	1118 (52.0)	1046 (51.5)	183 (56.3)	
Former	913 (42.5)	874 (43.0)	129 (39.7)	
Current	118 (5.5)	111 (5.5)	13 (4.0)	
Alcohol Intake (g/day)				0.24
Never	511 (27.9)	477 (27.5)	81 (29.7)	
≤median[2]	665 (36.2)	618 (35.7)	106 (38.8)	
>median	659 (35.9)	637 (36.8)	86 (31.5)	
Vitamin Supplement Use			**0.003**	
None	1263 (62.7)	177 (55.0)		
Calcium	334 (16.6)	61 (18.9)		
Vitamin D	259 (12.9)	43 (13.4)		
Both	158 (7.9)	41 (12.7)		
<0.0001				
No	1792 (88.2)	225 (78.5)		
≤6	165 (8.1)	50 (12.3)		
>6	76 (3.7)	30 (9.2)		
Any Fracture Before BC Diagnosis (years)			0.27	

Table 1. Cont.

	Overall	Postmenopausal Only		
	AI (Initial Use)	**AI (Initial Use)**	**TAM (Initial Use)**	**p value[1]**
	n = 2157	**n = 2033**	**n = 325**	
	n (%)	**n (%)**	**n (%)**	
No	1695 (83.4)	272 (83.7)		
≤6	179 (8.8)	23 (7.1)		
>6	159 (7.8)	30 (9.2)		
0.13				
No	1937 (95.3)	306 (94.2)		
≤6	60 (3.0)	11 (3.4)		
>6	36 (1.8)	8 (2.5)		

NOTE: Pharmacy data through December 31, 2013; Missing data for entire cohort: menopausal status (n = 9), BMI (n = 28), smoking (n = 13), alcohol (n = 552), vitamin supplements (n = 37).

[1] Logistic regression adjusted for age at breast cancer diagnosis as a continuous variable.

[2] Median (overall) = 3.10 g/day, median (postmenopausal women) = 2.90 g/day.

[3] Osteoporosis defined by ICD-9 code (733.00–733.09) or any prior bisphosphonate prescription.

[4] Major fracture includes fracture of spine, humerus, wrist, or hip.

known risk factors for fractures are also relevant in breast cancer patients, considering the paradoxical role of estrogens in promoting carcinogenesis yet maintaining bone health.

In a cross-sectional analysis of one of the largest contemporary cohorts of breast cancer patients, we describe history of osteoporosis and fracture and the prevalence of risk factors for fracture (age, race/ethnicity, body mass index (BMI), physical activity, smoking, alcohol intake, and calcium and vitamin D supplement use) before breast cancer diagnosis among initial AI users. We also compare prevalence of bone health history in postmenopausal AI users with postmenopausal TAM users. Lastly, we examine associations of these fracture risk factors with prior history of osteoporosis and fracture outcomes in AI users.

Materials and Methods

Study Population

The Pathways Study is a prospective study of 4,505 women with newly diagnosed invasive breast cancer who are members of Kaiser Permanente Northern California (KPNC), a large, integrated health care delivery system covering the San Francisco-Oakland Bay Area, Sacramento, and surrounding counties. Recruitment was from January 2006 to April 2013 through rapid case ascertainment procedures designed to enroll women prior to initiation of chemotherapy, as described elsewhere [17]. Eligibility criteria included: KPNC female members at least 21 years of age; had no previous history of malignancy other than non-melanoma skin cancer; spoke English, Spanish, Cantonese, or Mandarin; and resided within a 65-mile radius of a field interviewer. The mean time from diagnosis to enrollment was 2.0 (±0.7) months.

For this bone health sub-study, women were included if they had at least one hormonal therapy prescription of an AI or TAM that was indicated for treatment of their first primary breast cancer. A total of 1,159 women who had no hormonal therapy, 27 women who initiated hormonal therapy after recurrence of their original breast cancer, and 4 women who initiated hormonal therapy after their second primary breast cancer were excluded. The final study population consisted of 3,315 eligible women. Based on complete hormonal therapy prescription data through December 2013, 2,157 (65.1%) were initial AI users, and 1,158 (34.9%) were initial TAM users. For this analysis of baseline bone health history, only the initial AI users were included. In selected analyses, 325 postmenopausal women who received TAM as their initial hormonal therapy drug were also included as a comparison group to postmenopausal AI users (n = 2,033).

Clinicopathologic Characteristics

Clinical and diagnostic tumor characteristics were obtained from the KPNC Cancer Registry approximately four months post-diagnosis [18]. These included: stage at diagnosis, estrogen/progesterone receptor (ER/PR) positivity, HER2/neu (Her2) status, surgery type, and treatment received.

Self-reported Participant Information

The baseline interview was conducted at enrollment into the cohort approximately two months post-diagnosis, and included interviewer and self-administered questionnaires on sociodemographics, diet, physical activity, smoking, established breast cancer risk factors, health history, and use of vitamin/mineral supplements. Anthropometric measures were also obtained at baseline.

Information was collected on hysterectomy and oophorectomy and associated dates of the surgery, and age or date of last period. Menopause was defined as the absence of menses for 12 consecutive months or more relative to the date of the baseline interview, or having a complete hysterectomy or oophorectomy of both ovaries.

Physical activity was assessed using an activity frequency questionnaire based on the validated Arizona Activity Frequency Questionnaire (AAFQ) [19]. Activities in four main domains were asked: household, recreational, transportation, and sedentary. Diet was assessed using a 139-item modified version of the Block 2005 food frequency questionnaire (FFQ) (NutritionQuest, Berkeley, CA). Alcohol consumption (beer, wine, and liquor), including frequency and portion size, was obtained on the FFQ.

Pharmacy Data

Prescription drug data for nearly 100% of KPNC enrollees is recorded in the KPNC pharmacy database, including drug name,

Table 2. Baseline characteristics in relation to osteoporosis[1] before breast cancer diagnosis (BC) in aromatase inhibitor (AI) users.

	Osteoporosis Before BC Diagnosis - Yes	Osteoporosis Before BC Diagnosis - No	OR[2]	95% CI[2]	p for trend
	n = 242	n = 1915			
	n (%)	n (%)			
Age at BC Diagnosis (years)					**<0.0001**
<60	31 (12.8)	689 (36.0)	Ref		
60–69	95 (39.3)	796 (41.6)	**2.43**	**(1.58, 3.72)**	
≥70	116 (47.9)	430 (22.5)	**5.65**	**(3.68, 8.69)**	
Race/Ethnicity					–
White	182 (75.2)	1359 (71.0)	Ref		
African American	5 (2.1)	119 (6.2)	**0.38**	**(0.15, 0.94)**	
Asian	30 (12.4)	191 (10.0)	**1.82**	**(1.17, 2.81)**	
Hispanic	19 (7.9)	206 (10.8)	0.86	(0.52, 1.43)	
Other	6 (2.5)	40 (2.1)	1.46	(0.60, 3.54)	
BMI (kg/m²)					**<0.0001**
<25	114 (47.3)	528 (27.8)	Ref		
25–29.9	77 (32.0)	603 (31.8)	**0.55**	**(0.40, 0.76)**	
≥30	50 (20.8)	766 (40.4)	**0.32**	**(0.22, 0.45)**	
Mod-Vig Physical Activity (MET-hours/week)					–
Never	16 (6.7)	92 (4.8)	Ref		
≤median[3]	102 (42.5)	915 (48.2)	0.92	(0.51, 1.67)	
>median	122 (50.8)	893 (47.0)	1.25	(0.69, 2.27)	
Smoking History					–
Never	134 (55.4)	984 (51.6)	Ref		
Former	101 (41.7)	812 (42.6)	0.86	(0.65, 1.15)	
Current	7 (2.9)	111 (5.8)	0.62	(0.28, 1.39)	
Alcohol Intake (g/day)					–
Never	77 (34.8)	434 (26.9)	Ref		
≤median[3]	73 (33.0)	591 (36.6)	0.73	(0.51, 1.05)	
>median	71 (32.1)	589 (36.5)	0.72	(0.50, 1.04)	
Vitamin Supplement Use					–
None	146 (60.8)	1202 (63.5)	Ref		
Calcium	40 (16.7)	311 (16.4)	1.08	(0.73, 1.58)	
Vitamin D	34 (14.2)	235 (12.4)	1.06	(0.69, 1.63)	
Both	20 (8.3)	145 (7.7)	1.03	(0.61, 1.74)	

NOTE: Pharmacy data through December 31, 2013.
[1] Osteoporosis defined by ICD-9 code (733.00–733.09) or any prior bisphosphonate prescription.
[2] Logistic regression adjusted for age, race/ethnicity, menopausal status, and year of breast cancer diagnosis.
[3] Median (physical activity) = 20.9 metabolic equivalent (MET)-hours/week; median (alcohol intake) = 3.1 g/day.

National Drug Code, dosage and therapeutic class; prescription dates and cost; dispensing and refills; and prescribing physician, thus minimizing recall bias [20]. The pharmacy database was accessed to identify any outpatient prescriptions of AIs (anastrozole, letrozole, and exemestane) and TAM after breast cancer diagnosis. Prescriptions of bisphosphonates (BP) any time before breast cancer diagnosis were also captured. BPs are inhibitors of bone resorption and commonly prescribed to treat osteoporosis and other related conditions.

Prior Bone Outcomes

International Classification of Diseases, 9th edition (ICD-9) outpatient and hospitalization diagnoses of bone outcomes were obtained from the KPNC electronic medical record (EMR). These diagnosis codes include: (1) osteoporosis (733.00–733.09); (2) any prior fracture involving the neck, trunk, upper and lower extremities (805, 807–815, 817–825, 827–829, excluding open fractures, fractures involving spinal cord injury, fractures of the face/skull, fingers and toes, and those associated with major trauma); and (3) any major osteoporotic fracture of the spine, humerus, wrist, or hip (805.0, 805.2, 805.4, 805.8, 812.0, 812.2, 813.4, 813.5, 820.0, 820.2, 820.8, excluding those associated with major trauma) were ascertained as previously described [21].

Considering potential under-diagnosis or documentation of osteoporosis by clinicians [22,23], we assumed that if a woman was prescribed a BP prior to breast cancer diagnosis, and considering

Table 3. Baseline characteristics in relation to any fracture before breast cancer (BC) diagnosis in aromatase inhibitor (AI) users.

	Any Fracture Before BC Diagnosis – Yes	Any fracture Before BC Diagnosis – No	OR[1]	95% CI[1]	p for trend
	n = 352	n = 1805			
	n (%)	n (%)			
Age at BC Diagnosis (years)					**<0.0001**
<60	70 (19.9)	650 (36.0)	Ref		
60–69	143 (40.6)	748 (41.4)	**1.76**	**(1.27, 2.43)**	
≥70	139 (39.5)	407 (22.6)	**3.13**	**(2.24, 4.37)**	
Race/Ethnicity					–
White	268 (76.1)	1273 (70.5)	Ref		
African American	24 (6.8)	100 (5.5)	1.30	(0.81, 2.08)	
Asian	17 (4.8)	204 (11.3)	**0.50**	**(0.30, 0.84)**	
Hispanic	34 (9.7)	191 (10.6)	0.97	(0.66, 1.44)	
Other	9 (2.6)	37 (2.1)	1.37	(0.65, 2.90)	
BMI (kg/m²)					0.86
<25	93 (26.6)	549 (30.7)	Ref		
25–29.9	135 (38.6)	545 (30.5)	**1.43**	**(1.06, 1.92)**	
≥30	122 (34.9)	694 (38.8)	1.00	(0.74, 1.36)	
Mod-Vig Physical Activity (MET-hours/week)					–
Never	26 (7.5)	82 (4.6)	Ref		
≤median[2]	164 (47.0)	853 (47.6)	0.83	(0.51, 1.35)	
>median	159 (45.6)	856 (47.8)	0.84	(0.51, 1.37)	
Smoking History					–
Never	178 (50.7)	940 (52.3)	Ref		
Former	152 (43.3)	761 (42.3)	0.93	(0.73, 1.19)	
Current	21 (6.0)	97 (5.4)	1.24	(0.75, 2.07)	
Alcohol Intake (g/day)					–
Never	89 (30.4)	422 (27.4)	Ref		
≤median[2]	88 (30.0)	576 (37.4)	0.73	(0.52, 1.01)	
>median	116 (39.6)	544 (35.3)	1.00	(0.73, 1.38)	
Vitamin Supplement Use					–
None	203 (58.8)	1145 (64.0)	Ref		
Calcium	60 (17.4)	291 (16.3)	1.21	(0.88, 1.68)	
Vitamin D	49 (14.2)	220 (12.3)	1.12	(0.78, 1.61)	
Both	33 (9.6)	132 (7.4)	1.21	(0.79, 1.86)	
Osteoporosis Before BC Diagnosis					–
No	267 (75.9)	1648 (91.3)	Ref		
Yes	85 (24.2)	157 (8.7)	**2.86**	**(2.10, 3.89)**	

NOTE: Pharmacy data through December 31, 2013.
[1] Logistic regression adjusted for age, race/ethnicity, menopausal status, and year of breast cancer diagnosis.
[2] Median (physical activity) = 20.9 metabolic equivalent (MET)-hours/week; median (alcohol intake) = 3.1 g/day.

that BPs are usually indicated for clinical treatment of osteoporosis, she was most likely diagnosed with the condition. Therefore, we expanded our definition of osteoporosis to include any prescription of BP before breast cancer diagnosis regardless of whether or not an ICD-9 diagnosis code was present. Thus, osteoporosis was defined as having any relevant ICD-9 diagnosis code or any prior prescription of BP.

Statistical Analysis

Analyses of initial AI or TAM use in postmenopausal breast cancer patients by select characteristics, including prior history of osteoporosis and fracture, were conducted using logistic regression with adjustment for age at breast cancer diagnosis as a continuous variable.

In the overall initial AI user group, we calculated odds ratios (OR) and 95% confidence intervals (CI) using logistic regression to estimate the associations of lifestyle and clinical factors at breast

Table 4. Baseline characteristics in relation to major fracture[1] before breast cancer (BC) diagnosis in aromatase inhibitor (AI) users.

	Major Fracture Before BC Diagnosis – Yes	Major Fracture Before BC Diagnosis – No	OR[2]	95% CI[2]	p for trend
	n = 99	**n = 2058**			
	n (%)	**n (%)**			
Age at BC Diagnosis (years)					**<0.0001**
<60	16 (16.2)	704 (34.2)	Ref		
60–69	32 (32.3)	859 (41.7)	1.54	(0.81, 2.93)	
≥70	51 (51.5)	495 (24.1)	**4.23**	**(2.29, 7.83)**	
Race/Ethnicity					–
White	82 (82.8)	1459 (70.9)	Ref		
African American	3 (3.0)	121 (5.9)	0.52	(0.16, 1.70)	
Asian	4 (4.0)	217 (10.5)	0.47	(0.17, 1.30)	
Hispanic	6 (6.1)	219 (10.6)	0.59	(0.25, 1.37)	
Other	4 (4.0)	42 (2.0)	2.20	(0.76, 6.39)	
BMI (kg/m^2)					0.38
<25	28 (28.3)	614 (30.1)	Ref		
25–29.9	39 (39.4)	641 (31.4)	1.33	(0.80, 2.21)	
≥30	32 (32.3)	784 (38.5)	0.93	(0.55, 1.59)	
Mod-Vig Physical Activity (MET-hours/week)					–
Never	15 (15.5)	93 (4.6)	Ref		
≤median[3]	40 (41.2)	977 (47.8)	**0.33**	**(0.17, 0.64)**	
>median	42 (43.3)	973 (47.6)	**0.36**	**(0.18, 0.70)**	
Smoking History					–
Never	49 (49.5)	1069 (52.2)	Ref		
Former	48 (48.5)	865 (42.2)	1.05	(0.69, 1.60)	
Current	2 (2.0)	116 (5.7)	0.44	(0.11, 1.86)	
Alcohol Intake (g/day)					–
Never	24 (28.2)	487 (27.8)	Ref		
≤median[3]	24 (28.2)	640 (36.6)	0.76	(0.43, 1.38)	
>median	37 (43.5)	623 (35.6)	1.16	(0.67, 2.00)	
Vitamin Supplement Use					–
None	61 (63.5)	1287 (63.2)	Ref		
Calcium	13 (13.5)	338 (16.6)	0.82	(0.44, 1.53)	
Vitamin D	12 (12.5)	257 (12.6)	0.89	(0.46, 1.72)	
Both	10 (10.4)	155 (7.6)	1.20	(0.59, 2.45)	
Osteoporosis Before BC Diagnosis					–

Table 4. Cont.

	Major Fracture Before BC Diagnosis – Yes	Major Fracture Before BC Diagnosis – No	OR[2]	95% CI[2]	p for trend
	n = 99	n = 2058			
	n (%)	n (%)			
No	67 (67.7)	1848 (89.8)	Ref		
Yes	32 (32.3)	210 (10.2)	3.15	(1.98, 5.02)	

NOTE: Pharmacy data through December 31, 2013.
[1] Major fracture includes fracture of spine, humerus, wrist, or hip.
[2] Logistic regression adjusted for age, race/ethnicity, menopausal status, and year of breast cancer diagnosis.
[3] Median (physical activity) = 20.9 metabolic equivalent (MET)-hours/week; median (alcohol intake) = 3.1 g/day.

cancer diagnosis with prior history of 1) osteoporosis, 2) any fracture, and 3) any major osteoporotic fracture. All models were adjusted for age, race/ethnicity, menopausal status, and year of breast cancer diagnosis, and all p-values were two-tailed with a significance level of 0.05. Analyses were repeated after excluding those diagnosed with breast cancer before menopause. The results were similar to those from the overall initial AI user group and thus are not presented here.

All analyses were conducted in SAS version 9.3 (Cary, N.C.).

Ethics Statement

The study was approved by the KPNC institutional review board.

Results

As shown in **Table 1**, the mean age at breast cancer diagnosis among AI users was 64.4 years, with 2,033 (94.5%) initially diagnosed after menopause and 118 (5.5%) before menopause. As expected, the majority of the initial AI users were diagnosed with early stage disease (AJCC stage I–III) (98.4%). The study cohort was multi-ethnic, with 71.4% White, 10.4% Hispanic, 10.3% Asian, 5.8% African American, and 2.1% other race/ethnicity. The mean BMI at baseline was 29.0 kg/m^2, with 31.8% being overweight and 38.2% obese. The median (IQR) of moderate-vigorous physical activity at baseline was 19.5 (7.3–39.1) metabolic equivalent (MET)-hours/week. Over half of the patients were never smokers at baseline (52.0%), 42.5% were former smokers, and only 5.5% were current smokers. Alcohol intake was light at baseline, with 27.9% being never drinkers, and among those who drank, the median intake was 3.10 grams/day. Nearly two-thirds of the patients did not take either calcium or vitamin D supplements at baseline (63.2%), 16.5% took calcium, 12.6% took vitamin D, and 7.7% took both supplements.

Among the initial AI users, 11.2% had a prior history of osteoporosis, including 3.5% at 6 years or more before breast cancer diagnosis, and 7.7% within 6 years (**Table 1**). 16.3% of the patients had a prior history of any fracture, including 7.6% at 6 years or more before cancer diagnosis, and 8.7% within 6 years. For major fractures of the spine, humerus, wrist, or hip, 4.6% had a prior history of these fractures, including 1.7% at 6 years or more before cancer diagnosis, and 2.9% within 6 years.

Among postmenopausal patients with HR-positive breast cancer, the majority received AIs as their initial hormonal therapy (n = 2,033, 86.2%), and 325 patients (n = 13.8%) received TAM as their initial hormonal therapy. No apparent secular trend was found in the use of AIs relative to TAM during the study period (2005–2013). To explore whether bone health history or other known risk factors for fractures might affect the choice of hormonal therapy drugs, comparisons were conducted between postmenopausal initial AI users and postmenopausal initial TAM users. As shown among the postmenopausal women in **Table 1**, compared to initial AI users, women on TAM were younger (mean age 62.0 years vs. 65.2 years, $p<0.0001$), more likely to have stage I disease (67.1% vs. 55.1%, $p = 0.0003$), less obese (mean BMI 27.6 kg/m^2 vs. 29.0 kg/m^2, $p = 0.0001$), and more physically active (median 19.4 MET-hours/week vs. 24.4 MET-hours/week, $p = 0.03$). No differences in race/ethnicity, smoking history, or alcohol intake were found between the two groups. For bone health history prior to breast cancer diagnosis, although initial TAM users were younger, they had a significantly higher prevalence of prior osteoporosis than initial AI users (21.5% vs. 11.8%, $p<0.0001$), but a similar prevalence of any prior fracture (16.3% vs. 16.6%, $p = 0.27$) and major prior fracture (5.9% vs.

4.8%, p = 0.13). Consistent with a higher prevalence of prior osteoporosis compared with AI users, TAM users were more likely to take calcium and/or vitamin D than AI users (45.0% vs. 37.3%, p = 0.003).

In Tables 2–4, the associations of selected risk factors with prior history of osteoporosis and fractures among overall initial AI users are presented. In models adjusted for age, race/ethnicity, menopausal status, and year of breast cancer diagnosis, older age (60–69 y OR = 2.43; 95% CI: 1.58, 3.72; ≥70 y OR = 5.65; 95% CI: 3.68, 8.69; p for trend<0.0001) and being Asian (OR = 1.82; 95% CI: 1.17, 2.81) were associated with higher odds of prior osteoporosis, whereas increasing BMI (overweight OR = 0.55; 95% CI: 0.40, 0.76; obese OR = 0.32; 95% CI: 0.22, 0.45; p for trend<0.0001) and being African American (OR = 0.38; 95% CI: 0.15, 0.94) were associated with lower odds (**Table 2**).

Associations of patient characteristics and lifestyle factors with prior history of any fracture are given in **Table 3**. Older age was associated with higher odds of any prior fracture (p for trend< 0.0001), whereas being Asian (OR = 0.50; 95% CI: 0.30, 0.84) was associated with lower odds of any prior fracture. In contrast to associations with prior osteoporosis, no significant increasing BMI trend was found, yet being overweight was associated with increased odds of any prior fracture (OR = 1.43; 95% CI: 1.06, 1.92). Finally, as expected, prior history of osteoporosis was associated with increased odds of prior fracture (OR = 2.86; 95% CI: 2.10, 3.89). Associations of patient characteristics and lifestyle factors with prior major fracture were largely consistent with any prior fracture, but with wider CIs (**Table 4**). Unique to analyses of major fracture, however, any moderate-vigorous physical activity was associated with reduced odds of major fracture in the AI users (≤median 20.9 MET-hours/week OR = 0.33 95% CI: 0.17, 0.64; >median OR = 0.36; 95% CI: 0.18, 0.70).

Discussion

In a large contemporary cohort of breast cancer survivors who were initially treated with AIs, we found that 11.2% had a prior history of osteoporosis, 16.3% any fracture, and 4.6% major fracture before breast cancer diagnosis. Although the majority of postmenopausal women were initially treated with AIs, a sizable proportion (13.8%) was initially treated with TAM. Furthermore, these TAM users had nearly twice the prevalence of prior osteoporosis compared with initial AI users. Finally, the associations of selected risk factors with prior history of bone health outcomes in breast cancer patients initially treated with AIs were largely consistent with those expected from the healthy older population [13,14].

To our knowledge, our observational study is the largest to date to describe the use of AIs as primary hormonal therapy in conjunction with prior bone morbidity. A previous study of 343 women with early-stage breast cancer about to initiate AI therapy reported 22.2% with osteoporosis and 11.4% with any fracture [16]. Another study of 497 breast cancer patients also at the onset of AI therapy found 19.1% with non-vertebral fractures [15]. Compared with our prevalence findings of 11.2% osteoporosis and 16.3% any fracture, Servitja et al. reported a higher rate of osteoporosis but a lower rate of fracture, whereas Bouvard et al. reported a higher rate of fracture. While these studies were limited by small sample size, they did collect baseline bone health measures of BMD, spinal X-rays, and 25-hydroxyvitamin D [25-(OH)D] concentrations. Our current analysis does not consider these data, yet in future prospective analyses of fracture risk, we will be incorporating BMD measures and 25(OH)D concentrations around baseline entry into the cohort.

For postmenopausal women diagnosed with early stage, HR-positive breast cancer, AIs have been shown to have superior efficacy in lowering risk of recurrence compared with TAM, and thus have become the preferable choice for this patient subgroup. However, TAM remains a viable choice for initial hormonal therapy for those who seek to avoid AIs' musculoskeletal effects. This is likely true for women deemed to have low risk of recurrence but are susceptible to fractures, as suggested by our results. In postmenopausal patients in our study, initial TAM users were slightly younger than initial AI users, yet the former had significantly higher prevalence of osteoporosis history. However, initial TAM users were more likely to have stage I disease than initial AI users, suggesting their risk of recurrence was lower. A lower risk of recurrence coupled with a higher risk of fracture might have influenced physicians and patients to favor TAM over AIs as their first choice of initial hormonal therapy. This speculation was further strengthened by the findings of higher usage of calcium and/or vitamin D supplement and higher physical activity in the initial TAM users than in the initial AI users. As supplement use and physical activity were surveyed soon after breast cancer diagnosis, we could not assess whether these data represent exposure status before or after the diagnosis of osteoporosis. Higher usage of supplements and being more physically active might have been in response to being diagnosed with osteoporosis (reverse causality). It is also interesting to note that a small proportion of initial AI users were diagnosed with breast cancer before menopause. Most likely those patients experienced menopause due to chemotherapy or radiation therapy and were subsequently eligible for AI therapy.

Among initial AI users, we identified several risk factors associated with history of osteoporosis, including older age, Asian race, and lower BMI. Older age was also associated with fracture history and being physically active was associated with lower risk of major prior fracture. These associations were in the same direction as expected in a general healthy older population, suggesting common mechanisms for osteoporosis and fracture regardless of later breast cancer diagnosis. Although smoking and alcohol consumption are risk factors for osteoporosis and fracture in non-cancer patients, we did not find such associations in initial AI users, possibly due to the small proportion (5.5%) of current smokers in the study and light alcohol intake in the cohort (median intake of 3.10 grams/day among drinkers). We also found that Asian AI users had a higher risk of osteoporosis but lower risk of prior fracture than Whites. This observation potentially reflects known racial/ethnic differences of lower bone mineral density, yet decreased fracture risk, in healthy Asians compared with Whites [24,25,26].

When comparing our proportion of prior fracture to healthy postmenopausal women at a similar age in the Women's Health Initiative (WHI) [27], initial postmenopausal AI users were approximately two times less likely to have a history of fracture (16.6% vs. 34.4%, p = 0.0039). The lower rate of prevalent osteoporosis and fracture seen among breast cancer patients in our study may be explained by the paradoxical association between high BMD and breast cancer risk [28]. As estrogen plays a central role in bone growth and maintenance, it also drives the development of breast cancer. Therefore, at the time of diagnosis, women with breast cancer may have had higher lifetime estrogen exposure and associated BMD than non-cancer women at a similar age, which may explain the lower prevalence of osteoporosis and fracture among breast cancer patients seen in our study.

Our study was based on a large prospective breast cancer cohort from one of the nation's largest integrated healthcare delivery systems where complete electronic medical records and pharmacy information are available on all patients. This enabled us to accurately assess bone health history through their health insurance membership with Kaiser Permanente. Moreover, the cohort was established in 2005, a time concurrent with the widespread use of AIs. Our study was further strengthened by the availability of extensive demographic and lifestyle information collected at the time of diagnosis through in-person interviews.

Nevertheless, our study is not without limitations. Due to its cross-sectional nature, we could not infer causality of the selected risk factors for prevalent osteoporosis and fracture among breast cancer patients. In addition, osteoporosis was potentially underdiagnosed in our patient population. However, this is not a unique challenge to this study. Clinicians vary in their use and coding of the term osteoporosis such that it may be identified after BMD testing, after a primary care visit, at the time of a specialty visit, at the time of bisphosphonate initiation, or at the time of fracture. Further, a diagnosis may not always mean that the T-score is in the osteoporosis range, and a diagnosis could also be made in the presence of a fragility fracture while BMD is only in the osteopenic range. There have also been temporal changes in the frequency of osteoporosis diagnosis [29], which may explain the greater proportion of AI users with *a priori* osteoporosis diagnosis, as AIs did not become the preferential choice of hormonal therapy for postmenopausal breast cancer patients until the mid-2000's. To overcome this limitation, we classified patients with BP treatment but without an ICD-9 diagnosis of osteoporosis as osteoporotic. The results were similar when we relied only on osteoporosis ICD-9 diagnosis. Furthermore, the prevalence of prior spine fractures could have been underestimated due to asymptomatic fractures not being coded by the physician, but for our analyses, we considered spine fractures as clinically diagnosed. Finally, given our access to electronic medical records on the cohort, we estimate that only 35% had BMD measurements before breast cancer diagnosis based on Current Procedural Terminology (CPT) codes, thus precluding us from classifying osteoporosis status based on BMD data for the entire cohort. To note, the prevalence of prior BMD screening in our cohort is greater than 16% reported in a small study of BMD screening adherence among 342 breast cancer patients on AIs, and these women were also members of an integrated health care system [30].

To conclude, a small proportion of breast cancer patients initially treated with AIs had a positive history of osteoporosis or fracture before their cancer diagnosis. A history of osteoporosis might influence the choice of initial hormonal therapy drug among patients with low risk of recurrence. Risk factors for osteoporosis and fracture before breast cancer diagnosis were similar to those among healthy older women. Given that adverse effects on bone health is a common comorbidity concern for many cancer survivors [31], our findings may have wide clinical applicability beyond breast cancer that emphasize the importance of full consideration of prior bone health history before initiation of cancer treatment.

Author Contributions

Conceived and designed the experiments: MLK SY. Analyzed the data: CAL JMR MC CPQ MLK SY. Contributed reagents/materials/analysis tools: MLK SY. Contributed to the writing of the manuscript: MLK JCL LT JMR TEH CCH LSC DLH CPQ CBA LHK SY.

References

1. Geisler J, Haynes B, Anker G, Dowsett M, Lonning PE (2002) Influence of letrozole and anastrozole on total body aromatization and plasma estrogen levels in postmenopausal breast cancer patients evaluated in a randomized, cross-over study. J Clin Oncol 20: 751–757.
2. Chien AJ, Goss PE (2006) Aromatase inhibitors and bone health in women with breast cancer. J Clin Oncol 24: 5305–5312.
3. Boccardo F (2008) Switching to anastrozole after tamoxifen improves survival in postmenopausal women with breast cancer. Nat Clin Pract Oncol 5: 76–77.
4. Dowsett M, Cuzick J, Ingle J, Coates A, Forbes J, et al. (2010) Meta-analysis of breast cancer outcomes in adjuvant trials of aromatase inhibitors versus tamoxifen. J Clin Oncol 28: 509–518.
5. Burstein HJ, Prestrud AA, Seidenfeld J, Anderson H, Buchholz TA, et al. (2010) American Society of Clinical Oncology clinical practice guideline: update on adjuvant endocrine therapy for women with hormone receptor-positive breast cancer. J Clin Oncol 28: 3784–3796.
6. Hadji P (2009) Aromatase inhibitor-associated bone loss in breast cancer patients is distinct from postmenopausal osteoporosis. Crit Rev Oncol Hematol 69: 73–82.
7. Hillner BE, Ingle JN, Chlebowski RT, Gralow J, Yee GC, et al. (2003) American Society of Clinical Oncology 2003 update on the role of bisphosphonates and bone health issues in women with breast cancer. J Clin Oncol 21: 4042–4057.
8. Body JJ, Bergmann P, Boonen S, Boutsen Y, Devogelaer JP, et al. (2007) Management of cancer treatment-induced bone loss in early breast and prostate cancer – a consensus paper of the Belgian Bone Club. Osteoporos Int 18: 1439–1450.
9. Reid DM, Doughty J, Eastell R, Heys SD, Howell A, et al. (2008) Guidance for the management of breast cancer treatment-induced bone loss: a consensus position statement from a UK Expert Group. Cancer Treat Rev 34 Suppl 1: S3–18.
10. Gralow JR, Biermann JS, Farooki A, Fornier MN, Gagel RF, et al. (2013) NCCN Task Force Report: Bone Health In Cancer Care. J Natl Compr Canc Netw 11 Suppl 3: S1–50; quiz S51.
11. Siris ES, Genant HK, Laster AJ, Chen P, Misurski DA, et al. (2007) Enhanced prediction of fracture risk combining vertebral fracture status and BMD. Osteoporos Int 18: 761–770.
12. Nguyen ND, Eisman JA, Center JR, Nguyen TV (2007) Risk factors for fracture in nonosteoporotic men and women. The Journal of clinical endocrinology and metabolism 92: 955–962.
13. Cummings SR, Nevitt MC, Browner WS, Stone K, Fox KM, et al. (1995) Risk factors for hip fracture in white women. Study of Osteoporotic Fractures Research Group. The New England journal of medicine 332: 767–773.
14. Robbins J, Aragaki AK, Kooperberg C, Watts N, Wactawski-Wende J, et al. (2007) Factors associated with 5-year risk of hip fracture in postmenopausal women. Jama 298: 2389–2398.
15. Bouvard B, Hoppe E, Soulie P, Georgin-Mege M, Jadaud E, et al. (2012) High prevalence of vertebral fractures in women with breast cancer starting aromatase inhibitor therapy. Annals of oncology: official journal of the European Society for Medical Oncology/ESMO 23: 1151–1156.
16. Servitja S, Nogues X, Prieto-Alhambra D, Martinez-Garcia M, Garrigos L, et al. (2012) Bone health in a prospective cohort of postmenopausal women receiving aromatase inhibitors for early breast cancer. Breast 21: 95–101.
17. Kwan ML, Ambrosone CB, Lee MM, Barlow J, Krathwohl SE, et al. (2008) The Pathways Study: a prospective study of breast cancer survivorship within Kaiser Permanente Northern California. Cancer Causes Control 19: 1065–1076.
18. Oehrli MD, Quesenberry CP (2013) 2013 Annual Report on Trends, Incidence, and Outcomes. Kaiser Permanente, Northern California Cancer Registry.
19. Staten LK, Taren DL, Howell WH, Tobar M, Poehlman ET, et al. (2001) Validation of the Arizona Activity Frequency Questionnaire using doubly labeled water. Med Sci Sports Exerc 33: 1959–1967.
20. Selby JV, Smith DH, Johnson ES, Raebel MA, Friedman GD, et al. (2005) Kaiser Permanente Medical Care Program. In: BL S, editor. Pharmacoepidemiology. West Sussex: John Wiley & Sons, Ltd. 241–259.
21. Chau S, Chandra M, Grimsrud CD, Gonzalez JR, Hui RL, et al. (2014) Femur fracture classification in women with a history of breast cancer. Journal of Bone Oncology 3: 49–53.
22. Siris ES, Miller PD, Barrett-Connor E, Faulkner KG, Wehren LE, et al. (2001) Identification and fracture outcomes of undiagnosed low bone mineral density in postmenopausal women: results from the National Osteoporosis Risk Assessment. JAMA: the journal of the American Medical Association 286: 2815–2822.
23. Vestergaard P, Rejnmark L, Mosekilde L (2005) Osteoporosis is markedly underdiagnosed: a nationwide study from Denmark. Osteoporosis international: a journal established as result of cooperation between the European Foundation for Osteoporosis and the National Osteoporosis Foundation of the USA 16: 134–141.
24. Liu XS, Walker MD, McMahon DJ, Udesky J, Liu G, et al. (2011) Better skeletal microstructure confers greater mechanical advantages in Chinese-American

women versus white women. Journal of bone and mineral research: the official journal of the American Society for Bone and Mineral Research 26: 1783–1792.
25. Walker MD, Liu XS, Stein E, Zhou B, Bezati E, et al. (2011) Differences in bone microarchitecture between postmenopausal Chinese-American and white women. Journal of bone and mineral research: the official journal of the American Society for Bone and Mineral Research 26: 1392–1398.
26. Walker MD, Saeed I, McMahon DJ, Udesky J, Liu G, et al. (2012) Volumetric bone mineral density at the spine and hip in Chinese American and White women. Osteoporosis international: a journal established as result of cooperation between the European Foundation for Osteoporosis and the National Osteoporosis Foundation of the USA 23: 2499–2506.
27. Jackson RD, LaCroix AZ, Gass M, Wallace RB, Robbins J, et al. (2006) Calcium plus vitamin D supplementation and the risk of fractures. N Engl J Med 354: 669–683.
28. Eastell R (2007) Breast cancer and the risk of osteoporotic fracture: A paradox. The Journal of clinical endocrinology and metabolism 92: 42–43.
29. National Osteoporosis Foundation (2002) America's Bone Health: The State of Osteoporosis and Low Bone Mass in Our Nation. Available: http://noforg/files/nof/public/content/file/63/upload/49pdf. Accessed 2014 Jun 13.
30. Spangler L, Yu O, Loggers E, Boudreau DM (2013) Bone mineral density screening among women with a history of breast cancer treated with aromatase inhibitors. Journal of women's health 22: 132–140.
31. Lustberg MB, Reinbolt RE, Shapiro CL (2012) Bone health in adult cancer survivorship. Journal of clinical oncology: official journal of the American Society of Clinical Oncology 30: 3665–3674.

23

EPO Promotes Bone Repair through Enhanced Cartilaginous Callus Formation and Angiogenesis

Lin Wan[1], Fengjie Zhang[1,2], Qiling He[3], Wing Pui Tsang[1,2], Li Lu[1,4], Qingnan Li[4], Zhihong Wu[5], Guixing Qiu[5], Guangqian Zhou[6], Chao Wan[1,2]*

1 Ministry of Education Key Laboratory for Regenerative Medicine, School of Biomedical Sciences, Faculty of Medicine, The Chinese University of Hong Kong, Hong Kong SAR, China, **2** School of Biomedical Sciences Core Laboratory, Shenzhen Research Institute, The Chinese University of Hong Kong, Shenzhen, China, **3** Departments of Microbiology and Pathology, University of Alabama at Birmingham, Birmingham, Alabama, United States of America, **4** Guangdong Key Laboratory of Pharmaceutical Bioactive Substances, New Drug Function Research Center, School of Life Science and Biopharmacy, Guangdong Pharmaceutical University, Guangzhou, China, **5** Department of Orthopaedics, Peking Union Medical College Hospital, Peking Union Medical College and Chinese Academy of Medical Sciences, Beijing, China, **6** The Center for Anti-Ageing and Regenerative Medicine, Medical School, Shenzhen University, Shenzhen, China

Abstract

Erythropoietin (EPO)/erythropoietin receptor (EPOR) signaling is involved in the development and regeneration of several non-hematopoietic tissues including the skeleton. EPO is identified as a downstream target of the hypoxia inducible factor-α (HIF-α) pathway. It is shown that EPO exerts a positive role in bone repair, however, the underlying cellular and molecular mechanisms remain unclear. In the present study we show that EPO and EPOR are expressed in the proliferating, pre-hypertrophic and hypertrophic zone of the developing mouse growth plates as well as in the cartilaginous callus of the healing bone. The proliferation rate of chondrocytes is increased under EPO treatment, while this effect is decreased following siRNA mediated knockdown of EPOR in chondrocytes. EPO treatment increases biosynthesis of proteoglycan, accompanied by up-regulation of chondrogenic marker genes including SOX9, SOX5, SOX6, collagen type 2, and aggrecan. The effects are inhibited by knockdown of EPOR. Blockage of the endogenous EPO in chondrocytes also impaired the chondrogenic differentiation. In addition, EPO promotes metatarsal endothelial sprouting *in vitro*. This coincides with the *in vivo* data that local delivery of EPO increases vascularity at the mid-stage of bone healing (day 14). In a mouse femoral fracture model, EPO promotes cartilaginous callus formation at days 7 and 14, and enhances bone healing at day 28 indexed by improved X-ray score and micro-CT analysis of microstructure of new bone regenerates, which results in improved biomechanical properties. Our results indicate that EPO enhances chondrogenic and angiogenic responses during bone repair. EPO's function on chondrocyte proliferation and differentiation is at least partially mediated by its receptor EPOR. EPO may serve as a therapeutic agent to facilitate skeletal regeneration.

Editor: Domenico Ribatti, University of Bari Medical School, Italy

Funding: This work was supported by Hong Kong Research Grant Council General Research Fund (RGC GRF 475910), National Natural Science Foundation of China (NSFC 81130034), and NSFC-RGC Joint Research Scheme (CUHK445/10) to CW. The funders had no role in study design, data collection and analysis, decision to publish, or preparation of the manuscript.

Competing Interests: The authors have declared that no competing interests exist.

* Email: cwan@cuhk.edu.hk

Introduction

Impaired bone regeneration following injury or under pathological conditions causes severe pain to the patients and considerable financial burden to the society [1,2]. These conditions include delayed fracture union or non-union, osteoporotic fracture healing, impaired bone repair associated with diabetes, and large bone defects caused by trauma or surgical treatments [3,4,5,6]. Hallmarks of impaired bone repair in patients and animal models include the deficiency in vascular supply and cartilaginous callus formation at the site of injury, suggesting that impaired angiogenic and chondrogenic responses are major contributors to the pathology [7,8].

Bone regeneration is a complex process in which the recovery of skeletal tissue integrity relies upon close temporal and spatial coordination of molecular and cellular events involving resident bone cells, inflammatory cells, marrow stromal elements, and associated vascular structures [9,10,11,12] to achieve structural reconstitution and bone remodeling. The regeneration process has generally been characterized by four steps including inflammation phase with hematoma, cartilage callus formation, bony callus formation and bone remodeling [13,14]. During bone regeneration, angiogenesis is essential and depends on hypoxic stimuli and production of proangiogenic factors such as vascular endothelial growth factor (VEGF) [7], Erythropoietin (EPO) [15], fibroblast growth factor (FGF) [16], transforming growth factor-beta (TGF-beta) [17] and insulin like growth factor (IGF-1) [18].

The bone cells are readily located in a hypoxic microenvironment during development and regeneration. Hypoxia inducible factor-α (HIF-α) is identified as key mediator for cell adaptation to low oxygen tension. VEGF and EPO are established downstream targets of HIF-α. It is well established that VEGF is expressed in osteoblasts [19,20] and the HIF-α/VEGF pathway couples angiogenesis and osteogenesis during bone development and regeneration [7,21,22] while the study on the involvement of EPO in bone regeneration is just emerging.

EPO is a 34 kD circulating glycoprotein hormone which is initially recognized as the crucial growth factor that controls red blood cell development in bone marrow through binding to its high affinity receptor (EPOR) expressed on erythroid progenitor cells [23,24,25]. EPO is predominantly produced by the interstitial fibroblasts of the renal cortex and outer medulla in adult animals, and by Kuffer's cells in the liver during embryonic development [26,27,28,29], under the control of oxygen sensing HIF pathway [30]. In addition to its principal function in erythropoiesis, nonehematopoietic functions of EPO such as angiogenic [25], cardioprotective [31], neuroprotctive and neurotrophic [32,33] effects have raised great interest and been extensively studied, due to the findings that EPO is also produced in non-renal tissues such as brain [34], and that EPOR is present in a variety of non-hematopoietic cell types such as brain capillary endothelial cells [35], vascular smooth muscle cells [36], myocardial cells [37], neurons [38] and astrocytes [39]. The potential physiological effects of EPO on skeletal tissue were suggested by both clinical and animal studies that bone modulation was associated with erythropoiesis stimulation by systemic administration of EPO [40,41,42]. However, the underlying mechanism is largely unknown. It was reported that EPO activated JAK/STAT signaling in hematopoietic stem cells (HSCs) to produce bone morphogenetic proteins (BMPs) and thus exerted indirect function in bone formation [43]. Although there is one study showing that EPO indirectly increased bone turnover rate and induced trabecular bone loss [42], several other studies demonstrated that EPO improved bone healing [44,45,46], possibly through the proposed direct interaction between EPO with EPOR-expressed hypertrophic chondrocytes to promote endochondral ossification [45] or with EPOR-expressed bone marrow stromal cells to induce osteoblastic differentiation [43]. In addition, significant vascular expansion was also noted during bone healing when EPO was applied [44,46]. It is known that EPO and EPOR are expressed in the vasculature during embryogenesis, and exert a critical role for angiogenesis [25]. Therefore the improved bone healing may also be attributed to a better angiogenesis caused by EPO.

In the present study, we systemically examined the roles of EPO in regulating chondrogenesis and angiogenesis *in vitro* and *in vivo*. The promotive effects of EPO during the chondrogenic and angiogenic phases of femur fracture repair highlight its therapeutic potential in skeletal regenerative medicine.

Materials and Methods

Animals

C57BL/6 mice at age of three-days, fourteen-days and twelve-weeks were used in this study. Mice were housed in the controlled conditions with room temperature of 22±1°C and a light-dark cycle of 12:12 hour, and were fed with standard mouse chow and water ad libitum. Experimental procedures were carried out in accordance with the protocols approved by Animal Experimentation Ethics Committee from the Chinese University of Hong Kong and Animal (Control of Experiments) Ordinance from Department of Health, Hong Kong SAR.

Culture of primary chondrocytes from neonatal mice

The primary chondrocytes were isolated from growth plates following previous procedures [47]. Cells were cultured in minimum essential medium alpha (αMEM) supplemented with 10% fetal bovine serum (FBS), 2 mM L-glutamine and 100 U/ml penicillin and 100 μg/ml streptomycin (all from Gibco). The 1st and 2nd passage cells were processed in the below experiments.

Knockdown of EPOR in chondrocytes

Knockdown of EPOR in chondrocytes was performed by siRNA (Santa Cruz) method using lipofectamine2000 (Invitrogen) following standard protocol. 24 hours after transfection, cells were collected for real-time PCR and Western blot analysis to examine the efficiency of gene knockdown.

Bromodeoxyuridine (BrdU) incorporation assay

Chondrocytes were treated with 40 ng/ml or 80 ng/ml EPO (Sigma-Aldrich) for 2 days and compared with that without EPO treatment. The proliferation rate of chondrocytes was analyzed using the cell proliferation ELISA BrdU assay (Roche).

Cell mass culture

Cells were plated at density of 1×10^5 cells/10 μl and cultured for 3 hours to form the cell masses. Cell masses were then treated with no EPO, 40 ng/ml EPO or EPO block peptide (500 ng/ml, Santa Cruz) in chondrogenic medium supplemented with dexamethasone (100 nM, Sigma-Aldrich), ascorbic acid (50 μg/ml, Sigma-Aldrich), sodium pyruvate (100 μg/ml, Gibco), ITS+ Premix (50 mg/ml, BD) for 7 days following previous procedures [48].

Alcian blue staining

The Alcian blue staining was performed to examine proteoglycan synthesis during chondrocytes differentiation as previously described [49]. Briefly, the cell masses were rinsed with PBS after 7 days of culture, and stained with 1% acidic Alcian blue for 2 hours, followed by 5 times washing using 70% ethanol to remove the residual dyes. The proteoglycan was stained blue.

Quantitation of sulfated glycosaminoglycan (sGAG)

sGAG was quantitated using a dimethylmethylene blue colourimetric assay following established protocol (Blyscan sulfated glycosaminoglycan assay) [50,51]. DMB dye (1, 9-Dimethyl-Methylene Blue zinc chloride double salt) was added to measure the sGAG content in the digested substances.

RT PCR and real-time PCR

Total mRNA was extracted from primary chondrocytes using the TRIzol reagent (Life Technologies) following the manufacturer's instructions. First strand cDNA was synthesized from 1 μg of total RNA in the presence of oligo-dT$_{12-18}$ primer (Invitrogen) and MMLV reverse transcriptase according to manufacturer's instructions (Promega). Quantitative real-time PCR was performed with SYBR Premix Ex Taq (Takara) in ABI Fast Real-time PCR 7900HT System (Applied Biosystems). All samples were performed in triplicates. Primer sequences used for RT-PCR include: EPO-F, 5′-GCTGCTTTTACTCTCCTTGC-3′, EPO-R, 5′-C-TGTTCTTCCACCTCCATTC-3′; EPOR-F, 5′-CTCACCT-TCCAGCTTT-GAGT-3′, EPOR-R, 5′-TTCTCATAGGGGT-GGGAGTA-3′; β-actin-F, 5′-GTCCCT-CACCCTCCCAAA-AG-3′, β-actin-R, 5′-GCTGCCTCAACACCTCAACCC-3′. Primer sequences used for real-time PCR are: SOX9-F, 5′-AGGA-AGCTGGCAGACCAGTA-3′, SOX9-R, 5′-TCCAC-GAAGGGTCTCTTCTC; SOX5-F, 5′-CCAGGAGCTTG-TCTTTCCAG-3′, SOX5-R, 5′-CCCTGAAGCAGAGGAA-GATG-3′; SOX6-F, 5′-CTTCCTCTCCATC-CGCTGTA-3′, SOX6-R, 5′-ACCAGTGACTTCTGGGTGCT-3′; aggrecan-F,

5′-CTG-AAGTTCTTGGAGGAGCG-3′, aggrecan-R, 5′-CGC-TCAGTGAGTTG-TCATGG-3′; Col2α1-F, 5′-CTACGGTGT-CAGGGCCAG-3′, Col2α1-R, 5′-GCAAGA-TGAGGGCTTC-CATA-3′; EPOR-F, 5′-AAACTCAGGGTGCCCCTCTGGC-CT-3′, EPOR-R, 5′-GATGCGGTGATAGCGAGGAGAACC-3′; β-actin-F, 5′-CCCAGAGC-AAGAGAGG-3′, β-actin-R, 5′-GTCCAGACGCAGGATG-3′.

Western blot analysis

Cells were lysed and homogenized in RIPA lyses buffer with protease inhibitors (Gibco). Aliquots of protein extracts were separated by SDS-PAGE, and blotted on PVDF membrane (Millipore). The membrane was blocked by TBS-0.1% Tween 20 (TBST) containing 5% skim milk at room temperature for 1 hour, probed with anti-EPOR (Santa Cruz) primary antibody at 4°C overnight, washed in TBST, and then incubated with the appropriate horseradish peroxidase (HRP)-conjugated secondary antibody at room temperature for 1 hour. After intensive washing with TBST, immunoblots were developed using the ECL detection system.

In vitro fetal mouse metatarsal angiogenesis assay

The assay was performed according to established procedure [52,53]. Briefly, metatarsal bones were dissected from E17.5 embryos, cultured in 24-well plates in 150 μl αMEM containing 10% fetal calf serum, L-glutamine (2 mM) and penicillin (100 U/ml)/streptomycin (100 μg/ml) for 72 hours, and then changed to 250 μl of fresh medium. Medium was then replaced every two days. After 14 days, the explants were fixed in zinc formalin for 15 minutes and subsequently immunostained for endothelial marker CD31 using a rat polyclonal antiserum (BD Pharmingen).

Femur fracture model in mice

12-week-old mice were anesthetized by intraperitoneal injection of 0.1 ml xylene (2.6 mg/ml) and ketamine (17.4 mg/ml) cocktail. A 2 cm incision was performed between the greater trochanter and the knee joint. The quadriceps femoris muscles were mobilized anteriorly towards the knee and the hip. A hole was drilled on the intracondylar notch using a 21 gauge needle which was inserted into the intramedullary canal, and then pulled out. Subsequently, an osteotomy of the mid-shaft of the femur was made by a surgical saw and the fracture was stabilized by a needle inserting into the intramedullary cavity. The muscles and skin were closed with interrupted sutures. EPO (40 ng/mouse) was administered every other day directly at the fracture site from day 4 to day 12 post-surgery, with saline as non-treatment control.

Histology, histochemistry and immunohistochemistry

Paraffin sections of the long bones were dewaxed and processed for Safranin O staining. Briefly, the sections were stained with Weigert's iron hematoxylin working solution for 5 min, washed in running tap water for 10 min, and then stained with 0.05% fast green solution for 5 min. After quick rinse with 0.1% acetic acid solution for 2 min, the sections were stained in 0.1% Safranin O solution for 5 min (materials are all from Sigma-Aldrich) followed by rapid dehydration in graded ethanol, clearness and mounting in Permount mounting medium (SP15-100, Fisher Scientific). For preparation of cryosections, the femurs were fixed in 4% paraformaldhyde for 3 days at 4°C, and decalcified in 10% EDTA for 14 days at 4°Cwith gentle agitation followed by dehydration for cryoprotection in graded concentrations (15% and then 30%) of sucrose at 4°C until the femurs were fully sank in the sucrose. The femurs were then embedded in optimal cutting temperature (OCT) compound (Tissue-Tek, Sakura Finetek USA) and flash frozen in liquid nitrogen. 5 μm thick sections were cut on a cryostat. Immunostaining for EPO and EPOR was performed following established protocols.

MicroCT angiography analysis

At 14 days post-fracture, mice were anesthetized following above procedures. The abdominal cavity and heart were exposed. After opening the hepatic portal vein, the entire vascular system was completely flushed through injection of heparinized saline (20 U/ml, Sigma-Aldrich) into the left ventricle. Microfil (Flow Tech) was prepared immediately and injected into left ventricle. The specimens were then placed at 4°C overnight before the fractured femurs were harvested. The femurs were fixed in 10% formalin for 7 days, decalcified in 10% EDTA for 14 days with gentle agitation and were then processed for micro-CT scanning. Histomorphometric parameters of blood vessels including vessel volume (VV), total volume (TV), VV/TV, vessel surface (VS), vessel thickness (VTh), vessel separation (VSp), and vessel number (VN) were analyzed.

Radiological analysis of bone

The healing bones are examined by bench top digital X-ray system at day 28 post-surgery. The bone union at fracture site was quantified according to the X-ray scoring system described by Lane and Sandhu with modifications [54]. For analysis of the 3D microarchitecture of the healing bone, the femurs were scanned by the Scanco μCT40 desktop cone-beam micro-CT scanner [55]. In brief, the femurs were placed vertically in the scanning holder with diameter of 12 μm. The scans were performed at the following settings: 12 mm resolution, 55 kvp, 145 μA with an integration time of 200 ms. Images were automatically reconstructed into 2-D slices, and region of interest was outlined in every slice via micro-μCT Evaluation Program (v5.0A, Scanco Medical). Direct calculation of bone histomorphometric parameters is performed including bone volume (BV), total volume (TV), BV/TV, bone surface (BS), trabecular thickness (TbTh), trabecular separation (TbSp) and trabecular number (TbN).

Biomechanical test

Femurs were collected at 28 days post-fracture and fresh frozen. Specimens were thawed in PBS at room temperature for 3 h before mechanical testing. Specimens were tested to failure by three-point bending using the LR10K Plus Extended machine (Lloyd Instruments Ltd). Briefly, femurs were placed horizontally on two support rollers with a span of 7 mm while a vertical load was applied to the center of the diaphysis using a material testing apparatus until failure. Biomechanical parameters including peak load, elastic modulus, bend strain at maximum and bend strength at maximum were calculated from the force displacement data.

Statistics

For the quantitative real-time PCR, cell proliferation and colony formation assays, all the experiments were repeated at least three times unless otherwise stated. Data was presented as mean ± standard deviation (SD). Statistical analysis was performed using SPSS software. Two-tailed Student's *t* test, one-way ANOVA or two-way ANOVA were employed according to the experimental design. $P<0.05$ was considered as statistical significance.

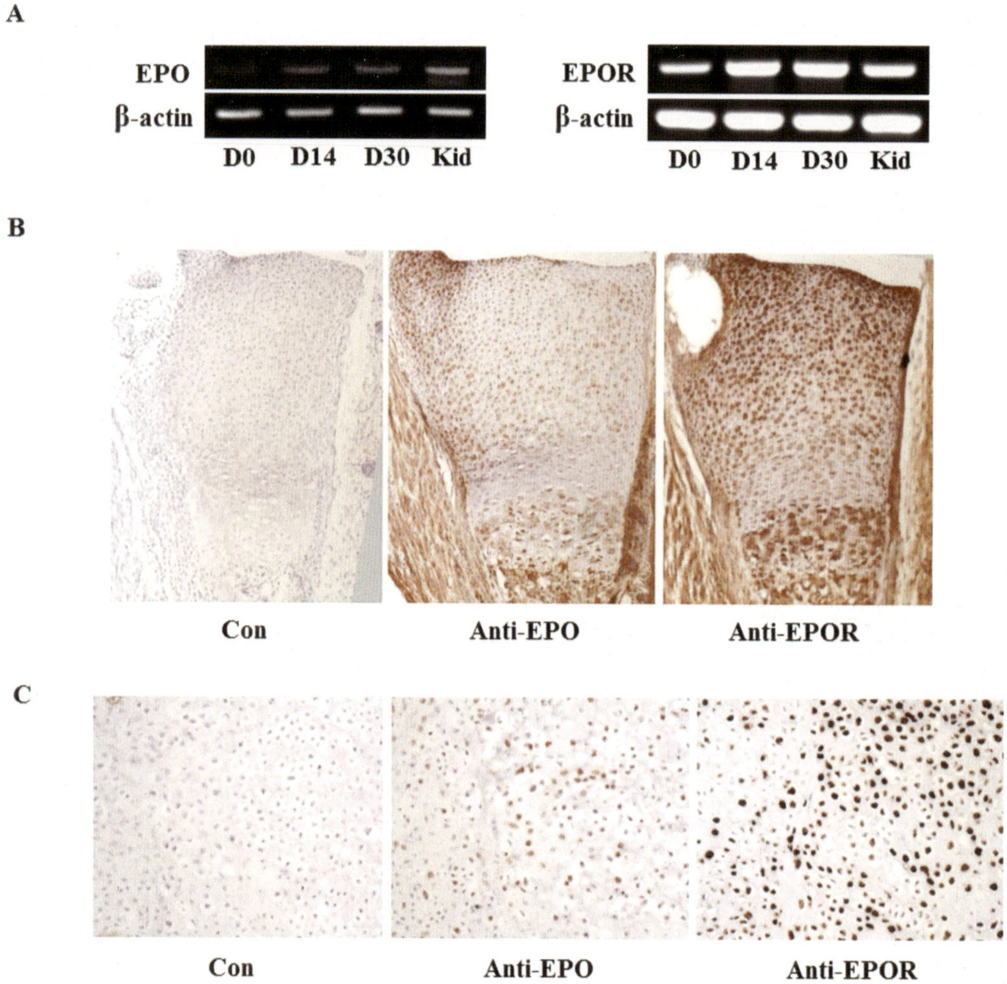

Figure 1. The expression and localization of EPO and EPOR in the developing bones. (A) mRNA expression of EPO and EPOR in the developing growth plates of tibiae by RT-PCR at indicated postnatal days. Tissues from kidney (Kid) of new born mice were used as positive control. (B) Immunohistochemistry for EPO and EPOR in growth plates of tibiae from new born mice. Con, non-primary antibody control. Magnification: 40×. (C) Immunohistochemistry for EPO and EPOR in cartilaginous callus of the bone healing in femoral fracture model of mouse. Con, non-primary antibody control. Magnification: 100×.

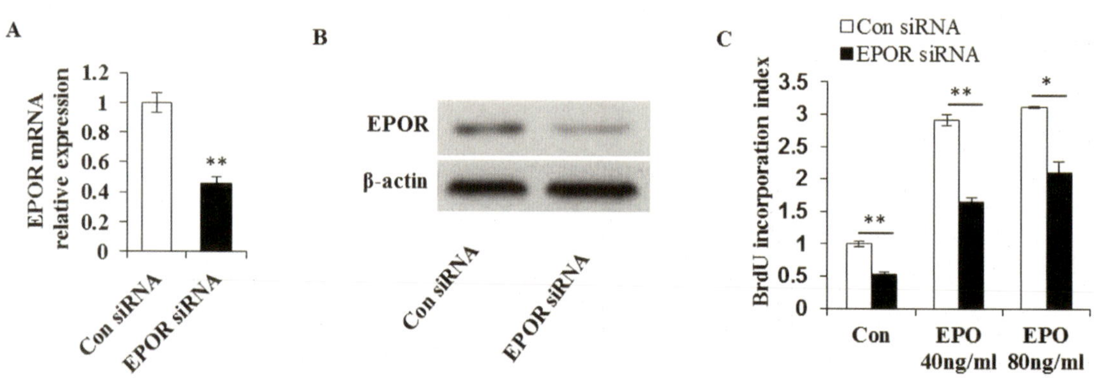

Figure 2. EPO promotes the proliferation of primary chondrocytes. (A) Examination of mRNA expression of EPOR in chondrocytes by real-time PCR after siRNA mediated knockdown of EPOR. (B) Western blot analysis of EPOR expression in primary chondrocytes with or without siRNA mediated knockdown of EPOR. (C) BrdU incorporation assay in primary chondrocytes with or without siRNA mediated knockdown of EPOR after 48 hours of EPO exposure. Con, non-treatment control. $^{*}P<0.05$; $^{**}P<0.01$; $n=3$.

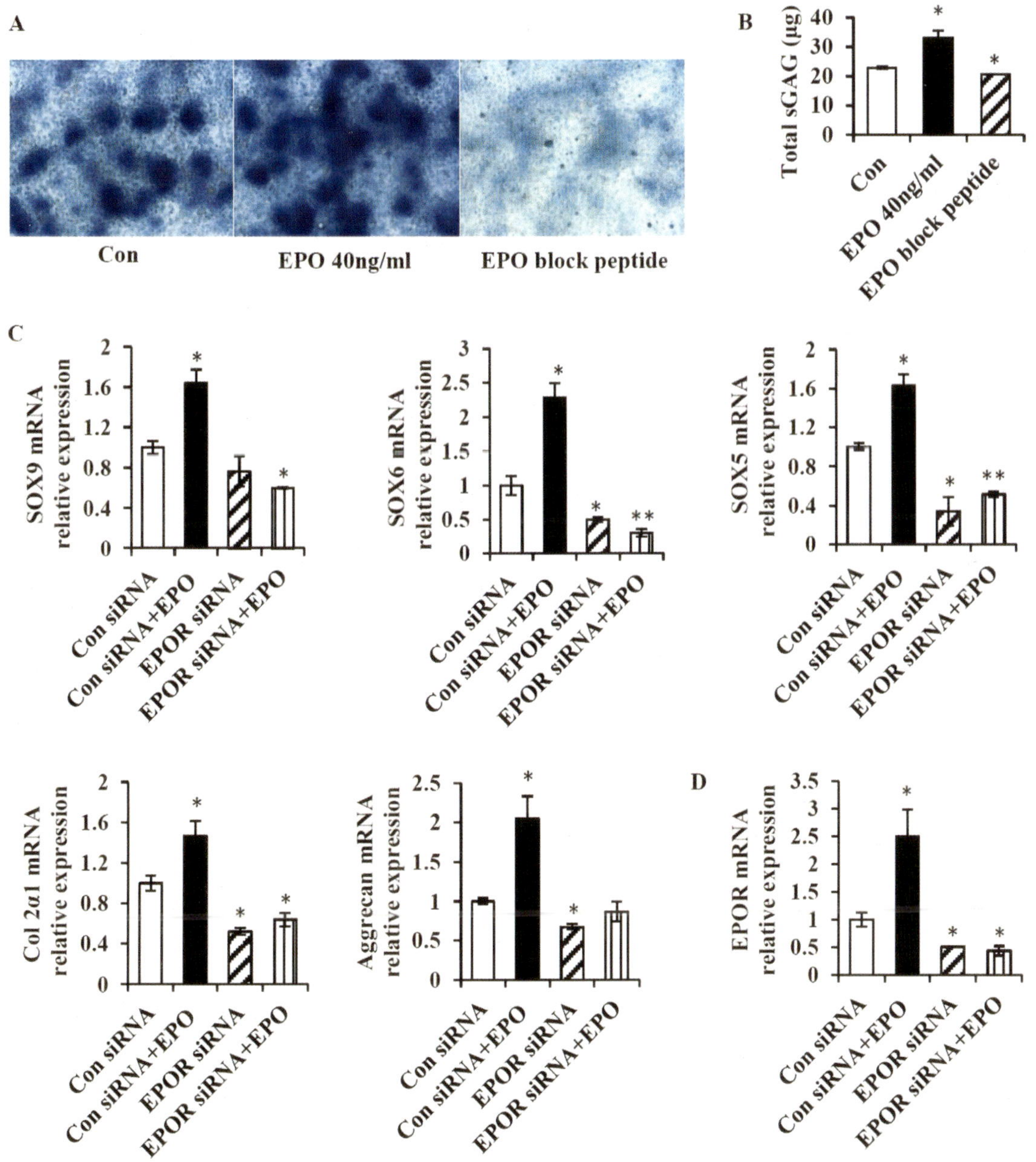

Figure 3. EPO increases biosynthesis of proteoglycan and upregulates chondrogenic marker genes expression during chondrogenic differentiation. (A) Alcian blue staining for preoteoglycan synthesis in the chondrogenic micromass culture supplemented with EPO, and with or without EPO block peptide for 7 days. Con, non-treatment control. Magnification: 10×. (B) Quantitation of total sGAG in the micromass culture by dimethylmethylene blue assay. (C) Detection of mRNA expression of chondrogenic marker genes including SOX9, SOX5, SOX6, Col2α1 and aggrecan by real-time PCR in chondrocytes in response to EPO treatment following siRNA mediated EPOR knockdown. (D) Real-time PCR quantification of EPOR mRNA expression in chondrocytes in response to EPO treatment following siRNA mediated EPOR knockdown. Con siRNA, control siRNA. *$P<0.05$; **$P<0.01$, $n=3$.

Results

The expression and localization of EPO and EPOR in the developing growth plate and the cartilaginous callus of healing bone

To examine the expression of EPO and EPOR in chondrocytes of the developing growth plates, we performed RT-PCR for EPO and EPOR using tissues obtained from the developing long bone growth plates of new born mice. EPO and EPOR mRNA was expressed in the growth plates derived from new born mice. Both of their expression in the growth plates was also detected at ages of day 14 and 30 (Fig. 1A). To identify the localization of EPO and EPOR in the growth plates, immunostaining for EPO and EPOR was performed in new borne mice. Our results showed that EPO and EPOR were abundantly present in proliferating, pre-hypertrophic and hypertrophic zones of growth plates of the developing bones (Fig. 1B). We next examined the localization of EPO and EPOR in the cartilaginous callus in the middle stage of bone healing. It showed that Both EPO and EPOR were localized in the proliferating, pre-hypertrophic and hypertrophic chondrocytes of the cartilaginous callus (Fig. 1C). These results suggested

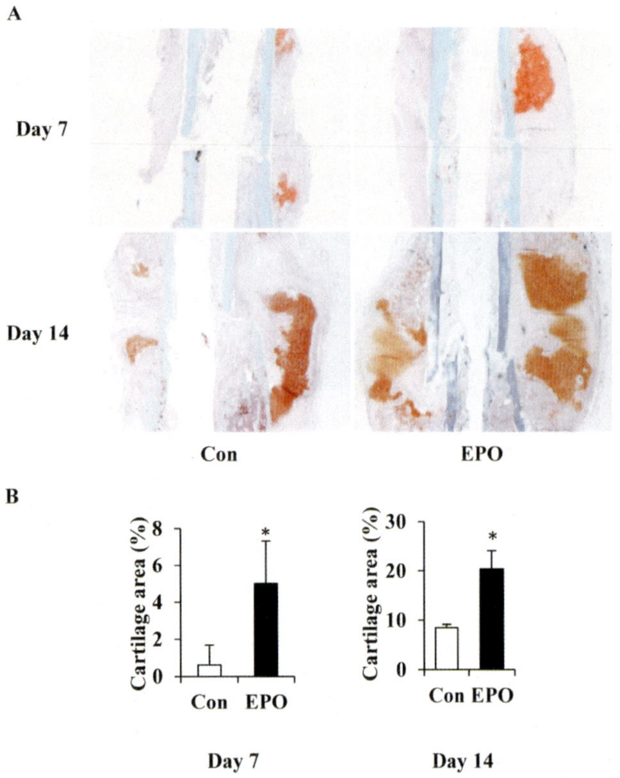

Figure 4. EPO enhances cartilaginous callus formation during bone healing. (A) Safranin O staining of the cartilaginous callus at days 7 and 14 post-surgery. Con, non-treatment control. Magnification: 2.5×. (B) Quantitation of the volume of cartilaginous callus formation at days 7 and 14 post-surgery. *$P<0.05$, $n=5$.

that EPO and EPOR might play an important role in the physiological development of the growth plate and cartilaginous formation during bone healing.

EPO increases the proliferation of primary chondrocytes

To elucidate EPO function in the development of growth plate, we first determined the effect of EPO treatment on the proliferation of primary chondrocytes with or without knockdown of EPOR. Using siRNA method, we achieved approximately 60% knockdown efficiency in the EPOR transcription level as shown by quantitative real-time PCR (Fig. 2A). Western blot verified the dramatically down-regulated EPOR protein level in chondrocytes following EPOR-siRNA transfection (Fig. 2B). We then added varied doses of EPO into the cultures of the primary chondrocytes transfected with control-siRNA or EPOR-siRNA, and cultured for two days followed by 6 hours of BrdU pulse labeling. In the cultures of the control-siRNA transfected chondrocytes, the BrdU incorporation index (indicating the numbers of BrdU incorporated cells) increased by (1.91±0.04) units in the 40 ng/ml EPO treatment group compared with that in the untreated group, and further increased by (2.12±0.02) units when 80 ng/ml EPO was applied (Fig. 2C), indicating that EPO may serve as a mitogenic factor for primary chondrocytes. We next asked whether the EPO-induced increase in the chondrocyte proliferation was EPOR dependent by looking at the effect of EPO on the chondrocytes following EPOR knockdown. Indeed, EPO's mitogenic effect on primary chondrocytes significantly decreased following siRNA mediated knockdown of EPOR. The increase of BrdU incorporation index induced by 40 ng/ml EPO and 80 ng/ml EPO dropped to (1.11±0.11) units and (1.57±0.08) units respectively in the chondrocytes transfected with EPOR-siRNA, which was significantly lower than what was observed in the control-siRNA groups (1.11 vs 1.91 and 1.57 vs 2.12; $P<0.05$). These results suggested that at least part of the proliferative effect of EPO on chondrocyte was mediated by its cognate receptor EPOR. Whether the elevation in BrdU incorporation index in EPOR-knockdown groups induced by the addition of EPO was caused by the interaction of EPO with the remaining EPOR, or by EPOR-independent function of EPO remains to be defined. Of interest, after knockdown of EPOR, the number of BrdU incorporated chondrocytes was significantly reduced when the cells were cultured in basal medium without exogenous EPO (Fig. 2C), suggesting that EPOR may be involved in the chondrocyte proliferation either independently or through its interaction with the endogenous EPO present in the chondrocytes.

EPO promotes chondrogenic differentiation *in vitro*

We then examined whether EPO also regulates chondrogenic differentiation by monitoring the proteoglycan biosynthesis in the extracellular matrix of chondrocyte micromass cultures following chondrogenic induction. After 7 days of chondrogenic induction. EPO (40 ng/ml) administration group showed more intense Alcian blue staining of chondrogenic nodules than the control group without EPO treatment (Fig. 3A), indicating increased amount of proteoglycan production. However, there appeared fewer and smaller Alcian blue stained nodules in the group where endogenous EPO was blocked by using EPO block peptide (Fig. 3A). The total amount of sGAG in chondrocytes was increased by 40% under EPO administration compared with the control group without EPO treatment, while there was a 20% decrease in the group treated with EPO block peptide (Fig. 3B). The reduction in proteoglycan levels after blockage of endogenous EPO and the increase of them following the addition of exogenous EPO implied the significance of both endogenous and exogenous EPO in chondrogenic differentiation.

To further understand the function of EPO in chondrogenic differentiation, mRNA expression of chondrogenic marker genes including SOX9, SOX5, SOX6, aggrecan, and Col2α1 was evaluated by quantitative real-time PCR in the micromass cultures of the EPOR-knockdown and control chondrocytes following 7 days of EPO treatment. The SOX family members SOX9, SOX5 and SOX6 have been demonstrated to be key transcription factors for chondrocyte specification [56,57]. EPO administration significantly up-regulated the above chondrogenic marker genes in the control chondrocytes by 1.5 to 2.5-fold while dramatic down-regulation of these marker genes was observed in EPOR-knockdown chondrocytes without EPO treatment (Fig. 3C), moreover, addition of EPO to the EPOR-knockdown chondrocyte cultures did not increase the expression of these genes to the levels that were comparable to what was achieved in the control chondrocytes treated with EPO (Fig. 3C). In addition, exogenous EPO significantly up-regulated EPOR mRNA level in chondrocytes (Fig. 3D). These results clearly demonstrated that EPO exerted a positive effect on chondrogenic differentiation, and this effect was mediated at least partially by EPOR.

EPO enhances cartilaginous callus formation during bone healing

We next determined the role of EPO in chondrogenesis *in vivo* using a femur fracture model in mouse. Direct delivery of EPO at

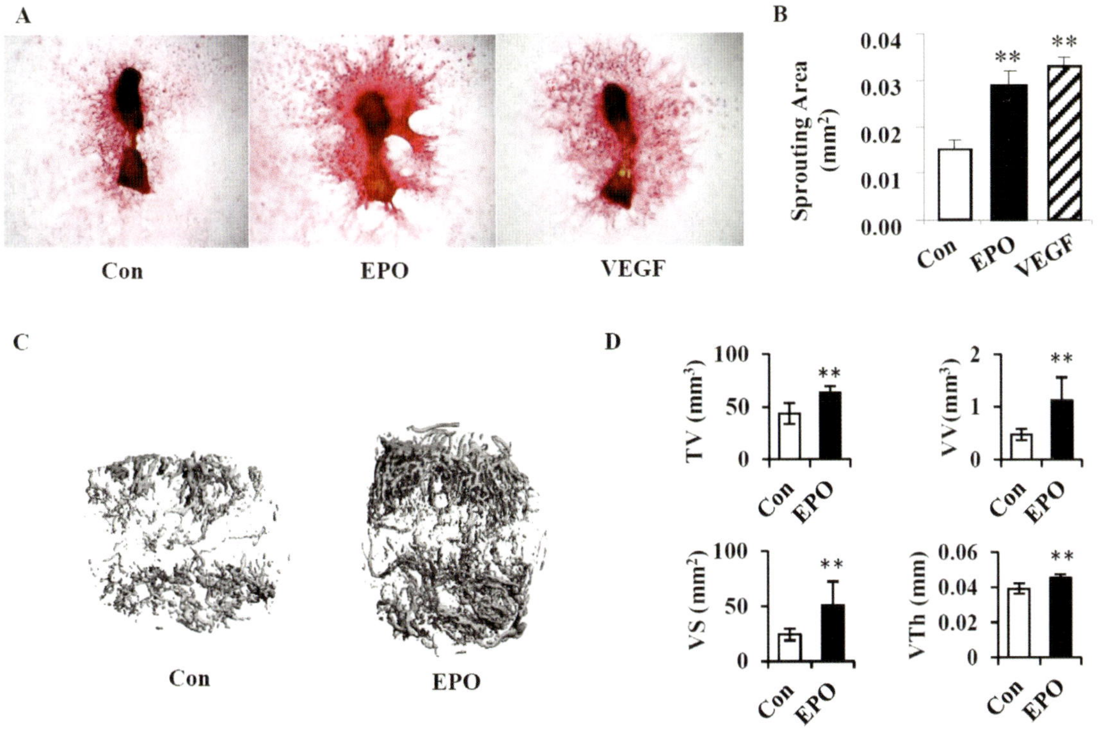

Figure 5. EPO stimulates angiogenesis *in vitro* and *in vivo*. (A) Representative images of endothelial sprouting from metatarsal bones of E17.5 embryos which were treated with different conditions as indicated. The endothelial sprouting was visualized by immunostaining for CD31. VEGF was used as positive control. Con, non-treatment control. Magnification: 2.5×. (B) Quantitation of the endothelial sprouting area for each group. (C) Representative micro-CT 3D reconstruction of vasculature at the fracture site following EPO treatment. The specimens were harvested for micro-CT scanning at day 14 post-surgery. Con, non-treatment control. (D) Quantitation of vascular parameters including the total volume (TV), vessel volume (VV), vessel surface (VS), and vessel thickness (VTh) by micro-CT angiography analysis. ** $P<0.01$, $n=5$.

the fracture site was performed every other day from day 4 to day 12 post-surgery. At days 7 and day 14 post-surgery, cartilaginous callus formed at the fracture sites was visualized by Safranin O staining (Fig. 4A). Histomorphometry analysis of cartilaginous callus of the healing bones showed that callus size and cartilage area in the EPO treatment group were larger than that in the saline control group (Fig. 4A). Upon EPO treatment, the ratios of cartilage volume to the total tissue volume were 5% and 20% respectively at day 7 and day 14 post-surgery, while the saline control group only gave rise to the ratios of 1% and 8%, which were significantly lower than the former (Fig. 4B). This result demonstrated that EPO enhanced cartilaginous callus formation during the early stage of bone healing.

EPO stimulates angiogenesis *in vitro* and *in vivo*

Besides the cartilage callus formation, angiogenesis is also a crucial factor during bone regeneration. To examine the role of EPO in angiogenesis, we isolated metatarsal bones from E17.5 mouse embryos and performed the endothelial sprouting assay in an *in vitro* culture system. As a result, the endothelial sprouting area was significantly increased by 1.9-fold in metatarsals treated with EPO 40 ng/ml compared with that of non-treatment controls, though this effect was not as dramatic as that of VEGF treatment (Fig. 5A and B). These results suggests that EPO may play a similar role like VEGF in stimulating endothelial sprouting from the metatarsal bones to form vessel like structure *in vitro*.

To further determine the effect of EPO in angiogenesis *in vivo*, we performed microCT angiography analysis in the middle stage of bone healing following local delivery of EPO at the fracture site. 3D reconstruction of newly formed vasculature at the fracture site showed more vascularity in the group treated with EPO than that of the control group (Fig. 5C). Microstructure parameters of the newly formed vessels including vessel volume (VV), vessel surface (VS) and vessel thickness (VTh) were all significantly increased following EPO administration compared with that of the control (Fig. 5D). And these changes were associated with the significantly enlarged total volume of callus area. These data demonstrated that EPO functioned as a proangiogenic factor during bone repair.

EPO enhances consolidation of bony callus during fracture healing

The observed positive effects of EPO on the cartilaginous callus formation and angiogenesis in the early and middle stages of bone healing led to an enhanced bone consolidation during facture healing. At day 28 post-surgery, the femurs from EPO treated group showed increased bone mass and density of the bony callus compared with the control group as evaluated by X-ray examination (Fig. 6A). X-ray score of the bony callus was increased by 1.5-fold in the EPO administrated group than that of the controls (Fig. 6B). Micro-CT 3D reconstruction of the bony callus clearly revealed a more robust bone formation in the EPO treated group than that of the controls (Fig. 6C), with the bone microstructure parameters of bone volume (BV), bone volume/total volume (BV/TV) and bone surface (BS) all significantly higher in the former than in the later (Fig. 6D). Further assessment of the biomechanical strength of the healing bones by three-point bending test showed that peak load, elastic modulus, bend strain at maximum, and bend strength at maximum were all significantly

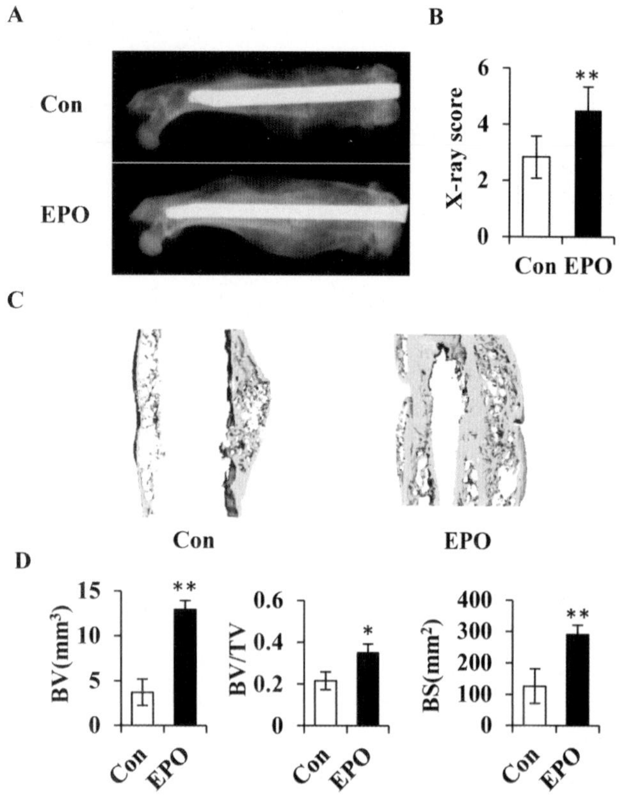

Figure 6. EPO increases the volume of the bony callus during consolidation of bone healing. (A) X-ray examination of the bony callus at day 28 post-surgery. Con, non-treatment control. (B) Quantitation of X-ray score of the bony callus at day 28 post-surgery. (C) Representative micro-CT 3D images of the new bone regenerates at day 28 post-surgery. (D) Quantitation of the bone microstructure parameters including bone volume (BV), bone volume/total volume (BV/TV), and bone surface (BS) by micro-CT analysis. $^{*}P<0.05$; $^{**}P<0.01$, $n=6$.

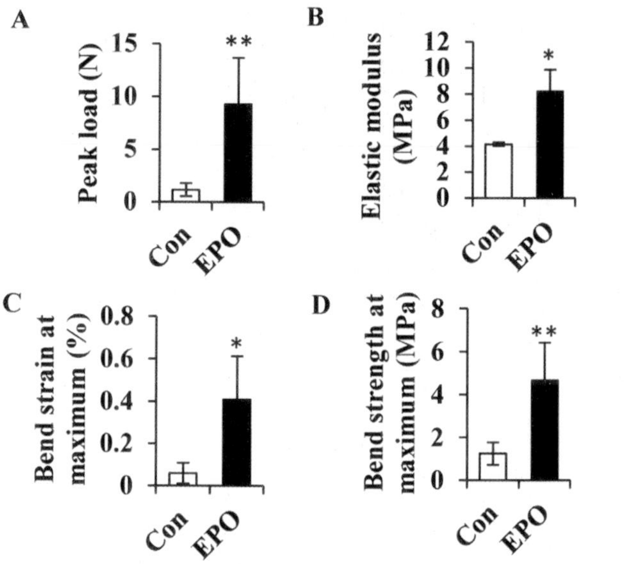

Figure 7. EPO improves biomechanical properties during consolidation of bone healing. Biomechanical parameters including peak load (A), elastic modulus (B), bend strain at maximum (C), and bend strength at maximum (D) were calculated at day 28 post-surgery. Con, non-treatment control. $^{*}P<0.05$; $^{**}P<0.01$, $n=3$.

increased in the group treated by EPO compared with the controls (Fig. 7A-D). Thus, local administration of EPO at the fracture site resulted in an increase in bony callus volume with improved biomechanical properties of the newly formed bone.

Discussion

Current procedures to promote skeletal regeneration include the applications of autografts, allografts, biocompatible implants, bioactive factors and mesenchymal stem cell-based therapy. However, the above approaches also face significant limitations due to insufficient supply, potential disease transmission, immuno-rejection, or less ability of functional engraftment. Thus, discovery of novel therapeutic approaches to improve skeletal repair and healing remains a great demand and clinical challenge in Orthopaedic regenerative medicine. In the present study, we demonstrated that local administration of EPO enhanced the consolidation and mechanical competence of the newly formed bone by promoting chondrogenic and angiogenic responses following injury, which can be explained by direct promotion effects of EPO on chondrocyte proliferation and differentiation, and on endothelial growth as shown in the *in vitro* studies. These findings expand the extent of EPO's tissue-specific functions and suggest that EPO may serve as a promising therapeutic agent for skeletal regeneration.

Previous study reported that EPOR was restrictedly expressed in hypertrophic chondrocytes during the cartilaginous callus stage of bone healing [45], and proposed that improved early endochondral ossification were mediated by EPO/EPOR signaling. In our study, knockdown of EPOR in primary chondrocytes resulted in a dramatic reduction of their responses to exogenous EPO in terms of cell proliferation (Fig. 2C) and chondrogenic marker genes expression upon chondrogenic differentiation (Fig. 3C). These evident reduction in EPO's effects on chondrocytes upon EPOR knockdown clearly demonstrated that EPO regulated the proliferation and differentiation of chondrocytes at least partially through EPOR.

Interestingly, EPO was also found to be present in chondrocytes in developing bones of new born mice as well as in newly formed cartilaginous callus of the healing bone in our study. Blockage of the endogenous EPO in primary chondrocytes using EPO block peptide impaired the chondrogenic differentiation, suggesting that endogenous EPO may function as an autocrine or paracrine factor for chondrocytes in normal bone development. Further clarifying the regulation of EPO production in chondrocytes in response to developmental and environmental cues will help better understanding its tissue-specific function in skeletal development and regeneration.

It is worthy to note that chondrocytes also produce VEGF [58,59], a well established angiogenic factor. Indeed, we observed a functional similarity of EPO and VEGF in the endothelial sprouting stimulation, indicating that both factors may exert overlapping but distinct roles in the angiogenic responses during bone healing. Given that EPO exerts versatile functions in varied tissues and cells and that bone regeneration is a complex process involving multiple cellular components or biological factors, the role of EPO in improving bone healing may also be versatile and complex. Direct and indirect signaling pathways may work coordinately to facilitate a better bone formation. For example, the increased volume of cartilaginous callus by EPO treatment may produce more VEGF and EPO to benefit angiogenesis and the increased vascularity by EPO administration may bring more blood and nutrient supply and osteoprogenitor cells to promote the consolidation of the healing bone. In addition, EPO may function as a coupling factor to coordinate haematopoiesis and the homeostasis of the skeleton, which deserves to be furthur defined.

In summary, EPO and EPOR are expressed in the neonatal developing growth plate and cartilaginous callus of healing bone. EPO may function as an autocrine or paracrine factor to regulate the spatial and temporal coordination among angiogenesis, chondrogenesis and osteogenesis during bone repair. EPO may serve as an effective agent to promote skeletal regeneration.

Acknowledgments

We are grateful for the assistance of the Core laboratories at School of Biomedical Sciences, the Chinese University of Hong Kong, and Small Animal Phenotyping Core at the University of Alabama at Birmingham.

Author Contributions

Conceived and designed the experiments: CW LW. Performed the experiments: LW FZ QH WPT CW. Analyzed the data: LW CW FZ QH. Contributed reagents/materials/analysis tools: LL QL ZW GQ GZ. Contributed to the writing of the manuscript: CW LW.

References

1. Einhorn TA (1995) Enhancement of fracture-healing. J Bone Joint Surg Am 77: 940–956.
2. Solomon DH, Patrick AR, Schousboe J, Losina E (2014) The Potential Economic Benefits of Improved Post-Fracture Care: A Cost-Effectiveness Analysis of a Fracture Liaison Service in the US Health Care System. J Bone Miner Res.
3. Hak DJ, Fitzpatrick D, Bishop JA, Marsh JL, Tilp S, et al. (2014) Delayed union and nonunions: Epidemiology, clinical issues, and financial aspects. Injury 45 Suppl 2: S3-7.
4. Richards JB, Rivadeneira F, Inouye M, Pastinen TM, Soranzo N, et al. (2008) Bone mineral density, osteoporosis, and osteoporotic fractures: a genome-wide association study. Lancet 371: 1505–1512.
5. Janghorbani M, Van Dam RM, Willett WC, Hu FB (2007) Systematic review of type 1 and type 2 diabetes mellitus and risk of fracture. Am J Epidemiol 166: 495–505.
6. Siddiqui NA, Owen JM (2013) Clinical advances in bone regeneration. Curr Stem Cell Res Ther 8: 192–200.
7. Wan C, Gilbert SR, Wang Y, Cao X, Shen X, et al. (2008) Activation of the hypoxia-inducible factor-1alpha pathway accelerates bone regeneration. Proc Natl Acad Sci U S A 105: 686–691.
8. Fassbender M, Strobel C, Rauhe JS, Bergmann C, Schmidmaier G, et al. (2011) Local inhibition of angiogenesis results in an atrophic non-union in a rat osteotomy model. Eur Cell Mater 22: 1–11.
9. Ferguson C, Alpern E, Miclau T, Helms JA (1999) Does adult fracture repair recapitulate embryonic skeletal formation? Mech Dev 87: 57–66.
10. Gerstenfeld LC, Cullinane DM, Barnes GL, Graves DT, Einhorn TA (2003) Fracture healing as a post-natal developmental process: molecular, spatial, and temporal aspects of its regulation. J Cell Biochem 88: 873–884.
11. Kanczler JM, Oreffo RO (2008) Osteogenesis and angiogenesis: the potential for engineering bone. Eur Cell Mater 15: 100–114.
12. Brandi ML (2013) Healing of the bone with anti-fracture drugs. Expert Opin Pharmacother 14: 1441–1447.
13. McKibbin B (1978) The biology of fracture healing in long bones. J Bone Joint Surg Br 60-B: 150–162.
14. Kolar P, Gaber T, Perka C, Duda GN, Buttgereit F (2011) Human early fracture hematoma is characterized by inflammation and hypoxia. Clin Orthop Relat Res 469: 3118–3126.
15. Sun H, Jung Y, Shiozawa Y, Taichman RS, Krebsbach PH (2012) Erythropoietin modulates the structure of bone morphogenetic protein 2-engineered cranial bone. Tissue Eng Part A 18: 2095–2105.
16. Kigami R, Sato S, Tsuchiya N, Yoshimakai T, Arai Y, et al. (2013) FGF-2 angiogenesis in bone regeneration within critical-sized bone defects in rat calvaria. Implant Dent 22: 422–427.
17. Warren SM, Steinbrech DS, Mehrara BJ, Saadeh PB, Greenwald JA, et al. (2001) Hypoxia regulates osteoblast gene expression. J Surg Res 99: 147–155.
18. Sheng MH, Lau KH, Baylink DJ (2014) Role of Osteocyte-derived Insulin-Like Growth Factor I in Developmental Growth, Modeling, Remodeling, and Regeneration of the Bone. J Bone Metab 21: 41–54.
19. Zelzer E, McLean W, Ng YS, Fukai N, Reginato AM, et al. (2002) Skeletal defects in VEGF(120/120) mice reveal multiple roles for VEGF in skeletogenesis. Development 129: 1893–1904.
20. Street J, Bao M, deGuzman L, Bunting S, Peale FV Jr, et al. (2002) Vascular endothelial growth factor stimulates bone repair by promoting angiogenesis and bone turnover. Proc Natl Acad Sci U S A 99: 9656–9661.
21. Wang Y, Wan C, Deng L, Liu X, Cao X, et al. (2007) The hypoxia-inducible factor alpha pathway couples angiogenesis to osteogenesis during skeletal development. J Clin Invest 117: 1616–1626.
22. Wan C, Shao J, Gilbert SR, Riddle RC, Long F, et al. (2010) Role of HIF-1alpha in skeletal development. Ann N Y Acad Sci 1192: 322–326.
23. Wu H, Liu X, Jaenisch R, Lodish HF (1995) Generation of committed erythroid BFU-E and CFU-E progenitors does not require erythropoietin or the erythropoietin receptor. Cell 83: 59–67.
24. Wu H, Klingmuller U, Besmer P, Lodish HF (1995) Interaction of the erythropoietin and stem-cell-factor receptors. Nature 377: 242–246.
25. Kertesz N, Wu J, Chen TH, Sucov HM, Wu H (2004) The role of erythropoietin in regulating angiogenesis. Dev Biol 276: 101–110.
26. Brines M, Grasso G, Fiordaliso F, Sfacteria A, Ghezzi P, et al. (2004) Erythropoietin mediates tissue protection through an erythropoietin and common beta-subunit heteroreceptor. Proc Natl Acad Sci U S A 101: 14907–14912.
27. Brines M, Cerami A (2006) Discovering erythropoietin's extra-hematopoietic functions: biology and clinical promise. Kidney Int 70: 246–250.
28. Tan CC, Eckardt KU, Ratcliffe PJ (1991) Organ distribution of erythropoietin messenger RNA in normal and uremic rats. Kidney Int 40: 69–76.
29. Fisher JW (1997) Erythropoietin: physiologic and pharmacologic aspects. Proc Soc Exp Biol Med 216: 358–369.
30. Yi C, Hak DJ (2012) Traumatic spinopelvic dissociation or U-shaped sacral fracture: a review of the literature. Injury 43: 402–408.
31. Tada H, Kagaya Y, Takeda M, Ohta J, Asaumi Y, et al. (2006) Endogenous erythropoietin system in non-hematopoietic lineage cells plays a protective role in myocardial ischemia/reperfusion. Cardiovasc Res 71: 466–477.
32. Kumral A, Tuzun F, Oner MG, Genc S, Duman N, et al. (2011) Erythropoietin in neonatal brain protection: the past, the present and the future. Brain Dev 33: 632–643.
33. Tsai PT, Ohab JJ, Kertesz N, Groszer M, Matter C, et al. (2006) A critical role of erythropoietin receptor in neurogenesis and post-stroke recovery. J Neurosci 26: 1269–1274.
34. Hak DJ, Makino T, Niikura T, Hazelwood SJ, Curtiss S, et al. (2006) Recombinant human BMP-7 effectively prevents non-union in both young and old rats. J Orthop Res 24: 11–20.
35. Acheson A, Richards JB, de Wit H (2007) Effects of sleep deprivation on impulsive behaviors in men and women. Physiol Behav 91: 579–587.
36. Cianferotti L, Brandi ML (2014) Muscle-bone interactions: basic and clinical aspects. Endocrine 45: 165–177.
37. Wright GL, Hanlon P, Amin K, Steenbergen C, Murphy E, et al. (2004) Erythropoietin receptor expression in adult rat cardiomyocytes is associated with an acute cardioprotective effect for recombinant erythropoietin during ischemia-reperfusion injury. FASEB J 18: 1031–1033.
38. Bernaudin M, Marti HH, Roussel S, Divoux D, Nouvelot A, et al. (1999) A potential role for erythropoietin in focal permanent cerebral ischemia in mice. J Cereb Blood Flow Metab 19: 643–651.
39. Sugawa M, Sakurai Y, Ishikawa-Ieda Y, Suzuki H, Asou H (2002) Effects of erythropoietin on glial cell development; oligodendrocyte maturation and astrocyte proliferation. Neurosci Res 44: 391–403.
40. Lee MY, Fukunaga R, Lee TJ, Lottsfeldt JL, Nagata S (1991) Bone modulation in sustained hematopoietic stimulation in mice. Blood 77: 2135–2141.
41. Takenaka T, Itaya Y, Ishikawa I, Kobayashi K, Tsuchiya Y (2003) Skeletal effects of erythropoietin in hemodialysis patients. Int Urol Nephrol 35: 407–413.
42. Singbrant S, Russell MR, Jovic T, Liddicoat B, Izon DJ, et al. (2011) Erythropoietin couples erythropoiesis, B-lymphopoiesis, and bone homeostasis within the bone marrow microenvironment. Blood 117: 5631–5642.
43. Shiozawa Y, Jung Y, Ziegler AM, Pedersen EA, Wang J, et al. (2010) Erythropoietin couples hematopoiesis with bone formation. PLoS One 5: e10853.
44. Garcia P, Speidel V, Scheuer C, Laschke MW, Holstein JH, et al. (2011) Low dose erythropoietin stimulates bone healing in mice. J Orthop Res 29: 165–172.
45. Holstein JH, Menger MD, Scheuer C, Meier C, Culemann U, et al. (2007) Erythropoietin (EPO): EPO-receptor signaling improves early endochondral ossification and mechanical strength in fracture healing. Life Sci 80: 893–900.
46. Mihmanli A, Dolanmaz D, Avunduk MC, Erdemli E (2009) Effects of recombinant human erythropoietin on mandibular distraction osteogenesis. J Oral Maxillofac Surg 67: 2337–2343.
47. Gosset M, Berenbaum F, Thirion S, Jacques C (2008) Primary culture and phenotyping of murine chondrocytes. Nat Protoc 3: 1253–1260.
48. Derks M, Sturm T, Haverich A, Hilfiker A (2013) Isolation and chondrogenic differentiation of porcine perichondrial progenitor cells for the purpose of cartilage tissue engineering. Cells Tissues Organs 198(3):179–189.
49. Ovchinnikov D (2009) Alcian blue/alizarin red staining of cartilage and bone in mouse. Cold Spring Harb Protoc 2009: pdb prot5170.
50. Lee YJ, Kong MH, Song KY, Lee KH, Heo SH (2008) The Relation Between Sox9, TGF-beta1, and Proteoglycan in Human Intervertebral Disc Cells. J Korean Neurosurg Soc 43: 149–154.

51. Enobakhare BO, Bader DL, Lee DA (1996) Quantification of sulfated glycosaminoglycans in chondrocyte/alginate cultures, by use of 1,9-dimethylmethylene blue. Anal Biochem 243: 189–191.
52. Deckers M, van der Pluijm G, Dooijewaard S, Kroon M, van Hinsbergh V, et al. (2001) Effect of angiogenic and antiangiogenic compounds on the outgrowth of capillary structures from fetal mouse bone explants. Lab Invest 81: 5–15.
53. Cackowski FC, Anderson JL, Patrene KD, Choksi RJ, Shapiro SD, et al. (2010) Osteoclasts are important for bone angiogenesis. Blood 115: 140–149.
54. Lane JM, Sandhu HS (1987) Current approaches to experimental bone grafting. Orthop Clin North Am 18: 213–225.
55. Casazza K, Hanks LJ, Clines GA, Tse HM, Eberhardt AW (2013) Diabetes-related impairment in bone strength is established early in the life course. World J Diabetes 4: 145–150.
56. Akiyama H, Lefebvre V (2011) Unraveling the transcriptional regulatory machinery in chondrogenesis. J Bone Miner Metab 29: 390–395.
57. Akiyama H, Chaboissier MC, Martin JF, Schedl A, de Crombrugghe B (2002) The transcription factor Sox9 has essential roles in successive steps of the chondrocyte differentiation pathway and is required for expression of Sox5 and Sox6. Genes Dev 16: 2813–2828.
58. Haigh JJ, Gerber HP, Ferrara N, Wagner EF (2000) Conditional inactivation of VEGF-A in areas of collagen2a1 expression results in embryonic lethality in the heterozygous state. Development 127: 1445–1453.
59. De Spiegelaere W, Cornillie P, Van den Broeck W (2010) Localization of erythropoietin in and around growing cartilage. Mol Cell Biochem 337: 287–291.

The Significance of Removing Ruptured Intervertebral Discs for Interbody Fusion in Treating Thoracic or Lumbar Type B and C Spinal Injuries through a One-Stage Posterior Approach

Qian-Shi Zhang, Guo-Hua Lü, Xiao-Bin Wang, Jing Li*

Department of Spine Surgery, The Second Xiangya Hospital of Central South University, Changsha, Hunan, P. R. China

Abstract

Objectives: To identify the negative effect on treatment results of reserving damaged intervertebral discs when treating type B and type C spinal fracture-dislocations through a one-stage posterior approach.

Methods: This is a retrospective review of 53 consecutive patients who were treated in our spine surgery center from January 2005 to May 2012 due to severe thoracolumbar spinal fracture-dislocation. The patients in Group A (24 patients) underwent long-segment instrumentation laminectomy with pedicle screw-rod fixators for neural decompression. In Group B (29 patients), the patients underwent long-segment instrumentation laminectomy with pedicle screw-rod fixators for neural decompression evacuating of the ruptured disc and inserting of a bone graft into the evacuated disc space for interbody fusion. The mean time between injury and operation was 4.1 days (range 2–15 days). The clinical, radiologic and complication outcomes were analyzed retrospectively.

Results: Periodic follow-ups were carried out until an affirmative union or treatment failure took place. A progressive kyphosis angle larger than 10°, loss of disc height, pseudoarthrosis, recurrence of dislocation or subluxation, or instrument failure before fusion were considered treatment failures. Treatment failures were detected in 13 cases in Group A (failure rate was 54.2%). In Group B, there were 28 cases in which definitive bone fusion was demonstrated on CT scans, and CT scans of the other cases demonstrated undefined pseudoarthrosis without hardware failure. There were statistically significant differences between the two groups ($p<0.001$ chi-square test). The neurologic recoveries, assessed by the ASIA scoring system, were not satisfactory for the neural deficit patients in either group, indicating there was no significant difference with regard to neurologic recovery between the two groups ($p>0.05$ Fisher's exact test).

Conclusion: Intervertebral disc damage is a common characteristic in type B and C spinal fracture-dislocation injuries. The damaged intervertebral disc should be removed and substituted with a bone graft because reserving the damaged disc in situ increases the risk of treatment failure.

Editor: Gwendolen Reilly, University of Sheffield, United Kingdom

Funding: The authors report no current external funding sources for this study.

Competing Interests: The authors have declared that no competing interests exist.

* E-mail: jingli1969@126.com

Introduction

In most type B and type C fracture-dislocations in the thoracic and lumbar spine, the intervertebral disc between the two separated segments is almost always injured. Its annular fibrosis is usually torn and ruptured leading to a nucleus pulposus leakage out of the disc space [1]. Furthermore, the anterior and posterior longitudinal ligaments are also ruptured in severe dislocation cases [2]. In many relevant literature reports, only a few authors discussed the ruptured intervertebral disc and its care [3]. If the injured disc is ignored and left in the spine, we hypothesized that it may have an adverse effect on the prognosis of the spinal fracture and dislocation. Although a few non-spine professionals have noticed the close relationship between spinal fractures or dislocations and disc injuries [4–6], there have been few clinical research reports specifically pertaining to the detrimental influence of ruptured discs on successful long-term bony fusion. It is well known that intervertebral discs do not have a blood supply in adults; their metabolism is extremely slow, and their growth potential for self-repair is very weak. Hence, once one is damaged, it has no opportunity to restore its pre-injury strength and function. Thus, the damaged disc interposes between two adjacent vertebrae (one or both of the vertebrae are also injured) and prevents the two vertebrae from contacting tightly, which is a major hindrance to bony fusion in the fracture-dislocation healing process. In our clinical practice, we found there were some recurrent dislocation and hardware breakage patients who suffered spinal fracture-dislocations and only underwent a posterior reduction, instrumentation, and posterolateral fusion without the

Table 1. Demographic characteristics of the two groups.

	Group A	Group B	Total
Patients	24	29	53
Male	18	19	37
Female	6	10	16
Mean age(range)*#	37.6±11.4(19–52)	38.1±10.7(22–54)	37.9±10.9(19–54)
Level of fracture			
upper thoracic spine	5	6	11
thoracolumbar	17	20	37
lumbar	2	3	5
Cause of injury			
vehicle accidents	8	11	19
falls from heights	7	6	13
violent blows from heavy objects	4	8	12
coal mine collapses	5	4	9
ASIA scale pre-operative			
A	14	17	31
B	6	6	12
C	2	4	6
D	2	2	4
E	0	0	0
AO classification			
B1	9	9	18
B2	6	4	10
B3	1	2	3
C1	2	4	6
C2	4	4	8
C3	2	6	8
Associated injuries			
rib fracture	13	12	25
pulmonary contusion	0	1	1
abrasion of skin	19	27	46
time between injury and operation #	3.9(range 3–15)	4.2(range 2–13)	4.1(range 2–15)

*Units: years.
#P>0.05 t test.

removal of the ruptured disc. The failed cases motivated us to determine their root causes. Therefore, we decided to add the procedure of removing the ruptured intervertebral discs during the latter part of our practice and conducted a comparative investigation to determine whether reserving the damaged intervertebral disc is a source of treatment failure.

Methods and Materials

Participants provided their written informed consent to participate in this study and this study was approved by the Institutional Review Board (IRB) of The Second Xiangya Hospital, Central South University.

General information and patient grouping

From January 2005 to May 2012, 53 patients (16 female and 37 male) from 19 to 55 years of age (mean 37.9 years of age), who suffered thoracic or lumbar type B or type C spine fracture-dislocation injuries were admitted to our spinal surgery center. The injuries were caused by a vehicle accident on a highway for 19 patients, falls from significant heights for 13 patients, violent blows from heavy objects for 12 patients, and coal mine collapses for 9 patients. The involved spinal segments included the upper thoracic spine in 11 cases, the thoracolumbar spine (T_{10}-L_2) in 37 cases, and the lumbar spine in 5 cases. The neurological injuries were evaluated according to the ASIA scale and the results were judged as follows: Grade A for 31, Grade B for 12, Grade C for 6, and Grade D for 4 patients. According to the AO classification for spine fractures and dislocations, there were 17 cases ascribed to subtype B_1, 10 cases to subtype B_2, 3 cases to subtype B_3, 8 cases to subtype C_1, 7 cases to subtype C_2, and 8 cases to subtype C_3.

We divided the patients into two groups according to whether the ruptured disc was removed and an intervertebral body fusion was performed. The patients in Group A (24 patients) underwent long-segment instrumentation laminectomy with pedicle screw-rod fixators, for neural decompression. In Group B (29 patients), the patients underwent long-segment instrumentation laminectomy with pedicle screw-rod fixators for neural decompression, evacuation of the ruptured disc, and insertion of a bone graft into the evacuated disc space for interbody fusion. The difference between these two surgical techniques lies in whether the ruptured disc is removed and an intervertebral body fusion with a posterolateral approach is performed. Periodic follow-ups were conducted until affirmative union or treatment failure occurred. The local kyphotic angle change, loss of disc height, instrument failure and non-fusion were recorded and analyzed in each case.

Patient demographics and spinal trauma severity in each group

In Group A, there were 18 males and 6 females of 19 to 52 years of age (mean 37.6 years of age). The injury types included B1 in 9 cases, B2 in 6, B3 in 1 case, C1 in 2 cases, C2 in 4 cases, and C3 in 2 cases. The neurologic status was judged as Grade A in 14 cases, Grade B in 6 cases, Grade C in 2 cases, and Grade D in 2 cases. The involved spinal segments were located in the upper thoracic levels for 5 cases, in T10-L2 for 17 cases, and in L3 for 2 cases. In Group B, there were 19 males and 10 females of 22 to 54 years of age (mean 38.1 years of age). The injury types included B1 in 9 cases, B2 in 4 cases, B3 in 2 cases, C1 in 4 cases, C2 in 4 cases, and C3 in 6 cases. The neurologic status was judged as Grade A in 17 cases, Grade B in 6 cases, Grade C in 4 cases, and Grade D in 2 cases. The involved spinal segments were located in the upper thoracic levels for 6 cases, in T10-L2 for 20 cases, and in L3 for 3 cases. The demographic characteristics of the two groups are shown in table 1.

Surgical treatment

The associated injuries included extremity fractures, rib fractures, pulmonary contusions (one patient), and abrasions of skin. The mean time between injury and operation was 4.1 days (range, 2–15 days). The vertebral segment was stabilized by bilateral pedicle fixation 2 or 3 levels above and 2 levels below the fracture. Five to six segments were fixed using 8 to 10 pedicle screws. There was no significant difference in the method of bilateral pedicle fixation between the two groups($p>0.05$) (Table 2). While exposing layer by layer, the local anatomic changes were observed and the existence of locked or jumped articular facets or articular process fractures was identified. After completing routine screw implantation and then releasing the locked facets by resecting the tip of articular processes, the rods were inserted into the screw ends, and the cap nuts were gradually screwed into the screw ends to lock the rods one after another from the most caudal to the most cephalic screw. In the process of tightening the cap nuts, a pulling force was produced spontaneously to lift the upper dislocated spine backward until it reduced completely. If complete reduction was not obtained at first reduction, then the depth of the pedicle screws was adjusted and/or the locked articular processes were further released, and good alignment was finally achieved. Because neurological injuries were present in all of the patients, exploration and decompression were performed routinely by resecting one upper lamina and one lower lamina adjacent to the displaced disc with a Kerrison rongeur, and the local autograft was saved for interbody fusion. If disc or bone fragments were detected in the spinal canal, they could be removed through a posterolateral approach. The patients in group A ($N=24$) only underwent posterolateral routine fusion. The patients in group B ($N=29$) underwent ruptured disc evacuation and interbody fusion using a posterolateral approach.

The concrete operative steps to remove the damaged disc and perform interbody fusion by a posterolateral approach were as follows: the decompression scope was extended by removing the relevant articular processes and facets on both sides to open the foramina and expose the lateral parts of the disc; the dura was gently moved from the working side slightly so that the ipsilateral half of the disc space could be visualized clearly; and if veins were covering the disc space, a bipolar coagulator was used to coagulate the vessels to prevent bleeding. Thus, the damaged disc was removed bilaterally through a posterolateral entry without over-traction of the dura tube. The disc tissue, including cartilage endplates and fracture fragments, was removed as thoroughly as possible by using a curette or small sharp osteotome until the cancellous bone was exposed to generate a well-prepared bone graft bed. Then, a local autologous bone graft was packed tightly into the prepared disc space to complete the interbody fusion.

Postoperative care

Rehabilitation treatment was initiated after 10 to 12 weeks of bed rest after the surgery. Sitting or standing training was initiated first, then the patients started active activities when they were capable under the protection of an external orthosis. The periodic follow-up interval was three months, but the patients could return sooner for further workups if an abnormal condition was felt. 3D CT scans were taken at 12 months postoperatively for the eventless patients to determine whether a solid fusion had been achieved.

Results

There were no significant differences between the two groups regarding age and time between injury and operation. The average operation time was 124 ± 19 minutes (range, 93–154 minutes) in group A and 195 ± 28 minutes (range, 168–232 minutes) in group B. The average amount of blood loss was 148 ± 66 mL (range, 50–225 mL) in group A and 480 ± 150 mL (range, 250–750 mL) in group B. There was a significant difference between the two groups with regards to the duration of the operation and the amount of blood loss ($p<0.001$, t test); the results are shown in Table 3.

The surgery was considered a failure if the implant was broken before union was achieved or if complications occurred in the patients, including pseudarthrosis and loss of disc height if the radiographs taken at follow-up demonstrated an increase of $\geq 10^\circ$ in the sagittal kyphosis compared to the local kyphotic angle measured immediately postoperatively [7], or if dislocation or subluxation was recurrent. Sagittal local kyphosis was measured from the superior endplate of the cephalic intact vertebra to the inferior endplate of the caudal intact vertebra.

In group A, there were 13 cases of sustained failure within one year, consisting of hardware breakage, pseudarthrosis formation, local kyphotic angle increase, or disc height loss. Spontaneous interbody bridging around the injured disc was achieved in 11 cases. The failure rate was as high as 54.2%; in group A, there were 8(33.3%) cases of loss of disc height, 13(54.2%) cases of implant failure, 1(4.2) case of pseudarthrosis, 6(25%) cases of local kyphotic angle change $\geq 10^\circ$ at follow-up compared to immediately after the operation, and 6(25%) cases of dislocation. Back pain was found in all of these failure cases and tuberositas of a fixation under the skin could be observed in 4 cases. In group B, there were 28 cases in which definitive bone fusion was demonstrated by CT scans and the fusion rate was 96.6%; the 1 other case (3.4% of group B) demonstrated doubtful pseudoarthrosis without hardware failure or local pain. There were no complications or mortality and back pain was relieved in all of the patients in group B. There are significant differences statistically between the two groups ($p<0.001$ chi-square test). The changes in

Table 2. Comparison of fixation segment in the two groups.

	Group A	Group B
Five segments	10	12
Six segments	14	17
Total	24	29

T test was used for statistical analysis showing there was no significant difference between the two groups, $p>0.05$.

kyphotic angle and disc space height in the failed patients in group A were measured and compared. The results shown in Table 4 demonstrate a significant difference between the two time-points of "immediately postoperative" and "initial detection of failure" for those two parameters.

Neurologic recoveries were not satisfactory for complete neural deficit patients in either group; in other words, 31 cases that were scored as Grade A prior to the surgery in both groups gained no measurable improvement at the final follow-up. 4 out of 6 Grade B cases in group A improved to Grade C, while the other 2 cases remained Grade B. 4 out of 6 Grade B cases in group B improved to Grade C, and the other 2 cases remained Grade B. 1 out of 2 Grade C cases in group A recovered to Grade D, and 2 cases of Grade C in group B improved to Grade D. 2 Grade D cases in group A recovered to Grade E, and 2 cases of Grade D in group B improved to Grade E. There was no significant difference between the two groups with regard to neurologic recovery ($p>0.05$ Fisher's exact test). The results are shown in Table 5.

Discussion

Except for the type B2.1 injury (according to the AO classification system), all other type B and C fracture-dislocations in the thoracic and lumbar spine are involved in intervertebral disc rupture and the dominant common feature in these types of injuries is the dislocation along the ruptured disc; that is to say the disc injury is an important component of spinal fracture-dislocations. Compared with type A spinal fractures, type B and C fracture-dislocations signify more severe trauma because of the accompanying complete disruption of the disco-ligamentous complexes, which contribute significantly to maintaining the dynamic stability of the spinal column. Greater violence or higher energy is needed to produce such crippling or devastating spinal column fracture-dislocations and results in a higher degree of neurological injury. Complete paralysis or spinal cord disruption, which is the most severe type of neural injury, is more common in type B and C than in type A injuries. The treatment goals and strategies are also different between these types of injuries and are worth further investigation and clarification because these issues are still controversial.

The treatment goals for type B and C spinal injuries include the following: 1. Re-aligning the dislocated spine to a normal arrangement by simple and effective methods and maintaining this restored alignment for an adequate duration until bony fusion. 2. Sufficient decompression of the spinal cord or cauda equina. 3. Reliable bone grafting to ensure bony fusion which is the ultimate goal — permanent stability should be achieved. A discussion about commonly used treatment strategies is developed below regarding the three goals.

Spinal dislocation and concomitant local kyphotic deformity are the dominant abnormal anatomic changes in type B and C injuries. Posterior surgery is indispensable in that only posterior instrumentation can provide sufficient pulling and lifting strength to reduce dislocation and correct the kyphotic deformity; this major advantage of the posterior approach has been verified by many authors [1,8,9]. The pedicle screw is the strongest and most powerful internal fixator available, it has been used since 1959 and is widely accepted. In the process of reducing the anteriorly or laterally dislocated upper part of the spine, a pulling force is needed to lift back the spine segment cephalic to the dislocation site for anatomical reduction by the upper screws and correspondingly, an enormous pullout stress is generated and concentrated on the lower screws. If only four screws are implanted when treating type B and C fracture-dislocations as is done with short-segment fixation in the posterior operation for type A fractures, each screw will sustain greater stress leading to a higher possibility of screw or rod breakage. In addition, four-screw short-segment fixation usually incurs incomplete reduction due to its weaker capability for reduction (Fig. 1). Yu et al reported a failure rate as high as 60% using a short-segment fixation technique [10]. Long-segment instrumentation is now a popular modality for treating such traumas because of its obvious advantages over short-segment fixation in mechanical strength [9]. The case illustrated in Figure 1 was treated by another hospital with 5 pedicle screws and an incomplete reduction was left, which suggests that the short-segment instrumentation was not a dependable method for the reduction of the spinal dislocation in that patient. In the current case series, 8 to 10 pedicle screws were implanted and a complete reduction was achieved in all cases (Fig. 2,3).

Sufficient decompression of the spinal cord or cauda equina can be obtained in several ways. The first method is complete

Table 3. Comparison of operation time and blood loss in the two groups.

	Group A(N = 24)	Group B(N = 29)	T test
operation time	124±19(range, 93–154 minutes)	195±28(range 168–232 minutes)	$P<0.001$
blood loss	148±66(range 50–225 mL)	480±150(range 250–750 mL)	$P<0.001$

T test was used for statistical analysis showing that there was a significant difference between the two groups according to the duration of operation and amount of blood loss, $p<0.001$.

Table 4. Complications in the failed patients in group A.

NO.	Hard ware breakage	Local kyphosis angle (°)			non-union	pseudarthrosis	Disc height (cm)		dislocation	pain
		Immediately postoperative	Initial detection of failure	>10°			Immediately postoperative	Initial detection of failure		
1	+	−12.9	−7.6	-	+	-	0.49	0.33	-	+
2	+	−8.0	−5.8	-	+	-	0.53	0.37	-	+
3	+	−12.8	3.8	+	+	-	0.43	0.28	+	+
4	+	−14.5	−7.5	-	+	-	0.48	0.43	-	+
5	+	−10.0	8.3	+	+	-	0.71	0.34	+	+
6	+	2.5	9.7	-	+	+	0.46	0.18	-	+
7	+	−3.3	12.6	+	+	-	0.38	0.32	+	+
8	+	−3.8	5.6	-	+	-	0.29	0.20	-	+
9	+	2.5	17.3	+	+	-	0.47	0.34	+	+
10	+	−17.2	5.8	+	+	-	0.47	0.39	+	+
11	+	−2.3	5.6	-	+	-	0.30	0.22	-	+
12	+	−11.6	2.0	+	+	-	0.48	0.25	+	+
13	+	−7.6	−5.4	-	+	-	0.41	0.17	-	+

Mann-Whitney test was used for statistical analysis showing significant difference in kyphotic angle and disc height changes between two time-points of "immediately postoperative" and "initial detection of failure", $P<0.001$.

Table 5. Neurologic recoveries in the two groups.

	Group A			Group B		
ASIA scale	Immediately postoperative	Initial detection of failure	Cases of improvement	Immediately postoperative	Initial detection of failure	Cases of improvement
A	14	14	0	17	17	0
B	6	2	4	6	2	4
C	2	1+4	1	4	2+4	2
D	2	0+1	2	2	0+2	2
E	0	2	0	0	2	0

Fisher's exact test was used for statistical analysis showing there was no significant difference between the two groups, $p>0.05$.

reduction to restore the continuity of the spinal canal, a fundamental step that can regain effective space and relieve tension on the neural structures. The second method is removing the posterior fracture fragments that collapsed into the spinal canal from the vertebral arch by resecting the lamina or articular processes. The third method is removing the anterior compression through a posterolateral approach. This is a demanding technique because anterior compression mainly originates from retropulsed fracture fragments or a ruptured disc located in the front of the neural elements, but it is still a good way to eliminate the anterior compression without additional injury and has been mastered by an increasing number of surgeons.

To stabilize the discontinuous spine into an integral column, the only permanent method is to achieve a solid bony fusion or reliable healing of the ruptured ligaments and discs to bridge the separated upper and lower segments. Spinal ligaments and discs are well known to have a minimal blood supply and without a blood supply, no human tissue can repair itself. Thus, the self-repair capabilities of disrupted discs and ligaments are weak and unreliable, so the restoration of spinal stability after dislocation cannot be dependent on the self-healing of soft tissues. Even if healing occurs, scar tissue connection is dominant and is not strong enough to maintain spinal stability [5]. At worst, the residual damaged disc within the intervertebral space continues to deteriorate because of accelerated desiccation and degeneration.

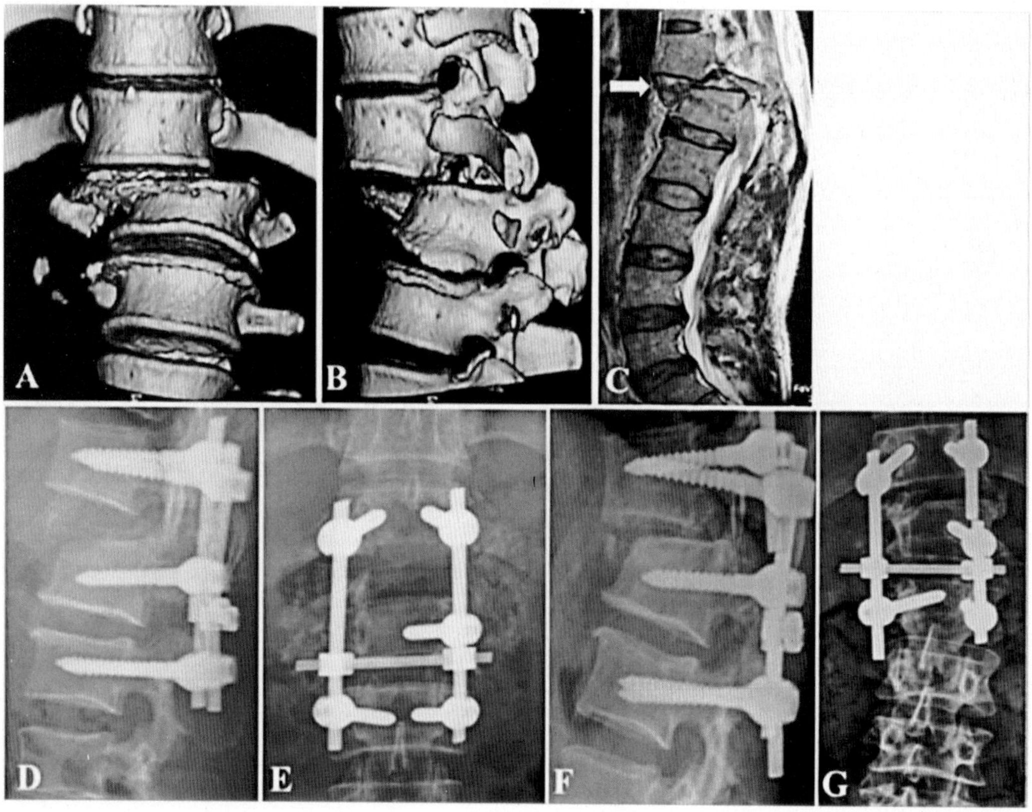

Figure 1. Type C2.2.2 fracture-dislocation in T12-L1 (A, B), the disruption crossing T12-L1 disc and the shattered disc(C, white arrow). Initial operative treatment was given by another hospital with posterior short-segment instrumentation, but the reduction was not complete (D). 9 months later, one rod was broken and disc space was collapsed; kyphosis and scoliosis occurred (F, C).

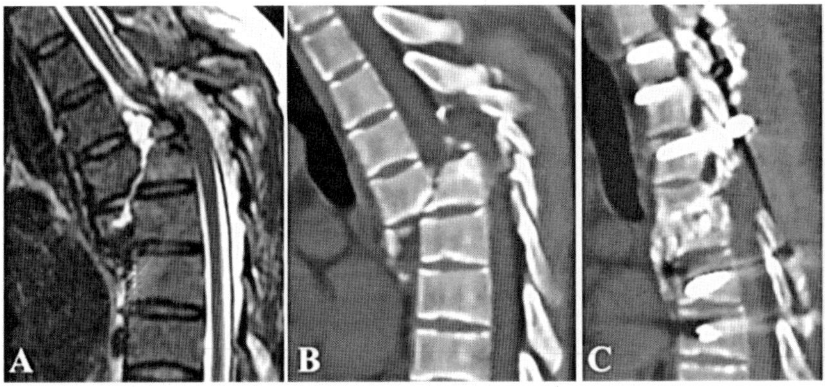

Figure 2. Type B1.2.3 severe fracture-dislocation involving T5-6; the disc was squeezed out of disc space posteriorly (black arrow) and anteriorly (white arrow) and intervened between two fractured vertebrae (A,B). Posterior reduction, instrumentation with 9 pedicle-screws, decompression, T5-6 disc excision, and bone graft in disc space were performed at one stage. One year later, follow-up CT showed good alignment and bony fusion (C).

This results in a greater disc space and height loss [11,12] which undermines the supportive function of the anterior spinal column and transfers the overloading to the internal fixators. Therefore, disc injury in spinal fracture-dislocation is not only an acute incident but also a chronic sequence of changes over time. Several authors have reported that in some conservatively treated cases, the injured discs collapsed and narrowed gradually, resulting in a late-onset kyphotic deformity because of rapid desiccation and biochemical changes in the nucleus pulposus secondary to the annulus fibrosus damage[5,13,14]. Thus, if a ruptured disc is left in situ rather than being removed, it will still interpose between the two separated segments and deter the natural post-traumatic healing process. An unstable spine is put at a disadvantage for fusion, so treatment failure is inevitable in these cases (Fig. 1, 4). Thus, leaving a severely damaged disc in situ is not reasonable; this is the main culprit for treatment failure in these spinal surgeries and it is wise to evacuate the damaged residual disc completely to eliminate its long-term negative effects. Another large benefit of radical disc excision is that it provides an adequate bone graft bed, which is a crucial prerequisite for reliable solid fusion. To best take advantage of this graft bed, adequate preparation should be undertaken in advance, including radically removing the upper and lower cartilage endplates to expose the subcortical cancellous bone in a large enough area (more than 75% of the disc area, or 2×2 cm^2). Thorough removal of the ruptured disc is a demanding technique because of the limited working field. Partially removing the disc tissue by laminectomy or laminotomy with a posterior approach is a routine operation of the lower lumbar spine; however, the complete removal of the disc by these techniques is difficult, especially for the removal of cartilage endplates, because the surgical field is limited and the surgical instruments, such as curettes and fine osteotomes, cannot be introduced into the disc space via the spinal canal. Thus, extended exposure is necessary by total laminectomy or even facet resection to enlarge the lateral exposure, allowing complete disc excision and avoiding violating the neural elements under direct vision. This approach is also more convenient for removing bone or retropulsing disc fragments to the spinal canal from the vertebral body or disc. We do not think diskectomy and associated facetectomy will increase the risk of instability of the spine in the immediate post-operative period. First, only a ruptured intervertebral disc, which is an unstable factor intrinsically, requires diskectomy. Second, most thoracic or

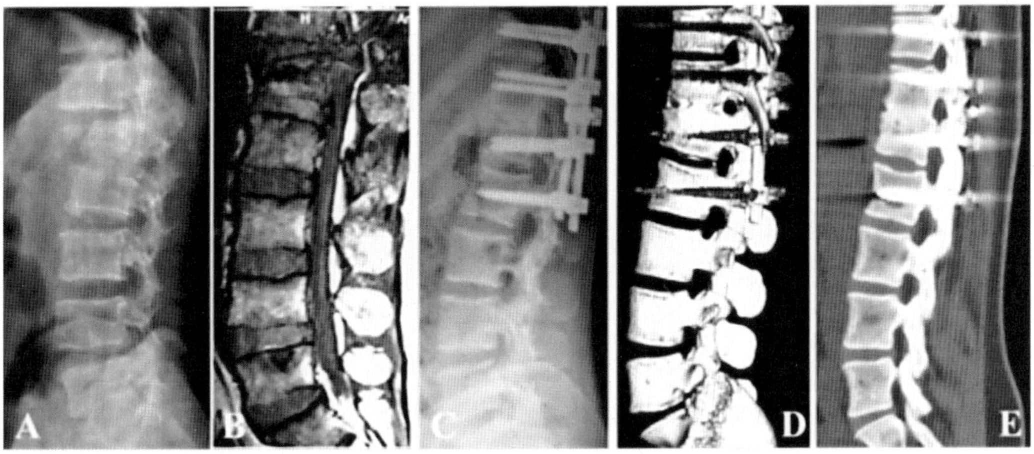

Figure 3. Type B1.2.2 fracture-dislocation in T12-L1 segment with disc rupture (A, B), posterior long-segment instrumentation, decompression, disc excision, and autologous local morselized bone graft in disc space in single-stage (C). Postoperatively 2 years, CT follow-up showing solid fusion in T12-L1 disc space (D, E).

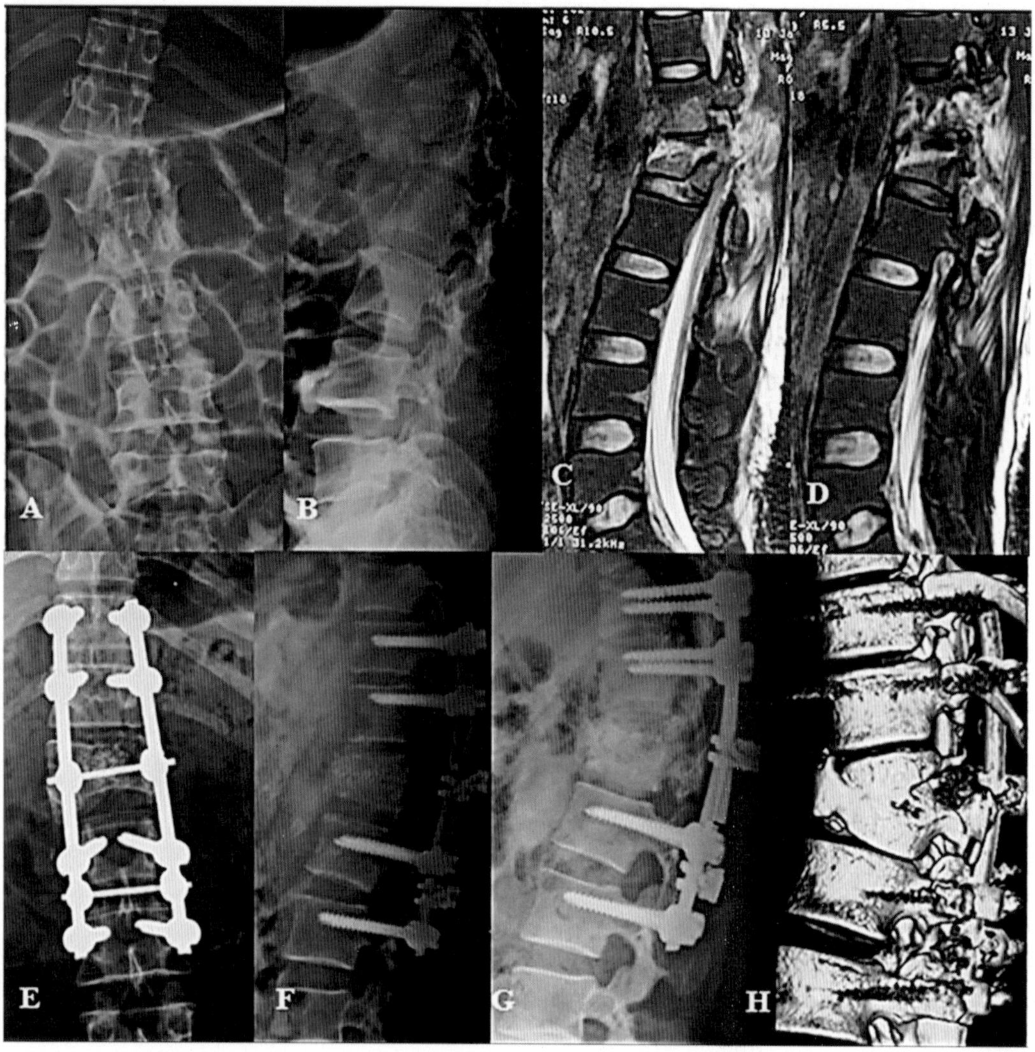

Figure 4. Type C1.3.1 fracture in L1 complicated with its two end-plates and T12-L1, L1-L2 disc rupture (A, B, C, D); excellent posterior reduction and instrumentation were achieved through the operation, but the ruptured discs were left untouched (E, F). Follow-up of 6 months after operation showed one rod was broken, two adjacent discs collapsed, and local kyphotic angle increased(G, H).

lumbar type B and C fractures have an intrinsically fractured posterior column. In some cases, we can even easily remove the processus articularis without a facetectomy. Lastly, rigid internal fixation can provide enough holding power before a rigid fusion has formed. There was an operative procedure introduced by Daniaux in 1986 of transpedicular intervertebral bone grafting after posterior stabilization of thoracolumbar fractures [15]; the intention of this technique was to remove the ruptured intervertebral disc and refill the space with a bone graft to obtain solid fusion and to prevent the late collapse of the intervertebral disc space, which would incur a recurrent kyphotic deformity and treatment failure. The notion itself was correct, but the clinical outcomes reported by many researchers were not improved compared with a simple posterior stabilization treatment [16,17]. Why were the results so frustrating? Why did this theoretically reasonable treatment not have better results? The main issue was that the disc could not be resected radically through the very limited transpedicular approach, so the cartilage endplates were not removed and as a consequence, the bone graft bed had a poor blood supply. Although a sufficiently sized bone graft was packed into the disc space, new bone growth could not be induced because of the isolation of the graft from the blood circulation. Naturally, this procedure was doomed to failure and was phased out. To overcome the issue of a poor blood supply to the bone graft bed, we undertook reliable measures for expanding the exposure to ensure an easy access to the injured disc from multiple directions and angles. This approach guaranteed that most of the disc was excised and a good bone graft bed with sufficient blood supply was prepared. By using this surgical procedure in our cases of group B cases, solid bony fusion between two vertebral bodies was achieved in 28 out of 29 patients (Fig. 2,3). However in group A, the ruptured disc was left in situ, and the prognosis of these patients was unsatisfactory with screw or rod breakage or recurrent kyphosis in 13 patients within 1 year postoperatively. There is some doubt regarding the osteogenic capacity and supporting function of the locally obtained autologous morselized bone because its growth into a solid mass from numerous separate, small-sized bone fragments can be a chronic and complicated process. In fact, we initially were not sure whether bony fusion would occur, but we believed it was worth trying. With the accumulation of cases and experience, we finally confirmed that the fusion was sure and solid with this procedure (Fig. 3). In some recent literature papers regarding the treatment of thoracolumbar fracture-dislocation, the authors still only emphasized reduction and instrumentation and did not mention the ruptured intervertebral disc and interbody fusion [18,19].

In severe thoracolumbar spinal fracture-dislocation cases, we preferred anterior decompression, reconstruction, and stabilization from a one-stage posterolateral approach to a combined anterior-posterior approach. Some authors have preferred a combined anterior-posterior approach because they believe that anterior reconstruction and bone grafting provided by a combined approach are more reliable [20]. In recent literature, authors compared the medium and long-term outcomes of anteroposterior versus posterior approach with corpectomy, decompression, and reconstruction of spine in the treatment of thoracolumbar fractures and showed that the two approaches were both adequate surgical treatments for thoracolumbar fractures. However, the one-stage posterolateral approach has the major advantages of less perioperative volume of blood loss, shorter operative duration, and better pulmonary function[21,22]. In addition, a combined anterior-posterior approach is more traumatic because of the additional incision, longer hospital stay, greater expense, and complications due to the anterior approach. Particularly in those patients who suffer from multiple traumas or internal diseases, a combined operation can increase mortality [23]. Although the one-stage posterolateral approach will make more damages to the processus articularis, it will not increase the risk of instability of the spine in the immediate post-operative period as mentioned above.

In fact, the surgical technique used for group B was neither advanced nor demanding. Our purpose in conducting this investigation was mainly to determine the negative influence of a damaged disc on long-term spinal stability if it is retained in situ. The aim of this paper is to increase awareness of the facts that the damaged intervertebral disc should not be ignored and that it is necessary to remove the damaged disc as completely as possible to complete a reliable interbody fusion.

Conclusions

The following conclusion can be drawn from this study: the residual ruptured intervertebral discs should be removed and replaced with a bone graft because reserving the damaged disc in situ is a high risk factor for treatment failure in thoracic and lumbar spinal type B and C fracture-dislocations. Although removing ruptured intervertebral discs leads to a longer operation time and more blood loss, it is still a reliable approach for operation.

Acknowledgments

IRB Approval Statement: This study has been approved from the Institutional Review Board (IRB) of The Second Xiangya Hospital, Central South University.

Author Contributions

Conceived and designed the experiments: QSZ GHL JL. Performed the experiments: QSZ XBW JL. Analyzed the data: QSZ JL. Contributed reagents/materials/analysis tools: GHL. Wrote the paper: QSZ JL.

References

1. Magerl F, Aebi M, Gertzbein SD, Harms J, Nazarian S (1994) A comprehensive classification of thoracic and lumbar injuries. Eur Spine J 3:184–201.
2. Elgafy H, Bellabarba C (2007) Three-column ligamentous extension injury of the thoracic spine: a case report and review of the literature. Spine (Phila Pa 1976) 32:E785–788.
3. Moore TA, Steinmetz MP, Anderson PA (2011) Novel reduction technique for thoracolumbar fracture-dislocations. J Neurosurg Spine 15:675–7.
4. Willen JA, Gaekwad UH, Kakulas BA (1989) Burst fractures in the thoracic and lumbar spine. A clinico-neuropathologic analysis. Spine (Phila Pa 1976) 14:1316–1323.
5. Oner FC, vd Rijt RH, Ramos LM, Groen GJ, Verbout AJ, et al. (1999) Correlation of MR images of disc injuries with anatomic sections in experimental thoracolumbar spine fractures. Eur Spine J 8:194–198.
6. Oner FC, der Rijt RR v, Ramos LM, Dhert WJ, Verbout AJ (1998) Changes in the disc space after fractures of the thoracolumbar spine. J Bone Joint Surg Br 80:833–839.
7. Alanay A, Acaroglu E, Yazici M, Oznur A, Surat A (2001) Short-segment pedicle instrumentation of thoracolumbar burst fractures: does transpedicular intracorporeal grafting prevent early failure? Spine 26:213–7.
8. Mikles MR, Stchur RP, Graziano GP (2004) Posterior instrumentation for thoracolumbar fractures. J Am Acad Orthop Surg 12:424–435.
9. Inamasu J, Guiot BH, Nakatsukasa M (2008) Posterior instrumentation surgery for thoracolumbar junction injury causing neurologic deficit. Neurol Med Chir (Tokyo) 48:15–21.
10. Yu SW, Fang KF, Tseng IC, Chiu YL, Chen WJ, et al. (2002) Surgical outcomes of short-segment fixation for thoracolumbar fracture dislocation. Chang Gung Med J 25:253–259.
11. Xu BS, Tang TS, Yang HL (2009) Long-term results of thoracolumbar and lumbar burst fractures after short-segmentpedicle instrumentation, with special reference to implant failure and correctionloss. Orthop Surg 1:85–93.
12. Speth MJ, Oner FC, Kadic MA, de Klerk LW, Verbout AJ (1995) Recurrent kyphosis after posterior stabilization of thoracolumbar fractures. 24 cases treated with a Dick internal fixator followed for 1.5–4 years. Acta Orthop Scand 66:406–410.
13. Przybyla A, Pollintine P, Bedzinski R, Adams MA (2006) Outer annulus tears have less effect than endplate fracture on stress distributions inside intervertebral discs: relevance to disc degeneration. Clin Biomech (Bristol, Avon) 21:1013–1019.
14. Mumford J, Weinstein JN, Spratt KF, Goel VK (1993) Thoracolumbar burst fractures. The clinical efficacy and outcome of nonoperative management. Spine (Phila Pa 1976) 18:955–970.
15. Daniaux H, Seykora P, Genelin A, Lang T, Kathrein A (1991) Application of posterior plating and modifications in thoracolumbar spine injuries. Indication, techniques, and results. Spine (Phila Pa 1976) 16:S125–133.
16. Knop C, Fabian HF, Bastian L, Blauth M (2001) Late results of thoracolumbar fractures after posterior instrumentation and transpedicular bone grafting. Spine (Phila Pa 1976) 26:88–99.
17. Knop C, Fabian HF, Bastian L, Rosenthal H (2002) Fate of the transpedicular intervertebral bone graft after posterior stabilisation of thoracolumbar fractures. Eur Spine J 11:251–257.
18. Moore TA, Steinmetz MP, Anderson PA (2011) Novel reduction technique for thoracolumbar fracture-dislocations—Technical note. J Neurosurg Spine 15:675–677.
19. Inamasu J, Guiot BH, Nakatsukasa M. (2008) Posterior instrumentation surgery for thoracolumbar junction injury causing neurologic deficit. Neurol Med Chir (Tokyo) 48:18–21.
20. Xia Q, Xu BS, Zhang JD, Miao J (2009) Simultaneous combined anterior and posterior surgery for severe thoracolumbar fracture dislocations. Orthop Surg 1:28–33.
21. Ma Y, Deng SC, Jia ZH, Hao YH (2013) Lateral position one-stage combined anteroposterior approach versus posterior approach with subtotal corpectomy, decompression, and reconstruction of spine in the treatment of thoracolumbar burst fractures. Zhonghua Yi Xue Za Zhi 93:2112–6.
22. Ayberk G, Ozveren MF, Altundal N, Tosun H, Kaplan M, et al. (2008) Three column stabilization through posterior approach alone: transpedicular placement of distractable cage with transpedicular screw fixation. Neurol Med Chir (Tokyo) 48:8–14.
23. P Oprel P, Tuinebreijer WE, Patka P, den Hartog D (2010) Combined anterior-posterior surgery versus posterior surgery for thoracolumbar burst fractures: a systematic review of the literature. Open Orthop J 4:93–100.

25

Relationship of Dickkopf1 (DKK1) with Cardiovascular Disease and Bone Metabolism in Caucasian Type 2 Diabetes Mellitus

Antonia Garcia-Martín[1,2], Rebeca Reyes-Garcia[1,3], Beatriz García-Fontana[1], Sonia Morales-Santana[1,4], Ana Coto-Montes[5], Manuel Muñoz-Garach[6], Pedro Rozas-Moreno[7], Manuel Muñoz-Torres[1]*

1 Bone Metabolic Unit (RETICEF), Endocrinology Division, Hospital Universitario San Cecilio, Instituto de Investigación Biosanitaria de Granada, Granada, Spain, **2** Endocrinology, Hospital Comarcal del Noroeste, Caravaca de la Cruz, Murcia, Spain, **3** Endocrinology Unit, Hospital General Universitario Rafael Mendez, Lorca, Murcia, Spain, **4** Proteomic Research Service, Fundación para la Investigación Biosanitaria de Andalucía Oriental -Alejandro Otero- (FIBAO), Granada, Spain, **5** Department of Morphology and Cellular Biology (RETICEF), Faculty of Medicine, University of Oviedo, Oviedo, Spain, **6** Critical Care and Emergencies Unit, Hospital Universitario San Cecilio, Granada, Spain, **7** Endocrinology Division, Hospital General de Ciudad Real, Ciudad Real, Spain

Abstract

Objectives: Dickkopf-1 (DKK1) is a potent inhibitor of Wnt signalling, which exerts anabolic effects on bone and also takes part in the regulation of vascular cells. Our aims were to evaluate serum DKK1 in type 2 diabetes (T2DM) patients and to analyze its relationships with cardiovascular disease (CVD). We also evaluated the relationship between DKK1 and bone metabolism.

Design: We conducted a cross-sectional study in which we measured serum DKK1 (ELISA, Biomedica) in 126 subjects: 72 patients with T2DM and 54 non-diabetic subjects. We analysed its relationship with clinical CVD, preclinical CVD expressed as carotid intima media thickness (IMT), and bone metabolism.

Results: T2DM patients with CVD ($P=0{,}026$) and abnormal carotid IMT ($P=0{,}038$) had higher DKK1 concentrations. DKK1 was related to the presence of CVD in T2DM, independently of the presence of risk factors for atherosclerosis. Therefore, for each increase of 28 pg/ml of serum DKK1 there was a 6,2% increase in the risk of CVD in T2DM patients. The ROC curve analysis to evaluate the usefulness of DKK1 as a marker for high risk of CVD showed an area under the curve of 0,667 (95% CI: 0,538–0,795; $P=0{,}016$). In addition, there was a positive correlation between serum DKK1 and spine bone mineral density in the total sample ($r=0{,}183$; $P=0{,}048$).

Conclusion: In summary, circulating DKK1 levels are higher in T2DM with CVD and are associated with an abnormal carotid IMT in this cross-sectional study. DKK1 may be involved in vascular disease of T2DM patients.

Editor: Rudolf Kirchmair, Medical University Innsbruck, Austria

Funding: This work was supported in part by Consejería de Salud y Bienestar Social, Junta de Andalucia (PI-0514-2012) and Red de Investigación Colaborativa en Envejecimiento y Fragilidad (RETICEF) (RD06/0013/1014-RD12/0043/0014). The funders had no role in study design, data collection and analysis, decision to publish, or preparation of the manuscript.

Competing Interests: The authors have declared that no competing interests exist.

* Email: mmt@mamuto.es

Introduction

Patients with type 2 diabetes mellitus (T2DM) have a higher risk of cardiovascular disease (CVD). This association has serious consequences on the morbidity and the mortality in this population. Atherosclerosis is the main pathological mechanism in macrovascular disease in T2DM, which causes the development of atheroma plaques and the major life-threatening events in atherosclerosis, including myocardial infarction and stroke [1].

Patients with osteoporosis have a higher prevalence of cardiovascular disease, and it has been proposed that both pathologies share common pathophysiologic pathways [2]. In T2DM there is an increased risk of fractures at any skeletal site even with greater bone mineral density (BMD) [3,4], and there are data from epidemiological studies supporting a relationship between low bone mineral density (BMD) and atherosclerosis in T2DM [5,6]. Thus, a better characterization of the pathways that could be involved in both processes is of interest, and may help in the development of new therapeutic tools.

The Wnt signalling pathways are involved in several developmental and physiological processes, including the cell differentiation and tissue/organ morphogenesis [7]. The discovery of the Wnt signaling pathway and its relevance in bone homeostasis has contributed to a better knowledge of the cellular and molecular mechanisms of bone biology [8]. The activation of this pathway results in an expansion of osteoprogenitor cells and also determines a reduction in the apoptosis of osteoblasts, which leads to anabolic effects on bone [8]. The canonical Wnt pathway is regulated by several families of secreted antagonists, such as the soluble frizzled-related receptors, dickkopf-1 (DKK1) and sclerostin. DKK1 regulates the Wnt signaling by binding to the Wnt co-receptor, the low-density lipoprotein-related receptor (LRP) 5/6. In addition to its binding to LRP 5/6, DKK1 binds to other trans-membrane molecules as proteins Kremen, which increases their inhibitory activity on the Wnt signaling pathway [9].

The role of Wnt signaling pathways in atherosclerosis it is a matter of growing interest. In preclinical studies the Wnt signaling pathways are involved in atherosclerosis-related processes as vascular calcification [10], inflammation [11], and the monocyte adhesion and its trans-endothelial migration [12]. In a recent study conducted in bovine aortic endothelial cells (ECs) [13], the authors found that Msx2 and Wnt7 family members stabilize the aortic ECs phenotype, whereas DKK1 promotes an endothelial–mesenchymal transition in cultured bovine aortic ECs, a process associated to the pathogenesis of myocardial fibrosis with ischemia [14] and valve calcification [15]. In addition, in animal models of CKD-MBD (chronic kidney disease-mineral bone disease) [16] there is an increased renal production of Wnt inhibitor family members and higher levels of circulating DKK1, sclerostin, and secreted klotho. In this model, the neutralization of DKK1 by administration of a monoclonal antibody after renal injury stimulated bone formation rates, corrected the osteodystrophy, and prevented CKD-stimulated vascular calcification. Besides, the neutralization of DKK1 suppressed aortic expression of the osteoblastic transcription factor Runx2, increased expression of vascular smooth muscle protein 22-α, and restored aortic expression of klotho"

There is also recent data showing a relationship between serum DKK1 and atherosclerosis in humans [17,18]. In a previous study from Register and colleagues, DKK1 concentrations were inversely related to coronary artery disease and aortic calcification. However, as the authors point, this study has been conducted in Afro-Americans (AAs) with T2DM, which has a different prevalence of atherosclerotic disease and osteoporosis compared to European populations. These differences make it interesting to explore this relationship in Caucasian type 2 diabetes. Besides, the relationship between DKK1 concentrations and bone mass has been explored with conflicting data [19–21], so its evaluation in a population with a high risk of bone fragility such as T2DM is of interest.

In this context, the objectives of our study were to evaluate serum DKK1 levels in a cohort of T2DM patients and to analyze its relationships with CVD and bone metabolism. In addition, we compared serum DKK1 concentrations between T2DM and non-diabetic subjects. Thus, our hypothesis was that DKK1 concentrations may be related to CVD and bone metabolism in T2DM patients.

Materials and Methods

Study population

Our study was a cross-sectional one that included 126 subjects. The estimated size of the sample considering an error of 5% and a statistical power of 80% was 84 subjects. The T2DM group included 72 patients with a diagnosis of diabetes according to the American Diabetes Association criteria (ADA, 2005). From January 2006 to December 2007 we consecutively recruited patients who had been referred to our outpatient clinic from community clinics for treatment of diabetes. The control group included 54 non-diabetic subjects who were consecutively recruited from the general community in the same period of time.

All participants were recruited according to the following criteria: Caucasian, free-living, aged 35 to 65 years and normal values for blood count, renal creatinine, hepatic function, calcium and phosphorus. We considered as exclusion criteria the presence of chronic diseases apart from T2DM in the non-diabetic group, the presence of diseases affecting bone (Paget's disease, rheumatoid arthritis, hyperparathyroidism, hypercortisolism, malignant tumors, renal bone disease, chronic liver disease and post-transplantation bone disease) and also previous or current treatment with drugs affecting bone metabolism (calcium supplements, vitamin D preparations, selective estrogen receptor modulators, calcitonin, estrogens therapy, antiresorptive therapy, thiazides, steroids, glucocorticoids or anticonvulsants). Patients treated with thiazolidinediones were also excluded.

The presence of cardiovascular disease was recorded by the medical history and after that it was checked in medical records. T2DM patients were classified into two groups according to the presence of clinical CVD: CVD group and non-CVD group. Inclusion criteria for patients with CVD were cerebrovascular disease (ischemic stroke or transient ischemic attack); coronary heart disease (previous myocardial infarction, diagnosed stable or unstable angina, or coronary revascularization surgery) or ischemic peripheral arterial disease (diagnosed by a positive Doppler ultrasound or arteriogram, or by a previous revascularization surgery).

The study was approved by the ethical review board of the Hospital Universitario San Cecilio and it was done conformed to the ethical guidelines for research in humans. All the participants in the study provided written informed consent after a full explanation of the purpose of the study and the nature of all the procedures that will be used in the study. Written informed consent was approved for the ethical review board of our hospital, and after that it was filed in the medical record of each patient.

Clinical evaluation

Height, weight, and waist circumference were measured at baseline according to standard procedures. Weight was measured to the nearest 100 grams using digital electronic scales. Height and waist circumference were measured to the nearest 1 mm using a stadiometer and a metal anthropometric tape, respectively. Body mass index (BMI) in Kg/m^2 was calculated as weight divided by the square of height in meters.

Blood pressure was measured in a standardized manner. The subjects remained at rest for at least 5 minutes, and after that blood pressure was measured twice using a standard mercury sphygmomanometer (12 centimeters long, 35 cm wide). The mean of the two values was used for analysis. We defined hypertension when blood pressure values were higher than 140/90 mmHg and/or where subjects were on antihypertensive treatment.

The participants reported their alcohol use, smoking status and their level of physical activity with a specific health questionnaire. Patients were classified as having a significant alcohol intake if it was higher than 40 grams/day in males and 24 grams/day in women; smoking status was categorized as no tobacco use or current tobacco use. Physical activity was collected through a specific questionnaire in which study subjects scored their physical activity on a scale from 0 (none) to 10 (sport more than one hour four times per week). Based on the results, the study sample was divided into two groups: sedentary (<5 on the scale) and no sedentary (≥5 on the scale).

Serum measurements

Samples of venous blood were taken in the morning after a fasting overnight. The sera were stored at −80°C until examina-

Table 1. Characteristics of the study population.

	Total Group (n = 126)	T2DM Group (n = 72)	Non-diabetic Group (n = 54)	P Value
Age (years)	57±6	58±6	55±7	0,018
Male/female (n)	62/64	39/33	25/29	0,472
Medical history				
Duration of diabetes (years)	-	13,7±7,6	-	
Hypertension (%)	53,2	80,6	46,3	<0,001
Dyslipidaemia (%)	65,9	94,4	70,4	<0,001
Albuminuria (%)	20,5	35,0	4,0	0,006
Chronic kidney disease (KDOQI stages) (%)				
Stage 1	51	52	52	0,938
Stage 2	46	44	48	0,815
Stage 3	3	4	0	0,155
Smoker or ex-smoker (%)	15,1	16,7	13	0,623
Alcohol (%)	8,7	6,9	11,1	0,104
Sedentarism (%)	47,6	55,6	37,0	0,048
Clinical evaluation:				
BMI (kg/m^2)	102,6±12,4	31,4±5,7	29,3±5,9	0,043
Waist circumference (cm)	130±20	106,4±11,4	97,4±11,9	<0,001
SBP (mm Hg)	80±13	134±97	124±17	0,002
DBP (mm Hg)	30,5±5,9	80±12	79±15	0,705
Serum parameters:				
FPG (mg/dL)	137,2±61,9	173±60,1	89,4±10,4	<0,001
HbA1$_c$ (%)	6,7±2,2	8±1,9	4,8±0,4	<0,001
GFR (MDR/CKD-EPI)(ml/min/1,73 m^2)	92±23	92±23	93±22	0,745
Calcium (mg/dL)	9,5±0,5	9,6±0,5	9,3±0,4	0,001
Phosphorus (mg/dL)	3,6±0,5	3,7±0,5	3,5±0,5	0,01
PTH (pg/mL)	43,6±19,5	38,5±18,4	50,4±19,1	<0,001
25(OH) D (ng/mL)	19,5±11,3	17,8±11,5	21,6±10,9	0,06
Triglyceride (mg/dl)	142±121	169,9±149,8	104,9±47,7	<0,001
HDL-c (mg/dl)	53,5±15,5	49±16	59,5±12,5	<0,001
LDL-c (mg/dl)	111,7±35,5	96,9±34,1	130,8±27,4	<0,001
DKK1 (pg/ml)	629±374	669±395	575±340	0,163
DXA parameters and VF:				
BMD LS (g/cm^2)	0,977±0,148	0,954±0,146	1±0,148	0,068
BMD FN (g/cm^2)	0,820±0,124	0,817±0,132	0,823±0,117	0,792
BMD TH (g/cm^2)	0,906±0,135	0,903±0,145	0,911±0,125	0,772
T-score LS	−1,08±1,36	−1,3±1,3	0,82±1,3	0,058
T-score FN	−0,55±1,01	−0,6±1,04	−0,49±0,99	0,565
T-score TH	−0,55±0,98	−0,62±1	−0,51±0,92	0,557
Osteoporosis (%)	15,9	24,6	9,4	0,047
Morphometric VF (%)	23,0	30,3	20,0	0,274
Cardiovascular disease:	35,7	58,3	5,6	<0,001
Cerebrovascular disease (%)	11,9	19,4	1,9	0,002
Coronary heart disease (%)	23,8	38,9	3,7	<0,001
Peripheral artery disease (%)	7,9	13,9	0	0,005
Abnormal intima-media thickness (%)	35,7	54,2	11,1	<0,001
Carotid plaques (%)	15,9	29,4	0	<0,001

Data for continuous variables are presented as mean ±SD. Data for categorical variables are presented as numbers and/or percentages. The comparison between groups was done by Student's t test (continuous variables) or Chi-square test (categorical variables).

T2DM: type 2 diabetes mellitus; BMI: body mass index; SBP: sistolic blood pressure; DBP: diastolic blood pressure; FPG: fasting plasma glucose; HbA1c: glycated hemoglobin; GFR: glomerular filtration rate; MDR/CKD-EPI: Chronic Kidney Disease Epidemiology Collaboration; PTH: parathormone; 25(OH) D: 25-hydroxyvitamin D; HDL-c: High-density lipoprotein; LDL-c: Low-density lipoprotein; BMD: bone mineral density; LS: lumbar spine; FN: femoral neck; TH: total hip; VF: vertebral fractures.

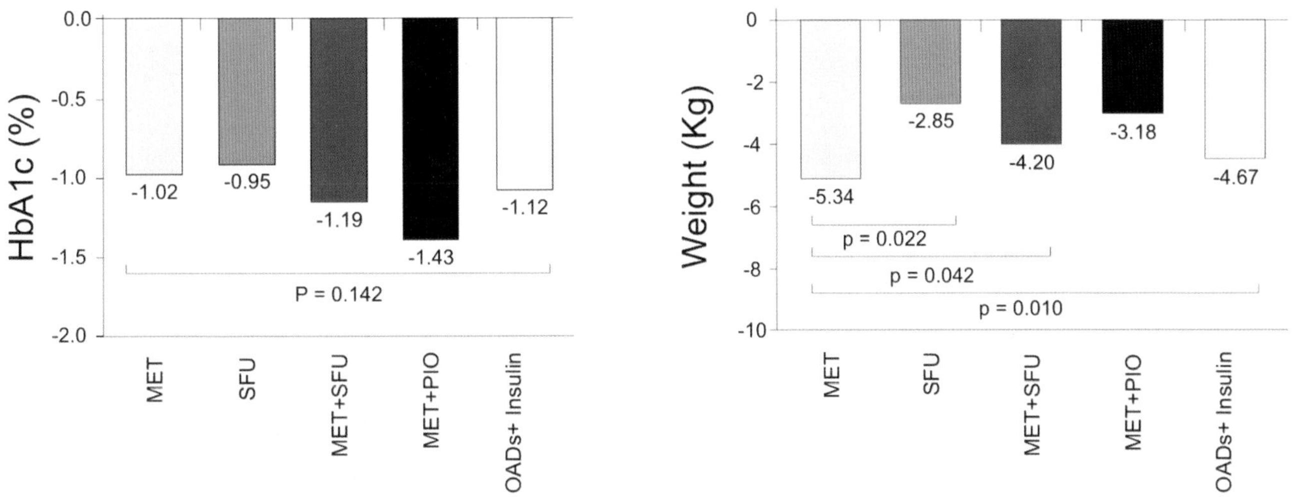

Figure 1. DKK1 serum levels in T2DM patients according to the presence of cardiovascular disease and abnormal intima-media thickness. Between groups differences are indicated through a bar with the P-value given above.

tion. Fasting plasma glucose (FPG), glycated hemoglobin (HbA1c), calcium, phosphorus and creatinine were measured using standard automated laboratory techniques. Glomerular filtration rate (GFR) was calculated by MDRD/CKD-EPI formula [22]. High-density lipoprotein (HDL), low-density lipoprotein (LDL) cholesterol and triglycerides (TGs) were measured by standard biochemical methods. Dyslipidemia was defined according to third report of the expert panel on detection, evaluation, and treatment of high blood cholesterol in adults (ATP-III) criteria or current treatment with statins.

Calciotropic hormones measurement included serum intact parathormone (Two-site immunoassay for iPTH, Roche Diagnostics SL, Barcelona, Spain; intra and interassay variability of 3%) and 25-hydroxyvitamin D (25-OH-D, radioimmunoassay, DiaSorin, Stillwater, Minnesota USA. Serum DKK1 was measured using quantitative sandwich enzyme-linked immunosorbent assay (ELISA) developed by Biomedica (Biomedica Medizinprodukte GmbH and Co. KG, Wien, Austria) according to the manufacturer's instructions. The Biomedica DKK-1 ELISA (BI-20412) detects free DKK-1. Intra-assay and interassay variability were of 7% and 9%, respectively. DKK1 measurements are reported throughout in pg/ml after conversion from pMol/L. 1 pMol/l is equivalent to 28,68 pg/ml.

Bone density measurement and vertebral fractures assessment

Bone mineral density at lumbar spine (LS) L2–L4, femoral neck (FN) and total hip (TH) was performed in all patients by dual-energy X-ray absorptiometry (DXA) using Hologic QDR 4500 densitometer (Whatman, MA; variation coefficient <1%). All the BMD measurements were done by the same experienced operator. We used the World Health Organization criteria for osteoporosis (Kanis JA, 1994).

Standardized spinal X-rays were taken for morphometric analysis of all participants of the study and they were interpreted according to the algorithm developed by McCloskey and colleagues [23].

Carotid intima-media thickness Ultrasonographic examination of the carotid arteries was performed with patients in supine position using Doppler ultrasonography (Toshiba PowerVision 6000). The maximum intima-media thickness (IMT) at the carotid bifurcation (BIF) was determined between the near and far walls of the carotid bifurcation on the right and left sides. Each part was measured from views of both longitudinal and vertical sections at the bifurcation. If a discrepancy was observed in the measured values between longitudinal and vertical sections, the smaller value was selected to avoid overestimation. BIF–IMT was defined as the mean of the measurements from the right and left sides. The value for each side was obtained from the mean of 10 wall measurements. The BIF–IMT, measured in millimeters (mm), was considered pathological if it was ≥0.9 mm, and was considered to be carotid atherosclerosis if the BIF–IMT was ≥ 1.2 mm or 50% greater than the BIF–IMT in the adjacent area [24]. Plaques were identified as calcified by findings of bright white echoes on sonography. A single trained sonographer performed the study in all subjects.

Statistical analysis

Data for continuous variables are presented as mean ± standard deviation (SD). Data for categorical variables are presented as numbers and/or percentages. Kolmogorov–Smirnov test was used to test the normality of distribution of continuous variables. The association between continuous variables was described by Pearson's or Spearman's correlation coefficients. The comparison of categorical variables among groups was performed using Chi-square test or Fisher test. The comparison of continuous variables among groups was performed using unpaired Student's *t* test or Mann-Whitney test. To determine the independent variables which correlated with DKK1 (dependent variable), the parameters that correlate significantly in univariate analysis and other which are biologically linked to DKK1 were tested in multiple backward model linear regression analysis. Multiple backward model of logistic regression analysis was performed to identify DKK1 as independent predictor for CVD (dependent variable) in T2DM patients. The model included established atherosclerotic risk factors (age, gender, body mass index, hypertension, dislipidaemia, smoking, sedentarism, HbA1c, GFR and intima-media thickness). CVD-defining parameters (cerebrovascular disease, coronary heart disease or ischemic peripheral arterial disease) were not included in the multiple logistic regression model. The usefulness of serum DKK1 as a marker of high risk of atherosclerotic disease in T2DM was

Table 2. DKK1 concentrations according to the presence of cardiovascular disease in the T2DM group.

	Yes	No	P value
Cardiovascular disease	757±416	547±333	0,026
Cerebrovascular disease	854±480	625±363	0,045
Coronary heart disease	694±379	654±408	0,677
Peripheral artery disease	634±247	675±415	0,762
Abnormal intima-media thickness	756±433	567±322	0,042
Carotid plaque	730±422	661±395	0,522

The comparison between groups was done by Student's t test.

analyzed using a receiver operating characteristic curve (ROC Curve). A p value of less than 0,05 was considered to be significant (two-tailed). Data were recorded and analyzed using SPSS version 18.0 software (SPSS Inc, Chicago, IL, USA).

Results

The clinical characteristics of the study population are summarized in Table 1. Serum DKK1 was significantly higher ($P = 0{,}026$) in T2DM patients with CVD (757±416 pg/ml) compared with those without CVD (547±333 pg/ml). (Figure 1 and Table 2). T2DM patients with abnormal IMT (756±433 pg/ml *vs* 563±322 pg/ml; $P = 0{,}042$) and cerebrovascular disease (854±480 pg/ml *vs* 625±363; $P = 0{,}045$) had higher DKK1 concentrations. (Figure 1 and Table 2). However, we did not find differences in DKK1 concentrations according to the presence of carotid plaque ($P = 0{,}522$), coronary heart disease ($P = 0{,}677$) or ischemic peripheral artery disease ($P = 0{,}762$).

A model of logistic regression analysis was performed using the presence of CVD as a dependent variable. Independent variables were serum DKK1 levels and risk factors for atherosclerosis (age, gender, body mass index, hypertension, dislipidaemia, smoking, sedentarism, HbA1c, GFR, and IMT). DKK1 levels were independently associated with the presence of CVD in T2DM (odds ratio: 1,062, 95% confidence interval: 1,003–1,125; $P = 0{,}04$). Therefore, for each increase of 28 pg/ml of serum DKK1 there was a 6,2% increased risk of CVD in T2DM patients.

In the ROC curve analysis to evaluate the usefulness of DKK1 as a marker for high risk of CVD, the area under the curve was 0,667 (95% confidence interval: 0,538–0,795; $P = 0{,}016$) (Figure 2). A concentration of 494 pg/ml or higher showed a sensitivity of 71,4% and a specificity of 60% to identify an increased risk of CVD.

We found no differences in DKK1 between study groups: T2DM 669±395 vs non-diabetic 575±340 pg/ml, $P = 0{,}163$. Serum DKK1 concentrations were significantly higher in females than in males in total sample (697±434 vs 563±293 pg/ml, $P = 0{,}046$) and in T2DM group (788±493 vs 569±255 pg/ml, $P = 0{,}025$) but were not significantly increased in control females (593±335 vs 553±349 pg/ml, $P = 0{,}682$).

Linear regression analysis was performed to determine the influence of independent factors identified in univariate correlation analysis, including group, gender, age, HbA1c, CVD and IMT as independent variables that explain serum DKK1 levels. The analysis demonstrated that gender ($\beta = -0{,}299$, $P = 0{,}002$) and CVD ($\beta = 0{,}292$, $P = 0{,}007$) were positively associated with serum DKK1.

Regarding bone metabolism, lumbar spine BMD was positively related to serum DKK1 in total sample ($r = 0{,}183$, $P = 0{,}048$). In contrast, we did not found a significant relationship with bone remodelling markers osteoporosis diagnosis or morphometric vertebral fractures (data not shown), in the total sample or in the study groups separately.

Discussion

To our knowledge, there is no previous study evaluating DKK1 concentrations and its relationship with CVD in Caucasian T2DM patients. There is also scarce data concerning the relationship between DKK1 and bone metabolism in T2DM. Our results show that higher levels of DKK1 are associated with clinical CVD and abnormal IMT in T2DM patients. These findings suggest that serum DKK1 are related to the presence of CVD in this population. However, our data showed no differences in serum DKK1 between T2DM patients and non-diabetic patients. Regarding bone metabolism, we found a significant relationship with bone mineral density.

In our study, higher DKK1 levels were positively related to cardiovascular disease in T2DM patients independently of the presence of others risk factors for atherosclerosis, and high concentrations of DKK1 were related to abnormal IMT in these patients. Our results are in accordance with previous reports showing the relationship between vascular disease and DKK1 in other populations. Patients with cerebrovascular disease have higher serum DKK1 levels compared with control subjects [25], and serum DKK1 correlated with coronary artery calcification and atherosclerotic plaques evaluated by coronary computed tomography and coronary artery calcium scoring [17]. Previously, Ueland and colleagues [26] demonstrated that DKK1 expression is enhanced in advanced carotid plaques and that DKK1 is a novel mediator in platelet-mediated endothelial cell activation, which could occur within the atherosclerotic lesions. Moreover, current data clearly demonstrate a novel role for Wnt proteins in the proliferation, migration, and survival of smooth muscle cells (SMCs) [27]. Regarding this, higher levels of DKK1 are present in advanced carotid plaques and DKK1 promotes platelet-mediated activation of endothelial cells. Thus, it has been proposed that this could lead to enhanced inflammation in the atherosclerotic lesion; however, it may also lead to a reduced survival, proliferation, and migration of SMCs, thereby reinforcing the potential complexity of the participation of Wnt proteins in atherosclerosis [27].

In contrast to our findings, DKK1 concentrations were negatively associated with atherosclerotic calcified plaque in African-Americans (AAs) patients with T2DM [18]. There are several reasons that might contribute to this discrepancy. As the authors point, AAs have lower rates of vascular calcification. It has

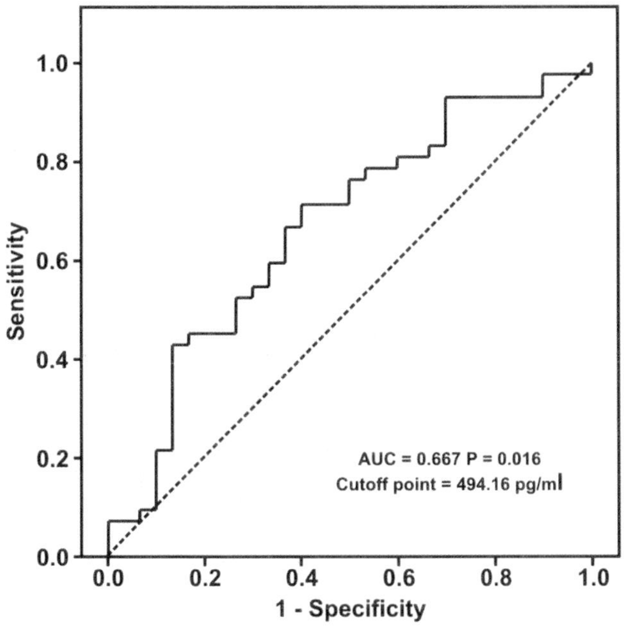

Figure 2. DKK1 ROC curve for cardiovascular disease.

been reported lower levels of coronary artery calcified plaque relative to European Americans (EAs) despite similar or more detrimental cardiovascular risk factor profiles [28,29]. This observation is consistent both in T2DM and subjects without diabetes [30,31], and suggests a differential impact of CV risk factors on atherosclerosis based on ethnicity although the underlying causes of ethnic differences in vascular calcification are not well established [32]. Reinforcing these ethnic differences, AAs are at lower risk for myocardial infarction based on less coronary artery calcification, and they have significantly lower rates of myocardial infarction than EAs, provided equal access to healthcare [33,34]. It has been suggested that AAs may be less susceptible than whites to hyperglycaemia–induced macrovascular disease [35]. Thus, these findings may explain the differences observed in the relationship between vascular disease and DKK1 between our study and the data from Register and colleagues.

Recent data suggest that the association between vascular calcification and osteoporosis is not simply a consequence of age, stressing that the co-incidence of vascular calcification with low bone activity and osteoporosis could be biologically linked. During the development of vascular calcification, there is a transition of vascular SMCs towards an osteoblast- like phenotype, which promotes the mineralization within these structures. In this process there are several players, including those related to mineral metabolism, like phosphorus, calcium or parathyroid hormone, which influences the expression of osteogenic factors [36]. There is emerging evidence suggesting that some inhibitors of the Wnt pathway, such as secreted frizzled Proteins 2 and 4 and DKK-1, may play a role linking vascular calcification and bone loss [26,27]. AAs manifest a skeletal resistance to the effects of parathyroid hormone [37,38] and exhibit opposite relationships between arterial calcification and serum vitamin D concentrations compared with Europeans [39]. In our opinion, these ethnic differences in the effects of calciotropic hormones on bone and vessels may indicate that differences in other pathways, as Wnt pathway, may be expected according to race. However, this hypothesis must be confirmed.

There are other differences between the study from Register and colleagues and ours, which may explain the discrepancy of results. First, the prevalence of cardiovascular disease is lower, 27%, compared to our study where a 58% of patients had previous cardiovascular disease. Second, in the study from Register and colleagues 28,3% of subjects were taking hormonal therapy while no women were on hormonal therapy in our study. Estradiol and progesterone has shown to regulate Wnt pathways in endometrial tissue [40] and brain [41], so an influence of hormonal therapy in DKK1 concentrations can not be excluded. Finally, despite the low expected incidence of arterial calcification in AAs, in the study from Register and colleagues there is a high prevalence of aortic calcification. Thus, differences between study populations apart from the ethnicity may influence the discrepancy of results.

There are no previous studies evaluating differences in serum DKK1 concentrations according to the presence of diabetes. We did not find differences in DKK1 between T2DM patients and subjects without diabetes. These results contrast with our previous data showing higher sclerostin concentrations in the same group of type 2 diabetes patients [42]. However, serum DKK1 and sclerostin have shown to be barely correlated [43], as we found in our sample (data not shown). In addition, the effects of DKK1 and sclerostin may differ due to differences in Kremen binding. While DKK1 is always an inhibitor of Wnt signaling, the effect of sclerostin is variable depending on context [44]. Unlike our previous results about sclerostin, women had higher DKK1 concentrations both in the total sample and in the T2DM group. Estradiol and progesterone have shown to take part in the regulation of the Wnt pathways in endometrial tissue [40] and brain [41], so a sex steroid-induced effect may explain gender differences in DKK1 although this hypothesis must be confirmed.

Regarding the relationship between bone metabolism and DKK1 we only found a weak correlation with BMD at lumbar spine in the total sample, and no relationship with bone turnover markers, osteoporosis or morphometric vertebral fractures (data not shown). In addition, lumbar spine BMD may be affected by aortic calcification. Our findings confirm previous data showing no relationship between DKK1 and bone turnover markers in postmenopausal osteoporosis [20]. The relationship between DKK1 and BMD is not totally established. It has been reported no relationship with volumetric BMD in Afro-American T2DM patients [18]. However, is also been described and inverse relationship between DKK1 and BMD, and higher DKK1 concentrations in patients with osteoporosis [19]. Therefore, in our opinion the data about serum DKK1 and bone metabolism are controversial and thus no clear conclusions can be drawn.

Our study has some limitations. First, the cross-sectional design does not allow to establishing a cause-effect relationship. Second, the sample size is relatively small and might affect the statistic power. Our study has also several strengths, as the evaluation of circulating serum DKK1 in Caucasian patients with T2DM for the first time, the comparison to non-diabetic subjects and the evaluation both of bone metabolism and atherosclerotic disease.

In summary, serum levels of DKK1 are elevated in Caucasian patients with T2DM presenting CVD. These findings suggest that Wnt signaling pathway is involved in vascular disease in diabetic subjects. However, the relations of DKK1 with bone metabolism are inconsistent.

Author Contributions

None. Conceived and designed the experiments: AGM PRM RRG MMT. Performed the experiments: BGF SMS. Analyzed the data: AGM RRG MMT. Contributed reagents/materials/analysis tools: BGF SMS. Wrote the paper: AGM RRG MMT PRM ACM MMG.

References

1. Madonna R, De Caterina R (2011) Cellular and molecular mechanisms of vascular injury in diabetes-part I: Pathways of vascular disease in diabetes. Vascular Pharmacology 54: 68–74.
2. Magnus JH, Brussard DL (2005) Relationship between bone mineral density and myocardial infarction in US adults. Osteoporosis International 16: 2053–2062.
3. Hofbauer LC, Brueck CC, Singh SK, Dognig H (2007) Osteoporosis in patients with diabetes mellitus. Journal of Bone and Mineral Research 22: 1317–1328.
4. Epstein S, Leroith D (2008) Diabetes and fragility fractures — A burgeoning epidemic? Bone 43: 3–6.
5. Carr JJ, Register TC, Hsu FC, Lohman K, Lenchik L, et al. (2008) Calcified atherosclerotic plaque and bone mineral density in type 2 diabetes: the diabetes heart study. Bone 42: 43–52.
6. Divers J, Register TC, Langefeld CD, Wagenknecht LE, Bowden DW, et al. (2011) Relationships between calcified atherosclerotic plaque and bone mineral density in AAs with type 2 diabetes. Journal of Bone and Mineral Research 26: 1554–1560.
7. Gordon MD, Nusse R (2006) Wnt signalling: multiple pathways, multiple receptors and multiple transcription factors. Journal of Biology and Chemistry 281: 22429–22433.
8. Huang H, He X (2008) Wnt/beta-catenin signaling: new (and old) players and new insight. Current Opinion in Cell Biology 20: 119–125.
9. Mao B, Wu W, Davidson G, Marhold J, Li M, et al. (2002) Kremen proteins are Dickkopf receptors that regulate Wnt/-catenin signalling. Nature 417: 664–667.
10. Shao JS, Cheng SL, Pingsterhaus JM, Charlton-Kachigian N, Loewy AP, et al. (2005) Msx2 promotes cardiovascular calcification by activating paracrine Wnt signals. Journal of Clinical Investigation 115: 1210–1220.
11. Sen M, Ghosh G (2008) Transcriptional outcome of Wnt-Frizzled signal transduction in inflammation: evolving concepts. Journal of Immunology 181: 4441–4445.
12. Christman MA 2nd, Goetz DJ, Dickerson E, McCall KD, Lewis CJ, et al. (2008) Wnt5a is expressed in murine and human atherosclerotic lesions. American Journal of Physiology and Heart Circulation and Physiology 294: H2864–2870.
13. Cheng SL, Shao JS, Behrmann A, Krchma K, Towler DA (2013) Dkk1 and MSX2-Wnt7b signaling reciprocally regulate the endothelial-mesenchymal transition in aortic endothelial cells. Arterioscler Thromb Vasc Biol 33: 1679–89.
14. Krenning G, Zeisberg EM, Kalluri R (2010) The origin of fibroblasts and mechanism of cardiac fibrosis. J Cell Physiol 225: 631–637.
15. Wylie-Sears J, Aikawa E, Levine RA, Yang JH, Bischoff J (2011) Mitral valve endothelial cells with osteogenic differentiation potential. Arterioscler Thromb Vasc Biol 31: 598–607.
16. Fang Y, Ginsberg C, Seifert M, Agapova O, Sugatani T, et al. (2014) CKD-Induced Wingless/Integration1 Inhibitors and Phosphorus Cause the CKD-Mineral and Bone Disorder. J Am Soc Nephrol 25: 1760–73.
17. Kim KI, Park KU, Chun EJ, Choi SI, Cho YS, et al. (2011) A novel biomarker of coronary atheroesclerosis: serum DKK1 concentration correlates with coronary artery calcification and atherosclerotic plaques. Journal of Korean Medical Science 26: 1178–1184.
18. Register TC, Hruska KA, Divers J, Bowden DW, Palmer ND, et al. (2013) Plasma Dickkopf (DKK1) concentrations negatively associate with atherosclerotic calcified plaque in african-americans with type 2 diabetes. Journal of Clinical Endocrinology and Metabolism 98: 60–65.
19. Butler JS, Murray DW, Hurson CJ, O'Brien J, Doran PP, et al. (2011) The role of Dkk1 in bone mass regulation: correlating serum Dkk1 expression with bone mineral density. Journal of Orthopaedic Research 29: 414–418.
20. Polyzos SA, Anastasilakis AD, Bratengeier C, Woloszczuk W, Papatheodorou A, et al. (2012) Serum sclerostin levels positively correlate with lumbar spinal bone mineral density in postmenopausal women-the six-month effect of risedronate and teriparatide. Osteoporosis International 23: 1171–1176.
21. Cejka D, Jäger-Lansky A, Kieweg H, Weber M, Bieglmayer C, et al. (2012) Sclerostin serum levels correlate positively with bone mineral density and microarchitecture in haemodialysis patients. Nephrology Dialysis Transplantion 27: 226–230.
22. Levey AS, Stevens LA, Schmid CH, Zhang YL, Castro AF 3rd, et al. (2009) CKD-EPI (Chronic Kidney Disease Epidemiology Collaboration). A new equation to estimate glomerular filtration rate. Ann Intern Med 150: 604–612.
23. McCloskey EV, Spector TD, Eyres KS, Fern ED, O'Rourke N, et al. (1993) The assessment of vertebral deformity: a method for use in population studies and clinical trials. Osteoporosis International 3: 138–147.
24. Junyent M, Gilabert R, Nuñez I, Corbella E, Vela M, et al. (2005) Carotid ultrasound in the assessment of preclinical atherosclerosis. Distribution of intima-media thickness values and plaque frequency in a Spanish community cohort. Medicina Clinica 125: 770–774.
25. Seifert-Held T, Pekar T, Gattringer T, Simmet NE, Scharnagl H, et al. (2011) Circulating Dickkopf-1 in acute ischemic stroke and clinically stable cerebrovascular disease. Atherosclerosis 218: 233–237.
26. Ueland T, Otterdal K, Lekva T, Halvorsen B, Gabrielsen A, et al. (2009) Dickkopf-1 enhances inflammatory interaction between platelets and endothelial cells and shows increased expression in atherosclerosis. Arteriosclerosis Thrombosis and Vascular Biology 29: 1228–1234.
27. Mill C, George SJ (2012) Wnt signalling in smooth muscle cells and its role in cardiovascular disorders. Cardiovascular Research 95: 233–40.
28. Bild DE, Detrano R, Peterson D, Guerci A, Liu K, et al. (2005) Ethnic differences in coronary calcification: the Multi-Ethnic Study of Atherosclerosis (MESA). Circulation 111: 1313–20.
29. Lee TC, O'Malley PG, Feuerstein I, Taylor AJ (2003) The prevalence and severity of coronary artery calcification on coronary artery computed tomography in black and white subjects. J Am Coll Cardiol 41: 39–44.
30. Freedman BI, Hsu FC, Langefeld CD, Rich SS, Herrington DM, et al. (2005) The impact of ethnicity and sex on subclinical cardiovascular disease: the Diabetes Heart Study. Diabetologia 48: 2511–8.
31. Wade AN, Fedyna S, Mehta NN, St. Clair C, Ginwala N, et al. (2011) Type 2 diabetes does not attenuate racial differences in coronary calcification. Diabetes Res Clin Pract 91: 101–7.
32. Divers J, Palmer ND, Lu L, Register TC, Carr JJ, et al. (2013) Admixture mapping of coronary artery calcified plaque in African Americans with type 2 diabetes mellitus. Circ Cardiovasc Genet; 6: 97–105.
33. Karter AJ, Ferrara A, Liu JY, Moffet HH, Ackerson LM, et al. (2002) Ethnic disparities in diabetic complications in an insured population. JAMA 287: 2519–27.
34. Young BA, Maynard C, Boyko EJ (2003) Racial differences in diabetic nephropathy, cardiovascular disease, and mortality in a national population of veterans. Diabetes Care 26: 2392–9.
35. Freedman BI, Hsu FC, Langefeld CD, Rich SS, Herrington DM, et al. (2005) The impact of ethnicity and sex on subclinical cardiovascular disease: the Diabetes Heart Study. Diabetologia 48: 2511–8.
36. Cannata-Andia JB, Roman-Garcia P, Hruska K (2011) The connections between vascular calcification and bone health. Nephrol Dial Transplant 26: 3429–36.
37. Bell NH, Williamson B, Hollis B, Riggs BL (2001) Effects of race on diurnal patterns of renal conservation of calcium and bone resorption in premenopausal women. Osteoporos Int 12: 43–8.
38. Aloia J, Vaswani A, Yeh J, Flaster E (1996) Risk for osteoporosis in black women. Calcif Tissue Int 59: 415–23.
39. Freedman BI, Register TC (2012) Effect of race and genetics on vitamin D metabolism, bone and vascular health. Nature Review Nephrology 8: 459–466.
40. Wang Y, Hanifi-Moghaddam P, Hanekamp EE, Kloosterboer HJ, Franken P, et al. (2009) Progesterone inhibition of Wnt/beta-catenin signaling in normal endometrium and endometrial cancer. Clinical Cancer Research 15: 5784–5793.
41. Scott EL, Brann DW (2012) Estrogen regulation of Dkk1 and Wnt/β-Catenin signaling in neurodegenerative disease. Brain Research 1514: 63–74.
42. García-Martín A, Rozas-Moreno P, Reyes-García R, Morales-Santana S, García-Fontana B, et al. (2012) Circulating levels of sclerostin are increased in patients with type 2 diabetes mellitus. Journal of Clinical Endocrinology and Metabolism 97: 234–241.
43. Thambiah S, Roplekar R, Manghat P, Fogelman I, Fraser WD, et al. (2012) Circulating sclerostin and Dickkopf-1 (DKK1) in predialysis chronic kidney disease (CKD): relationship with bone density and arterial stiffness. Calcified Tissue International 90: 473–480.
44. Kawano Y, Kypta R (2003) Secreted antagonists of the Wnt signalling pathway. J Cell Sci 116: 2627–34.

Moderate-Intensity Rotating Magnetic Fields Do Not Affect Bone Quality and Bone Remodeling in Hindlimb Suspended Rats

Da Jing[1]☯, Jing Cai[2]☯, Yan Wu[3]☯, Guanghao Shen[1], Mingming Zhai[1], Shichao Tong[1], Qiaoling Xu[4], Kangning Xie[1], Xiaoming Wu[1], Chi Tang[1], Xinmin Xu[5], Juan Liu[1], Wei Guo[1], Maogang Jiang[1], Erping Luo[1]*

1 Department of Biomedical Engineering, Fourth Military Medical University, Xi'an, China, **2** Department of Endocrinology, Xijing hospital, Fourth Military Medical University, Xi'an, China, **3** Institute of Orthopaedics, Xijing hospital, Fourth Military Medical University, Xi'an, China, **4** Department of Nursing, Fourth Military Medical University, Xi'an, China, **5** Department of Medical Engineering, PLA No. 323 Hospital, Xi'an, China

Abstract

Abundant evidence has substantiated the positive effects of pulsed electromagnetic fields (PEMF) and static magnetic fields (SMF) on inhibiting osteopenia and promoting fracture healing. However, the osteogenic potential of rotating magnetic fields (RMF), another common electromagnetic application modality, remains poorly characterized thus far, although numerous commercial RMF treatment devices have been available on the market. Herein the impacts of RMF on osteoporotic bone microarchitecture, bone strength and bone metabolism were systematically investigated in hindlimb-unloaded (HU) rats. Thirty two 3-month-old male Sprague-Dawley rats were randomly assigned to the Control ($n = 10$), HU ($n = 10$) and HU with RMF exposure (HU+RMF, $n = 12$) groups. Rats in the HU+RMF group were subjected to daily 2-hour exposure to moderate-intensity RMF (ranging from 0.60 T to 0.38 T) at 7 Hz for 4 weeks. HU caused significant decreases in body mass and soleus muscle mass of rats, which were not obviously altered by RMF. Three-point bending test showed that the mechanical properties of femurs in HU rats, including maximum load, stiffness, energy absorption and elastic modulus were not markedly affected by RMF. μCT analysis demonstrated that 4-week RMF did not significantly prevent HU-induced deterioration of femoral trabecular and cortical bone microarchitecture. Serum biochemical analysis showed that RMF did not significantly change HU-induced decrease in serum bone formation markers and increase in bone resorption markers. Bone histomorphometric analysis further confirmed that RMF showed no impacts on bone remodeling in HU rats, as evidenced by unchanged mineral apposition rate, bone formation rate, osteoblast numbers and osteoclast numbers in cancellous bone. Together, our findings reveal that RMF do not significantly affect bone microstructure, bone mechanical strength and bone remodeling in HU-induced disuse osteoporotic rats. Our study indicates potentially obvious waveform-dependent effects of electromagnetic fields-stimulated osteogenesis, suggesting that RMF, at least in the present form, might not be an optimal modality for inhibiting disuse osteopenia/osteoporosis.

Editor: Robert Lafrenie, Sudbury Regional Hospital, Canada

Funding: The authors acknowledge support from the National Natural Science Foundation of China (No. 51077128 and 31270889), Shaanxi Provincial Natural Science Foundation (No. 2014JQ4139), and the Doctoral Thesis Foundation of the Fourth Military Medical University (No. 2012D01). The funders had no role in study design, data collection and analysis, decision to publish, or preparation of the manuscript.

Competing Interests: The authors have declared that no competing interests exist.

* Email: luoerping@fmmu.edu.cn

☯ These authors contributed equally to this work.

Introduction

Osteoporosis, a progressive 'silent bone disease' caused by age, disuse or disease, is characterized by loss of bone mass and deterioration of bone microarchitecture, resulting in pain and deformity and increased risk of bone fracture [1,2]. Bone loss due to the removal of weight-bearing physical activities, which occurs during therapeutic bed rest, limb immobilization and spaceflight, has become a non-negligible health concern in clinics and space medicine. Mechanical unloading induces negative skeletal calcium homeostasis, uncoupling of osteoclast and osteoblast activities, and resultant bone mineral loss [3]. Studies have shown that astronauts experienced loss of bone mineral density (BMD) with approximately 1.5% per month during spaceflight, equaling to that for postmenopausal women in 1 year [4,5,6]. It has been proved that individuals subjected to long-term bed rest or immobilization exhibited dramatic bone mass loss, deterioration of cancellous and cortical bone microarchitecture, and increased risk of falls and bone fracture [7,8]. In view of the side effects or high cost of anti-osteoporosis drugs (e.g., bisphosphonates, calcitonin and hormones) [9,10,11], safe and noninvasive biophysical stimuli for the prevention and treatment of disuse osteoporosis might be more promising in clinical application, and especially favorable for the use of spaceflight.

Our growing understanding of the intricate piezoelectric and electromagnetic properties of bone tissues raised the possibility that exogenous electric or magnetic stimulation might regulate the activities and functions of bone cells. Since the 1970s when Bassett et al. for the first time promoted fracture healing in clinics using pulsed electromagnetic fields (PEMF) [12], abundant evidence has substantiated that electromagnetic fields (EMF) therapy was capable of producing satisfying therapeutic effects in a diverse range of bone diseases in the past four decades [13,14]. The EMF has been approved by the FDA as a safe noninvasive treatment method in 1979. Basically, the three most common EMF application modalities well documented thus far include PEMF, static magnetic fields (SMF) and rotating magnetic fields (RMF). A large body of evidence has shown that PEMF displayed strong osteogenic potential both experimentally and clinically [15,16,17,18], which was primarily associated with the induction of electric currents in tissues to initiate a battery of biological cascades. Several investigators also reported that SMF exposure was able to stimulate *in vivo* skeletal anabolic responses and increase BMD [19,20]. Unlike PEMF, SMF induced no remarkable electrical potential in tissues and might directly affect bone cells through magnetic actions [20]. In recent years, several commercial therapeutic devices with RMF exposure are available on the market. Several previous studies have reported the beneficial effects of RMF on the musculoskeletal system [21,22]. Zhang and colleagues found that 0.4 T RMF increase BMD and serum calcium and phosphatase (ALP) in ovariectomized (OVX) rats [21]. Pan et al. reported that 0.4 T RMF exposure mitigated hyperlipidaemia and steroid-induced necrosis of femoral head in rabbits [22]. However, to date the possible impacts of RMF on disuse-induced osteopenia/osteoporosis remain unknown. Thus, systemic assessment of the regulatory effects of RMF exposure on bone mass, bone microarchitecture, bone strength and bone metabolism in animal models of disuse-induced osteopenia is of great significance for the scientific application of RMF.

One of the best-recognized animal models to study disuse osteoporosis is the hindlimb unloading (HU) model via tail suspension [23,24], which could induce decreased bone formation and increased bone resorption, and thus lead to the loss of bone mass and reduction of bone mechanical strength [25,26]. Therefore, in the present investigation, the efficiency of RMF exposure on disuse-induced bone loss was systematically evaluated via analyses for serum biochemical, bone biomechanical, µCT and histomorphometric parameters in rats subjected to tail suspension.

Materials and Methods

Animals and experimental design

Thirty two mature 3-month-old male Sprague-Dawley rats (276.8±13.5 g, Vital River Laboratory Animal Technology, Beijing, China) were used in the present study. All procedures in the experiment were in strict accordance with the guiding principles of Institutional Animal Ethical Committee (IAEC), Committee for the Purpose of Control and Supervision of Experiments on Animals (CPCSEA), and the Guide for the Care and Use of Laboratory Animals published by the National Institutes of Health [NIH Publication.85–23]. The animal protocol was approved by the Institutional Animal Care and Use Committee of Fourth Military Medical University. All efforts were made to minimize the number of animals used. Animals were housed at 23±1°C temperature, 50%–60% relative humidity, 12:12 h light-dark cycle. Rats were randomly assigned to the Control ($n = 10$), HU ($n = 10$) and HU with RMF exposure (HU+RMF, $n = 12$) groups. The disuse of rat hindlimbs was induced by the tail-suspension technique according to the previously described protocol [27,28]. Briefly, the tail after cleaned with 70% ethanol, was coated with a thin layer of liquid-like benzoin and resin dissolved in 99% ethanol. Then, a strip of adhesive tape was firmly attached laterally along the proximal portion of the tail and allowed thorough air dry, forming a loop close to the end of the tail. The adhesive tape was subsequently secured by three tape strips in its perpendicular direction. A plastic paperclip was employed to attach the loop of the surgical tape to a swivel hoop mounted at the top of a custom-designed plexiglass cage (length = 35 cm, width = 30 cm, height = 45 cm). The rat was maintained in an approximately 30° head-down-tilt position with its hindlimbs unloaded. Rats were caged individually and allowed free access to tap water and chow. The rats in the HU+RMF group were exposed to daily 2 h/day whole-body RMF for 4 weeks. Animals were intramuscularly injected with 25 mg/kg tetracycline (Sigma-Aldrich, Louis, MO, USA) at 14 and 13 days and 5 mg/kg calcein (Sigma-Aldrich) at 4 and 3 days before sacrifice, respectively. Rats were euthanatized with an overdose of chloral hydrate at the end of 4-week experiment. Serum samples were obtained via abdominal aorta puncture, centrifuged for 20 min and stored at −70°C for biochemical analysis. Bilateral femora were harvested, wrapped in saline-soaked gauze and stored at −70°C, which were used for mechanical testing and µCT analysis, respectively. Right tibiae were also harvested for bone histomorphometric analysis.

RMF treatment

As shown in **Fig. 1**, a commercial treatment system with RMF exposure (CRSMART-C, Chaoruishi Medical Supplies Co., Ltd, Zibo, China) was used in the present study. The therapeutic device mainly consisted of a treatment table, two opposite anti-parallel arrays of NdFeB permanent magnets, and a signal display and control module. Each magnet array comprised a total of 20 disc-shaped NdFeB magnets. The maximum magnetic flux density for each magnet was 400 mT. The network topology of the lower NdFeB permanent magnet array is shown in **Fig. 1B**. The lower magnet array was rotated at 7 Hz driven by a high-power spinning motor. The upper magnet array was also rotated accordingly at the same frequency driven by the upper motor. The rotation of both magnet arrays generated non-uniform RMF in the space between the arrays. The cage was placed coaxially with the upper and lower magnet arrays. A Gaussmeter (Model 455, Lake Shore Cryotronics, Westerville, OH, USA) with a transversal Hall Probe (HMFT-3E03-VF) was used to determine the spatial distribution of the magnetic field intensity. The determined magnetic flux density distribution in the position of the cage region ranged from 0.60 T to 0.38 T. The measured environmental background electromagnetic field was 0.5±0.02 Gs.

Serum biochemical analysis

Commercial ELISA kits were employed for quantifying serum biochemical markers, including bone formation-associated osteocalcin (OC) and N-terminal propeptide of type 1 procollagen (P1NP), bone resorption-related tartrate-resistant acid phosphatase (TRAcP5b) and C-terminal cross-linked telopeptides of type I collagen (CTX-I) (Biomedical Technologies, Stoughton, MA, USA). ELISA kits were also used to determine the serum concentrations of two essential osteogenesis-associated cytokines, including prostaglandin E_2 (PGE_2) and transforming growth factor-β1 (TGF-β1) (JRDUN Biotechnology Co., Ltd., Shanghai, China). Assays were performed according to the manufacturers' instructions.

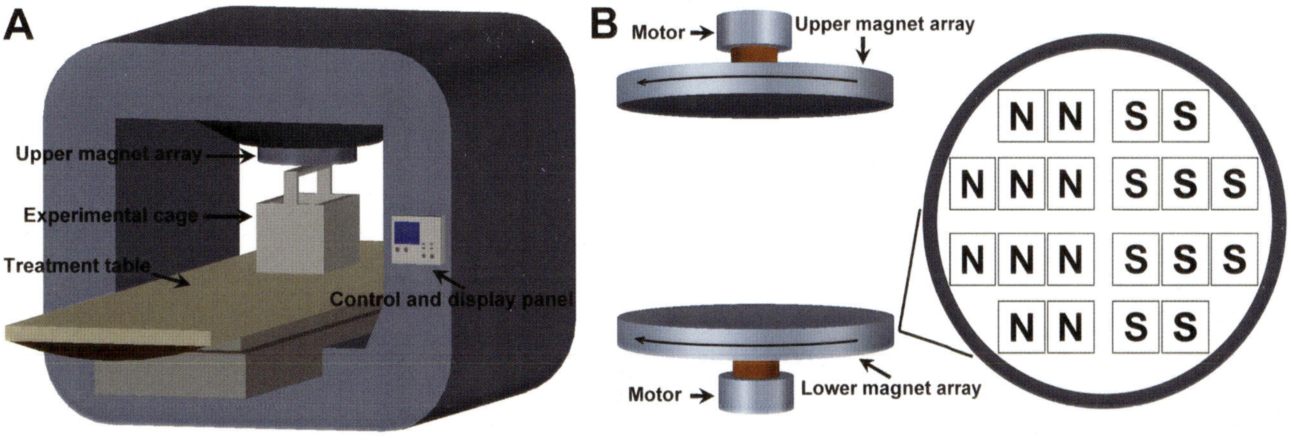

Figure 1. Schematic representation of the treatment device with RMF exposure used in the present study. (**A**) The therapeutic device mainly consists of a treatment table, two opposite anti-parallel arrays of NdFeB permanent magnets, and a signal display and control module. (**B**) Each magnet array comprises a total of 20 disc-shaped NdFeB magnets. The maximum magnetic flux density for each magnet is 400 mT. The right panel in (**B**) shows the network topology of the lower NdFeB permanent magnet array (**N** and **S** in the figure indicate the north pole and south pole of the magnet, respectively). The lower magnet array is rotated at 7 Hz driven by a high-power spinning motor, and thus driving the rotation of the upper magnet array. The rotation of both magnet arrays generates non-uniform RMF in the space between the arrays. The cage is placed coaxially with the upper and lower magnet arrays. The magnetic flux density distribution in the position of the cage region was determined to be 0.60–0.38 T.

Biomechanical examination

The left femora after thawing in phosphate buffer solution (PBS) at room temperature were used for three-point bending test. The mechanical properties were evaluated at the femoral mid-diaphysis using a commercial mechanical testing system (*AGS-10 kNG, Shimadzu*, Kyoto, Japan). The femur with its physiological curvature facing up was stabilized on a supporter with two fixed loading points with 20-mm distance. A stabilizing preload with 2 N was applied on the femoral medial surface using a steel cross-bar plate, which was oriented perpendicularly to the long axis of the sample and at the midpoint between the lower loading points. The bending load was applied at a constant displacement rate of 2 mm/min until fracture occurred. Then, the internal and external major axis and minor axis lengths of the femur at the fracture point were immediately measured using a vernier caliper. The following indices were determined from the load-deformation curve: maximum load (the maximum tensile load that the femur can sustain before failure), stiffness (slope of the linear part of the curve representing elastic deformation), and energy absorption (area under the load-deformation curve). Elastic modulus was calculated according to the formula: $E = FL^3/48dI$, where F is the maximum load, L is the distance between supporting points, d is the displacement, I is the moment of inertia of the cross-section in relation to the horizontal axis.

µCT analysis

The right femora of rats were scanned at a spatial resolution of 16 µm/slice using a high-resolution µCT system (GE healthcare, Madison, WI, USA). The femoral samples were placed in a 20-mm-diameter tube perpendicularly to the scanning axis with a total of 12-mm reconstruction height. After scanning, the 2-D image sequences were transferred to a workstation and 3-D images were reconstructed. For analyses of trabecular bone microarchitecture, a volume of interest (VOI) with 2.0-mm height was selected. The VOI started at a distance of 0.4 mm from the lowest end of the growth plate of the distal femur and extended to the proximal end with a distance of 2.0 mm, which excluded all the primary spongiosa and only contained the second spongiosa. The trabecular bone parameters, including trabecular BMD, trabecular number (Tb.N), trabecular thickness (Tb.Th), trabecular separation (Tb.Sp), bone volume per tissue volume (BV/TV), and structure model index (SMI) were automatically quantified using the MicroView program (GE healthcare, Madison, WI, USA). Moreover, the mid-diaphyseal cortical bone was manually traced by another VOI. The cortical bone parameters, including cortical thickness (Ct.Th) and cortical area (Ct.Ar) were also determined.

Histology and histomorphometry

Right tibiae were immediately cut longitudinally into two pieces along the sagittal plane after animal dissection. One piece was fixed in 4% paraformaldehyde (PFA), decalcified in 10% ethylenediaminetetraacetic acid (EDTA), and embedded in paraffin. Five-µm-thick sections were stained with toluidine blue to visualize osteoblasts, and stained with tartrate resistant acid phosphatase (TRAP) to label osteoclasts. Static bone histomorphometric parameters, including osteoblast numbers per millimeter of trabecular bone surface (N.Ob/BS) and osteoclast numbers per millimeter of trabecular bone surface (N.Oc/BS) were quantified. The other piece was fixed in 80% ethanol for 24 h, and then embedded in methylmethacrylate. Eighty-µm-thick unstained sections were imaged with fluorescence microscope (LEICA DM LA, Leica Microsystems, Heidelberg, Germany) to observe and calculate the distance between the tetracycline and calcein labels divided by the labeling intervals of 10 days. Then, the dynamic bone histomorphometric parameters were quantified, including mineral apposition rate (MAR) and bone formation rate per bone surface (BFR/BS).

Statistical analysis

All data presented in this study were expressed as the mean ± standard deviation (S.D.). Statistical analyses were performed using SPSS version 13.0 for Windows software (SPSS, Chicago, IL, USA). One-way analysis of variance (ANOVA) was employed for evaluating the existence of differences among the three groups and once a significant difference was detected, Bonferroni's post hoc analysis was used to determine the significance between every two groups. The significance level was set at 0.05.

Results

Effects of RMF on body mass and soleus muscle mass in HU rats

The results of body mass and soleus muscle mass of rats before and after RMF exposure are shown in **Table 1**. No significant difference in body mass was observed between the Control, HU and HU+RMF groups before RMF exposure ($P>0.05$). HU for 4 weeks induced dramatic loss in body mass ($P<0.01$), soleus muscle mass ($P<0.01$) and soleus muscle mass normalized with body mass ($P<0.01$) as compared with the Control group; nevertheless, 4-week RMF exposure did not significantly alter the body mass, soleus muscle mass, or normalized soleus muscle mass in HU rats ($P>0.05$).

Effects of RMF on serum biochemical indices in HU rats

As shown in **Fig. 2**, bone formation markers, including serum OC and P1NP in the HU group were significantly lower than those in the Control group ($P<0.01$). Serum TRAcP5 b and CTX-I, two serum markers for bone resorption, were remarkably higher in the HU group than those in the Control group ($P<0.01$). However, no significant difference in serum OC, P1NP, TRAcP5 b or CTX-I levels was found between the HU and HU+RMF groups ($P>0.05$). Moreover, serum levels of PGE_2 and TGF-β1 in the HU group were lower than those in the Control group ($P<0.05$), whereas RMF did not significantly increase serum PGE_2 or TGF-β1 concentrations ($P>0.05$).

Effects of RMF on the biomechanical properties of bone in HU rats

The results of biomechanical testing of three-point bending are shown in **Fig. 3**. HU resulted in prominent decreases in the biomechanical properties of femora, including maximum load, stiffness, energy absorption and elastic modulus ($P<0.01$), whereas RMF exposure for 4 weeks exerted no significant impacts on maximum load, stiffness, energy absorption or elastic modulus in HU rats ($P>0.05$).

Effects of RMF on bone microarchitecture in HU rats

Representative 3-D and 2-D μCT images in the Control, HU and HU+RMF groups are shown in **Fig. 4**. The rat femur in the HU group exhibited notable reductions in the trabecular number, trabecular area and cortical thickness as compared with that in the Control group. RMF exposure did not exhibit remarkable effects on trabecular bone microarchitecture and cortical bone thickness in HU rats. The statistical results for the μCT analysis of trabecular and cortical bone structure in rat femora are shown in **Fig. 5**. Four-week skeletal disuse by HU caused significant decreases in trabecular BMD, Tb.N, Tb.Th and BV/TV ($P<0.01$), and increase in Tb.Sp and SMI ($P<0.01$). Moreover, HU induced significant deterioration in cortical bone structure of rat femora, as evidenced by decreased Ct.Ar and Ct.Th ($P<0.01$). However, no significant difference was observed in any trabecular or cortical bone parameter between the HU and HU+RMF groups, including BMD, Tb.N, Tb.Th, Tb.Sp, BV/TV, SMI, Ct.Ar or Ct.Th ($P>0.05$).

Effects of RMF on bone remodeling in HU rats

As shown in **Fig. 6**, the HU rats exhibited significant decrease in N.Ob/BS ($P<0.01$) and increase in N.Oc/BS ($P<0.01$) comparing to those in the Control group; nevertheless, RMF exposure did not alter N.Ob/BS or N.Oc/BS in HU rats. Furthermore, HU for 4 weeks also led to significant decreases in MAR and BFR/BS ($P<0.01$). However, no significant difference in MAR or BFR/BS was found between the HU and HU+RMF groups ($P>0.05$).

Effects of RMF on bone microstructure and bone turnover in normal rats

The descriptions for the methods for evaluating the effects of RMF on bone microstructure and bone turnover in normal rats are shown in File S1. As shown in **Fig. S1 in File S1**, RMF exposure did not significantly affect the parameters of bone microstructure in normal rats, including trabecular BMD, trabecular BV/TV or Cr.Ar ($P>0.05$). Moreover, no significant difference was observed in serum OC (the bone formation marker), and serum TRAcP5b (the bone resorption marker) between the Control and RMF groups ($P>0.05$).

Discussion

Accumulating evidence has demonstrated the promotional effects of PEMF and SMF on osteogenesis both *in vivo and in vitro*, whereas few studies have reported the efficiency of RMF in the musculoskeletal system. A previous study has demonstrated that moderate-intensity RMF was able to increase BMD and regulate bone metabolism in OVX rats [21]. However, the impacts of RMF on disuse-induced osteopenia/osteoporosis have never been previously investigated. Therefore, in the present study, we systematically evaluated the effects of RMF on HU-induced bone loss in rats subjected to tail suspension. Our findings clearly demonstrated that 4-week RMF exposure did not obviously affect soleus muscle mass, bone mass, bone microarchitecture, bone mechanical strength or bone remodeling in HU rats.

In the present study, soleus muscle atrophy and deceased body mass in rats were induced by 4-week HU. Disturbed balance between protein synthesis and protein degradation are regarded to

Table 1. Comparisons of body mass and soleus muscle mass of rats in the three experimental groups.

	Control ($n=10$)	HU ($n=10$)	HU+RMF ($n=12$)
Body Mass Day 0 (g)	275.6±12.9	275.6±12.6	279.4±16.4
Body Mass Day 29 (g)	354.3±20.9	293.6±16.7*	291.4±14.4*
Body Mass Change (g)	78.6±14.5	18.0±12.5*	12.0±17.6*
Soleus Mass (mg)	174.9±15.7	79.0±13.3*	89.8±13.5*
Soleus Mass/Body Mass (μg/g)	494.3±42.7	270.4±51.1*	308.6±48.3*

Values are expressed as mean ± S.D.
*Significant difference from Control group with $P<0.05$.

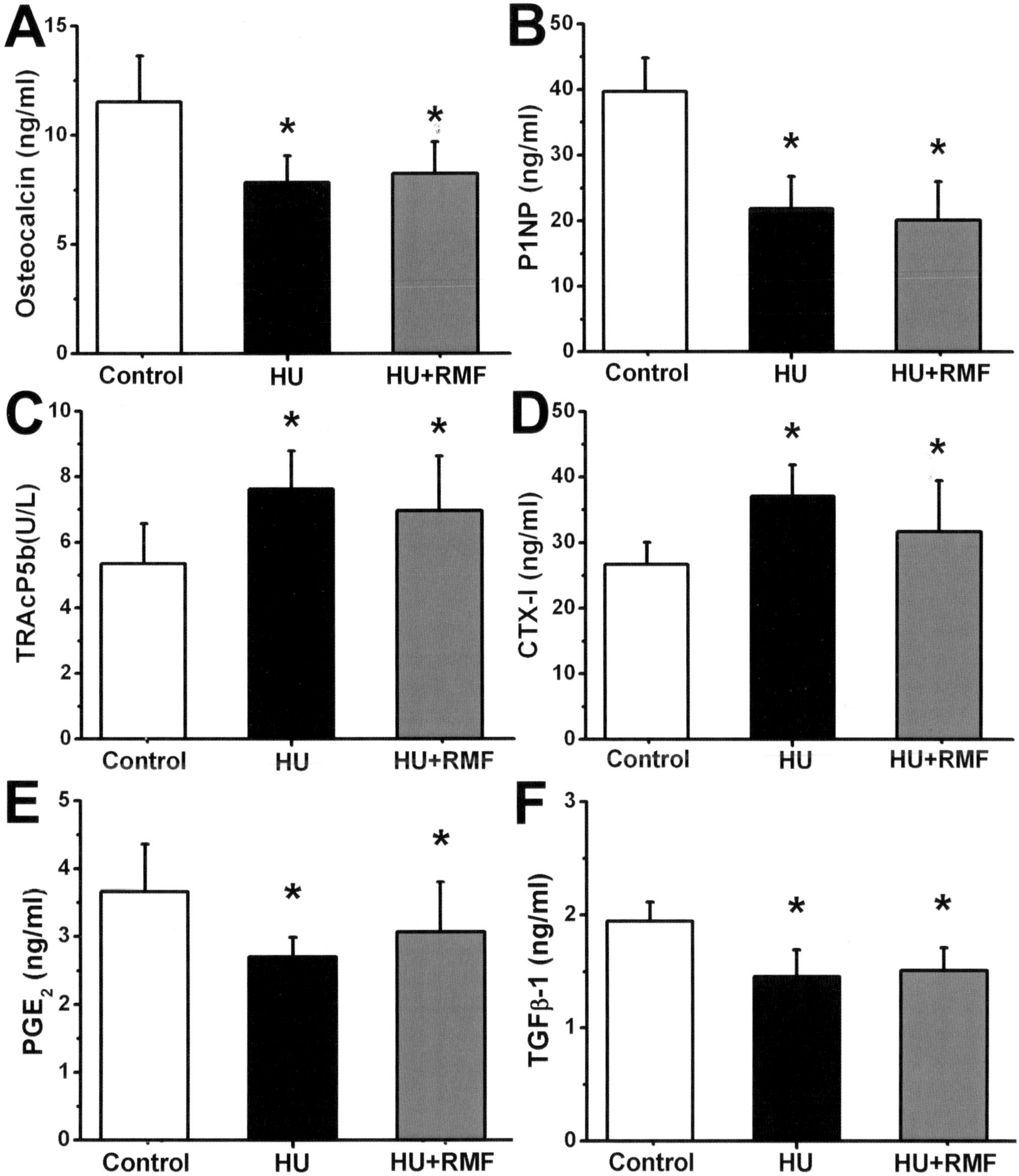

Figure 2. Effects of 4-week RMF exposure on serum biochemical indices (bone turnover markers and osteogenesis-associated cytokines) in HU rats, including bone formation markers (A) serum osteocalcin (OC) and (B) serum N-terminal propeptide of type 1 procollagen (P1NP), bone resorption markers (C) serum tartrate-resistant acid phosphatase (TRAcP5b) and (D) serum C-terminal cross-linked telopeptides of type I collagen (CTX-I), (E) prostaglandin E_2 (PGE_2), and (F) transforming growth factor-β1 (TGF-β1). Control, the control group ($n=10$); HU, the hindlimb unloading group ($n=10$); HU+RMF, the hindlimb unloading with RMF exposure group ($n=12$). Values are all expressed as mean ± S.D. *Significant difference from the Control group with $P<0.05$.

be the major mechanism of HU-induced muscle atrophy [29], although the exact signaling pathways and molecular mechanisms remain elusive. Previous investigation has demonstrated that pulsed electrical stimulation with 20 Hz has the potency to inhibit

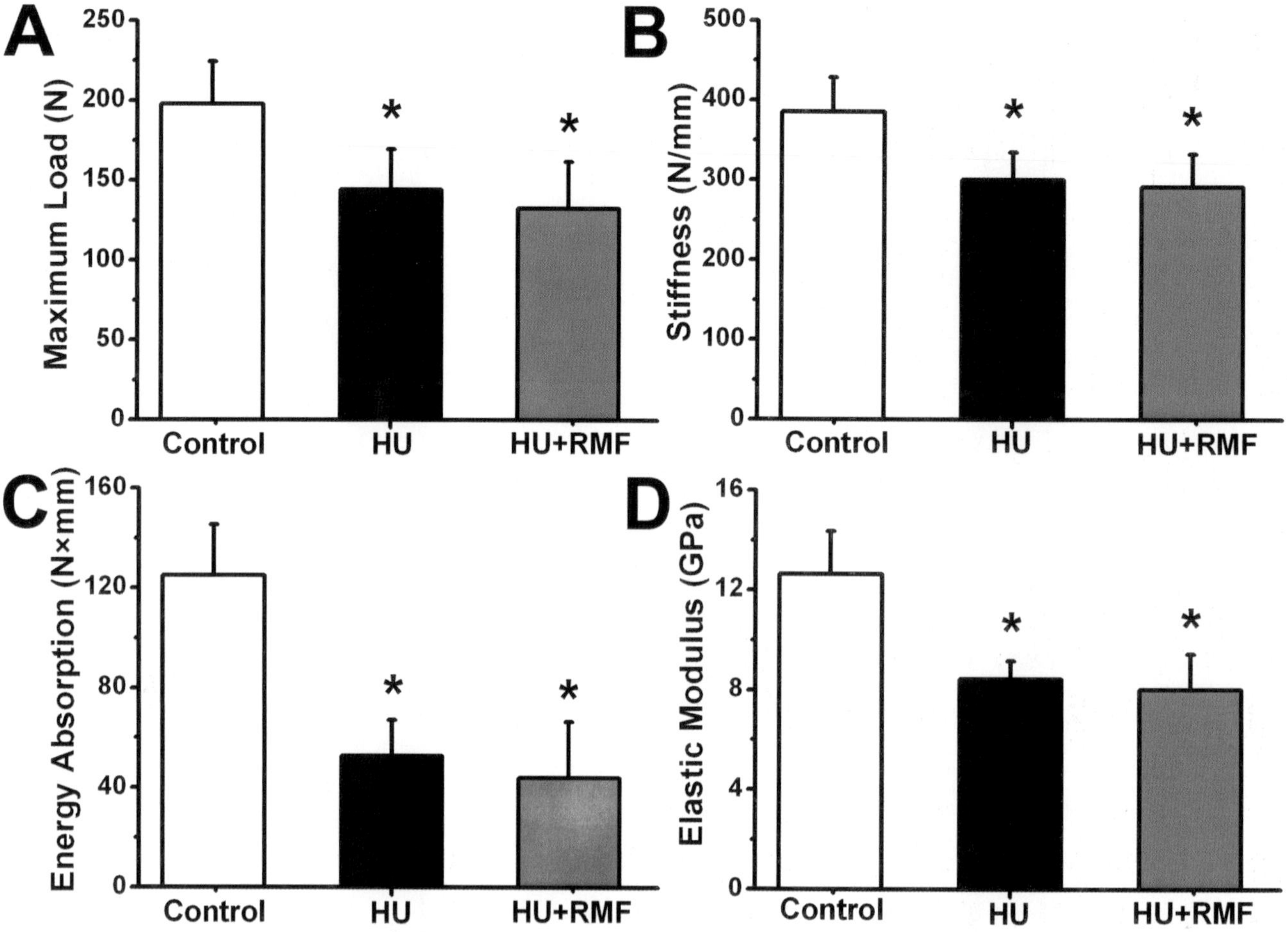

Figure 3. Effects of 4-week RMF exposure on femoral biomechanical parameters in HU rats, including (A) maximum load (B) stiffness (C) energy absorption and (D) elastic modulus. Control, the control group ($n = 10$); HU, the hindlimb unloading group ($n = 10$); HU+RMF, the hindlimb unloading with RMF exposure group ($n = 12$). Values are all expressed as mean ± S.D. *Significant difference from the Control group with $P<0.05$.

muscle atrophy by rescuing myonuclei and satellite cells [30]. It has also been shown that SMF exposure contributed significantly to the promotion of myogenic differentiation and myoblast alignment [31]. However, no obvious attenuation of soleus muscle atrophy in HU rats was observed after 4-week exposure to RMF in the present study.

The skeleton is a highly mechanoadaptive system, and insufficient mechanical stimuli to weight-bearing regions of the skeleton lead to bone mass loss [32,33]. In line with previous studies [34,35], HU resulted in marked deterioration in trabecular bone microarchitecture, as evidenced by decreased trabecular BMD, Tb.N, Tb.Th and BV/TV, and increased Tb.Sp. More importantly, increased trabecular SMI was also observed in HU rats, revealing a potentially dramatic reduction of trabeculae with plate-like structures [36]. Moreover, in accordance with previous findings [35], skeletal disuse by HU caused lower cortical bone thickness in the present study. Further observations by mechanical testing demonstrated that the skeletal extrinsic mechanical properties (maximum load, stiffness and energy absorption) and intrinsic mechanical properties (elastic modulus) were decreased in HU rats, implying the impaired mechanical integrity and declining capacity of fracture toughness [37]. However, RMF exposure did not obviously contribute to the improvement of trabecular bone microarchitecture, cortical bone thickness or bone mechanical strength.

To further evaluate whether RMF regulated osteoblastic and osteoclastic activities in HU rats, systemic analyses of serum biomarkers and bone histomorphometry for bone remodeling were performed. Similar with previous investigations [33], dramatically reduced bone formation was observed in HU rats, as evidenced by decreased serum markers (OC and P1NP) and histomorphometric parameters in trabecular bones (MAR, BFR/BS and N.Ob/BS). Our results also showed elevated serum TRAcP5b, serum CTX-I and N.Oc/BS in trabecular bones, revealing remarkably enhanced bone resorption induced by HU. However, we found no obvious regulatory effects of RMF on either serum markers or bone histomorphometric parameters for bone turnover, implying no direct impacts of RMF on skeletal anabolic or catabolic activities in HU rats. Moreover, many cytokines have proven to play essential roles in regulating the process of bone remodeling, such as PGE_2 and TGF-β1. PGE_2 is the most extensively produced prostanoid and has the capacity of stimulating bone formation and promoting fracture healing [38,39]. Chang et al. showed that PEMF inhibited osteopenia in OVX rats and stimulated serum PGE_2 secretions [40]. Significant evidence has demonstrated that TGF-β1 was able to regulate osteoblastic and osteoclastic functions [41]. More importantly,

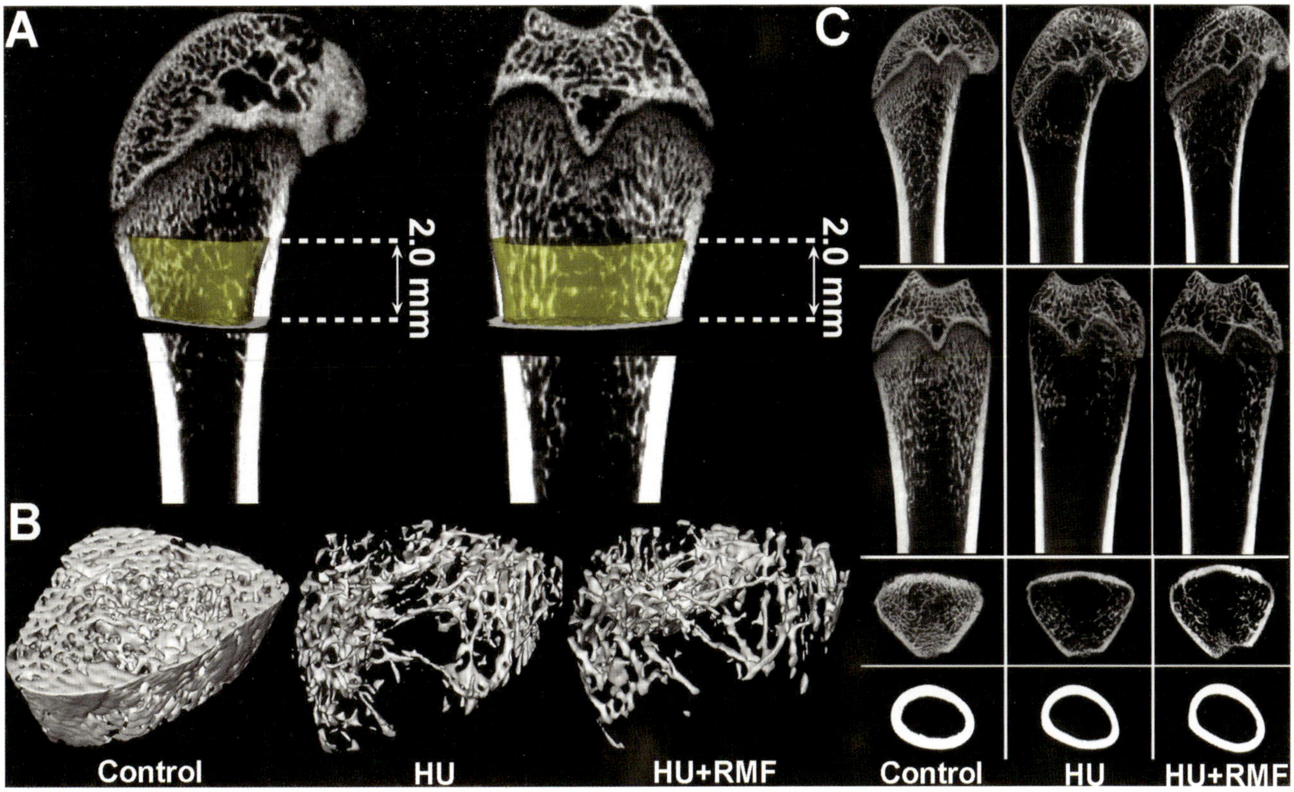

Figure 4. Effects of 4-week RMF exposure on trabecular bone microarchitecture in the distal femora and cortical bone thickness in the mid-diaphyseal femora. (**A**) The selected trabecular volume of interest (VOI) with yellow color in 2.0 mm height, which is represented with yellow color and only contains the secondary spongiosa. (**B**) 3-D μCT images of trabecular bone microarchitecture determined by the VOI. (**C**) 2-D μCT images of trabecular bone microarchitecture from the axial, coronal and sagittal plane observation in the distal femora, and cortical bone images in the femoral mid-diaphysis. The rat femur in the HU group exhibited significant decrease in the trabecular number, trabecular area and cortical thickness as compared with that in the Control group, whereas RMF exposure did not exhibit remarkable effects on trabecular bone microarchitecture and cortical bone thickness in HU rats.

TGF-β1 has also proven to be an essential mediator for the coupling of dynamic bone resorption and bone formation [42,43]. Our present study showed that serum PGE_2 and TGF-β1 secretions were decreased in the absence of regular mechanical stimulation. However, 4-week RMF exposure did not significantly change the concentrations of serum PGE_2 or TGF-β1.

The discovery of the skeletal piezoelectric effect by Fukada et al. in 1957 raised the possibility of the application of exogenous electrical stimulus on bone repair [44]. Subsequent studies have confirmed the osteogenic effects of electrical stimulation [45,46]. Bassett et al. for the first time found that PEMF treatment, a more accessible and affordable non-contact modality, was able to dramatically accelerate fracture healing in patients [12]. Numerous studies have further proved that PEMF could promote potently osteogenesis and enhance bone mineralization both *in vivo* and *in vitro* [15,16,47]. Clinical investigations revealed that PEMF produced satisfying therapeutic effects on fresh and nonunion fractures and osteoporosis [14,17]. It should be noted that the positive effects derived from PEMF stimulation revealed by Bassett et al. and other investigators were based on low-intensity and low-frequency non-thermal exposure levels, which were anticipated to primarily induce weak low-frequency electric current inside bone tissues. Moreover, these PEMF waveforms previously used were unidirectional single pulse or pulse burst. Several previous studies demonstrated that time-varying electromagnetic fields, e.g., sinusoidal wave, led to marked decreases of BMD and mechanical strength in rats [48]. Zhang et al. also demonstrated that sinusoidal EMF treatment decreased the osteoblasts proliferation and suppressed mineralized nodules formation, which exhibited opposite effects by unidirectional PEMF stimulation [47]. In the present study, moderate-intensity RMF we used could also induce spatial time-varying bidirectional electric fields in body tissues. However, different exposure waveforms, intensities and directionalities may contribute to the dramatically distinct effects between PEMF and RMF on the skeleton.

The beneficial effects of moderate-intensity and high-intensity SMF on osteogenesis have also been well documented thus far. Previous investigation has demonstrated that SMF promoted the differentiation and activation of osteoblasts *in vitro* [49]. It has been shown that SMF have the potency to enhance the local BMD in osteoporotic rats and accelerate fracture healing [19,50,51]. More interestingly, Kotani et al. found that high-intensity SMF exposure stimulated skeletal anabolic responses, and the orientation of bone formation and osteoblast growth was parallel to the magnetic field both *in vivo* and *in vitro* [20]. Thus, SMF may only induce a direct magnetic field to regulate osteoblast orientation, proliferation, differentiation, and bone formation, which shows distinct osteogenic mechanism with PEMF. However, unlike SMF with constant magnetic field direction, time-varying spatial magnetic fields generated by RMF we used in the present study might not facilitate the orientation of bone cells and

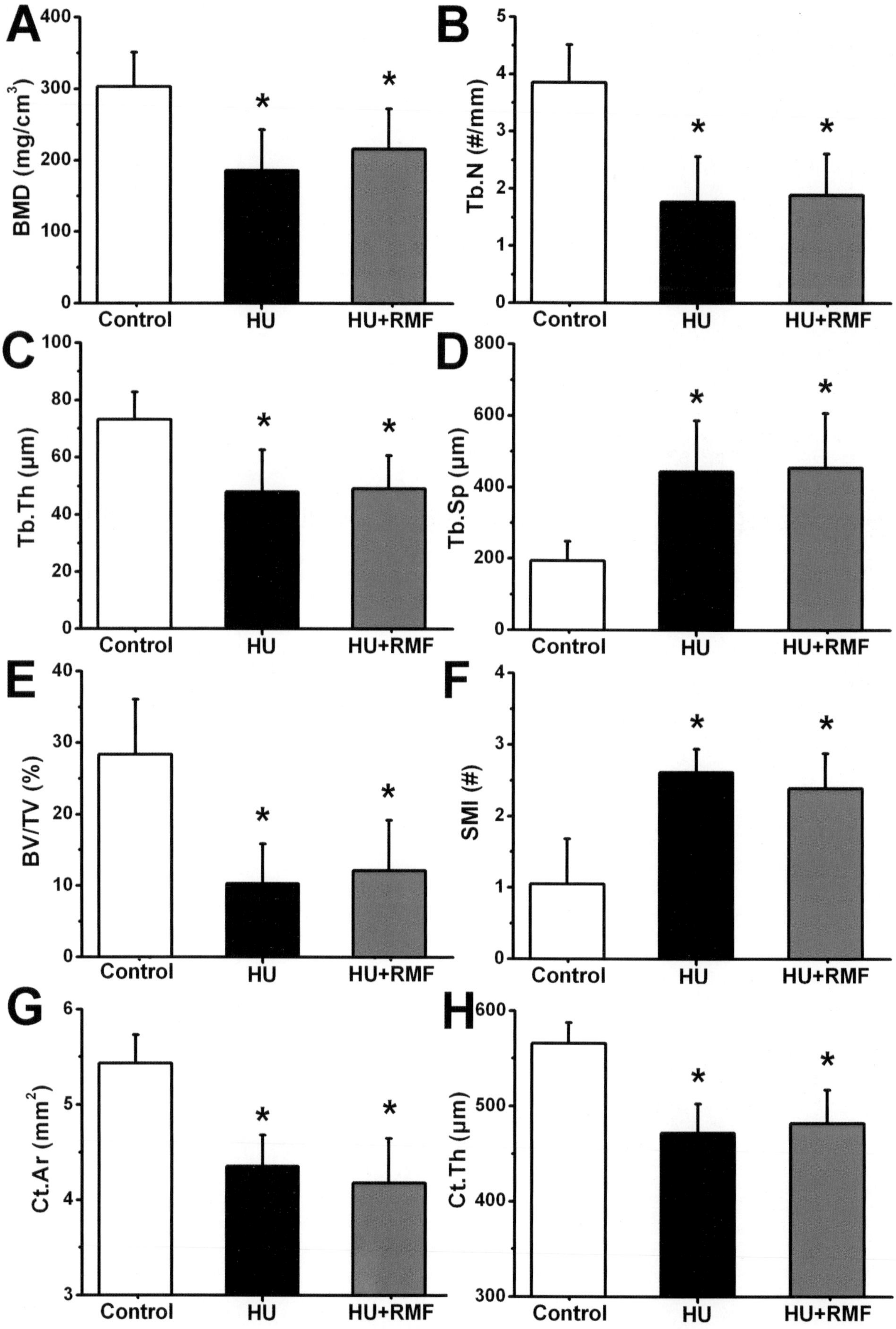
A
BMD (mg/cm^3)
400
300
200
100
0
Control
HU
HU+RMF
B
Tb.N (#/mm)
5
4
3
2
1
0
Control
HU
HU+RMF
C
Tb.Th (μm)
100
80
60
40
20
0
Control
HU
HU+RMF
D
Tb.Sp (μm)
800
600
400
200
0
Control
HU
HU+RMF
E
BV/TV (%)
40
30
20
10
0
Control
HU
HU+RMF
F
SMI (#)
4
3
2
1
0
Control
HU
HU+RMF
G
Ct.Ar (mm^2)
6
5
4
3
Control
HU
HU+RMF
H
Ct.Th (μm)
600
500
400
300
Control
HU
HU+RMF

Figure 5. Effects of 4-week RMF exposure on μCT indices of femoral trabecular and cortical bone microstructure in HU rats, including (A) trabecular bone mineral density (BMD), (B) trabecular number (Tb.N), (C) trabecular thickness (Tb.Th), (D) trabecular separation (Tb.Sp), (E) bone volume per tissue volume (BV/TV), (F) structure model index (SMI), (G) cortical area (Ct.Ar) and (H) cortical thickness (Ct.Th). Control, the control group ($n=10$); HU, the hindlimb unloading group ($n=10$); HU+RMF, the hindlimb unloading with RMF exposure group ($n=12$). Values are all expressed as mean ± S.D. *Significant difference from the Control group with $P<0.05$.

their cytoskeletons, and thus might not facilitate stimulating bone formation in one particular direction. This might be one of the possible reasons for the minor impacts of RMF on bone quality and bone metabolism in HU rats in the present study.

Another interesting aspect for helping decipher the mechanism of RMF on the tissues is the quantification of the electromagnetic energy absorbed by the tissues and the heat effect because of the energy absorption. According to the previous description, the Specific Absorption Rate (SAR) of the tissue is calculated in the following equation [52]: $SAR = \sigma \cdot E^2/\rho$, where σ is the conductivity of the tissue, ρ is the tissue mass, and E is the electric field intensity inside the tissue. The temperature alterations due to the energy absorption are able to be numerically quantified by analyzing the bioheat transfer equation based on the obtained SAR value [53]. A systematic numerical calculation based on finite element analysis will be performed in our following studies to obtain comprehensive understanding for the electromagnetic energy absorption in the tissues.

In conclusion, the present study demonstrated that exposure with moderate-intensity RMF at 7 Hz did not affect bone mass, bone microstructure, bone mechanical strength and bone remodeling in HU-induced osteoporotic rats, as evidenced by systemic evaluation for the serum biochemical, bone biomechanical, μCT and histomorphometric analyses. Although RMF stimulation may yield both a time-varying magnetic field and an electric current inside tissues, the RMF exposure was indeed not an optimal modality for regulating bone quality and bone remodeling, at least in its present form. It is regarded that treatment with EMF on various disorders probably exists "biological windows" of stimulus parameters. Thus, further investigations for the regulatory effects of high-intensity and low-intensity RMF on bone loss in HU rats are necessary to obtain a more comprehensive understanding for

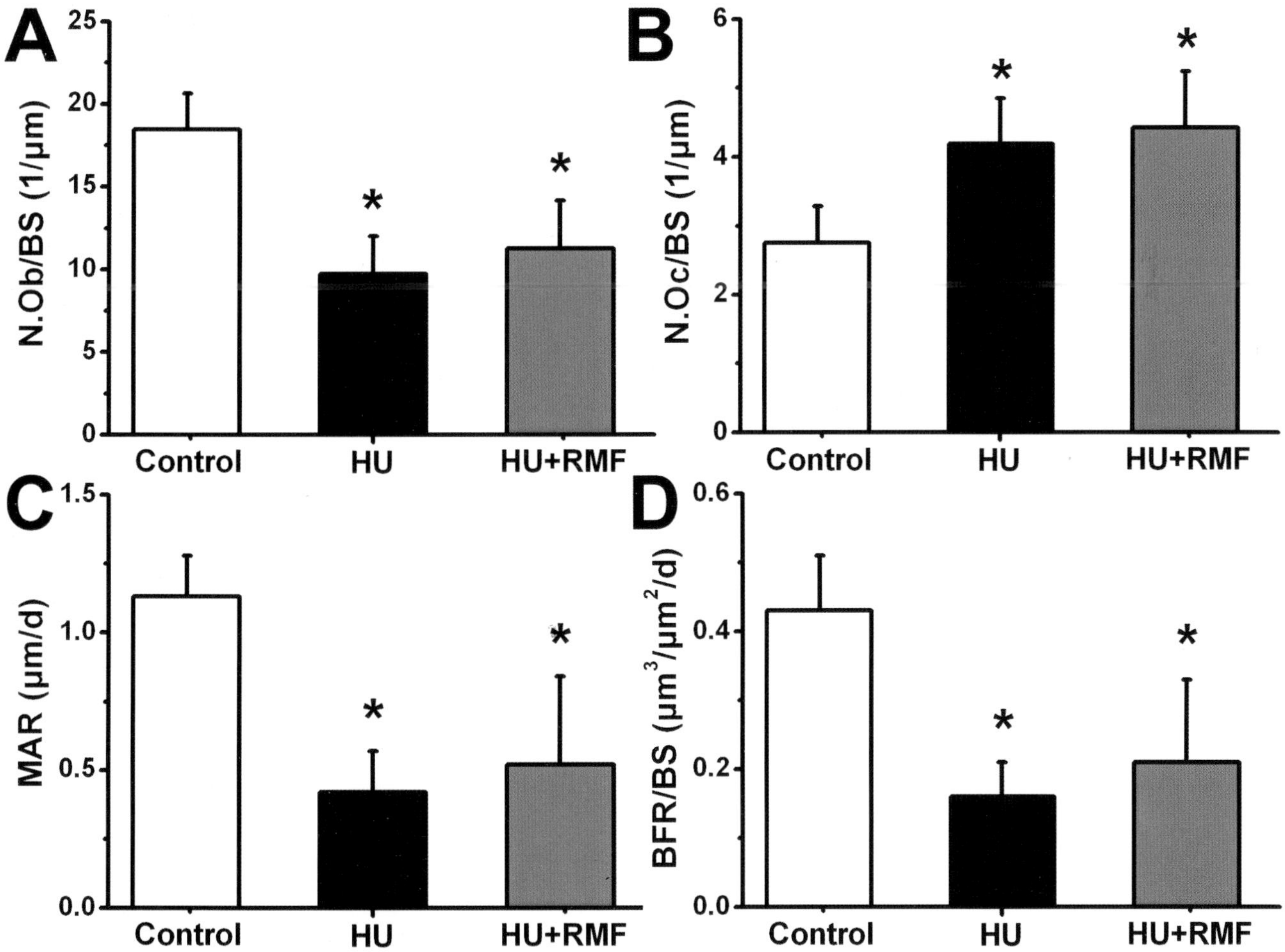

Figure 6. Effects of 4-week RMF exposure on tibial static and dynamic bone histomorphometric parameters in HU rats, including (A) osteoblast numbers per millimeter of trabecular bone surface (N.Ob/BS), (B) osteoclast numbers per millimeter of trabecular bone surface (N.Oc/BS), (C) mineral apposition rate (MAR) and (D) bone formation rate per bone surface (BFR/BS). Control, the control group ($n=10$); HU, the hindlimb unloading group ($n=10$); HU+RMF, the hindlimb unloading with RMF exposure group ($n=12$). Values are all expressed as mean ± S.D. *Significant difference from the Control group with $P<0.05$.

the osteogenic effects of RMF, which may be helpful for more scientific evaluation of RMF stimulation on osteopenia/osteoporosis in clinics.

Supporting Information

File S1 Combined file containing supporting materials and methods and Figure S1. Figure S1: Effects of 4-week RMF exposure on femoral trabecular and cortical bone microarchitecture and serum markers for bone turnover in normal rats, including **(A)** trabecular bone mineral density (BMD), **(B)** trabecular bone volume per tissue volume (BV/TV), **(C)** cortical area (Ct.Ar), the bone formation marker **(D)** serum osteocalcin (OC), and bone resorption marker **(E)** serum tartrate-resistant acid phosphatase (TRAcP5b). Control, the control group; RMF, the RMF exposure group. Values are all expressed as mean ± S.D. ($n = 8$).

Acknowledgments

The authors sincerely thank Dr. Yaochun Wang (Department of Aerospace Biodynamics, Fourth Military Medical University, Xi'an, China) for his assistance in the establishment of animal model.

Author Contributions

Conceived and designed the experiments: DJ EL JC. Performed the experiments: DJ JC YW ST. Analyzed the data: DJ JC YW GS QX KX XW MJ. Contributed reagents/materials/analysis tools: MZ CT XX JL WG. Wrote the paper: DJ.

References

1. Heaney RP, Abrams S, Dawson-Hughes B, Looker A, Marcus R, et al. (2000) Peak bone mass. Osteoporos Int 11: 985–1009.
2. McCombs JS, Thiebaud P, McLaughlin-Miley C, Shi J (2004) Compliance with drug therapies for the treatment and prevention of osteoporosis. Maturitas 48: 271–287.
3. Takata S, Yasui N (2001) Disuse osteoporosis. J Med Invest 48: 147–156.
4. LeBlanc A, Schneider V, Shackelford L, West S, Oganov V, et al. (2000) Bone mineral and lean tissue loss after long duration space flight. J Musculoskelet Neuronal Interact 1: 157–160.
5. Lang TF, Leblanc AD, Evans HJ, Lu Y (2006) Adaptation of the proximal femur to skeletal reloading after long-duration spaceflight. J Bone Miner Res 21: 1224–1230.
6. Riggs BL, Khosla S, Melton LJ 3rd (1998) A unitary model for involutional osteoporosis: estrogen deficiency causes both type I and type II osteoporosis in postmenopausal women and contributes to bone loss in aging men. J Bone Miner Res 13: 763–773.
7. Thomsen JS, Morukov BV, Vico L, Alexandre C, Saparin PI, et al. (2005) Cancellous bone structure of iliac crest biopsies following 370 days of head-down bed rest. Aviat Space Environ Med 76: 915–922.
8. Lazo MG, Shirazi P, Sam M, Giobbie-Hurder A, Blacconiere MJ, et al. (2001) Osteoporosis and risk of fracture in men with spinal cord injury. Spinal Cord 39: 208–214.
9. Mahavni V, Sood AK (2001) Hormone replacement therapy and cancer risk. Curr Opin Oncol 13: 384–389.
10. Musette P, Brandi ML, Cacoub P, Kaufman JM, Rizzoli R, et al. (2010) Treatment of osteoporosis: recognizing and managing cutaneous adverse reactions and drug-induced hypersensitivity. Osteoporos Int 21: 723–732.
11. Rizzoli R, Reginster JY, Boonen S, Breart G, Diez-Perez A, et al. (2011) Adverse reactions and drug-drug interactions in the management of women with postmenopausal osteoporosis. Calcif Tissue Int 89: 91–104.
12. Bassett CA, Pawluk RJ, Pilla AA (1974) Augmentation of bone repair by inductively coupled electromagnetic fields. Science 184: 575–577.
13. Bassett CA, Mitchell SN, Gaston SR (1982) Pulsing electromagnetic field treatment in ununited fractures and failed arthrodeses. JAMA 247: 623–628.
14. Assiotis A, Sachinis NP, Chalidis BE (2012) Pulsed electromagnetic fields for the treatment of tibial delayed unions and nonunions. A prospective clinical study and review of the literature. J Orthop Surg Res 7: 24.
15. Jing D, Cai J, Shen G, Huang J, Li F, et al. (2011) The preventive effects of pulsed electromagnetic fields on diabetic bone loss in streptozotocin-treated rats. Osteoporos Int 22: 1885–1895.
16. Rubin CT, McLeod KJ, Lanyon LE (1989) Prevention of osteoporosis by pulsed electromagnetic fields. J Bone Joint Surg Am 71: 411–417.
17. Tabrah F, Hoffmeier M, Gilbert F Jr, Batkin S, Bassett CA (1990) Bone density changes in osteoporosis-prone women exposed to pulsed electromagnetic fields (PEMFs). J Bone Miner Res 5: 437–442.
18. Jing D, Cai J, Wu Y, Shen G, Li F, et al. (2014) Pulsed Electromagnetic Fields Partially Preserve Bone Mass, Microarchitecture, and Strength by Promoting Bone Formation in Hindlimb-Suspended Rats. J Bone Miner Res. doi:10.1002/jbmr.2260.
19. Yan QC, Tomita N, Ikada Y (1998) Effects of static magnetic field on bone formation of rat femurs. Med Eng Phys 20: 397–402.
20. Kotani H, Kawaguchi H, Shimoaka T, Iwasaka M, Ueno S, et al. (2002) Strong static magnetic field stimulates bone formation to a definite orientation in vitro and in vivo. J Bone Miner Res 17: 1814–1821.
21. Zhang XY, Xue Y, Zhang Y (2006) Effects of 0.4 T rotating magnetic field exposure on density, strength, calcium and metabolism of rat thigh bones. Bioelectromagnetics 27: 1–9.
22. Pan X, Xiao D, Zhang X, Huang Y, Lin B (2009) Study of rotating permanent magnetic field to treat steroid-induced osteonecrosis of femoral head. Int Orthop 33: 617–623.
23. Morey-Holton ER, Globus RK (1998) Hindlimb unloading of growing rats: a model for predicting skeletal changes during space flight. Bone 22: 83S–88S.
24. Swift JM, Nilsson MI, Hogan HA, Sumner LR, Bloomfield SA (2010) Simulated resistance training during hindlimb unloading abolishes disuse bone loss and maintains muscle strength. J Bone Miner Res 25: 564–574.
25. Halloran BP, Bikle DD, Wronski TJ, Globus RK, Levens MJ, et al. (1986) The role of 1, 25-dihydroxyvitamin D in the inhibition of bone formation induced by skeletal unloading. Endocrinology 118: 948–954.
26. Machwate M, Zerath E, Holy X, Hott M, Godet D, et al. (1995) Systemic administration of transforming growth factor-beta 2 prevents the impaired bone formation and osteopenia induced by unloading in rats. J Clin Invest 96: 1245–1253.
27. Morey-Holton ER, Globus RK (2002) Hindlimb unloading rodent model: technical aspects. J Appl Physiol 92: 1367–1377.
28. Zhang LN, Zhang LF, Ma J (2001) Simulated microgravity enhances vasoconstrictor responsiveness of rat basilar artery. J Appl Physiol 90: 2296–2305.
29. Fitts RH, Riley DR, Widrick JJ (2000) Physiology of a microgravity environment invited review: microgravity and skeletal muscle. J Appl Physiol (1985) 89: 823–839.
30. Guo BS, Cheung KK, Yeung SS, Zhang BT, Yeung EW (2012) Electrical stimulation influences satellite cell proliferation and apoptosis in unloading-induced muscle atrophy in mice. PLoS One 7: e30348.
31. Coletti D, Teodori L, Albertini MC, Rocchi M, Pristera A, et al. (2007) Static magnetic fields enhance skeletal muscle differentiation in vitro by improving myoblast alignment. Cytometry A 71: 846–856.
32. Kazakia GJ, Tjong W, Nirody JA, Burghardt AJ, Carballido-Gamio J, et al. (2014) The influence of disuse on bone microstructure and mechanics assessed by HR-pQCT. Bone.
33. Spatz JM, Ellman R, Cloutier AM, Louis L, van Vliet M, et al. (2013) Sclerostin antibody inhibits skeletal deterioration due to reduced mechanical loading. J Bone Miner Res 28: 865–874.
34. Hu M, Cheng J, Qin YX (2012) Dynamic hydraulic flow stimulation on mitigation of trabecular bone loss in a rat functional disuse model. Bone 51: 819–825.
35. Lloyd SA, Bandstra ER, Willey JS, Riffle SE, Tirado-Lee L, et al. (2012) Effect of proton irradiation followed by hindlimb unloading on bone in mature mice: a model of long-duration spaceflight. Bone 51: 756–764.
36. Parkinson IH, Badiei A, Stauber M, Codrington J, Muller R, et al. (2012) Vertebral body bone strength: the contribution of individual trabecular element morphology. Osteoporos Int 23: 1957–1965.
37. Sun Y, Shuang F, Chen DM, Zhou RB (2013) Treatment of hydrogen molecule abates oxidative stress and alleviates bone loss induced by modeled microgravity in rats. Osteoporos Int 24: 969–978.
38. Li M, Thompson DD, Paralkar VM (2007) Prostaglandin E(2) receptors in bone formation. Int Orthop 31: 767–772.
39. Keila S, Kelner A, Weinreb M (2001) Systemic prostaglandin E2 increases cancellous bone formation and mass in aging rats and stimulates their bone marrow osteogenic capacity in vivo and in vitro. J Endocrinol 168: 131–139.
40. Chang K, Chang WH (2003) Pulsed electromagnetic fields prevent osteoporosis in an ovariectomized female rat model: a prostaglandin E2-associated process. Bioelectromagnetics 24: 189–198.
41. Janssens K, ten Dijke P, Janssens S, Van Hul W (2005) Transforming growth factor-beta1 to the bone. Endocr Rev 26: 743–774.
42. Tang Y, Wu X, Lei W, Pang L, Wan C, et al. (2009) TGF-beta1-induced migration of bone mesenchymal stem cells couples bone resorption with formation. Nat Med 15: 757–765.
43. Buijs JT, Stayrook KR, Guise TA (2012) The role of TGF-beta in bone metastasis: novel therapeutic perspectives. Bonekey Rep 1: 96.
44. Fukada E, Yasuda I (1957) On the Piezoelectric Effect of Bone. J Phys Soc Jpn 12: 1158–1162.

45. O'Connor BT, Charlton HM, Currey JD, Kirby DR, Woods C (1969) Effects of electric current on bone in vivo. Nature 222: 162–163.
46. McElhaney JH, Stalnaker R, Bullard R (1968) Electric fields and bone loss of disuse. J Biomech 1: 47–52.
47. Zhang X, Zhang J, Qu X, Wen J (2007) Effects of different extremely low-frequency electromagnetic fields on osteoblasts. Electromagn Biol Med 26: 167–177.
48. Gurgul S, Erdal N, Yilmaz SN, Yildiz A, Ankarali H (2008) Deterioration of bone quality by long-term magnetic field with extremely low frequency in rats. Bone 42: 74–80.
49. Yamamoto Y, Ohsaki Y, Goto T, Nakasima A, Iijima T (2003) Effects of static magnetic fields on bone formation in rat osteoblast cultures. J Dent Res 82: 962–966.
50. Xu S, Okano H, Tomita N, Ikada Y (2011) Recovery Effects of a 180 mT Static Magnetic Field on Bone Mineral Density of Osteoporotic Lumbar Vertebrae in Ovariectomized Rats. Evid Based Complement Alternat Med 2011.
51. Puricelli E, Ulbrich LM, Ponzoni D, Filho JJ (2006) Histological analysis of the effects of a static magnetic field on bone healing process in rat femurs. Head Face Med 2: 43.
52. Shiba K, Nukaya M, Tsuji T, Koshiji K (2008) Analysis of current density and specific absorption rate in biological tissue surrounding transcutaneous transformer for an artificial heart. IEEE Trans Biomed Eng 55: 205–213.
53. Pennes HH (1998) Analysis of tissue and arterial blood temperatures in the resting human forearm. 1948. J Appl Physiol (1985) 85: 5–34.

Permissions

All chapters in this book were first published in PLOS ONE, by The Public Library of Science; hereby published with permission under the Creative Commons Attribution License or equivalent. Every chapter published in this book has been scrutinized by our experts. Their significance has been extensively debated. The topics covered herein carry significant findings which will fuel the growth of the discipline. They may even be implemented as practical applications or may be referred to as a beginning point for another development.

The contributors of this book come from diverse backgrounds, making this book a truly international effort. This book will bring forth new frontiers with its revolutionizing research information and detailed analysis of the nascent developments around the world.

We would like to thank all the contributing authors for lending their expertise to make the book truly unique. They have played a crucial role in the development of this book. Without their invaluable contributions this book wouldn't have been possible. They have made vital efforts to compile up to date information on the varied aspects of this subject to make this book a valuable addition to the collection of many professionals and students.

This book was conceptualized with the vision of imparting up-to-date information and advanced data in this field. To ensure the same, a matchless editorial board was set up. Every individual on the board went through rigorous rounds of assessment to prove their worth. After which they invested a large part of their time researching and compiling the most relevant data for our readers.

The editorial board has been involved in producing this book since its inception. They have spent rigorous hours researching and exploring the diverse topics which have resulted in the successful publishing of this book. They have passed on their knowledge of decades through this book. To expedite this challenging task, the publisher supported the team at every step. A small team of assistant editors was also appointed to further simplify the editing procedure and attain best results for the readers.

Apart from the editorial board, the designing team has also invested a significant amount of their time in understanding the subject and creating the most relevant covers. They scrutinized every image to scout for the most suitable representation of the subject and create an appropriate cover for the book.

The publishing team has been an ardent support to the editorial, designing and production team. Their endless efforts to recruit the best for this project, has resulted in the accomplishment of this book. They are a veteran in the field of academics and their pool of knowledge is as vast as their experience in printing. Their expertise and guidance has proved useful at every step. Their uncompromising quality standards have made this book an exceptional effort. Their encouragement from time to time has been an inspiration for everyone.

The publisher and the editorial board hope that this book will prove to be a valuable piece of knowledge for researchers, students, practitioners and scholars across the globe.

List of Contributors

Petra Benzinger, Kilian Rapp and Jochen Klenk
Department of Clinical Gerontology and Rehabilitation, Robert Bosch Krankenhaus Stuttgart, Stuttgart, Germany

Kilian Rapp, Andrea Jaensch, Jochen Klenk and Gisela Büchele
Institute of Epidemiology and Medical Biometry, Ulm University, Ulm, Germany

Walter Maetzler
Hertie-Institute for Clinical Brain Research, University Hospital Tuebingen, Tuebingen, Germany

Walter Maetzler
DZNE, German Center for Neurodegenerative Diseases, Tuebingen, Germany

Hans-Helmut König
Department of Health Economics and Health Services Research, Hamburg Center for Health Economics,University Medical Center Hamburg-Eppendorf, Hamburg, Germany

Stefan Döbele, Steffen Schröter, Dankward Höntzsch, Ulrich Stöckle and Thomas Freude
BG Trauma Center, Eberhard Karls Universitaet Tuebingen, Tübingen, Germany

Michael Gardner
Department of Orthopaedic Surgery, Washington University School of Medicine, St.Louis, Missouri, United States of America

Tyler J. O'Neill, Laura Rivera, Vladi Struchkov and Hla-Hla Thein
Dalla Lana School of Public Health, University of Toronto, Toronto, Ontario, Canada

Hla-Hla Thein
Ontario Institute for Cancer Research/Cancer Care Ontario, Toronto, Ontario,Canada

Vladi Struchkov and Ahmad Zaheen
Faculty of Medicine, University of Toronto, Toronto, Ontario, Canada

Ahmed E. Elbanna
Department of Physics, University of California Santa Barbara, Santa Barbara, California, United States of America
Department of Civil and Environmental Engineering,University of Illinois at Urbana-Champaign, Urbana, Illinois, United States of America

Jean M. Carlson
Department of Physics, University of California Santa Barbara, Santa Barbara,California, United States of America

Hsuan-Ni Lin and J. Patrick O'Connor
Department of Biochemistry and Molecular Biology, Graduate School of Biomedical Sciences, Rutgers, The State University of New Jersey, Newark, New Jersey, United States of America

J. Patrick O'Connor
Department of Biochemistry and Molecular Biology, New Jersey Medical School, Rutgers, The State University of New Jersey, Newark, New Jersey, United States of America

Christopher L. Newman and Matthew R. Allen
Department of Anatomy and Cell Biology, Indiana University School of Medicine, Indianapolis, Indiana, United States of America

Sharon M. Moe and Neal X. Chen
Division of Nephrology, Department of Medicine, Indiana University School of Medicine, Indianapolis, Indiana, United States of America

Sharon M. Moe
Roudebush VA Medical Center, Indianapolis, Indiana, United States of America

Max A. Hammond and Joseph M. Wallace
Weldon School of Biomedical Engineering, Purdue University, West Lafayette, Indiana, United States of America

Jeffry S. Nyman
Department of Orthopaedic Surgery and Rehabilitation and Vanderbilt Center for Bone Biology, Vanderbilt University Medical Center, Nashville, Tennessee, United States of America
Department of Veterans Affairs, Tennessee Valley Healthcare System, Nashville, Tennessee, United States of America

Li Mao, Naoyuki Kawao, Yukinori Tamura, Kiyotaka Okada, Masato Yano, Osamu Matsuo and Hiroshi Kaji
Department of Physiology and Regenerative Medicine, Kinki University Faculty of Medicine, Osaka, Japan

Katsumi Okumoto
Life Science Research Institute, Kinki University, Osaka, Japan

Charlotte Salter, Lisa McDaid, Richard Holland and Amanda Howe
Norwich Medical School, Faculty of Medicine and Health Science, University of East Anglia, Norwich, Norfolk, United Kingdom

Debi Bhattacharya
School of Chemistry and Pharmacy,University of East Anglia, Norwich, Norfolk. United Kingdom

Tarnya Marshall
Rheumatology Department, Norfolk and Norwich University Foundation Trust Hospital. Norwich, Norfolk. United Kingdom

Jannike Øyen, Clara Gram Gjesdal and Margrete Apalset
Department of Rheumatology, Haukeland University Hospital, Bergen, Norway

Jannike Øyen and Margrete Apalset
Department of Global Public Health and Primary Care, University of Bergen, Bergen, Norway

Clara Gram Gjesdal, Ottar Kjell Nygård, Per Magne Ueland and Eva Ringdal Pedersen
Department of Clinical Science, University of Bergen, Bergen, Norway

Ottar Kjell Nygård
Department of Heart Disease, Haukeland University Hospital, Bergen, Norway

Stein Atle Lie
Department of Clinical Dentistry, University of Bergen, Bergen, Norway

Haakon E. Meyer
Section for Preventive Medicine and Epidemiology, University of Oslo, Oslo, Norway,
Norwegian Institute of Public Health, Division of Epidemiology, Oslo

Per Magne Ueland
Laboratory of Clinical Biochemistry, Haukeland University Hospital, Bergen, Norway

Øivind Midttun
Bevital AS, Bergen, Norway

Dongfeng Zhao and Yongjun Wang
Longhua Hospital, Shanghai University of Traditional Chinese Medicine, Shanghai, People's Republic of China

Dongfeng Zhao, Zhenqi Shi, Ping Qiao, Huixian Hong and Xu Feng
Department of Pathology, University of Alabama at Birmingham, Birmingham, Alabama, United States of America

Amy H. Warriner
Department of Medicine, University of Alabama at Birmingham, Birmingham, Alabama, United States of America

Li Zhang, Dong Zhang, Ying Zheng and Xiangmei Chen
State Key Laboratory of Kidney Disease, Department of Nephrology, Chinese PLA General Hospital and Military Medical College, Beijing, China

Minggang Zhao, Wenhao Fu and Xinqiang Gao
National Health and Family Planning Commission of the People's Republic of China, Beijing, China

Ji Shen, Zuyun Zhang, Ming Xian,Yunzhi Jiao, Jian Jiang and Jinqian Wang
Health and Family Planning Commission of Sichuan Province, Chengdu, China

Guomin Gao, Bin Tang and Liang Chen
Department of Health, United Logistic Ministry, Chengdu Military Region, Chengdu, China

Weimin Li
West China Hospital, Sichuan University, Chengdu, China

Changhua Zhou
Public Health Bureau of Yaan City, Yaan, China

Shaoping Deng
Sichuan Provincial People's Hospital, Chengdu, China

Jianwen Gu
General Hospital of Chengdu Military Command, Chengdu, China

Li Tan., Ying Wang, Lingling Zhou, Yun Shi, Fan Zhang, Li Liu and Shaofa Nie
Department of Epidemiology and Biostatistics, School of Public Health, Tongji Medical College, Huazhong University of Science and Technology, Wuhan, P. R. China

Xianye Tang, Gang Liu, Jian Kang, Yang Hou, Wen Yuan and Jiangang Shi
Orthopaedic Department, Changzheng Hospital, Second Military Medical University, Shanghai, China

Fungui Jiang
Department of Orthopaedics, People's Hospital of Wujiang City,Wujiang, China

Matthew L. Brown, Kiminori Yukata, Christopher W. Farnsworth, Ding-Geng Chen, Hani Awad, Matthew J. Hilton, Regis J. O'Keefe, Lianping Xing, Robert A. MooneyMichael J. Zuscik
Center for Musculoskeletal Research, University of Rochester Medical Center, Rochester, New York, United States of America

Matthew L. Brown
School of Medicine and Dentistry,University of Rochester Medical Center, Rochester, New York, United States of America

Ding-Geng Chen
Department of Biostatistics and Computational Biology, University of Rochester Medical Center, Rochester, New York, United States of America

Hani Awad, Matthew J. Hilton, Regis J. O'Keefe and Michael J. Zuscik
Center for Musculoskeletal Research, University of Rochester Medical Center, Rochester, New York, United States of America

Matthew L. Brown
School of Medicine and Dentistry,University of Rochester Medical Center, Rochester, New York, United States of America

Ding-Geng Chen
Department of Biostatistics and Computational Biology, University of Rochester Medical Center, Rochester, New York, United States of America

Hani Awad, Matthew J. Hilton, Regis J. O'Keefe and Michael J. Zuscik
Department of Orthopaedics and Rehabilitation, University of Rochester Medical Center, Rochester, New York, United States of America

Hani Awad
Department of Biomechanical Engineering, University of Rochester, Rochester, New York, United States of America

Christopher W. Farnsworth, Lianping Xing and Robert A. Mooney
Department of Pathology and Laboratory Medicine, University of Rochester Medical Center, Rochester, New York, United States of America

Albrecht W. Popp and Helene Buffat
Department of Osteoporosis, Inselspital, Berne University Hospital and University of Berne, Berne, Switzerland

Ursula Eberli, Manuela Ernst, R. Geoff Richards,Vincent A. Stadelmann and Markus Windolf
AO Research Institute Davos, Davos, Switzerland

Robert J. Losey, Erin Jessup and Tatiana Nomokonova
Department of Anthropology, University of Alberta, Edmonton, Alberta, Canada

Mikhail Sablin
Zoological Institute, Russian Academy of Science, Saint-Petersburg, Russia

Christoph Wölfl, Daniela Schweppenhäuser, Thorsten Gühring, Caner Takur and Paul Alfred Grützner
Department for Traumatology and Orthopaedic Surgery, BG Traumacenter Ludwigshafen, Ludwigshafen, Germany

Bernd Höner
SRH Hochschule Heidelberg, Dpt. Of Social Sciences and Law, Heidelberg, Germany

Ulrich Kneser and Leila Kolios
Department for Plastic-, Reconstructive and Handsurgery, Burn Care Centre, Department of Plastic Surgery of Heidelberg University, BG Traumacenter Ludwigshafen, Ludwigshafen, Germany

Jin Zhu, Aixi Yu, Baiwen Qi, Zonghuan Li and Xiang Hu
Department of Micro-Orthopedics, Zhongnan Hospital of Wuhan University, Wuhan, China

Marie-Soleil Dubois, Samantha Morello, Kelsey Rayment, Mark D. Markel, Vicki L. Kalscheur, Zhengling Hao,Patricia Marquis and Peter Muir
Comparative Orthopaedic Research Laboratory, School of Veterinary Medicine, University of Wisconsin-Madison, Madison, Wisconsin, United States of America

Ray Vanderby Jr and Ronald P. McCabe
Department of Orthopedics and Rehabilitation, School of Medicine and Public Health, University of Wisconsin-Madison, Madison, Wisconsin, United States of America

Patricia Marquis
Gulfstream Park, Hallandale Beach, Florida, United States of America

Wen Zhang, Yanjie Liu, Yao Pan, Wei Zhang, Changqing Zhang, Bingfang Zeng and Yunfeng Chen
Department of Orthopaedic Surgery, Shanghai Jiao Tong University Affiliated Sixth People's Hospital, Shanghai Jiao Tong University, Shanghai, China

Langqing Zeng
Department of Orthopaedics, Zhuhai People's Hospital, Jinan University Affiliated Zhuhai Hospital, Guangdong, China.

Ming Chen and Ming Ling
Department of Orthopedics, Shaanxi Provincial Peoples Hospital, Xían, Shaanxi, China

Qun Huang, Wei Xu, Chang She, Zong-Gang Xie, Yong-Tao Mao and Qi-Rong Dong
Department of Orthopedics, Second Affiliated Hospital of Soochow University, Suzhou, Jiangsu, China

Ulrike Ritz, Volker Spies, Isabella Mehling, Dominik Gruszka, Pol Maria Rommens and Alexander Hofmann
BiomaTiCS-Group, University Medical Centre of the Johannes Gutenberg University, Center of Orthopaedic and Trauma Surgery, Mainz, Germany

Anna Shipov, Gilad Segev, Hagar Meltzer, Moran Milrad, Ayelet Atkins and Ron Shahar
Koret School of Veterinary Medicine, Hebrew University of Jerusalem, Rehovot, Israel

Ori Brenner
Department of Veterinary Resources, Weizmann Institute, Rehovot, Israel

Xiong Liu, Wei-dong Wu, Ya-feng Fang, Mei-chao Zhang and Wen-hua Huang
Department of Anatomy, Southern Medical University, Guangdong Provincial Key Laboratory of Medical Biomechanics, Guangzhou, Guangdong, P.R. China

Xiong Liu
Department of Orthopaedics, Shilongboai Hospital (The Eight People's Hospital of Dongguan), Dongguan, Guangdong, P.R. China

Wei-dong Wu
Department of Orthopaedics, Wuzhou Red Cross Hospital, Wuzhou, Guangxi, P.R. China

Marilyn L. Kwan, Joan C. Lo, Cecile A. Laurent, Janise M. Roh, Malini Chandra, Charles P. Quesenberry Jr. and Lawrence H. Kushi
Division of Research, Kaiser Permanente Northern California, Oakland, California, United States of America

Li Tang, Theresa E. Hahn, Chi-Chen Hong, Lara Sucheston-Campbell, Christine B. Ambrosone and Song Yao
Department of Cancer Prevention and Control, Roswell Park Cancer Institute, Buffalo, New York, United States of America

Dawn L. Hershman
Department of Medicine and the Herbert Irving Comprehensive Cancer Center, Columbia University, New York, New York, United States of America

Lin Wan, Fengjie Zhang, Wing Pui Tsang,Li Lu and Chao Wan
Ministry of Education Key Laboratory for Regenerative Medicine, School of Biomedical Sciences, Faculty of Medicine, The Chinese University of Hong Kong, Hong Kong SAR, China

Fengjie Zhang, Wing Pui Tsang and Chao Wan
School of Biomedical Sciences Core Laboratory, Shenzhen Research Institute, The Chinese University of Hong Kong, Shenzhen, China

Qiling He
Departments of Microbiology and Pathology, University of Alabama at Birmingham, Birmingham, Alabama, United States of America

Li Lu and Qingnan Li
Guangdong Key Laboratory of Pharmaceutical Bioactive Substances, New Drug Function Research Center, School of Life Science and Biopharmacy, Guangdong Pharmaceutical University, Guangzhou, China

Zhihong Wu and Guixing Qiu
Department of Orthopaedics, Peking Union Medical College Hospital, Peking Union Medical College and Chinese Academy of Medical Sciences, Beijing, China

Guangqian Zhou
The Center for Anti-Ageing and Regenerative Medicine, Medical School, Shenzhen University, Shenzhen, China

Qian-Shi Zhang, Guo-Hua Lü and Xiao-Bin Wang, Jing Li
Department of Spine Surgery, The Second Xiangya Hospital of Central South University, Changsha, Hunan, P. R. China

Antonia Garcia-Martín, Rebeca Reyes-Garcia, Beatriz García-Fontana, Sonia Morales-Santana and Manuel Muñoz-Torres
Bone Metabolic Unit (RETICEF), Endocrinology Division, Hospital Universitario San Cecilio, Instituto de Investigación Biosanitaria de Granada, Granada, Spain

Antonia Garcia-Martín
Endocrinology, Hospital Comarcal del Noroeste, Caravaca de la Cruz, Murcia, Spain

Rebeca Reyes-Garcia
Endocrinology Unit, Hospital General Universitario Rafael Mendez, Lorca, Murcia,Spain

Sonia Morales-Santana
Proteomic Research Service, Fundación para la Investigación Biosanitaria de Andalucía Oriental -Alejandro Otero- (FIBAO), Granada, Spain

Ana Coto-Montes
Department of Morphology and Cellular Biology (RETICEF), Faculty of Medicine, University of Oviedo, Oviedo, Spain

Manuel Muñoz-Garach
Critical Care and Emergencies Unit, Hospital Universitario San Cecilio, Granada, Spain

Pedro Rozas-Moreno
Endocrinology Division, Hospital General de Ciudad Real, Ciudad Real, Spain

Da Jing, Guanghao Shen, Mingming Zhai, Shichao Tong, Kangning Xie, Xiaoming Wu, Chi Tang, Juan Liu, Wei Guo, Maogang Jiang and Erping Luo
Department of Biomedical Engineering, Fourth Military Medical University, Xían, China

Jing Cai
Department of Endocrinology, Xijing hospital, Fourth Military Medical University, Xían, China

Yan Wu
Institute of Orthopaedics, Xijing hospital, Fourth Military Medical University, Xían, China

Qiaoling Xu
Department of Nursing, Fourth Military Medical University, Xían, China

Xinmin Xu
Department of Medical Engineering, PLA No. 323 Hospital, Xían, China

Index